Cellular and Molecular Neurobiology

Edited by

Constance Hammond

Directeur de Recherches
INSERM U. 159
Paris
France

ACADEMIC PRESS

San Diego London Boston New York
Sydney Tokyo Toronto

This book is printed on acid-free paper.

Copyright © 1996 by ACADEMIC PRESS

Original version in French, DOIN Publishers, Paris © DOIN ASO

This version has received an award from the French Academy of Sciences

Academic Press, Inc.
525 B Street, Suite 1900, San Diego, California 92101-4495, USA
http://www.apnet.com

Academic Press Limited
24–28 Oval Road, London NW1 7DX, UK
http://www.hbuk.co.uk/ap/

ISBN 0-12-322040-8

Library of Congress Cataloging-in-Publication Data

A catalogue record for this book is available from the British Library

Typeset by Wyvern Typesetting Limited, Bristol
Printed in Great Britain at The Bath Press, Colour Books, Glasgow.

96 97 98 99 00 01 EB 9 8 7 6 5 4 3 2 1

Contents

Chapter 4 *The Nervous Tissue*
C. Hammond

PART II Neurons are Excitable and Secretory Cells

Chapter 5 *The Neuronal Plasma Membrane*
C. Hammond

Chapter 6 *Basic Properties of Excitable Cells at Rest*
A. Nistri and A. Gutman

Chapter 7 *The Voltage-Gated Channels of Action Potentials*
C. Hammond

PART III Ionotropic Receptors in Synaptic Transmission and Sensory Transduction

Chapter 10 *The GABA$_A$ Receptor*
C. Hammond

Chapter 11 *Ionotropic Glutamate Receptors*
C. Hammond

Chapter 12 *Ionotropic Mechanoreceptors: The Mechanosensitive Channels*
C. Bourque

PART IV Metabotropic Receptors in Synaptic Transmission and Sensory Transduction

Chapter 13 *The GABA$_B$ Receptor*
D. Mott

PART V Integration of Post-synaptic Currents and Synaptic Plasticity

Chapter 16 *The Integration of Synaptic Currents*
C. Hammond

Chapter 17 *Subliminal Voltage-Gated Currents*
C. Hammond

Chapter 18 *Firing Patterns of Neurons*
C. Hammond

Chapter 19 *Synaptic Plasticity*
C. Hammond

Contributors

C Hammond, U. 159 INSERM, Paris, France (Chapters 1–5, 7–11, 15–19)

A Nistri, Biophysics Sector, International School for Advanced Studies (SISSA), 34014 Trieste, Italy (Chapter 6)

A Gutman, Laboratory of Neurophysiology, Kaunas Medical Academy, Kaunas, Lithuania (Chapter 6)

C Bourque, Centre for Research in Neuroscience, Montreal General Hospital and McGill University, Montréal, PQ H3G 1A4, Canada (Chapter 12)

D Mott, Department of Pharmacology, Emory University School of Medicine, Atlanta, Georgia 30322, USA (Chapter 13)

R W Gereau, Molecular Neurobiology Laboratory, The Salk Insitute for Biological Studies, La Jolla, California, CA 92037, USA (Chapter 14)

P J Conn, Department of Pharmacology, Emory University School of Medicine, Atlanta, Georgia, USA (Chapter 14)

Y Tan, Biomedical Engineering Institute, Bogazici University, P.K.2 Bebek Istanbul, Turkey (Appendix 11.1)

Acknowledgements

I wish to thank Drs B. Barbour, P.Y. Coté, J. Golowash, K. Grant, L. Hazrati, Y. de Koninck and Y. Smith for the traduction of some of the French Chapters and Drs Y. Ben Ari, F. Crépel, H. Daniel, J.L. Galzi, J. Johnson, K. Krnjevic, M. Mallat, E. Seward and A. Triller for their helpful comments.

I am particularly thankful to Philippe Ascher for his constant support in the initial French version of this book.

We are grateful to the French Ministry of Culture and to Sandoz (Switzerland) for financial support for the translation.

Constance Hammond

Part I

General Properties of Neurons in the Nervous Tissue

Neurons

By using the silver impregnation method developed by Golgi (1873) Ramon y Cajal studied neurons, and their connections, in the nervous system of numerous species. Based on his own work (1888) and that of others (including Forel, His, Kölliker and Lenhossék) he proposed the concept that neurons are isolated units connected to each other by contacts formed by their processes: 'The terminal arborizations of neurons are free and are not joined to other terminal arborizations. They make contacts with the cell bodies and protoplasmic processes of other cellular elements'.

As proposed by Cajal, neurons are independent cells making specific contacts, named synapses, with hundreds or thousands of other neurons sometimes greatly distant from their cell bodies. The neurons connected together form circuits and so the nervous system is composed of neuronal networks which transmit and process information (see Chapters 1 and 2). In the nervous system there is another class of cells, the glial cells, which surround the different parts of neurons and cooperate with them. Glial cells will be considered in Chapter 3.

According to the information received, neurons generate electrical signals and propagate them along their processes. This capacity is due to the presence of particular proteins in their plasma membrane which allow the selective passage of ions: the ion channels.

The neurons are also secretory cells. Their secretory product is called a neurotransmitter. The release of a neurotransmitter only occurs in restricted regions, the synapses. The neurotransmitter is released in the extracellular space. The synaptic secretion is highly focalized and directed specifically on cell regions to which the neuron is connected. The synaptic secretion is thus different (with only a few exceptions) from other secretions such as hormonal cell or exocrine cell secretions which, respectively, release their secretory product into the general circulation (endocrine secretion) or the external environment (exocrine secretion).

1.1 Neurons Have a Cell Body from Which Emerge Two Types of Processes: The Dendrites and the Axon

Although neurons have various morphologies, they all share features that identify them as neurons. The cell body gives rise to processes that define the neuron's functions, polarity and capacity to connect to other neurons, sensory cells or effector cells; neurons are excitable cells, which are triggered by afferent stimuli; when lesioned, most neurons cannot be replaced, thus they renew their constituents during their entire life, involving the precise targeting of mRNAs and proteins to particular intracellular domains or membrane areas.

1.1.1 The Somato-dendritic Tree is the Neuron's Receptive Pole

The cell body or soma of the neuron contains the nucleus and its surrounding cytoplasm (or perikaryon). Its shape is variable: pyramidal soma for pyramidal cells in the cerebral cortex and hippocampus; ovoid soma for Purkinje cells in the cerebellar cortex; granular soma for small multipolar cells in the cerebral cortex, cerebellar cortex and hippocampus; fusiform soma for neurons in the pallidal complex; and stellar or multipolar soma for motoneurons in the spinal cord (Figure 1.1). One function of the soma is to ensure the synthesis of many of the components required for the structure and function of a neuron. Indeed, the soma contains all the organelles responsible for the synthesis of macromolecules. Most neurons in the central nervous system cannot further divide or regenerate after birth, and the cell body must maintain the structural integrity of the neuron throughout the individual's entire life.

The neurons have one or several processes emerging from the cell body and arborizing more or less pro-

Figure 1.1   The neurons of the central nervous system present different dendritic arborizations. (a) Photomicrographs of neurons in the central nervous system as observed under the light microscope: A, Purkinje cell of the cerebellar cortex; B, pyramidal cell of the hippocampus; C, soma of a motoneuron of the spinal cord. Golgi (A and B) and Nissl (C) staining. The Golgi technique is a silver staining which allows observation of dendrites, somas and axon emergence. Nissl staining is a basophile staining which displays neuronal regions (soma and primary dendrites) containing Nissl bodies (parts of the rough endoplasmic reticulum). (b) Camera lucida drawings of neurons in the central nervous system of primates, revealed by the Golgi silver impregnation technique and reconstructed from serial sections: A, pyramidal cell of the cerebral cortex; B, spiny neurons of the striatum; C, local circuit neurons of the striatum; D, neurons of the pallidal complex; E, neurons of the thalamus (ventralis intermedialis nucleus); F, neurons of the inferior olivary complex. All these neurons are illustrated at the same magnification. Photomicrographs: Olivier Robain (aA and aB) and Paul Derer (aC). Drawings: Jérôme Yelnik.

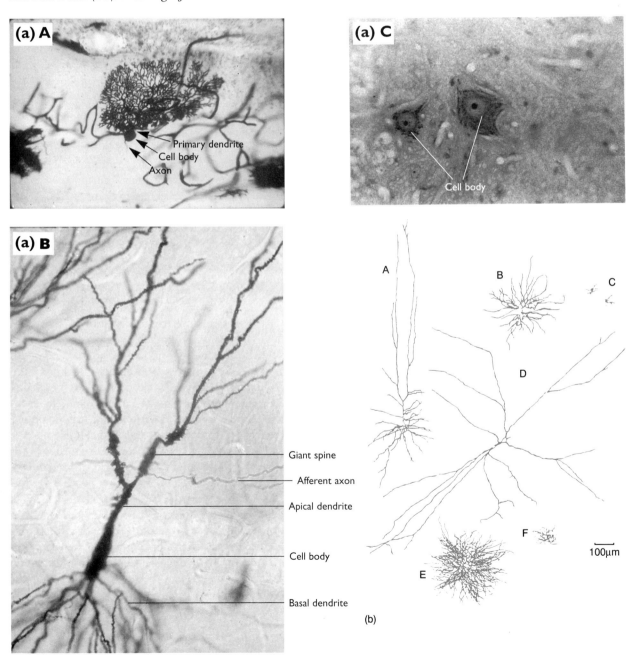

fusely. The two types of neuronal processes are the dendrites and the axons (Figures 1.1 and 1.3). This division is based on morphological, biochemical and functional criteria.

The dendrites, when they emerge from the soma, are simple perikaryal extensions, the primary dendrites. On average, one to nine primary dendrites emerge from the soma and then divide successively to give a dendritic tree with specific characteristics (number of branches, volume, etc.) for each neuronal population (Figures 1.1 and 1.2).

The dendrites are morphologically distinct from axons by their irregular outline, by their diameter which decreases along their branches, by the acute angles between the branches and by their ultrastructural characteristics (Figures 1.1, 1.3 and 1.7). The irregular outline of dendrites is related to the presence of numerous appendices of various shapes and dimensions at their surface. The more frequently observed are the dendritic spines, which are lateral expansions with ovoid heads binding to the dendritic branches by a peduncle of variable length (Figure 1.3).

Figure 1.2   Tridimensional illustration of a dendritic arborization. Computer drawing of a neuron of the subthalamic nucleus injected intracellularly with horseradish peroxidase (HRP) and reconstructed in three dimensions from serial sections. At 0°, the dendritic arborization of this neuron is represented in its principal plane, i.e. in the plane where it has its largest surface. In this plane, the dendritic field is almost circular (859 μm long and 804 μm wide). 30°, 60° and 90° rotations from the principal plane around the horizontal (horizontal column) and vertical (vertical column) axis show that the dendritic field has a flattened ovoid form (230 μm thick). (From Hammond C and Yelnik J, 1983. Intracellular labeling of rat subthalamic nucleus with horseradish peroxidase: computer analysis of dendrites and characterization of axon arborization, *Neuroscience* 8, 781–790, with permission.)

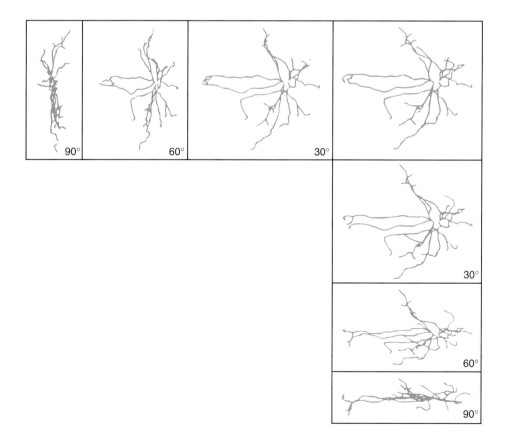

Some neurons are termed 'spiny' because there are 40 000 to 100 000 spines on the surface of their dendrites (e.g. pyramidal neurons of the cerebral cortex and hippocampus, the medium-sized neurons of the striatum and the Purkinje cells of the cerebellar cortex). However, other neurons with only a few spines on their dendritic surface are termed smooth (e.g. neurons of the pallidal complex) (Figure 1.1).

Dendrites and soma receive numerous synaptic contacts from other neurons and constitute the main receptive area of neurons (Figure 1.5 and Section 2.2). In response to this afferent information, they generate electrical signals such as post-synaptic potentials (Figure 1.5) or calcium action potentials and integrate this afferent information (spines are implicated in the segregation of this information).

The mechanisms underlying the small depolarizations and hyperpolarizations are called, respectively, the excitatory post-synaptic potential (EPSP) and inhibitory post-synaptic potential (IPSP) and are generated in the post-synaptic membrane in response to afferent activity. We shall consider this problem in Chapters 9, 10 and 11.

Although dendrites are generally a receptive zone there are certain exceptions: some dendrites are connected with other dendrites and act as a transmitter area by releasing neurotransmitters (Figure 2.2d).

1.1.2 The Axon and Axonal Collaterals are the Neuron's Transmitter Pole

The axon is morphologically distinct from dendrites in having a smooth appearance, a uniform diameter along its entire extent and by its ultrastructural characteristics (Figures 1.3 and 1.7). It generally emerges at the level of a conical expansion of the soma, the emerging cone, but sometimes at the level of a primary dendrite. After the emerging cone, an initial segment with a smaller diameter is observed and is followed by the true axon. The axon is not a single process; it is divided into one or several collaterals which form right angles with the main axon. Some collaterals return toward the cell body area; these are recurrent axon collaterals. The axon and its collaterals may be surrounded by a sheath, the myelin sheath. Myelin is formed by glial cells (see Sections 3.2 and 3.5.1).

The length of an axon varies. Certain neurons in the central nervous system have axons that project to one

Figure 1.3 Dendrite and axon of a subthalamic nucleus neuron (rat). (a) A distal dendrite. Dendritic spines of various shapes are present on its surface. (b) The axon. It has a smooth surface and gives off an axonal collateral. The pro-cesses of this neuron are stained by an intracellular injection of horseradish peroxidase. To follow the dendrites and axon along their trajectories, each figure is a photomontage of numerous photomicrographs of serial sections. (From Hammond C and Yelnik J, 1983. Intracellular labeling of rat subthalamic nucleus with horseradish peroxidase: computer analysis of dendrites and characterization of axon arborization, *Neuroscience* 8, 781–790, with permission.)

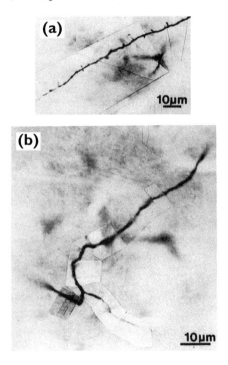

or several structures of the central nervous system that are distant from their cell bodies (Figure 1.4) whereas other neurons have short axons (a few microns in length) that are confined to the structure where their cell bodies are located (see also Figures 1.13). Thus projection neurons, or Golgi type I neurons, and local circuit neurons, or Golgi type II neurons, can be differentiated (Figure 1.1b, C). In Golgi type I neurons, the length of the axon is variable: certain projection neurons are directed to one structure only (e.g. corticothalamic neurons, see Figure 1.14) whereas other projection neurons have numerous axon collaterals which project to several cerebral structures (Figure 1.4).

Figure 1.4 Neuron of the reticular formation (brainstem) showing a complex axonal arborization. This cat reticulo-spinal neuron is stained by intracellular injection of peroxidase and drawn in a parasagittal plane obtained from serial sections. The axon (ax) gives off numerous collaterals along its rostrocaudal trajectory, making contacts with different neuronal populations (broken lines). (From Grantyn, A 1987. Reticulo-spinal neurones participating in the control of synergic eye and head movement during orienting in the cat, *Exp. Brain Res.* **66**, 355–377, with permission.)

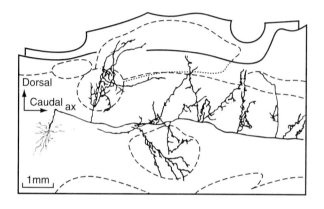

The axon and axonal collaterals in certain neurons end in a terminal arborization, i.e. numerous thin branches whose extremities, the synaptic boutons, make synaptic contacts with target cells (Figure 1.5). In other neurons the axon and its collaterals have enlargements or varicosities which contact target cells along their way: these are 'boutons en passant'. It can be noted that both types of boutons are named axon terminals although 'boutons en passant' are not the real endings of the axon (see Chapter 2).

The main characteristic of axons is their capacity to trigger sodium action potentials and to propagate them over considerable distances without any decrease in their amplitude (Figure 1.5 left, 3). It is generally accepted that action potentials are generated at the initial segment level in response to synaptic information transmitted by the somato-dendritic tree. Action potentials are then propagated along the axon and its collaterals toward the axon terminals (synaptic boutons or boutons en passant). When action potentials reach the axon terminals they trigger calcium action potentials which may cause the release of the neurotransmitter(s) contained in axon terminals in a specific compartment, the synaptic vesicles. This release or secretion is localized only at the synaptic contact levels. Overall, the axon is considered to be the transmitter pole of the neuron.

- What are the mechanisms underlying the abrupt, large and transient depolarizations called (sodium) action potentials? (see Chapter 7).
- How are they triggered? (see Chapters 7 and 17).
- How do they propagate? (see Chapter 7).
- How do they trigger the entry of calcium in synaptic terminals and the secretion of transmitter molecules? (See Chapter 8).

Certain regions, such as the initial segment, nodes of Ranvier (zones between two myelinated segments, Figure 1.5) and axon terminals, can also act as receptive areas for synaptic contacts from other neurons (see Section 2.2).

1.2 Ultrastructural Characteristics of the Different Regions of the Neuron

The organelles and cytoplasmic elements present in neurons are the same organelles found in other cells of the body. However, some elements such as cytoskeletal elements are more abundant in neurons. The non-homogeneous distribution of organelles in their soma and processes is one of the most distinguishing characteristics of neurons.

1.2.1 The Cytoskeletal Elements are Particularly Abundant in Neurons Where They Contribute to Organelle Transport

The cytoskeletal filaments present in neurons are protein polymers that form a tridimensional network, which acts as the inner structure of the entire intracellular area and forms a specialized architecture in different parts of the neuron: soma, dendrites, dendritic spines, axon and axon terminals. Three principal types of filaments exist (Figure 1.6):

- microtubules (24 nm in diameter): polymers of tubulin α and β and associated proteins, the MAPs (microtubule-associated proteins);
- microfilaments (7 nm in diameter): polymers of actin G;

Figure 1.5   Comprehensive schematic drawing of neuron polarity. The somato-dendritic compartment of a neuron receives a large amount of information from other neurons that establish synapses with it. At each synapse level the neuron generates post-synaptic potentials in response to the released neurotransmitter (1, EPSP; 2, IPSP). These post-synaptic potentials propagate and summate in the somato-dendritic compartment, then they propagate to the initial segment of the axon where they generate (or not) action potential(s) (3a). The action potentials propagate along the axon (3b, 3c) and its collaterals up to the axon terminals where they evoke (or not) the entry of calcium (4) and neurotransmitter release. Note the different voltage and time calibrations.

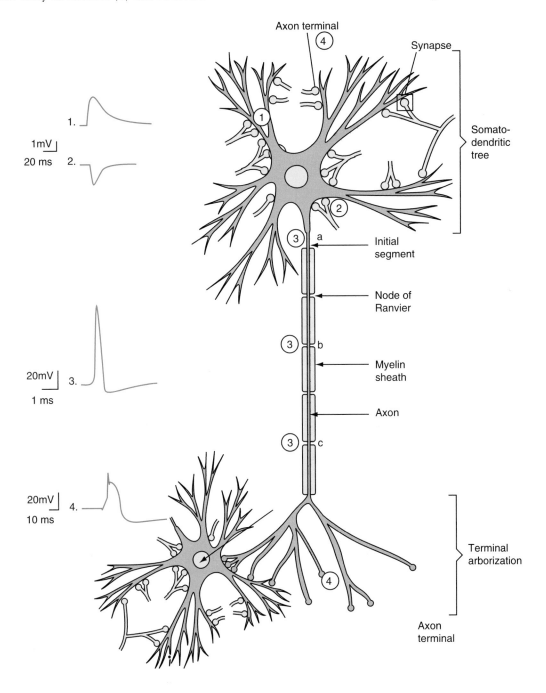

Figure 1.6   The cytoskeletal elements. (a) The micro-tubules are composed of 13 rows of tubulin polymers (tubulin is a heterodimer, αβ). In presence of guanosine triphosphate (GTP), the dimers of tubulin are continuously assembled and disassembled at their two ends but with different speeds. The net result is a polymerization of microtubules at the (+) end and a depolymerization at the (−) end. (b) The microfilaments are polymers formed by two-stranded helices of actin. (c) The intermediate filaments or neurofilaments are formed by three fibrous polypeptides arranged in superhelices. (a: From Margolis RL and Wilson L, 1981. Micro-tubule treadmills: possible molecular machinery, *Nature* **293**, 705–711, with permission.) (b: From Alberts B *et al*, 1986. *Biologie moléculaire de la Cellule*, Flammarion Médecine-Sciences, Paris, with permission.) (c: From Steinert PM, 1978. Structure of the three-chain unit of the bovine epidermal keratin filament, *J Mol Biol*; **123**, 49–70, with permission.)

ments is much more stable. The microtubules are polarized structures which polymerize and depolymerize both their ends at different rates: as a result, the end denoted (+) polymerizes whereas the end denoted (−) depolymerizes (Figure 1.6a).

The three types of cytoskeletal filaments are joined to each other and to mitochondria, smooth endoplasmic reticulum and vesicles by protein bridges. The network of filaments forms the neuronal skeleton, which gives the neuron its shape and a certain rigidity mostly at the level of its processes. Furthermore, microtubules support the fast anterograde and retrograde axonal transport (Section 1.3). Their associated proteins, the MAPs, have numerous roles including a motor role in anterograde and retrograde axonal transport.

1.2.2 The Soma: Main Site of Macromolecule Synthesis in Neurons

The soma contains the same organelles and cytoplasmic elements that exist in other cells: cellular nucleus, Golgi apparatus, mitochondria, polysomes, cytoskeletal elements and lysosomes.

The soma is the main site of synthesis of macromolecules since it is the one compartment containing all the required organelles. Compared with other types of cells, the neuron differs at the nuclear level and more specifically at the chromatin and nucleolus levels. The chromatin is light and sparsely distributed: the nucleus is in interphase. Indeed, in humans, most neurons cannot divide after birth since they are post-mitotic cells. The nucleolus is the site of ribosomal synthesis and ribosomes are essential for translating messenger RNA into proteins. The large size of the nucleolus indicates a high level of protein synthesis in these cells.

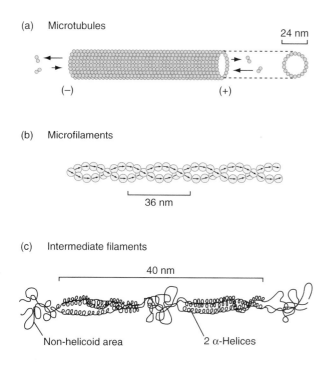

(a)   Microtubules

24 nm

(−)   (+)

(b)   Microfilaments

36 nm

(c)   Intermediate filaments

40 nm

Non-helicoid area   2 α-Helices

1.2.3 The Dendrites Contain Free Ribosomes and Synthesize Some of Their Proteins

In dendrites we find smooth endoplasmic reticulum, elongated mitochondria, free ribosomes or polysomes and numerous cytoskeletal elements including microtubules which are oriented parallel to the long axis of the dendrites (Figure 1.7). One of the MAPs, the MAP-2 proteins (more precisely the high molecular weight MAP-2A and MAP-2B), are more common to

- neurofilaments or intermediate filaments, which have an intermediate diameter (7–11 nm) compared with the two other types. They are formed by three fibrous polypeptides.

The microtubules and microfilaments are unstable, dynamic polymers whereas the structure of neurofila-

Figure 1.7   Photomicrograph of a tissue section of the central nervous system at the hippocampal level (see Figures 1.1 and 4.3a) showing the ultrastructure of a dendrite, numerous axons and their synaptic contacts (observed under the electron microscope). The apical dendrite of a pyramidal neuron contains mitochondria, microtubules, ribosomes *en rosettes* or in polysomes and smooth endoplasmic reticulum. It is surrounded by fascicles of unmyelinated axons with mitochondria and microtubules but no ribosomes. The axons' trajectory is perpendicular to the section plane. Two synaptic boutons (Ax Term) with synaptic vesicles make synaptic contacts (arrows) with the dendrite. (Photomicrograph: Olivier Robain.)

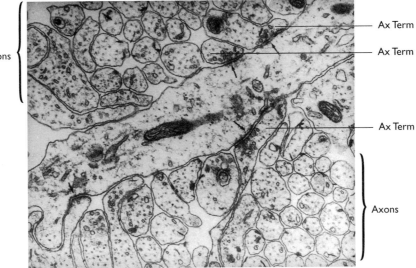

dendrites compared with axons. For this reason MAP-2A or 2B antibodies coupled to fluorescent molecules are useful for labeling dendrites, particularly for dendrite identification in cell cultures. Since dendrites have ribosomes they can, at least in part, synthesize their own proteins (when they are not glycosylated). This is possible only if the messenger RNA (mRNA) synthesized in the nucleus is transported into the dendrites up to the polysomes where they are translated. In hippocampal neuron cultures, RNA labeled with tritiated uridine was shown to be transported at a rate of 250–500 μm per day. This transport was blocked by metabolic poisons and the RNA in transit appeared to be bound to the cytoskeleton, since much of it remained following detergent extraction of the cells. Therefore, this energy-dependent transport seems to be associated with the dendrite cytoskeleton. However, the following questions still remain: which proteins are synthesized in dendrites beneath synaptic sites, and which mRNAs are present in dendrites? If we assume that the proteins synthesized in the dendrites are not

glycosylated because of the absence of the Golgi apparatus, they would be essentially cytoskeletal proteins and cytoplasmic proteins (but not protein channels).

Dendritic spines contain ribosomes and smooth endoplasmic reticulum of a particular shape. Electron microscopy studies show them to be associated with dense material formed by neurofilaments: this is the spiny apparatus and its functions are not fully understood.

1.2.4 The Axon is Characterized by the Absence of Structures Responsible for the Synthesis of Macromolecules

The axoplasm is devoid of ribosomes associated with the reticulum or in polysomal form. It contains thin, elongated mitochondria, numerous cytoskeletal elements and transport vesicles (Figure 1.7). Axons therefore cannot restore the macromecules from which they are made, neither can they alone ensure the synthesis of the neurotransmitter(s) that they release since they are unable to synthesize proteins. This problem is resolved by the existence of a continuous supply of macromolecules from the cell body to the axon through anterograde axonal transport (Section 1.3).

1.2.5 Hypothesis on the Origin of Selective Transport of Ribosomes to One or Other Neuronal Processes

The dendritic compartment contains ribosomes whereas the axon does not. What is the origin of this ribosomal selective distribution? This question is particularly important since this compartmentalization could lead to different properties of dendrites and axons: dendrites could synthesize proteins locally in response to synaptic information thus allowing either the stability of the synaptic transmission or a modulation of it.

The microtubules are implicated in the distribution of organelles: in the non-neuronal cells, the introduction of agents blocking the polymerization of microtubules completely disturbed the distribution of organelles in the different cellular regions. By studying axonal transport (Section 1.3) we now know that microtubules act as the substrate for vesicle transport and that their polarity influences the polarity of this transport.

What is the direction of ribosomal transport with regard to the microtubule's polarity?

This has been studied in the nutritive tubules of developing ovarioles in insects. These ovarioles contain nurse cells and oocytes connected to one another by cytoplasmic bridges. The nurse cells synthesize numerous components including ribosomes that are transported into the oocytes through the cytoplasmic bridges. In these bridges, we find a network of microtubules with a uniform polarity: the (+) end is located on the nutritive cell side and the (−) end on the oocyte side. Since the ribosomes are closely related to microtubules at the electron microscopic level, the following hypothesis has been proposed for this model: ribosomes are transported from the (+) end toward the (−) end of microtubules.

What is the polarity of the microtubules in dendrites and axons?

By using the hook procedure (see Figure 1.8 caption) in cultured neurons, it has been shown that the polarity of microtubules is uniform in the axon, meaning all (+) ends are oriented toward the axon terminals. In dendrites the situation is more complex: about half of the microtubules are oriented as in the axons whereas the other half are in the opposite direction (Figure 1.8). By combining these data with our information on the polarity of ribosomal transport in the ovariole of insects, it can be noted that ribosomes in neurons can be transported only toward dendrites since they are the only process containing microtubules with somatofugal (−) ends. This situation corresponds to what is observed. A general hypothesis has been proposed: the organelles transported from the (+) ends to the (−) ends of microtubules are present in dendrites but are absent in axons.

1.3 Axonal Transport Allows Bidirectional Communication Between the Cell Body and the Axon Terminals

1.3.1 Demonstration of Axonal Transport

Weiss and Hiscoe (1948) first demonstrated the existence of material transport in growing axons (during development) as in mature axons. Their work consisted of placing a ligature on the chicken sciatic nerve, and then examining the change in diameter of the axons over several weeks. They showed that these neurons become enlarged in their proximal part and presented degenerative signs in their distal part (Figure 1.9). The authors thus suggested that material from the cell body had accumulated above the ligature and ensured the survival of the distal part.

Later Lubinska *et al.* (1964) elaborated the concept of anterograde and retrograde transport. These authors placed two ligatures on a dog sciatic nerve and divided the isolated part of the nerve into short segments in order to analyze their acetylcholinesterase content. This enzyme is responsible for acetylcholine degradation and was used as a marker. They showed that it accumulates at the level of both ligatures. This result therefore suggested the existence of two types of transport: an

Figure 1.8   Microtubule polarity in neuronal processes. The polarity of microtubules is defined by the hook procedure: neurons are lysed in the presence of exogenous tubulin. When this is added to endogenous microtubules, hook-like structures are formed as observed on transverse sections at electron microscopic level. The orientation of hooks in a clockwise direction indicates the (+) ends of microtubules. (From Black MM and Baas PW, 1989. The basis polarity in neurons, *TINS*; **12**, 211–214, with permission.)

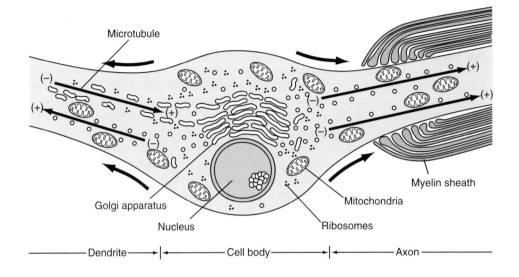

anterograde transport (from cell body to terminals) and a retrograde transport (from terminals to cell body). Moreover, it appeared that these types of transport are distributed along the entire extent of the axon.

We presently know of three types of axonal transport: fast transport (anterograde and retrograde), slow anterograde transport and mitochondrial transport.

1.3.2 Fast Anterograde Axonal Transport Allows the Turnover of Membrane Proteins of the Axon

Fast anterograde axonal transport consists of the movement of vesicles along the axonal microtubules at a rate of 100–400 mm/day. These transport vesicles, 40–60 nm in diameter, are formed by the Golgi apparatus in the cell body (Figure 1.10a). They transport, among other things, proteins required to renew plasma membrane and internal axonal membranes, neurotransmitter synthesis enzymes and neurotransmitter precursors when the neurotransmitter is a peptide. This transport is independent of the type of axon (central, peripheral, etc.)

Figure 1.9   Experiment by Weiss P *et al.* demonstrating anterograde axonal transport. Schematic drawing of a chicken motoneuron (1). When a ligature is placed on the axon (2) an enlargement of the axon's diameter above the ligature is noted after several weeks (3). When this ligature is removed, the enlargement progressively disappears (4). (From Weiss P and Hiscoe HB, 1948. Experiments on the mechanism of nerve growth, *J Exp Zool*. **107**, 315–396, with permission.)

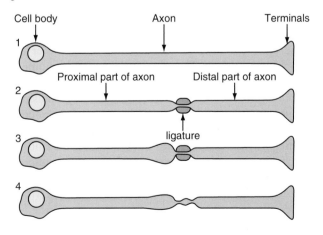

Figure 1.10   Fast axonal transport. (a) Schematic illustration of fast anterograde axonal transport (antero-grade movement of vesicles) and retrograde axonal transport (retrograde movement of plurivesicular bodies). These two transports use microtubules as substrate. (Inset) Recycling of small synaptic vesicles. Vesicles syn-thesized in the cell body and transported to the axon terminals are loaded with cytoplasmic neurotransmitter and targeted to the pre-synaptic plasma membrane. In response to Ca^{2+} entry, they fuse with the plasma mem-brane and release their content into the synaptic cleft (exocytosis); then they are recycled via an endosomal compartment. (b) Schematic illustration of mitochondrial transport. Note that the neuron representation is extremely schematic since axons do not give off *one* axon terminal. (a: adapted from Allen R, 1987. Les trot-toirs roulants de la cellule, *Pour la Science*, **April** 52–66 and from Südhof TC and Jahn R, 1991. Proteins of synaptic vesicles involved in exocytosis and membrane recycling, *Neutron* **6**, 665–677, with permission.) (b: from Lasek RJ and Kartz M, 1987. Mechanisms at the axon tip regulate metabolic processes critical to axonal elogation, *Prog. Brain Res.* **71**, 49–60, with permission.)

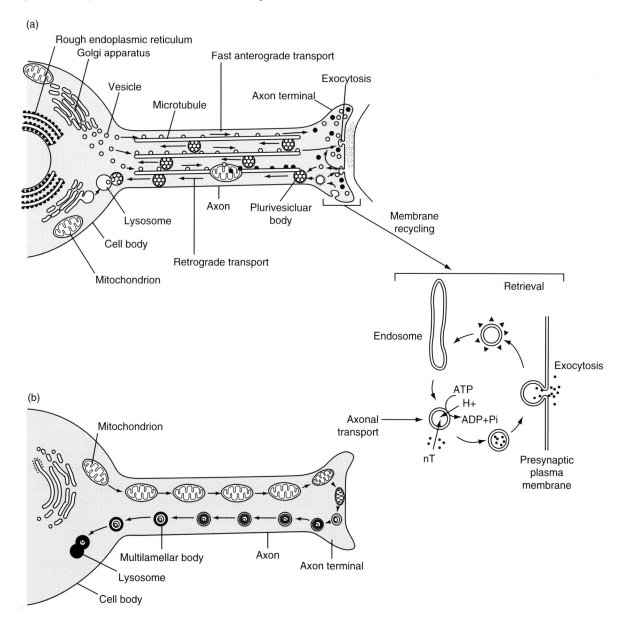

The most currently used preparation

The squid's giant axon is most commonly used for these observations since its axoplasm can easily be extruded and a translucent cylinder of axoplasm devoid of its membrane is thus obtained. This living extruded axon keeps its transport properties for several hours. The absence of plasma membrane allows a precise control of the experimental conditions and entry into the axoplasm of several components that cannot usually pass through the membrane barrier *in vivo* (e.g. antibodies). The improvement of video techniques applied to light microscopy allowed the first observations of the movement of a multitude of small particles along the microtubules in a living extruded axon.

Identification of the moving organelles and their substrates

Analysis of the particles that accumulate on each side of the 1.0–1.5 mm long isolated frozen segments of the squid axon has permitted the identification of moving organelles in axons. Correlation between video and electron microscopy images of these axonal segments has shown that the particles moving anterogradely on video images are small vesicles (Figure 1.10a). Indeed, when a purified fraction of small labeled vesicles (with fluorescent dyes) is placed in an extruded axon, these vesicles and also native vesicles are transported essentially in the anterograde direction. Evidence demonstrating the implication of microtubules in fast anterograde transport came from experiments with antimitotic agents (colchicine, vinblastine) which prevent the elongation of microtubules and block this transport. Finally video techniques have also demonstrated that the vesicles are associated with microtubules by long arms 16–18 nm in length (Figure 1.11a).

Role of ATP and kinesin

By analogy to actin–myosin movements in muscle cells, scientists tried to isolate in neurons an ATPase (the enzyme responsible for the hydrolysis of ATP) associated with microtubules and able to generate the movement of vesicles. To demonstrate molecular components responsible for interactions between vesicles and microtubules, the vesicle–microtubule complex

Figure 1.11 The motors of fast anterograde axonal transport and retrograde axonal transport. (a) Hypothetical model of the anterograde movement of vesicles along a microtubule. (b) Hypothesis to explain anterograde transport of vesicles and retrograde transport of plurivesicular bodies along one microtubule: kinesin and dynein (MAP-1C) bind to only one type of vesicle. (a: From Filliatreau G, 1988. Les moteurs moléculaires du transport axonal, *Médecine Sciences*, **6**,370, with permission.) (b: From Vallee RB, Shpetner HS and Paschal BM, 1989. The role of dynein in retrograde axonal transport, *TINS* **12**, 66–70, with permission.)

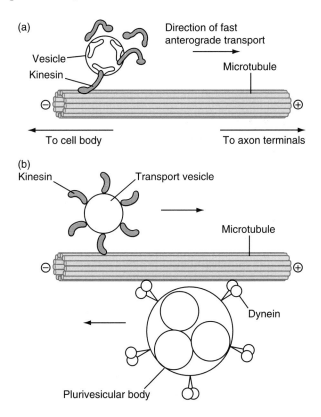

system has been reconstituted *in vitro*: isolated vesicles from squid giant axons are added to a preparation of purified microtubules and placed on a glass coverslip. These vesicles occasionally move in the presence of ATP. If an extract of solubilized axoplasm is then added to this system the number of transported vesicles is considerably increased.

In order to determine the factor present in the solubilized fraction responsible for vesicle movement, a nonhydrolyzable ATP analog has been used: 5'-adenylyl imidophosphate (AMP-PNP). In the presence of AMP-

PNP the vesicles associate with the microtubules but then stop. In these conditions vesicles are bound to the microtubules and also, consequently, to the transport factor. When an overdose of ATP is added to this vesicle–microtubule complex isolated by centrifugation, the AMP-PNP is removed and so vesicles are released and the transport factor is solubilized. Kinesin has been thus isolated and purified. It is a soluble microtubule-associated ATPase that translocates vesicles. As we have already seen, microtubules have a polarity determined by the orientation of their tubulin dimers: one end is marked (+) and the other end is marked (–). In axons, all microtubules are identically oriented, their (+) end being distally located from the cell body. It has been shown that kinesin moves vesicles in one direction only: from the (–) end toward the (+) end. This protein is obviously responsible for anterograde transport. In mammals, kinesin is composed of two identical heavy chains associated with light chains.

In proposed mechanism models, the arms observed between vesicles and microtubules *in vitro* would be kinesin. Each arm or kinesin would be associated with vesicles by the intermediate of a membrane protein and the vesicle movement implicates the hydrolysis of ATP and a cycle: association–movement–dissociation (Figure 1.11a). Kinesin is a microtubule-associated protein (MAP) belonging to the family of mechano-chemical ATPases.

The effects of mutations of the kinesin heavy chain gene were studied on the physiology and ultrastructure of *Drosophila* larval neurons. Motoneuron activity and corresponding synaptic (junctional) excitatory potentials of the muscle cells they innervate were recorded in control and mutant larvae in response to segmental nerve stimulation. The mutations dramatically reduced the evoked motoneuron activity and synaptic responses. The synaptic responses were reduced even when the terminals were directly stimulated. However, there was no apparent effect on the number of axons in the nerve bundle or of synaptic vesicles in the nerve terminal cytoplasm. These observations show that kinesin mutations impair the function of action potential propagation and neurotransmitter release at nerve terminals. Thus kinesin appears to be required for axonal transport of material other than synaptic vesicles: for example, ion channels of axonal and axon terminal membranes (see Chapter 5) or proteins responsible for exocytosis (see Chapter 8) involved in these functions.

1.3.3 Slow Anterograde Axonal Transport Allows the Turnover of the Axonal Cytoskeleton

The cytoskeleton (microtubules, neurofilaments and microfilaments) and cytosoluble proteins (intermediate metabolic enzymes including glycolysis enzymes) are transported anterogradely at a rate of 0.1–2 mm/day. This transport ensures the renewal of 80% of the total proteins present in the axon. In the elongating axon, i.e. during development or regeneration, the function of slow transport is to supply axoplasm required for axonal growth. In mature neurons its function is to renew continuously the cytoskeleton and to act as a substrate for anterograde and retrograde axonal transport.

Contrary to fast anterograde transport, slow transport is specific to the axon type. For example, the nature of the transported components is different in peripheral and central axons. The mechanisms responsible for slow transport are actually unknown. This gives rise to several questions: (i) in which state are cytoskeletal proteins transported in the axons: as soluble proteins or as polymers? (ii) in which axonal region(s) is the cytoskeleton (i.e. the complex network of filaments) assembled? and (iii) how are the assembly and the interactions between different cytoskeletal elements regulated?

The following are a few of the proposed hypotheses.

- The different cytoskeletal elements are assembled and connected by bridges in the cell body. They then progress as a whole (a matrix) in the axon. However, studies have demonstrated that cross-bridges between the different cytoskeletal elements are weak and unstable. Moreover, numerous cytoskeletal discontinuities exist along the axon as seen in the nodes of Ranvier. Thus, the hypothesis of a continuous elaboration of a stable matrix of assembled cytoskeletal elements explaining the ultrastructure of the axon is very unlikely.
- The cytoskeletal proteins are transported in a soluble form or as isolated fibrils and are assembled during their progression. When they are assembled some become stationary and would be renewed on site (Figure 1.12). This was demonstrated by pulse-labeling studies and particularly those coupled with photobleaching experiments. Purified subunits of cytoskeletal proteins (tubulin or actin) coupled to a fluorescent dye molecule are introduced into living

Figure 1.12 Model of slow axonal transport. The cytoskeletal elements would be present in the axon as two forms in equilibrium with one another: a stationary (or in very slow movement) form and a form in slow movement. (a) Soon after their synthesis insoluble neurofilament proteins are in polymeric or oligomeric form and move toward the axon terminals interchanging with a pool of neurofilaments in the polymeric and stationary form. The transition between both pools depends on the phosphorylation state of the neurofilament proteins. (b) A pool of tubulin in dimeric or insoluble oligomeric form and a pool of polymerized tubulin progress at different rates. The passage from one pool to another is made by addition of tubulin dimers at the (+) end of the microtubules (or by depolymerization of the (−) end). (From Hollenbeck PJ, 1989. The transport and assembly of the axonal cytoskeleton, *J. Cell. Biol.*; **108**: 223–227, reproduced with permission of The Rockfeller University Press.)

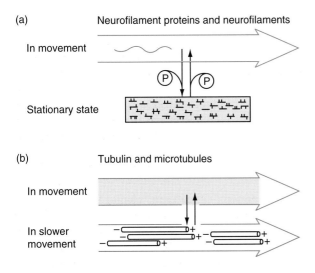

(a) Neurofilament proteins and neurofilaments
In movement
Stationary state

(b) Tubulin and microtubules
In movement
In slower movement

neurons in culture by injection into their soma. The observation with fluorescent microscopy shows that these labeled subunits are gradually incorporated into the polymer pool of the corresponding cytoskeletal proteins (microtubules and microfilaments) throughout the axon. A highly focused light source is then used to extinguish or bleach the fluorescence of the molecules contained within a discrete axonal segment. The fate of the bleached zone is followed over a period of hours. The bleached zone does not move along the axon or widen and recovers a low level of fluorescence within seconds. This latter effect is ascribed to the diffusion of free fluorescent subunits from the neighbouring fluorescent regions

into the bleached region. These observations suggest that microtubules and microfilaments are essentially stationary and are exchanging subunits.

1.3.4 Axonal Transport of Mitochondria Allows the Turnover of Mitochondria in Axons and Axon Terminals

The mitochondria recently formed in the cell body are transported in axons up to axon terminals at a rate of 10–40 mm/day. The transport of axonal mitochondria, as observed with video techniques, consists of saccadic backward and forward movements. A retrograde movement of mitochondria showing degenerative signs is also observed. The mitochondrial transport mechanism remains unknown (Figure 1.10b).

1.3.5 Retrograde Axonal Transport Allows Debris Elimination and Could Represent a Feedback Mechanism for Controlling the Metabolic Activity of the Soma

The vesicles transported retrogradely are larger (100–300 nm) than those transported anterogradely. Structurally they resemble pre-lysosomal structures: they are pluricellular bodies (Figure 1.10a). In the squid extruded axoplasm, vesicles move onto each filament in both directions and frequently cross each other without apparent collisions or interactions. *In vitro* experiments with purified kinesin show that this protein allows the vesicles to move in only one direction, i.e. from the (−) end to the (+) end.

It would be interesting to know if the filaments used for the fast transport of vesicles form a complex made up of several distinct filaments where certain filaments would be implicated in fast anterograde transport and others in retrograde transport. By using a monoclonal antibody raised against α-tubulin (a specific component of microtubules) it has been demonstrated that all the filaments implicated in anterograde or retrograde axonal transport contain α-tubulin. Moreover by using a toxin binding actin (and so consequently binding microfilaments) one can observe that filaments used for fast anterograde transport or retrograde transport are devoid of actin in their structure. Thus it appears that filaments used for the movement of vesicles in both directions are microtubules.

Which are the factor(s) that determine the direction of the transport on one microtubule?

Morphometric analysis of the arms between retrograde vesicles (pluricellular bodies) and microtubules demonstrated that these are similar to the arms between anterograde vesicles and microtubules. Studies looking for a factor different from, but homologous to, kinesin and responsible for retrograde transport were undertaken. This factor present in axoplasm homogenate might be lost during kinesin purification procedures since no retrograde vesicle movement was observed *in vitro* with kinesin. This factor has been isolated and described as having a high molecular weight. It is a microtubule-stimulated ATPase, a cytoplasmic form of dynein (also called MAP-1C). It is composed of subunits forming a tridimensional structure which presents two heads (the parts associated with the microtubules) and a stalk (the part associated with the membrane vesicles) (Figure 1.11b).

How does the cell determine which vesicles undergo anterograde transport and which undergo retrograde transport

It can be hypothesized that kinesin and dynein are bound to one type of vesicle since specific receptors present at their surface recognize only one of the two proteins (Figure 1.11b). Alternatively, both motor proteins are located on vesicles but by a regulation mechanism only one type is active and so transport takes place in only one direction.

Functions

Retrograde axonal transport allows the return of membrane molecules to cell bodies where they are degraded by acidic hydrolases found in lysosomes. Retrograde axonal transport may not only be a means of transporting cellular debris for their elimination but also a way of communicating information from the axon terminals to the soma. The retrogradely transported molecules would inform the cell body about activities taking place at the axon terminal level or they may even have a neurotrophic action on the neuron. Nerve growth factor (NGF), a trophic substance released by cells and taken up by endocytosis at the axon terminal level, is transported to the cell body where it has a trophic function. This uptake seems to be the major entry of NGF into neurons.

Moreover, it allows the transport of tetanus toxin or cholera toxin macromolecules that are taken up by axon terminals. These substances have a toxic effect on the cell body. These toxins, as well as horseradish peroxidase (HRP), an enzyme taken up by the axon terminals, are used for the retrograde labeling of neuronal pathways.

1.4 Neurons Connected by Synapses Form Networks or Circuits

1.4.1 The Circuit of the Withdrawal Medullary Reflex

Sensory stimuli (including visual, auditory, tactile, gustatory, olfactory, proprioceptive and nociceptive stimuli) are detected by specific sensory receptors and transmitted to the central nervous system (encephalon and spinal cord) by networks of neurons. These stimuli are analyzed at the encephalic levels. They can also evoke movements such as motor reflexes on their way to higher central structures.

Thus, when a noxious stimulus (i.e. a stimulus provoking tissue damage, for example pricking or burning) is applied to the skin of the right foot, it induces a withdrawal reflex consisting of the removal of the affected foot (contraction of flexor muscles of the right inferior limb) to protect itself against this stimulus. The noxious stimulus activates nociceptors, which are the peripheral endings of primary sensory neurons whose cell bodies are located, in this case, where injury is located at the body level, in dorsal root ganglia. Action potentials are then generated (or not, if the intensity of the noxious stimulus is too small) in primary sensory neurons and propagate to the central nervous system (spinal cord). Local circuit neurons of the dorsal horn of the spinal cord (Figure. 1.13a) relay the sensory information. Sensory information is thus transmitted to motoneurons (neurons innervating skeletal striated muscles and located in the ventral horn) through a complex network of local circuit neurons (Golgi type II neurons) which have either an excitatory or inhibitory effect. It results on the stimulus side (ipsilateral side) in an activation of the flexor

Figure 1.13   Withdrawal medullary reflex pathway. (a) Schematic illustration of a horizontal section through the spinal cord and of connections between a primary nociceptive sensory neuron, medullary local circuit neurons and ipsi- and contralateral motoneurons innervating inferior limb muscles. See text for details. (b) Anterograde inhibitory circuit. (c) Recurrent inhibitory circuit.

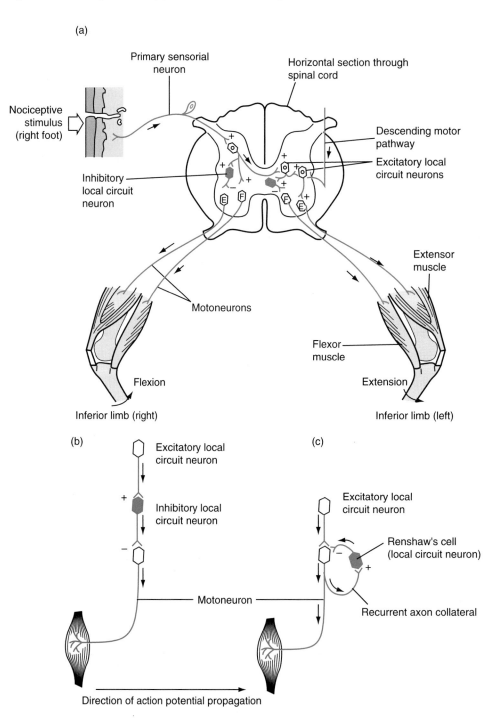

motoneurons (F) and an inhibition of the extensor motoneurons (E): the right inferior limb is being withdrawn (is in flexion). The opposite limb is extended to maintain posture.

This pathway illustrates peculiarities present in numerous other circuits.

- *Divergence of information.* Primary sensory information is distributed to several types of neurons in the medulla: local circuit neurons connected to motoneurons that innervate posterior limb muscles and also projection neurons that relay sensory information to higher centers where they are analyzed.
- *Convergence of information.* Motoneurons receive sensory information via local circuit neurons and also descending motor information via descending neurons whose cell bodies are located in central motor regions (motor commands elaborated at the encephalic level) (Figure 1.13a).
- *Anterograde inhibition* (feed forward inhibition). A neuron inhibits another neuron by the activation of an inhibitory interneuron (Figure 1.13b).
- *Recurrent inhibition.* A neuron inhibits itself by a recurrent collateral of its own axon which synapses on an inhibitory interneuron. The inhibitory interneuron establishes synapses on the motoneuron (Figure 1.13c). This recurrent inhibition allows the rapid cessation of the motoneuron's activity.

The last two circuits described are also called microcircuits, since they are included in a larger circuit or macrocircuit. In this selected example, all the neurons forming the microcircuit enable precise regulation of motoneuron activity.

1.4.2 The Spinothalamic Tract or Anterolateral Pathway, a Somatosensory Pathway

Noxious stimuli (temperature and sometimes touch) are detected at the skin level by free nerve endings (see above), transducted (or not) in action potentials and conveyed to the somatosensory cortex via relay neurons. Information from the body reaches the dorsal horn neurons of the spinal cord and information from the face reaches the trigeminal nuclei in the brain stem, both via primary sensory neurons whose cell bodies are located in dorsal root ganglia or cranial

ganglia, respectively. They relay on projection neurons whose cell bodies are located in dorsal horns or trigeminal nuclei and which send axons to the thalamus. These axons cross the midline, form a tract in the anterolateral part of the white matter and terminate in non-specific thalamic nuclei. Thalamic neurons then send the sensory information to cortical areas specialized in somatic senses (somatosensory cortex). At each level of synapses (dorsal horn or trigeminal nucleus, thalamus, cortex), the somatosensory information is not simply relayed, it is also processed through local microcircuits receiving afferent sensory information and descending information from higher centers which modulate incoming sensory information.

When superimposing horizontal sections through the spinal cord of Figures 1.13a and 1.14, it becomes clear that a noxious stimulus applied to the skin of the right inferior limb is transmitted to motoneurons where it can evoke a withdrawal reflex and also reaches the somatosensory cortex where it is analyzed. The reflex is evoked before consciousness of the stimulus because of the longer distance to brain areas than to the ventral horn of the spinal cord.

1.5 In Summary, a Neuron is an Excitable and Secretory Cell Presenting an Extreme Functional Regionalization

In this chapter we have learnt that the different functions of neurons, such as their metabolism, excitability and secretion, are localized to specific regions of the neuron. These regions are sometimes located at great distances from each other and so neurons have to resolve the problems of communication between these regions and harmonization of their activities.

Regionalization of metabolic functions

The essential synthesis activity of a neuron is localized in its cell body, since dendrites can only synthesize some of their proteins and axons are unable to synthesize any. In this cell, where the axon's volume represents up to a thousand times the volume of the cell body, the structural and functional integrity of the axon and its terminals requires an important and continuous supply of macromolecules. This supply is ensured by anterograde axonal transport. In dendrites, RNA transport from the

Figure 1.14   The spinothalamic tract or anterolateral ascending sensory pathway. This pathway integrates and conveys sensory information such as nociception, temperature and some touch. From bottom to top, horizontal sections through the spinal cord, the pons and frontal section through the diencephalon. See text for explanations.

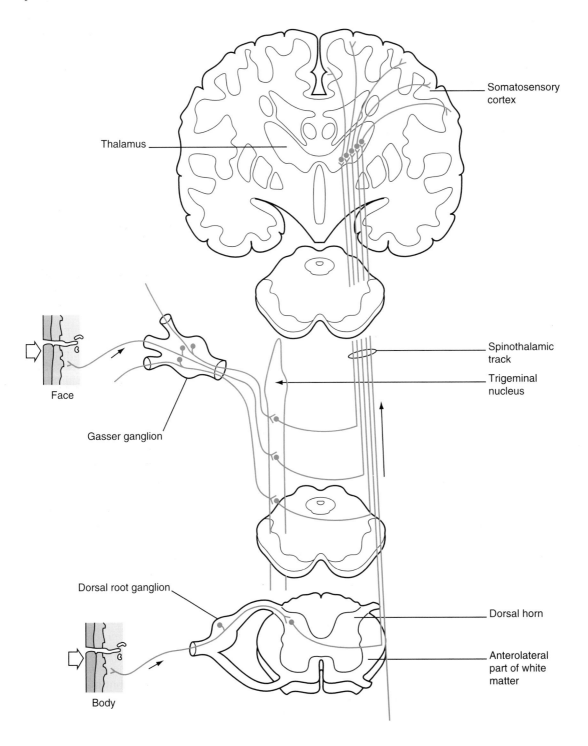

cell body to the polysomes has been demonstrated, which would allow the synthesis of some of their proteins. Transport of macromolecules from the cell body toward its dendrites, similar to axonal transport, has not yet been described.

The degradation of cellular metabolism debris and non-neuronal elements taken up from the external environment by endocytosis (e.g. uptake of viruses) takes place in the lysosomes of the cell body. They are transported from axon terminals to the cell body via retrograde axonal transport. Finally, to coordinate synthesis activity in the cell body with the needs of the axon terminals, the existence of a feedback mechanism (from terminals to cell body) seems essential. This could take place through retrograde axonal transport.

Regionalization of functions implicated in reception and transmission of electrical signals

The neuronal regions receiving synapses are mainly the dendritic (primary segments, branches and spines of dendrites) and somatic regions but also axonal regions. These receptive regions, named post-synaptic elements, have a restricted surface and contain in their plasma membrane, proteins specialized in the recognition of neurotransmitters: the neurotransmitter receptors (receptor channels and receptors coupled to G-proteins). These proteins synthesized in the cell body are then transported toward the dendritic or axonal post-synaptic membranes to be incorporated. Similarly, the proteins specialized in the generation and propagation of action potentials (voltage-dependent channels) are synthesized in the soma and have to be transported and incorporated in the axonal membrane.

Regionalization of secretory function

This function is localized in regions making synaptic contacts and more generally in pre-synaptic regions such as axon terminals (and sometimes in dendritic and somatic regions). At the level of pre-synaptic structures, the neurotransmitter is stored in synaptic vesicles and released. The secretory function implicates the presence of specific molecules and organelles in the pre-synaptic region: neurotransmitter synthesis enzymes, synaptic vesicles, microtubules and associated proteins, voltage-dependent channels, etc.

In conclusion, because of its extensive regionalization and the length and volume of its processes, the neuron has the challenge of delivering the proteins synthesized in the soma to the appropriate sites (targeting) at appropriate times.

Further Reading

Andressen, C., Blümcke, I. and Celio, M.R. (1993) Calcium-binding proteins: selective markers of nerve cells. *Cell Tiss. Res.* **271**, 181–208.

Azhderian, E.M., Hefner, D., Lin, C.H., Kaczmarek, L.K. and Forscher, P. (1994) Cyclic AMP modulates fast axonal transport in aplysia bag cell neurons by increasing the probability of single organelle movement. *Neuron* **12**, 1223–1233.

Brady, S., Sperry, A.O. (1995) Biochemical and functional diversity of microtubule motors in the nervous system. *Curr. Opin. Neurobiol.* **5**, 551–558.

Craig, A.M. and Banker, G. (1994) Neuronal polarity. *Ann. Rev. Neurosci.* **17**, 267–310.

Palay, S.L. and Chan-Palay, V. (1977) General morphology of neurons and neuroglia. In: Brookhart, I.M., Mountcastle, V.B., Kandel, E.R. and Geiger, S.R. (Eds), *Handbook of Physiology*, Vol 1, Part 1, pp. 5–37: American Physiological Society, Bethesda, MD.

Ramon Y. Cajal (1911) *Histologie du Système Nerveux de l'Homme et des Vertébrés*, Vols I and II, Maloine, Paris.

Gho, M., McDonald, K., Ganetsky, B. and Saxton, W.M. (1992) Effects of kinesin mutations on neuronal functions. *Science* **258**, 313–316.

2

The Chemical Synapses

In 1888, Ramon y Cajal suggested that the contacts between the axon terminals of a neuron and the dendrites or the perikaryon of another neuron are the points at which the information flows from one neuron to the other: 'Les articulations ou contacts utiles et efficaces entre neurones ne s'effectuent qu'entre cylindre-axiles, collatérales ou terminales d'un neurone et les prolongements ou le corps cellulaire d'un autre neurone'. The term 'synapse' was introduced by Sherrington (1897) to describe these zones of contact between neurons, specialized in the transmission of information.

In fact, the term synapse is not only used to describe connections between neurons (interneuronal connections) but also those between neurons and effector cells such as muscle and glandular cells (neuro-effector synapses) and those between receptive cells and neurons (Figure 2.1). These contacts are the points where the information is transmitted from one cell to the other: the synaptic transmission.

According to morphological and functional criteria, there are various types of synapses, including:

- The *chemical synapses*, which are characterized morphologically by the existence of a space between the plasma membranes of the connected cells. These spaces are called synaptic clefts. In this case, a molecule, the neurotransmitter, conveys the information between the pre-synaptic cell and the post-synaptic cell. These synapses will be described in this chapter (Figure 2.2a). Some of the chemical synapses have particular characteristics:
  - (i) the *reciprocal synapses* formed by the juxtaposition of two chemical synapses oriented in the reverse direction to each other (Figure 2.2d);
  - (ii) the *glomeruli* formed by a group of chemical synapses. In some cases, a group of dendrites form chemical synapses with the axon they surround (Figure 2.2e). In other cases, numerous axon terminals form synapses with the dendrite they surround.

- The *electrical synapses* or gap junctions are characterized by the apposition of the plasma membranes of the connected cells. In this case, the ions flow directly from one cell to the other without the use of a chemical transmitter. Gap junctions also allow the exchange of small-diameter intracellular molecules such as second messengers and metabolites. The gap junctions are described in more detail in Section 5.4.4 (Figure 2.2b). These synapses are common between glial cells in the mammalian central nervous system.

- The *mixed synapses* are formed by the juxtaposition of a chemical synapse and a gap junction (Figure 2.2c). In mammals, between neurons, these synapses are more common than the electrical synapses.

2.1 The Synaptic Complex Includes Three Components: The Pre-synaptic Element, Synaptic Cleft and Post-synaptic Element: It Has a Structural and Functional Asymmetry

In this paragraph we will take as an example the interneuronal chemical synapses. When we observe under the electron microscope a section of brain tissue taken from a region of the central nervous system rich in cell bodies and dendrites (gray matter, see Section 4.1.2), we see at the surface of a dendritic shaft or a dendritic spine one or many synaptic contacts (Figure 2.3, arrows). One of these synaptic contacts represents the synaptic complex (Figure 2.4). The synaptic complex includes three components: the pre-synaptic element, the synaptic cleft and the post-synaptic element. The synaptic complex is the *non-reducible basic unit* of each chemical synapse since it includes the minimal requirement for an efficient chemical synaptic transmission.

Figure 2.1 Different types of cells connected by chemical synapses. (a) Interneuronal synapses. Example of synapses between a spinal motoneuron (Golgi type I neuron that innervates striated muscle fibers) and a Renshaw cell (a local circuit neuron in the spinal cord). Neuromuscular junction: synapse between a motoneuron and a striated muscle cell. (b) Synapse between a sensory receptor and a neuron. Example of synapses between an auditory receptive cell (ciliary cell in the cochlea) and a primary sensory neuron whose cell body is located in the spiral ganglion. This neuron is free of dendrites and has a T-shaped axon that drives sensory information from the periphery to the central nervous system. (a: From Eckert R, Randall D and Augustine G, 1988. *Animal Physiology* p. 683, W.A. Freeman, New York, with permission.)

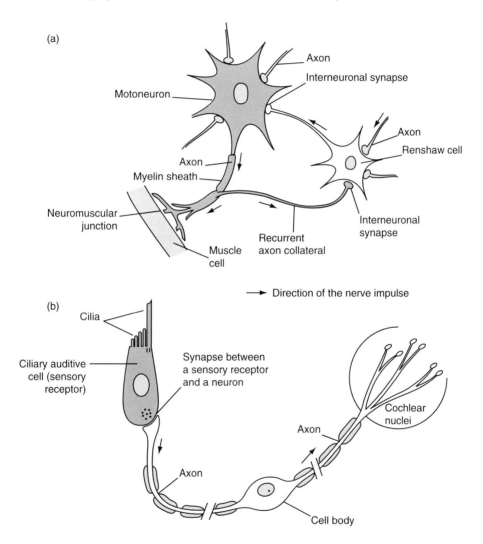

2.1.1 The Pre- and Post-synaptic Elements are Morphologically and Functionally Specialized

The pre-synaptic element is characterized by the presence of numerous mitochondria and synaptic vesicles which store the neurotransmitter (Figures 2.3 and 2.4). Two types of synaptic vesicles are described: clear vesicles (40–50 nm in diameter) and dense-core vesicles or dense granules, which have an electron-dense core (40–60 nm in diameter). Occasionally, we see under the pre-synaptic membrane an electron-dense zone with a geometry more or less distinguishable, the pre-synaptic grid (Figure 2.8). It corresponds to a particular organization of the cytoskeleton which

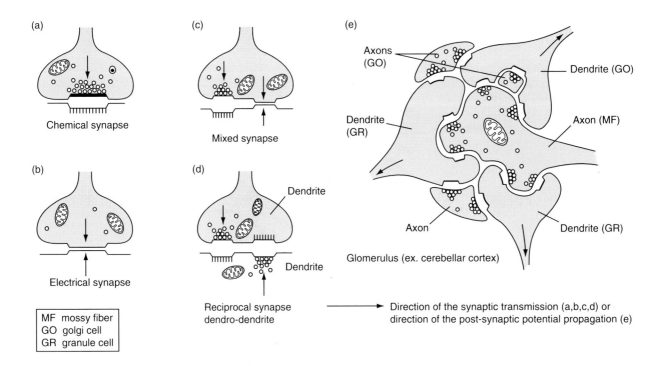

Figure 2.2 Different types of synapses. See text for explanation. MF, mossy fiber, axon of pontine nuclei neurons; Go, Golgi cell; GR, granule cell. (a to d: From Bodian D, 1972. Neuronal junctions: a revolutionary decade, *Anat. Rec.* **174**, 73–82, with permission. e: From Steiger U, 1967. Uber den Feinbau des Neuropils im Corpus pedunculatum des Waldaneise, *Z. Zelforsch*, **81**, 511–536, with permission.)

Figure 2.3 Axo-spinous synapses, one of which (center) is a 'perforated' synapse. Microphotography of a section of the hippocampus (molecular layer of the fascia dentata) observed under the electron microscope. Two synaptic boutons (Ax. Term.), filled with synaptic vesicles (Ves) and forming one or many asymmetric synaptic contacts (arrows, see also Figure 2.8) with dendritic spines (Sp) of pyramidal neurons, can be visualized. (Microphotography: Olivier Robain.)

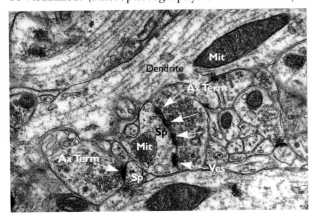

might be related to the exocytosis of synaptic vesicles.

The post-synaptic element in the interneuronal synapses is characterized by a sub-membranous electron-dense zone, which most probably corresponds to the region where the post-synaptic receptors are anchored. In cases where the post-synaptic element is non-neuronal, we shall see that various other post-synaptic specializations exist.

The synaptic complex displays a particular asymmetric structure, the synaptic vesicles being present only in the pre-synaptic element. This structural asymmetry suggests a functional asymmetry, which we will describe.

2.1.2 General Functional Model of the Synaptic Complex

A general functional model of chemical synaptic transmission would be as follows (Figure 2.4a): the newly

Figure 2.4   Pre- and post-synaptic specializations. (a) Schematic representation of the synaptic transmission (see text for explanation). (b) Electron photomicrographs of transverse sections at the level of synaptic complexes (inhibitory synapse afferent to the motorneuron in the spinal cord of the rat). Left: Exocytosis (arrow) between two dense projections and a coated vesicle (crossed arrow) characteristic of the recycling of the membrane. Right: localization of the glycine receptor associated gephyrin visualized with gold particles associated to a specific monoclonal antibody (arrows); with this pre-embedding technique the gold particles are localized on the intracellular side of the postsynaptic membrane. Gephyrin is a non-glycosylated protein which contributes to aggregation and/or stabilization of the glycine receptor to the postsynaptic microdomain (double headed arrow). (see Appendixes 2.2 and 2.3). AP, action potential. (Top: From Triller A and Korn H, 1985. Activity dependent deformations of presynaptic grids at central synapses, *J. Neurocytol.* **14**, 177–192, with permission. From Triller A, Cluzeaud F, Pfeiffer F and Korn H, 1986. Distribution and transmembrane organization of glycine receptor at central synapses: an immunocytochemical touch, In: Levi-Montalcini R. *et al.* eds, *Molecular Aspects of Neurobiology*, pp. 101–105, Springer-Verlag, Berlin, with permission.)

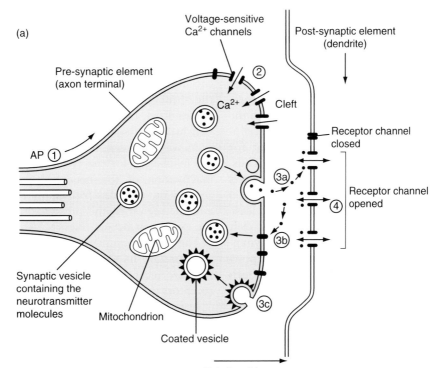

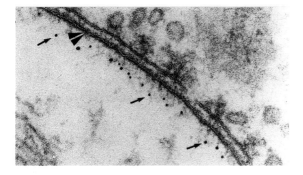
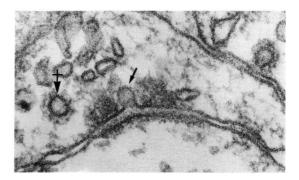

synthesized neurotransmitter molecules are stored in the synaptic vesicles present in the pre-synaptic element. The exocytosis of synaptic vesicles is triggered by an increase in the intracellular Ca^{2+} concentration ($[Ca^{2+}]_i$) (see Chapter 8). In a non-depolarized pre-synaptic element, the voltage-sensitive Ca^{2+} channels (see Section 7.5) are closed and Ca^{2+} ions cannot enter the intracellular space. Then, while the pre-synaptic membrane is at rest, i.e. as long as it is not depolarized by the arrival of an action potential, the probability of exocytosis of a synaptic vesicle and the release of its contents into the synaptic cleft is low. The neurotransmitter molecules are not released in significant quantities into the synaptic cleft: there is no synaptic transmission.

The propagation of action potentials to the pre-synaptic terminal (1) induces a depolarization of the pre-synaptic membrane. This results in the opening of the voltage-sensitive Ca^{2+} channels present in the pre-synaptic membrane (2). The entry of Ca^{2+} through the opened channels evokes an increase in the intracellular Ca^{2+} concentration, an indispensable factor for triggering exocytosis of synaptic vesicles (3a). Thus, the probability of exocytosis of synaptic vesicles is strongly increased. This results in fusion of a vesicle(s) with the pre-synaptic plasma membrane and release of the neurotransmitter molecules in the synaptic cleft (extracellular medium). Once released into the synaptic cleft, neurotransmitter molecules bind to post-synaptic (4), pre-synaptic and glial receptors, which are specific for them. By binding to post-synaptic receptor channels (4) or to post-synaptic receptors coupled to G-proteins (see Chapter 5), the neurotransmitter will induce the movement of ions through post-synaptic channels. At that stage, the synaptic transmission is completed. Simultaneously, the neurotransmitter molecules present in the synaptic cleft, which have already been bound to a receptor or not, are recaptured in the pre-synaptic element (3b) and/or the glial cells and/or degraded in the synaptic cleft by specific enzymes. In these ways the neurotransmitter is eliminated from the synaptic cleft. In the pre-synaptic element, the neurotransmitter is taken back into vesicles or degraded. The membrane is recycled by an endocytotic process (3c).

To refill the stores, the neurotransmitter has to be synthesized *de novo*. Neurotransmitters are generally synthesized in axon terminals from a precursor present in the axon terminals or taken up from the blood.

The enzymes necessary for its synthesis are synthesized in the soma and carried via anterograde axonal transport to the axon terminals. However, neurotransmitters that are peptides are synthesized as an inactive precursor form in the neuronal soma and carried to the axonal terminals via anterograde axonal transport. The question about the factors involved in the regulation of neurotransmitter synthesis, i.e. how the terminals or the soma are instructed to synthesize more or less neurotransmitter molecules, is still under study.

This general scheme is of course oversimplified. The pre-synaptic element can contain more than a single neurotransmitter: we speak of the coexistence of neurotransmitters; the intracellular concentration of Ca^{2+} ions can also be increased by the release of Ca^{2+} ions from intracellular stores (Figure 18.5) and this can induce the exocytosis of synaptic vesicles without the opening of voltage-sensitive Ca^{2+} channels. Finally, we omitted the role of pre-synaptic receptors for which there is evidence in most synapses.

As we have seen, the *pre-synaptic element* contains the machinery for the synthesis, storage, release and inactivation of the neurotransmitter(s). The active zone is the complex formed by the synaptic vesicles and the region of the pre-synaptic membrane where the exocytosis occurs (Figure 2.4b).

The *post-synaptic element* is specialized to receive information. Its plasma membrane contains proteins that are receptors for the neurotransmitter: channel receptors (Figure 2.4b) and G-protein linked receptors.

In most cases the synaptic transmission is unidirectional (or polarized): it is propagated only from the pre-synaptic element, which contains the neurotransmitter, to the post-synaptic element at the surface of which are located receptors for the neurotransmitter (Figure 2.4b).

In the case of dendro-dendritic synapses (olfactory bulb of the rat), we recognize two juxtaposed synaptic complexes that work in opposite polarities; these are the reciprocal synapses (Figure 2.2d). However, it is worth noting that, here also, the synaptic transmission is polarized in each of the synaptic complexes.

2.1.3 Complementarity Between the Neurotransmitter Stored and Released by the Pre-synaptic Element and the Nature of Receptors in the Post-synaptic Membrane

In general, there is a complementarity between the neurotransmitter stored and released by the pre-synaptic element and the receptor proteins which occur in high density in the membrane of the post-synaptic element, and even when the pre- and post-synaptic cells have a different embryonic origin (as in the nerve–muscle junction, for example). This complementarity is essential for an efficient synaptic transmission.

Various methods are used to characterize the neurotransmitter(s) present in a pre-synaptic element and the receptors present in the post-synaptic membrane. More specifically, there is:

- To identify a neurotransmitter: immunohistochemical methods that identify the synthesis enzyme of the neurotransmitter in various parts of the neuron and the *in situ* hybridization technique that identifies the mRNA coding for the synthesis enzyme of the neurotransmitter. With this technique, only the somata of the positive neurons are labeled (Appendix 2.2). However, the identification of a substance as a neurotransmitter requires the experimental proof of several other criteria (Appendix 2.1). If these criteria are not satisfied, the substance is called a putative neurotransmitter.
- To identify the receptors: radioautographic techniques, with monoclonal antibodies or, more rarely, anti-idiotype antibodies (Appendix 2.3).

In order to obtain a match between the neurotransmitter and its receptors, the genes coding for the complementary proteins of the pre- and post-synaptic elements (neurotransmitter synthesis enzymes, receptors) must be expressed in the two connected cells. It is important to remember that the post-synaptic neuron receives numerous afferents and therefore must synthesize a large pool of receptors. These receptors are then directed to different post-synaptic regions of the plasma membrane so that they match with the corresponding afferent neurotransmitter. This specificity between the receptor and the neurotransmitter is a problem that generally occurs in regionalized functions and which is solved by the specific targeting of proteins.

Various hypotheses have been suggested to explain the complementarity between the pre- and post-synaptic elements. The different types of receptors would at first be synthesized by the post-synaptic cell and randomly inserted in the plasma membrane before functional synaptic contacts are formed. Then an anterograde signal (from the pre-synaptic element to the post-synaptic element) would contribute to selection at the transcriptional level of the receptors expressed by the post-synaptic cell and inserted in the post-synaptic membrane. This signal, which does not seem to be the neurotransmitter, might be a peptide released simultaneously with it.

In the same way, a retrograde signal would be given by the post-synaptic cell once the synaptic contact is established. This signal would control the type of neurotransmitter present in the pre-synaptic element. Therefore, the complementarity between the pre- and post-synaptic element would result from the reciprocal selection of the genes expressed by the cells in contact.

However, the pre-/post-synaptic complementarity not only involves the nature of the neurotransmitter and the receptors for this neurotransmitter but also the occurrence, in the pre-synaptic element, of a membrane specialized in exocytosis (for the release of the neurotransmitter) and in the recycling of membrane. Exocytosis of the synaptic vesicles occurs in a very small area of the pre-synaptic membrane. This phenomenon implies the recognition between the vesicular membrane and the plasma membrane in the pre-synaptic element. The hypothetical mechanisms involved in this recognition are described in Sections 5.7.1 and 8.2. Moreover, after each exocytosis the surface of the pre-synaptic membrane increases because of the addition of vesicular membrane. This excess in membrane surface is corrected by a compensatory mechanism of recycling of the plasma membrane. This process corresponds to the formation of new synaptic vesicles by endocytosis (see Section 5.7.2). The mechanisms of recycling are still hypothetical and many questions remain to be answered, including the following: the protein content of the vesicular membrane is different from that of the plasma membrane, so what is the protein content of the recycled membrane? Is it similar to vesicular membrane or to any other membrane in the pre-synaptic element? In the first case, the recycled membrane would be the vesicular membrane itself before it is completely mixed with the plasma membrane. In the second case, the recycled

Figure 2.5   Different types of interneuronal synapses. (a) Terminal boutons forming axo-somatic synapses. (b, from top to bottom) Synapses between terminal boutons and a smooth dendritic branch (axo-dendritic synapse) and two examples of indented synapses between terminal boutons and a dendritic spine (axo-spinous synapses). (c) Synapse between an axon terminal and a terminal axon collateral (axo-axonic synapse). The 'post-synaptic' axon terminal is itself 'pre-synaptic' to a dendrite. (From Hamlyn LH, 1972. The fine structure of the mossy fiber endings in the hippocampus of the rabbit, *J. Anat.* **96**, 112–120, with permission.)

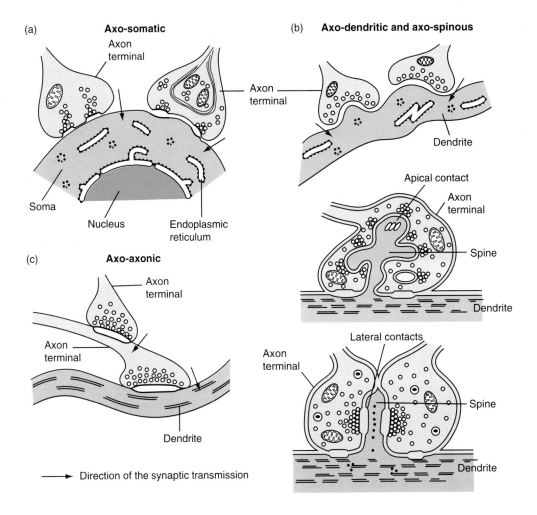

membrane would be any region of the pre-synaptic membrane. Various steps to transform the recycled membrane in vesicular membrane able to store the neurotransmitter would then take place. The answer to this question can be obtained by the use of specific markers of the vesicular and plasma membranes.

2.2 The Interneuronal Synapses

2.2.1 In the Central Nervous System, the Most Common Synapses are Those Where the Axon Terminal is the Pre-synaptic Element

As we have seen in the previous chapter (Section 1.1.2), the axon terminals are *terminal boutons* (Figure 2.5), which are terminals of axonal branches, and *'boutons en passant'* (see Figure 2.13), which appear as swellings located along the non-myelinated axons and at the nodes of Ranvier along myelinated axons. These two types of axon terminals form synaptic contacts with various neuronal post-synaptic elements: a dendrite (axo-dendritic synapse), a soma (axo-somatic synapse) or an axon (axo-axonic synapse) (Figure 2.5). More rarely, there are synapses in which the pre-synaptic element is a dendrite (dendro-dendritic synapse, see Figures 2.2d) or a soma (soma-somatic or soma-dendritic synapses).

2.2.2 At Low Magnification, the Axo-dendritic Synaptic Contacts Display Various Features: These Various Features Imply Different Functions

We will consider as an example the cerebellar cortex, a layered structure in which the cells and their afferents are well characterized. The Purkinje cells are the single 'output' cells of the cerebellar cortex (Golgi type I neurons) which send their axon to the deep cerebellar nuclei. They have a cell body with a large diameter (20–30 µm) from which emerges a single dendritic trunk that gives rise to numerous spiny dendritic branches which arborize in the molecular layer. The dendritic tree is planar, and the dendritic branches extend mainly in the transverse plane (Figure 2.6). The neurotransmitter of Purkinje cells is γ-aminobutyric acid (GABA) (Appendix 2.1).

Purkinje cells receive two types of excitatory afferents: the climbing fibers (axons of the neurons in the inferior olivary nucleus) and the parallel fibers (axons of the granule cells in the cerebellar cortex). The inhibitory afferents arise mainly from the numerous local circuit neurons in this structure: the basket cells, the stellate cells and the Golgi cells (Figure 2.6).

A single climbing fiber innervates each single Purkinje cell. The climbing fiber gives rise to numerous axon collaterals that 'fit' the shape of the post-synaptic dendritic tree: the axon collaterals 'climb' along the dendrites (Figure 2.7a, b) forming numerous synaptic contacts with the soma and the dendrites of the Purkinje cell. These contacts are axo-dendritic or axo-spinous, the pre-synaptic element being a terminal bouton. Such a synaptic organization implies that this excitatory afferent is very efficient: a single action potential along the climbing fiber can induce a response in the Purkinje cell (see Section 18.3).

The axons of the granule cells form very different synaptic contacts with the Purkinje cells. The axons enter the molecular layer where they bifurcate and extend for 2 mm in a plane perpendicular to the plane of the dendritic tree of the Purkinje cell and form what are called parallel fibers (Figure 2.6). Parallel fibers form a few 'en passant' synapses (axo-spinous synapses between axonal varicosities and distal dendritic spines) with the numerous Purkinje cells (about 50). Therefore, each Purkinje cell receives synaptic contacts from about 200 000 parallel fibers. The consequence of such a synaptic organization is as follows: the activation of a parallel fiber cannot induce a Purkinje cell response since the activation of one or a few of these excitatory synapses cannot trigger post-synaptic action potentials; numerous parallel fibers converging onto a single Purkinje cell must be activated to induce a response in this cell.

The basket cells are local circuit neurons (Golgi type II neurons) which inhibit the activity of Purkinje cells. The axons of these neurons project to a large number of Purkinje cells and give rise to numerous axon collaterals which form 'baskets' around the soma of Purkinje cells. The axonal branches extend further and terminate 'en pinceau' around the initial segment of the Purkinje cells' axon (Figures 2.6 and 2.7a, c). Such an organization allows the inhibition of the Purkinje cells at a strategic point where the sodium action potentials arise. This represents an efficient way to counteract the excitatory potentials propagating along the dendritic branches to the initial axonal segment.

2.2.3 The Interneuronal Synapses Display Ultrastructural Characteristics that Vary Between Two Extremes: Types 1 and 2

A classification of the synapses on the basis of the form of their synaptic complex was proposed by Gray (1959). This author described two types of synaptic complexes in the cerebral cortex, which he named types 1 and 2 (Figure 2.8). Type 1 synapses are asymmetrical because they have a prominent accumulation of electron-dense material on the post-synaptic side. These synapses are found more often on dendritic spines or distal dendritic branches. The pre-synaptic element contains round vesicles and the synaptic cleft is about 30 nm wide. Type 2 synapses

Figure 2.6   Synaptic connections in the cerebellar cortex. In a section of the cerebellar cortex the different layers are depicted: below the surface (pia mater) we can see the molecular layer (mol), the layer of Purkinje cells (Pc), the granular layer (gr) and the white matter (wm). In the sagittal plane, bottom left, are four granular cells localized in the granular layer that send their axons to the molecular layer where they bifurcate in a T to form the parallel fibers. These fibers travel in parallel to the large axis of the folium in the transverse plane. Two Purkinje cells and a basket cell with an axon that gives numerous collaterals surrounding the soma (basket) of many Purkinje cells. A climbing fiber that arborizes along the dendrites of one of the Purkinje cells is shown. By comparing the Purkinje cells in the sagittal plane with those in the transverse plane, we notice that the dendritic tree of the Purkinje cells is plane. (From Chan-Palay V and Palay S, 1974. *Cerebellar Cortex. Cytology and Organization*, Springer-Verlag, Berlin, with permission.)

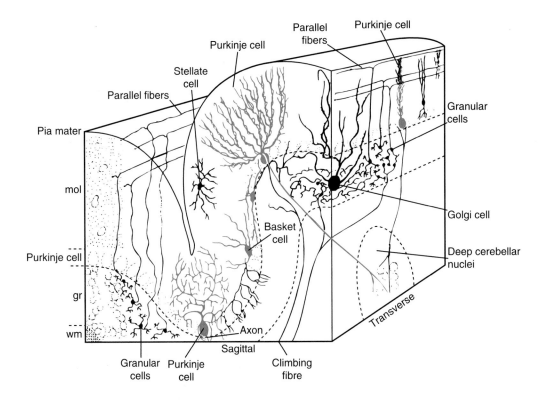

are symmetrical because they have electron-dense zones of the same size in both the pre- and post-synaptic elements. The pre-synaptic element contains oval-shaped vesicles and the synaptic cleft is narrow. These synapses are more commonly found at the surface of dendritic trunks and soma. On the basis of correlations between physiological and morphological data obtained in the cerebellar cortex, Gray proposed that type 1 synapses are excitatory whereas type 2 synapses are inhibitory.

The electron-dense zones located on the cytoplasmic side of the pre-synaptic membrane form the pre-synaptic grid. When they are examined in transverse section at the level of a synapse, these dense zones have a triangular shape, their base being apposed against the plasma membrane. They are linked to each other by filamentous bridges. In a section parallel to the plane of the synapse, they appear to be organized as a 'triagonal' network and the closest synaptic vesicles to the plasma membrane are embedded between these dense zones as 'eggs in an egg box'. The pre-synaptic grid might be a dynamic structure involved in exocytosis.

In the central nervous system, types 1 and 2 synapses are the extremes of a morphological continuum since synaptic complexes may have intermediate forms and display features that characterize both types of synapses, e.g. a large synaptic cleft (type 1)

Figure 2.7 Varieties of synaptic arrangements at the level of a Purkinje cell. Representation on a single drawing (a) and in two separate schematic drawings (b and c) of the synaptic arrangements between a climbing fiber and a Purkinje cell (a and b) and between a basket cell and a Purkinje cell (a and c). (a: From Chan-Palay V and Palay S, 1974. *Cerebellar Cortex. Cytology and Organization*, Springer-Verlag, Berlin, with permission. b: From Scheibel ME and Scheibel AB, 1958. *Electroencephalogr. Clin. Neurophysiol.* **Suppl 10**, 43–50, with permission. c: From Hamori J and Szentagothai J, 1965. The Purkinje cell baskets: ultrastructure of an inhibitory synapse, *Acad. Biol. Hung.* **15**, 465–479, with permission.)

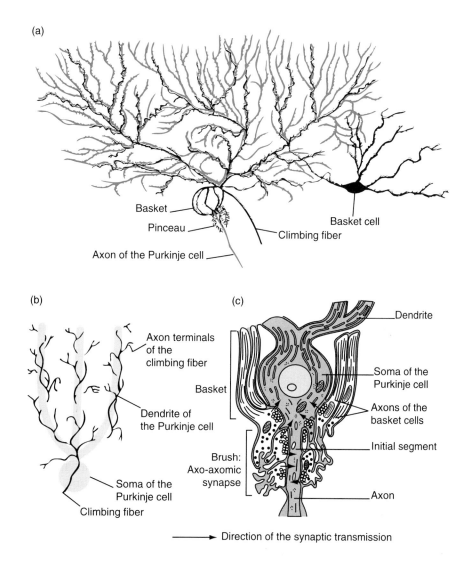

(a)

Basket
Pinceau
Axon of the Purkinje cell
Basket cell
Climbing fiber

(b)

Axon terminals
of the
climbing fiber

Basket

Dendrite of
the Purkinje cell

Soma of the
Purkinje cell

Climbing fiber

(c)

Dendrite

Soma of the
Purkinje cell

Axons of the
basket cells

Initial segment

Brush:
Axo-axomic
synapse

Axon

Direction of the synaptic transmission

Figure 2.8 Schematic representation of type 1 (asymmetric) and type 2 (symmetric) synapses according to Gray.

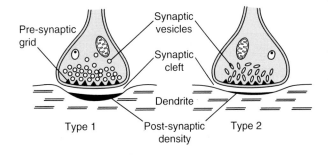

Type 1   Type 2

Figure 2.9 The neuromuscular junction. Photograph of a rat neuromuscular junction observed in the scanning electron microscope. The terminal part of the axon (ax) is detached from the muscle cell (m) in order to show the synaptic gutter (g); c, capillary; n, motor nerve; s, nucleus of a Schwann cell. (From Matsuda Y *et al*, 1988. Scanning electron microscopic study of denervated and reinnervated neuromuscular junction, *Muscle Nerve* **11**, 1266–1271, with permission.)

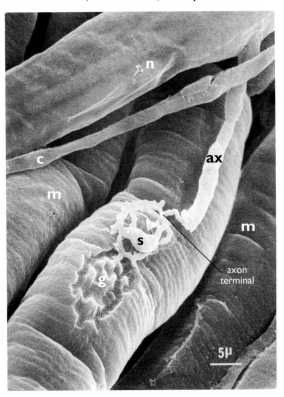

and a narrow post-synaptic density (type 2). In addition, it has been shown that the form of synaptic vesicles is dependent on the fixation technique used.

2.3 The Neuromuscular Junction is the Group of Synaptic Contacts Between the Terminal Arborization of a Motor Axon and a Striate Muscle Fiber

The motoneurons or motor neurons have their cell body located in motor nuclei of the brainstem or in the ventral horn of the spinal cord. The axons of these neurons are myelinated and form the cranial and spinal nerves that innervate the skeletal striate muscles (see Figures 1.13a and 4.5a). In general, a single striated muscle fiber is innervated by one motoneuron but a single motoneuron can innervate many muscle fibers. The myelin sheath of each axon is interrupted at the zone where the axon arborizes at the surface of the muscle fiber. At this point, the thin non-myelinated axonal branches possess numerous varicosities which are located in the depression at the surface of the muscle fiber: the synaptic gutter. The axon terminals are covered by the non-myelinating Schwann cells (Figure 2.9).

2.3.1 In the Axon Terminals the Synaptic Vesicles are Concentrated at the Level of the Electron-dense Bars: They Contain Acetylcholine (Figure 2.10)

The neuromuscular junction is formed by the juxtaposition of the terminals of a motor axon and the corresponding sub-synaptic domains of a striated muscle fiber, these two elements being separated by a 50–100 nm wide cleft.

In a transverse section of a neuromuscular junction, we observe by electron microscopy a particular organization. The vesicles in the pre-synaptic element are small (40–60 nm in diameter), clear and contain acetylcholine, the neurotransmitter of all the neuromuscular junctions (Appendix 2.1). Other larger vesicles (80–120 nm in diameter) that contain an electron-dense material are also present but in a much lower proportion (1% of the total population). The vesicles are aggregated in the pre-synaptic zones where an electron-dense material is present, the dense bars. These dense bars are functionally homologous to the pre-synaptic grid of interneuronal synapses. They are 100 nm wide and are located perpendicularly to the largest axis of each axonal branch. The vesicles are aligned along each side of these bars. The complex of dense bar and synaptic vesicles forms a pre-synaptic active zone (Couteaux 1960). There are many active zones per varicosity. They are located opposite to the folds of the post-synaptic plasma membrane. Each active zone with the folds of the sarcolemma in front of them forms a synaptic complex. Therefore, the neuromuscular junction contains numerous synaptic complexes.

The synthesis of acetylcholine takes place in the cytoplasm of the pre-synaptic element from two precursors: choline and acetylcoenzyme A (acetyl CoA). The reaction is catalyzed by choline acetyltransferase (CAT). Acetylcholine is transported actively into synaptic vesicles where it is stored. The protein responsible for this active transport is a transporter which uses the energy of the proton (H^+) gradient. This gradient of protons is established by the active transport of H^+ ions from the cytoplasm towards the interior of the vesicles by an H^+/ATPase pump (see Sections 5.5.2). The vesicles contain, apart from acetylcholine, ATP and a negatively charged mucopolysaccharide, vesiculine, whose role is still unknown. In the axon terminals, acetylcholine is present in the vesicular compartment but also in the cytoplasmic compartment, these two compartments being in equilibrium with one another (see Appendix 8.1).

2.3.2 The Synaptic Cleft is Narrow and Occupied by a Basal Membrane Which Contains the Degradative Enzyme for Acetylcholine, Acetylcholinesterase

The post-synaptic muscular membrane (sarcolemma) is covered, on the extracellular surface, with a layer of electron-dense material, the basal membrane (Figure 2.10). This membrane, which follows the folds of the sarcolemma, is a conjunctive tissue secreted by the non-myelinating Schwann cells covering the axon terminals. It contains, among others, collagen, proteoglycans and laminin (see Section 4.1.4).

One form of the degradative enzyme of acetylcholine, the asymmetric form of acetylcholinesterase (A), is anchored in the basal lamina (Figure 2.10). Acetylcholinesterases are glycoproteins synthesized in the soma and carried to the terminals via anterograde axonal transport. They are then inserted into the pre-synaptic membrane and the basal membrane. The molecules of acetylcholine released in the synaptic cleft, when the neuromuscular junctions are activated, cross the basal membrane which comprises loose stitches and a part of these acetylcholine molecules is thus degraded before being fixed to post-synaptic receptors. The other part is quickly degraded after its fixation. Acetylcholinesterases hydrolyze acetylcholine into acetic acid and choline. Choline is taken up by pre-synaptic terminals for the synthesis of new molecules of acetylcholine. This degradation system of acetylcholine is a very efficient system for inactivation of the neurotransmitter.

2.3.3 The Nicotinic Receptors for Acetylcholine are Abundant in the Crests of the Folds in the Post-synaptic Membrane

The plasma membrane of muscle, the sarcolemma, presents numerous folds in mammalian neuromuscular junctions. By using a radioactive ligand for a type of acetylcholine nicotinic receptor, α-bungarotoxin labeled with a radioactive isotope or a fluorescent molecule, it has been shown that the radioactive material accumulates predominantly in the crests of the folds in the sarcolemma. Immunocytochemical techniques produce similar results. These results indicate that acetylcholine receptors of the neuromuscular junction are nicotinic and accumulate in the post-synaptic muscular membrane, more precisely at the level of the folds in the membrane. Other studies have shown that they are anchored to the underlying cytoskeleton.

The nicotinic receptor is a transmembranous glycoprotein comprising four homologous subunits assembled into a heterologous $\alpha_2\beta\gamma\delta$ pentamer. It is a receptor channel permeable to cations whose activation results in the net entry of positively charged ions and in depolarization of the post-synaptic membrane. The structure and functional characteristics of muscular nicotinic receptors are discussed in Chapter 9.

Figure 2.10   Ultrastructure of a neuromuscular junction and the location of acetylcholinesterases. (a) Micro-photography of the neuromuscular junction of a batrachian visualized in the electron microscope. In the axon terminal, we can see mitochondria and numerous vesicles. The axonal plasma membrane displays signs of exocytosis (active zones). The basal membrane is located in the synaptic cleft. The post-synaptic muscular membrane has numerous folds. (b) Schematic representation of the asymmetric (A12) and globular (G2) forms of acetylcholinesterase (AChE). The index number of A or G indicates the number of catalytic subunits. The asymmetric forms consist of a collagen tail, three peptide parts and catalytic subunits. The globular forms consist of one or more catalytic subunits (hydrophilic domain) and a glycolipid part (hydrophobic domain) which permit their insertion in the lipid bilayer. Location of acetylcholinesterase in the neuromuscular junction (see page 33). The A forms are synthesized in the motoneurons and secreted into the synaptic cleft where they are associated with the basal lamina. The globular forms are synthesized in the motoneurons and inserted into the pre-synaptic plasma membrane or secreted into the synaptic cleft. (a: microphotography: Pécot-Dechavassine.) (b: After Berkaloff A, Naquet R and Demaille J, eds, 1987. *Biologie 1990, Enjeux et Problématiques*, p. 80, CNRS, Paris, with permission.)

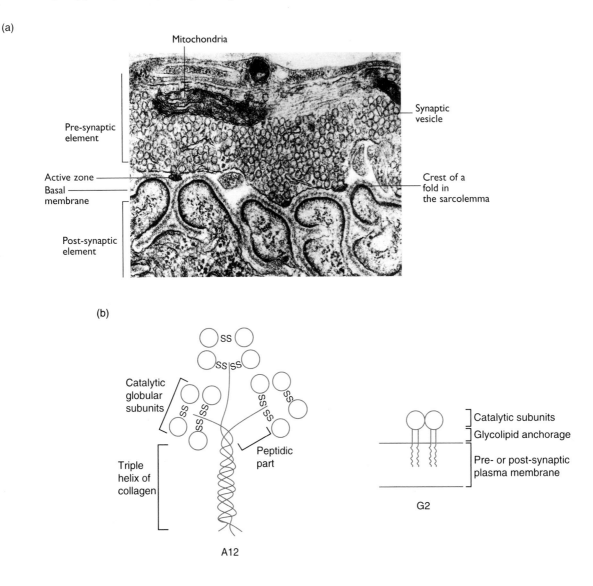

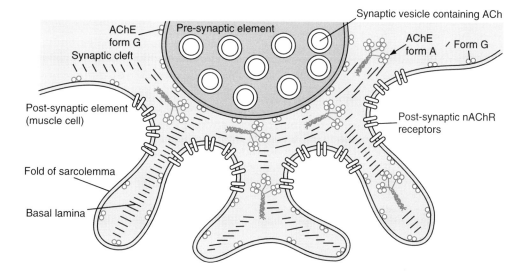

2.3.4 Mechanisms Involved in the Accumulation of Post-synaptic Receptors in the Folds of the Post-synaptic Muscular Membrane

The acetylcholine nicotinic receptors are, in the adult neuromuscular junction, localized at a high density (about 10 000 molecules/μm^2) in the post-synaptic regions and occur at a much lower density in the non-synaptic muscular membrane (extrajunctional membrane). Under the nerve terminal, the muscle cell is free of the myofilaments actin and myosin. At this level, four to eight cell nuclei are found, the fundamental nuclei (Ranvier 1875). The cell nuclei located outside the post-synaptic region are the sarcoplasmic nuclei. The formation of this well-organized sub-synaptic domain, which not only concerns the nicotinic receptors but also the Golgi apparatus and the cytoskeleton (it also comprises the organization of the basal lamina and the distribution of the asymmetric form of acetylcholinesterase in the synaptic cleft), occurs in numerous steps. During maturation of the neuromuscular junction (Figure 2.11) we observe:

- An increase in the number of nicotinic receptors (1 and 2) during fusion of the myoblasts to form myotubes owing to neosynthesis of these receptors. They have an even distribution over the membrane surface. This phenomenon is independent of neuro-

muscular activity since it is not affected by the injection *in ovo* of nicotinic antagonists such as curare.
- The formation of aggregates of nicotinic receptors (nAChR) under the nerve terminal (3–5) and the disappearance of extrajunctional receptors (5). Upon innervation, nAChR rapidly accumulate under the nerve endings. *In situ* hybridization experiments with a genomic coding probe (Appendix 2.2) have shown that in innervated 15-day-old chick muscle, the nAChR α-subunit mRNAs accumulate under the nerve endings. More precisely, accumulation of the mRNAs increases around the sub-synaptic (fundamental) nuclei and decreases around the sarcoplasmic nuclei. This can be interpreted as a differential expression of the α-subunit gene in the fundamental and sarcoplasmic nuclei. The presence of motor nerve and muscle activity are both crucial for the regulation of nAChR mRNA levels in the developing fiber.

The distribution of the Golgi apparatus, studied by using a monoclonal antibody directed against it, shows a similar evolution. In cultured myotubes, the Golgi apparatus is associated with every nucleus. Conversely, in 15-day-old innervated chick muscle, the Golgi apparatus is now restricted to discrete, highly focalized regions that appear to co-distribute with end plates (revealed by fluorescein isothiocyanate conjugated α-bungarotoxin, a labeled ligand of nAChR).

Figure 2.11　Expression of the nicotinic receptor during formation of the neuromuscular junction. The black dots indicate the nicotinic receptor (nAChR). (1, 2) Fusion of myoblasts to form myotubes and approach of the axon growth cone; (3) the growth cone forms contact with the myotube and induces the clustering of nicotinic receptors at this level; (4) numerous motor terminals converge towards a single aggregate of nicotinic receptors; but (5) a single terminal stabilizes and the folds of the sarcolemma develop. (From Laufer R and Changeux JP, 1989. Activity dependent regulation of gene expression in muscle and neuronal cells, *Mol. Neurobiol.* 3, 1–53, with permission.)

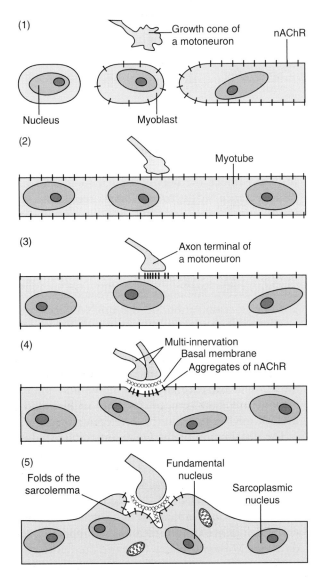

These observations raise the question about the nature of the signaling pathways which underlie such a reorganization: activation of second messengers by anterograde signals from the nerve endings that would lead to positive regulation of nicotinic receptor expression in the junctional regions and negative regulation in the extrajunctional regions? The existence of retrograde signals too?

- Stabilization of the nicotinic receptors in the post-synaptic membrane (5). Many factors seem to contribute to the focal increase in nAChR density in end plates: the compartmentalization of nAChR expression (confined to the sub-synaptic part), its synthesis rate, its metabolic stabilization in the membrane end plate (where its half-life is about 10 days compared with 1 day in extrajunctional membrane).

These results provide a basis for the study of the mechanisms involved in the formation and maintenance of the pre-/post-synaptic complementarity in other types of synapses.

2.4 The Synapse Between the Vegetative Post-ganglionic Neuron and the Smooth Muscle Cell

Smooth muscle cells are present in most of the visceral organs (digestive system, uterus, bladder, etc.) but also in the wall of blood vessels and around the hair follicles. They are innervated by post-ganglionic neurons of the autonomic nervous system (orthosympathetic neurons and parasympathetic neurons, Figures 2.12 and 4.5b,c).

2.4.1 The Pre-synaptic Element is a Varicosity of the Post-ganglionic Axon

The axons of the post-ganglionic neurons are not myelinated. Before contacting the smooth muscles, the axons divide into numerous thin filaments 0.1–0.5 μm in diameter which travel alone or in fascicles over long distances along the smooth muscle cells (Figure 2.13a). Each of these filaments has swellings or varicosities 0.5–2.0 μm in diameter spaced 3–5 μm apart. The varicosities contain mitochondria and numerous synaptic

Figure 2.12 The efferent neurons of the orthosympathetic (a) and parasympathetic (b) systems and the synapses between post-ganglionic neurons and smooth muscle fibres. The axon terminals of post-ganglionic neurons are varicosities and the synaptic contacts are of the 'boutons en passant' type. ACh, acetylcholine, NA, noradrenaline; arrows, direction in which the action potentials propagate (see also Figure 4.5B, C).

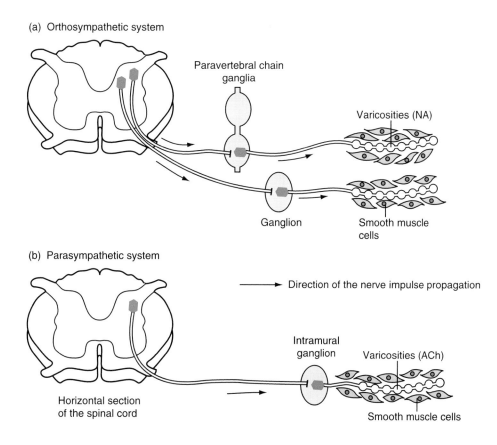

vesicles whereas the intervaricose segments contain mainly elements of the cytoskeleton (Figure 2.13b). The varicosities are the pre-synaptic elements. There are no electron-dense regions in the pre-synaptic membrane, which suggests the absence of a preferential zone for exocytosis (active zone) in these synapses.

The axonal varicosities contain a large number of small granular synaptic vesicles, i.e. with an electron-dense central core (30–50 nm in diameter), but also some large granular vesicles (60–120 nm in diameter) and small agranular vesicles. The neurotransmitter of the orthosympathetic post-ganglionic neurons is noradrenaline (Figure 2.12a). It is stored in small and large granular vesicles. Noradrenaline is a catecholamine (like dopamine and adrenaline) synthesized from the amino acid tyrosine. The first step, the

hydroxylation of tyrosine by tyrosine hydroxylase, is the limiting step. The activity of tyrosine hydroxylase is regulated by the product of the terminal synthesis, in this case noradrenaline.

Long-term regulation (in the order of hours to a few days) of tyrosine hydroxylase activity by trans-synaptic induction has also been reported. Studies on the superior cervical ganglion of the rat showed that depolarization of catecholaminergic neurons (induced by an extracellular medium highly concentrated in K^+ ions) after 2 days results in an increase in the quantity of tyrosine hydroxylase mRNA in these neurons. As a result there is an increase in the apparent activity of the enzyme owing to an increase in its transcription and translation. This result can be reproduced by the electrical stimulation of the afferents of

Figure 2.13 A nerve–smooth muscle synapse. (a) Microphotography of smooth muscle cells of the intestine (M) and post-ganglionic axon fascicles (parasympathetic nervous system, Ax) which are half covered by a Schwann cell (S), sectioned in the transverse plane and observed in the electron microscope. Note the width of the synaptic cleft. (b) Longitudinal section of a post-ganglionic axon showing a varicosity filled with vesicles and an intervaricose region. The post-synaptic smooth muscle cell contains numerous mitochondria. (Microphotographs: Jacques Taxi.)

(a)

(b)

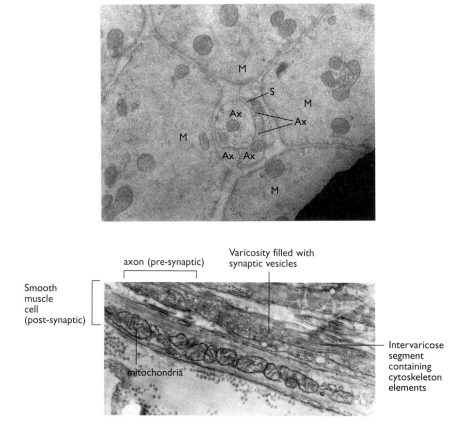

catecholaminergic neurons. In the orthosympathetic nervous system, the first event that leads to trans-synaptic induction of tyrosine hydroxylase in post-ganglionic neurons is the activation of their nicotinic receptors by acetylcholine released by the preganglionic neuron (Figure 2.12). The goal of trans-synaptic induction is the adjustment of the synthesis of catecholamines to the activity and needs of catecholaminergic neurons.

The noradrenaline receptors present in the post-synaptic membrane of smooth muscle cells are named α and β noradrenergic receptors; they are G-protein coupled receptors (see Section 5.4.2).

The inactivation of noradrenaline released from nerve terminals is, to a large extent, achieved by reup-

take by the catecholaminergic neurons or the nearby glial cells. It is recycled into the synaptic vesicles or degraded by specific enzymes such as the monoamine oxidases (MAO). Some of the catecholamines are degraded in the synaptic cleft by catechol-O-methyl-transferase (COMT).

Acetylcholine is the neurotransmitter of the parasympathetic post-ganglionic neurons (Figure 2.12b). The varicosities of these axons contain mainly small agranular vesicles but also large granular vesicles. Acetylcholine is stored in small agranular vesicles. The acetylcholine receptors present in the post-synaptic membrane of smooth muscle cells are cholinergic muscarinic receptors (mAChR or M receptors); they are G-protein coupled receptors (see Section 5.4.2).

2.4.2 The Width of the Synaptic Cleft is Very Variable

Where the synaptic cleft is narrowest, in the vas deferens or in the pupil for example, it measures between 15 and 20 nm. However, in the wall of blood vessels, the closest contacts are spaced 50–100 nm apart.

2.4.3 The Autonomous Post-ganglionic Synapse is Specialized to Ensure a Greater Effect of the Neurotransmitter

The large width of the synaptic cleft results in a greater effect of the neurotransmitter on a post-synaptic membrane surface than in the neuromuscular junction or in central synapses, where secretion of the neurotransmitter is focused on a small post-synaptic region. Moreover, in some autonomous synapses there is no distinguishable specialization of the pre-synaptic membrane, which suggests that the vesicles have no preferential site for exocytosis. The formation of a dense plexus by the post-ganglionic axons also contributes to the extended diffusion of pre-synaptic messages. Therefore, the activation of a post-ganglionic neuron results in the activation of numerous post-synaptic cells. Finally, the presence of numerous gap junctions which connect smooth muscle cells allows the synaptic response to spread to neighboring muscle cells, even those not innervated.

2.5 An Example of a Neuroglandular Synapse: The Synapse Between an Orthosympathetic Pre-ganglionic Neuron and the Chromaffin Cell of the Adrenal Medulla (Figure 2.14)

The adrenal medulla is the central part of the adrenal gland, the endocrine gland located above each kidney. It is formed by secretory cells, which are called chromaffin cells since they are colored by chromium salts. The adrenal medulla is innervated by orthosympathetic pre-ganglionic neurons which have axons that form the splanchnic nerve. When this nerve is stimulated, the chromaffin cells secrete mainly adrenaline but also noradrenaline and enkephalins (an endogenous opioid peptide). These hormones are then transported via the blood to numerous target tissues and mainly the heart and blood vessels.

The *pre-synaptic element* of this synapse is the axon

Figure 2.14   Synapses between an orthosympathetic pre-ganglionic neuron and chromaffin cells in the adrenal medulla. (a) The cell bodies of pre-ganglionic neurons are localized in the spinal cord and their axons form the orthosympathetic splanchnic nerve. These neurons innervate the chromaffin cells. (b) Post-ganglionic axon terminal forming numerous synapses with chromaffin cells. (From Coupland RE, 1965. Electron microscopic observations on the structure of the rat adrenal medulla. II. Normal innervation, *J. Anat. (Lond.)* **99**, 255–272, with permission.)

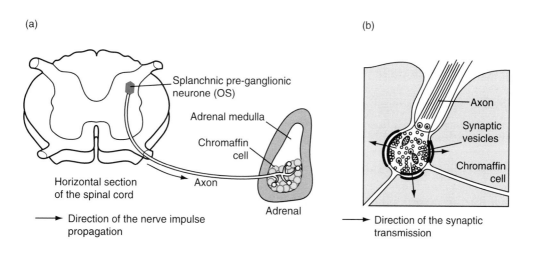

(a)

Splanchnic pre-ganglionic neurone (OS)

Adrenal medulla

Chromaffin cell

Horizontal section of the spinal cord

Axon

→ Direction of the nerve impulse propagation

Adrenal

(b)

Axon

Synaptic vesicles

Chromaffin cell

→ Direction of the synaptic transmission

terminal of the splanchnic orthosympathetic pre-ganglionic neurons. Their cell bodies are located in the intermediate horn of the spinal cord. Most of the axons are non-myelinated and are surrounded by the extensions of the non-myelinating Schwann cells. This glial sheath is present until the axon collaterals penetrate the junctional space. The axon terminals are mainly terminal boutons with a diameter ranging between 1 and 3 μm. They contain clear vesicles (10–60 nm in diameter) as well as some dense-core and granular vesicles (25–115 nm in diameter). Acetylcholine is the neurotransmitter of this synapse.

The terminal boutons form a large variety of synaptic contacts with the chromaffin cells. They are characterized by a narrow synaptic cleft (15–20 nm) and the presence of electron-dense pre- and post-synaptic zones similar to those observed at the level of the central interneuronal synapses.

In the *post-synaptic region*, the cytoplasm of the chromaffin cells is free of chromaffin granules, organelles that store hormones in the adrenal medulla. The acetylcholine receptors present in the post-synaptic membrane are cholinergic nicotinic receptor channels (N1 type). In the rest of the chromaffin cell cytoplasm we observe numerous chromaffin granules. These granules are colored by chromium salts which react with adrenaline to form a yellow-brown precipitate.

Appendix 2.1
Neurotransmitters, Agonists and Antagonists

Neurotransmitters are molecules of varied nature: quaternary amines, amino acids, catecholamines or peptides, which are released by neurons at chemical synapses. They transmit a message from a neuron to another neuron, or to an effector cell, or a message from a sensory cell to a neuron. Though each neurotransmitter has its characteristics, one can still define a general scheme of synaptic transmission (see Figure 2.4a).

A2.1.1 Different Criteria Have to Be Satisfied Before a Molecule Can Be Identified as a Neurotransmitter

The identification of a substance as a neurotransmitter requires the experimental proof of several criteria. If these criteria are not satisfied, the term putative neurotransmitter is used:

- *Presence* of the putative neurotransmitter in the pre-synaptic element.
- *Synthesis*: the precursors and the enzymes necessary for the synthesis of the putative neurotransmitter are present in the pre-synaptic neuron.
- *Release*: the putative neurotransmitter is released in response to activation of the pre-synaptic neuron and in a quantity sufficient to produce a post-synaptic response. This release should be dependent on Ca^{2+} ions.
- *Binding to specific post-synaptic receptors*:
  (i) specific receptors of the neurotransmitter are present in the post-synaptic membrane;
  (ii) application of the substance at the level of the post-synaptic element reproduces the response obtained by stimulation of the pre-synaptic neuron;
  (iii) drugs, which specifically block or potentiate the post-synaptic response, have the same effects on the response induced by the application of the putative neurotransmitter.
- *Inactivation*: the elements of the synaptic nervous tissue (pre- or post-synaptic elements, glial cells, basal membrane) possess one or several mechanisms for inactivation of the putative neurotransmitter.

Until now, few molecules have satisfied all these criteria and could be firmly identified as a neurotransmitter at a particular synapse: for example, acetylcholine at the neuromuscular junction and GABA (γ-aminobutyric acid) in the lateral vestibular nucleus (nucleus of Deiter, GABA is the neurotransmitter of the synapse between the axon terminals of Purkinje cells and vestibular neurons). In most cases there is no more than fragmentary evidence owing to technical limitations.

A2.1.2 The Different Types of Neurotransmitters

Neurotransmitters are molecules of varied chemical nature. In vertebrate neurons, we find the following.

A *quaternary amine*: acetylcholine. In the peripheral nervous system, acetylcholine is the neurotransmitter of all the synapses between motoneurons and striated muscle cells, of all the synapses between pre-ganglionic and post-ganglionic neurons of the para- and orthosympathetic systems and of all the synapses between parasympathetic post-ganglionic neurons and effector cells (see Figures 2.10, 2.12 and 2.13). It is also a neurotransmitter in the central nervous system. Choline acetyltransferase (CAT), the enzyme required for acetylcholine synthesis, is a specific marker of cholinergic neurons. Using immunocytochemical or *in situ* hybridization techniques (Appendix 2.2), one can visualize cholinergic neuronal pathways by labeling choline acetyl transferase or its mRNA. At the same time, the acetylcholine receptors (Appendix 2.3) can be localized. This holds true for all the pathways studied.

Amino acids: glutamate, aspartate, GABA (γ-aminobutyric acid) and glycine. Glutamate represents the major 'excitatory' and GABA the major 'inhibitory' neurotransmitters in the central nervous system. This classification as excitatory or inhibitory amino acids is not precise since a neurotransmitter is not excitatory or inhibitory by itself: this depends on the type of receptor(s) it activates. However, no example of glutamate or aspartate having an inhibitory action on post-synaptic neurons has yet been shown. For GABA, the situation is different and some examples of an excitatory action of GABA have been demonstrated, notably during development. In contrast to other neurotransmitters, glutamate and aspartate also play an important role in cellular metabolism (in intermediary metabolism, in the synthesis of proteins and as precursor of GABA). They are, therefore, present in all neurons and their identification as neurotransmitters poses several problems. In fact, evidence for the enzymes of their synthesis or degradation cannot represent a valid criterion for the identification of these neurons. These difficulties can be overcome as glutamate and aspartate are present in much higher concentrations in neurons where they play a neurotransmitter role. In addition, these neurons have the property of recapturing selectively glutamate and aspartate with the help of a high-affinity transport system, and localization of this transport system could be used to identify glutamate and aspartate neurons. Glutamic acid decarboxylase, the enzyme required for GABA synthesis, is a good marker of GABAergic neurons.

Monoamines: These are classified as catecholamines (adrenaline, noradrenaline, dopamine), indolamine (serotonin) and imidazole (histamine). Adrenaline, noradrenaline and dopamine are all catecholamines. Their structure has a common part, the catechol nucleus (a benzene ring with two adjacent substituted hydroxyl groups). They are synthesized in catecholaminergic neurons and glandular cells of the adrenal medulla (or chromaffin cells) from a common precursor: tyrosine.

Serotonin or 5-hydroxytryptamine (5HT) is synthesized from tryptophan, a neutral amino acid. The key step in this synthesis is the hydroxylation of tryptophan by tryptophan hydroxylase.

The monoaminergic neurons have the following properties: their cell bodies are grouped in very localized regions of the mammalian central nervous system but they send numerous axonal projections to several central structures. Thus, a restricted number of monoaminergic cell bodies is sufficient to innervate a very large number of central structures.

Neuropeptides. Peptides that are present in neurons with a supposed role in synaptic transmission are called neuropeptides. They are, for example, opioid peptides (enkephalins, dynorphin, β-endorphin) or they are peptides that have already been identified in the gastrointestinal tract (substance P, cholecystokinin, vasoactive intestinal peptide (VIP)) or in the hypothalamo-hypophyseal complex (luteinizing hormone releasing hormone (LHRH), somatostatin, adrenocorticotropic hormone (ACTH), vasopressin) or they are also circulating hormones (corticotropin or ACTH, insulin), before they were suggested as neurotransmitters in the central nervous system. It seems reasonable that other neuropeptides await discovery. These peptides were proposed to be neurotransmitters on the basis of their presence and synthesis in the neurons as well as by their release from axonal terminals by a Ca^{2+}-dependent mechanism. For some peptides other criteria have also been demonstrated.

The differences in the chemical nature of neurotransmitters have a fundamental consequence. Non-peptidic neurotransmitters are synthesized in axonal terminals: a precursor (or precursors) synthesized by the neuron or taken up from the extracellular medium is transformed into a neurotransmitter via an enzymatic reaction in axon terminals. The synthesis enzyme(s) is (are) synthesized in the cell body and transported to axon terminals via axonal transport. The newly synthesized neurotransmitter is then actively transported inside the synaptic vesicles (Figure A2.1a). Peptidic neurotransmitters are synthesized in the cell body since axon terminals, being deprived of the organelles responsible for protein synthesis, cannot themselves synthesize neuropeptides (Figure A2.1b). These are synthesized in cell bodies in the form of larger peptides called precursors. These precursors are then transported to the axon terminals by fast axonal transport. Cleavage of the precursors into neuroactive peptides (Figure A2.1b) is carried out by vesicular peptidases during anterograde axonal transport. Since these precursors have no biological activity, regulation of peptidase activity seems to be an important factor in the regulation of the synthesis of peptidic neurotransmitters.

Concerning their mode of inactivation, most of the neurotransmitters are taken up by axon terminals or glial cells via specific transporters. The major exception is acetylcholine, which is degraded in the synaptic cleft by acetylcholinesterases. Since enzymatic degradation is more rapid than a transporter reaction, acetylcholine is much more rapidly inactivated than the other neurotransmitters.

A2.1.3 Agonists and Antagonists

An *agonist* is a molecule (drug, neurotransmitter, hormone) that binds to a specific receptor, activates the receptor and thus elicits a physiological response:

$$A + R \underset{k_{-1A}}{\overset{k_{+1A}}{\rightleftharpoons}} AR \rightleftharpoons AR^* \dashrightarrow \text{physiological response}$$

where A is the agonist, R is the free receptor, AR is the agonist–receptor complex and AR^* is the activated state of the receptor bound to the agonist. k_{+1} and k_{-1} measure the rate at which association and dissociation occur. An agonist (and an antagonist) is defined in relation to a receptor and not to a neurotransmitter. For example, an agonist of nicotinic acetylcholine receptors such as nicotine is not an agonist of muscarinic acetylcholine receptors though both receptors are activated by acetylcholine.

An *antagonist* is a molecule that prevents the effect of the agonist. A *competitive antagonist* (I) is a receptor antagonist that acts by binding reversibly to agonist receptor site (R). It does not activate the receptor and thus does not elicit a physiological response:

$$B + R \underset{k_{-1B}}{\overset{k_{+1B}}{\rightleftharpoons}} BR \dashrightarrow \text{no physiological response}$$

The effect of a reversible competitive antagonist can be reversed when the agonist concentration is increased since the agonist (A) and the reversible competitive antagonist (B) compete for the same receptor site (R). Competition means that the receptor can bind only one molecule (A or B) at a time.

An *irreversible competitive antagonist* is a receptor antagonist that dissociates from the receptor slowly or not at all. For this reason its effect cannot be reversed when the agonist concentration is increased.

Appendix 2.2
Identification and Localization of Neurotransmitters Synthesized by a Neuron

A2.2.1 Immunocytochemical Techniques

These techniques are based on the antigen–antibody reaction, and consist of the detection of an antigen linked to its specific antibody in histological sections.

Principle

The *antigen* is an endogenous protein such as a synthesis enzyme for a neurotransmitter, a neuroactive peptide or a receptor for a neurotransmitter. The antigens are extracted from the nervous tissue, purified and injected into a host, usually a rabbit. In the case of peptides, they are not necessarily purified because they can be chemically synthesized. To increase the antigenicity of peptides, they are conjugated to a protein or a polysaccharide before being injected into the host.

Figure A2.1   Synthesis of (a) a non-peptidic neurotransmitter (example, acetylcholine) and (b) a peptidic neurotransmitter (example, opioid peptides). The synthesis reaction of acetylcholine from acetylcoenzyme A is shown in the left side. CAT, choline acetyl transferase; HSCoA, coenzyme A. Precursors of endomorphines are pro-opiomelanocortin, proenkephalin A and prodynorphin and the peptide they contain (shown on right side). The numbers indicate the position of the peptides along the protein. MSH, melanocyte stimulating hormone; ACTH, corticotropin: enk, enkephalin, SP: substance P.

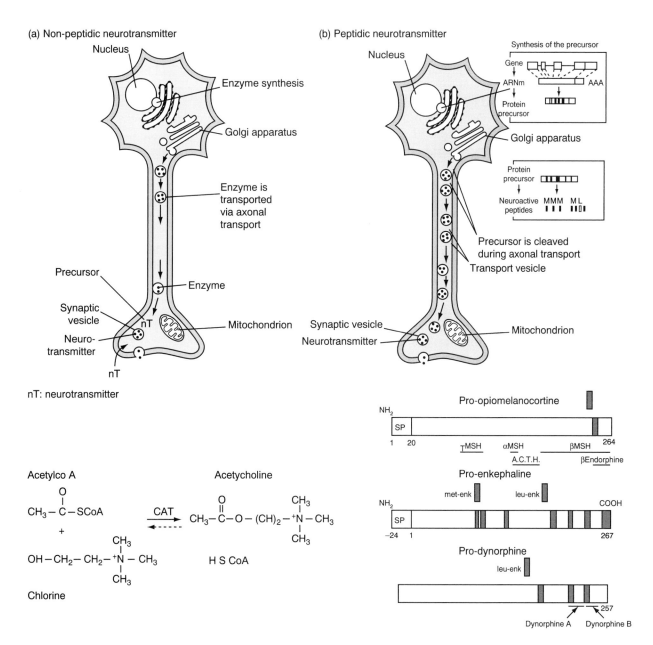

The *antibody* is a type G immunoglobulin (IgG) which, in general, has two recognition sites for the antigen. The antibody that recognizes the antigenic determinant is the 'primary antibody'. This is a monoclonal antibody, i.e. raised from a single parent cell. It is generally labeled immunologically, the label being conjugated to a secondary antibody that recognizes the primary antibody.

The *antigen–antibody reaction*. When they are in the presence of each other, the antigen and its specific antibody form a stable conjugate. This antigen–antibody reaction is revealed by labeling the antibody with a second antibody conjugated to a marker that can be visualized under light or electron microscopy. Therefore, this marker will localize the antigen.

Applications

Localization of neurons synthesizing a specific neurotransmitter

If we want to localize, for example, the cholinergic neurons in a section of brain tissue, the approach is to reveal the neurons that contain the synthesis enzyme for acetylcholine, choline acetyltransferase (ChAT). The labeled anti-ChAT antibodies are applied to sections of brain tissue. They form a stable antigen–antibody reaction only in the neurons that contain ChAT. The sections are then washed to remove the antibodies that did not link with the antigen. Therefore, only the cholinergic neurons (ChAT-positive) are labeled.

Localization of neurotransmitter receptors

See Appendix 2.3.

The Different Immunocytochemical Techniques

Direct labeling with monoclonal antibodies

The antibodies are conjugated with chemicals that can be visualized under the light microscope (e.g. a fluorescent molecule) or electron microscope (electron-dense compounds). Such a technique needs only one step (Figure A2.2): the serum containing the labeled

monoclonal antibodies is applied to sections of brain tissue. These sections are then observed under the light microscope after washing away the antibodies that are not conjugated with the antigen. However, labeling of the antibody reduces significantly its capacity to recognize the antigen. Moreover, there is only one molecule of marker for a single antigen–antibody complex. Therefore, this technique cannot be used to localize peptides or enzymes that are present in small quantities in neurons. In addition, for each antigen studied, it is necessary to label the corresponding antibody. For these reasons, this technique is not used. We have explained it in order to understand better the following techniques.

Figure A2.2 Direct labeling of antibodies directed against a neuronal antigen.

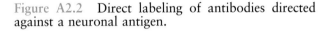
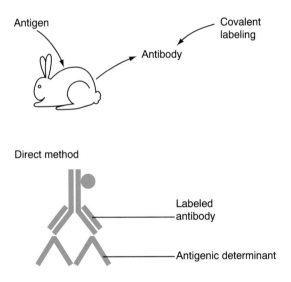

Immunological labeling of monoclonal antibodies

The primary antibody is recognized by a secondary antibody raised in another species (Figure A2.3a). The secondary antibody is labeled. The secondary antibodies recognize numerous antigenic sites on the primary antibody, and therefore amplify the labeling.

Immunofluorescent labeling: the secondary antibody is conjugated to a fluorescent molecule that can be visualized with a microscope equipped with an epifluorescence system. Many fluorochromes are conjugated to a single secondary antibody and many secondary antibodies recognize a single primary antibody

Figure A2.3   Synthesis and indirect labeling of monoclonal antibodies raised against a neuronal antigen.

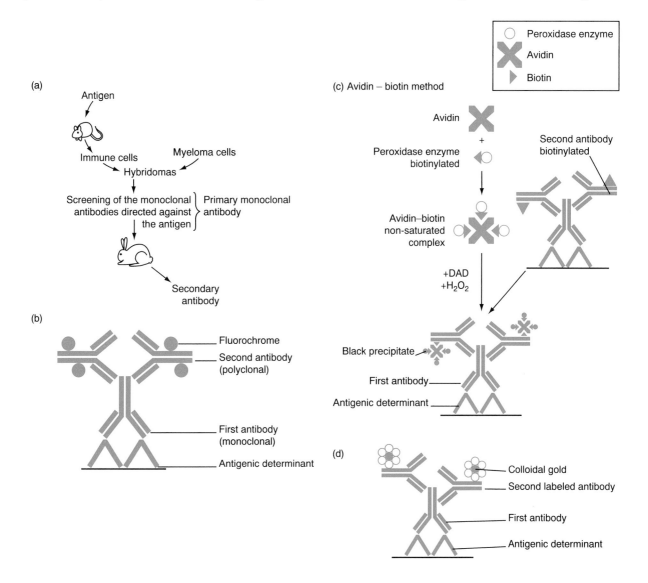

(Figure A2.3b). This technique allows an increase in the labeling and consequently a better visualization of the antigen.

Immunoenzymatic labeling: the most frequently used approach is labeling with peroxidase (HRP). This enzyme oxidizes, in the presence of hydrogen peroxide, a soluble chromogen (diaminobenzidine) which precipitates once oxidized. This oxidized molecule adsorbs onto non-soluble elements and can then be visualized under the electron microscope because heavy metallic salt deposits are formed after fixation with osmium tetroxide. Labeling with the avidin–biotin complex is an amplification method that is frequently used. In this case, the secondary antibody is biotinylated and a non-saturated complex of avidin and biotin conjugated to peroxidase is prepared. The classic peroxidase reaction (DAB + H_2O_2) reveals the peroxidase and consequently the complex (avidin–biotin–secondary antibody) conjugated with the complex (antigen–primary antibody) (Figure A2.3c).

Labeling with colloidal gold particles: these spheric electron-dense metallic elements are adsorbed with protein A. This complex links with the Fc (Fragment c) part of the primary or secondary antibody, which increases the signal (Figure A2.3d).

A2.2.2 In Situ Hybridization

The aim of this technique is to localize the cells that transcript a particular messenger RNA (mRNA).

Principle

The *in situ* hybridization technique aims at detecting a specific sequence of nucleic acids present in cells on histological sections or in culture. The sequence of nucleic acids recognized may correspond to *chromosomal DNA*, called hybridization on chromosomes. In general the term *in situ* hybridization relates to the detection of *messenger RNA* (mRNA). This detection or recognition is made possible by the use of a *probe* that corresponds to a sequence of nucleic acids complementary to the DNA or RNA that is to be detected. The probe is labeled with a marker that can be visualized under the light microscope. When they are in the presence of each other, the specific probe and the endogenous RNA (or DNA) recognized by the probe will conjugate and form hybrids (because of the complementary sequences). The marker incorporated into the probe is revealed by autoradiographic technique, fluorescence or cytochemistry in order to visualize the hybrids that have been formed.

Applications

The *in situ* hybridization technique can be applied in various experiments since it allows visualization of the transcription of a gene and, therefore, localization of the potential site of synthesis for the protein or the peptide coded by this gene. In the case of nerve cells, this technique can localize the neurons that express a gene coding for a neurotransmitter (if it is a peptide), a synthesis or degradative enzyme of a specific neurotransmitter or a receptor for a neurotransmitter. For example, this technique has been used to localize neurons that transcribe the mRNA coding for the precursors of the enkephalins in the mammalian central nervous system. A detailed map of the neurons synthesizing the enkephalins and other opioid peptides has thus been established. Moreover, the role of various factors that act on the expression of these peptides has been studied because this technique can be used to analyze variations in the level of transcribed mRNA in relation to the activity of the neuron, the presence of hormonal factors, etc.

- *Preparation of sections of nervous tissue*. The tissue is fixed with a fixative in order to preserve its structural integrity. The fixation can be done before or after tissue sectioning.
- *The probes have different characteristics*. There are single-strand RNA probes, single-strand DNA probes or double-strand probes. The RNA probes are obtained by the use of RNA polymerase to transcribe a double-strand DNA sub-cloned in a vector that possesses a promoter for the RNA polymerase. The double-strand DNA probes are synthesized from a family of RNA by the use of a reverse transcriptase, followed by that of a DNA polymerase. After screening, the cDNAs are incorporated into vectors and amplified in bacteria. The cDNA, always included in the vector, is then extracted from the bacteria and excised from the vector by the use of appropriate enzymes.
- *Labeling of the probe*. Labeling of the single-strand RNA probe is obtained during transcription by the incorporation of labeled nucleotides. Labeling of the double-strand DNA probe: this probe is mixed with DNAse which induces cuts in the double-strand DNA. These cuts are repaired by the incorporation of labeled and non-labeled deoxynucleotides in the presence of DNA polymerase.
- In situ *hydization reaction*. The probe is applied to each section of brain tissue during an incubation period.
- *Detection of the hybrids*. For example, for a radioactive probe, the slide is placed in contact with X-ray film. If the results of the film are considered satisfactory, the slides are covered with a liquid photographic emulsion and developed; the slides are then stained with toluidine blue and observed under the microscope.

Appendix 2.3
Identification and Localization of the Receptors of a Neurotransmitter

A2.3.1 Use of a Radioactive Ligand

The radioactive ligand must be recognized specifically by only one type of receptor and dissociate from this receptor with a slow speed constant. Detection of radioactivity on sections of brain tissue allows the localization of the receptors recognized by the ligand (e.g. labeling of the nicotinic receptors of acetylcholine by labeled alpha-bungarotoxin).

A2.3.2 Use of an Antibody Directed Against a Receptor

Three types of anti-receptor antibodies can be used:

- *Conventional anti-receptor antibodies.* These are monoclonal antibodies raised against a purified receptor. They are labeled according to one of the methods described in Section A2.2.1 and the receptor–antibody complex is visualized under the light or electron microscope. With this method a particular type of receptor can be localized on sections of brain tissue.
- *Anti-ligand antibodies.* These are monoclonal antibodies directed against a specific ligand for a receptor. These antibodies are labeled (Section A2.2.1) and the receptor–ligand–antibody complex is visualized under the light or electron microscope.
- *Anti-idiotype antibodies.* In this technique, as in the preceding one, the primary antibodies are directed against a specific ligand for a receptor. Antibodies against this primary antibody (called secondary antibodies) are then used and some of those will directly label the receptor. In fact, with such a method, secondary antibodies presenting a molecular structure similar to that of a specific ligand for the receptor under study can be obtained.

What is an idiotype?

Among the antigenic determinants of an antibody, some are localized in the recognition site for the ligand (the antibody site) or close to it. These particular determinants are called idiotypes and they define the idiotype of the antibody.

What is an anti-idiotype antibody?

Secondary antibodies raised in another rabbit and having the same allotypic specificities are anti-idiotype antibodies. Of these anti-idiotype antibodies, those that recognize the determinants localized inside the antibody site of the primary antibodies will be selected since they must have structural similarities with the ligand itself, of which they constitute a type of 'molecular' image. This property allows them to bind to the recognition site for the ligand on the biological receptor.

Example of anti-idiotype antibodies to substance P for the visualization of substance P receptors (Figure A2.4)

The first aim of the technique is to obtain a specific antibody directed against substance P (anti-substance P antibody or primary antibody). The substance P receptors and the anti-substance P antibody are both able to recognize substance P; these antibodies are therefore likely to have similar structural characteristics. Using the substance P antibody, secondary antibodies directed against the substance P antibody are obtained from another rabbit. Some of the secondary antibodies are likely to have strong structural similarities with the endogenous substance P. These anti-idiotype antibodies are labeled indirectly (Section A2.2.1) and their link with substance P receptors is visualized under the microscope. With this approach, substance P receptors can be localized on sections of brain tissue.

Interests and applications of this technique

This technique enables receptor antibodies to be obtained without a pre-purification of the receptor. The receptor can therefore be localized and its stereospecificity studied, and it is also more easily purified.

Figure A2.4 Synthesis of anti-idiotype antibodies for substance P (SP).

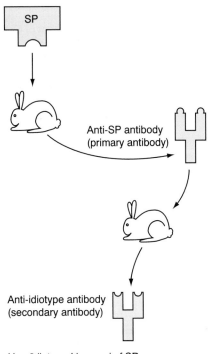

SP receptor   SP

Conjugated BSA far from the
site recognized by the receptor

SP

Anti-SP antibody
(primary antibody)

Anti-idiotype antibody
(secondary antibody)

Has 2 'internal images' of SP

Limitation of the technique

The technique depends on the specificity of the anti-idiotype antibodies that have been obtained.

Further Reading

Bowe, M.A. and Fallon, J.R. (1995) The role of agrin in synapse formation. *Ann. Rev. Neurosci.* **18**, 443–462.

Carbonetto, S. and Lindenbaum, M. (1995) The basement membrane at the neuromuscular junction: a synaptic mediatrix. *Curr. Opin. Neurobiol.* **5**, 596–605.

Harris, K.M. and Kater, S.B. (1994) Dendritic spines: cellular specializations imparting both stability and flexibility to synaptic function. *Ann. Rev. Neurosci.* **17**, 341–371.

Heuser, J.E. and Reese, T.S. (1977) Structure of the synapses. In: Brookhart, J.M. Mountcastle, V.B., Kandel, E.R. and Geiger, S.R. (Eds), *Handbook of Physiology*, Vol 1, Part 1, American Physiological Society, Bethesda, MD.

Scheller, R.H. (1995) Membrane trafficking in the presynaptic nerve terminal. *Neuron* **14**, 893–897.

3

Glial Cells

There are roughly twice as many glial cells as there are neurons in the central nervous system. They occupy the space between neurons and neuronal processes and separate neurons from blood vessels. As a result, the extracellular space between the plasma membranes of different cells is narrow, of the order of 15–20 nm.

Virchow (1846) was the first to propose the existence of non-neuronal tissue in the central nervous system. He named it nevroglie (nerve glue), because it appeared to stick the neurons together. Following this, Deiters (1865) and Golgi (1885) identified glial cells as making up the nevroglie and distinguished them from neurons.

There are several categories of glial cells. Depending on their anatomical position they are classed as:

- *Central glia* are found in the central nervous system, and comprise four cell types: astrocytes, oligodendrocytes, microglia (these three types are also known as interstitial glia, because they are found in interneuronal spaces) and ependymal cells which form the epithelial surface covering the walls of the cerebral ventricles and of the central canal of the spinal cord.
- *Peripheral glia* comprise a single type: Schwann cells. These cells ensheath the axons and encapsulate the cell bodies of neurons. In the latter case, they are also called satellite cells.

Glial cells, excluding microglia, have an ectodermal origin. Those of the central nervous system derive from the germinal neural epithelium (neural tube), while peripheral glia (Schwann cells) are derived from the neural crest. Microglia, in contrast, have a mesodermal origin.

Glial cells have morphological as well as functional and metabolic characteristics that distinguish them from neurons:

- They do not generate or conduct action potentials. Thus, although they extend processes, these are only of one type and are neither dendrites nor axons.
- They do not form chemical synapses between themselves, with neurons, or with any other cell type.
- Unlike most neurons in humans, glial cells are capable of division for at least several years post-natally.

Nervous tissue is made compact by glial cells and for this reason they are often ascribed the role of supporting tissue. However, as we will see in this chapter, they have additional functions.

3.1 Astrocytes Form a Vast Cellular Network or Syncytium Between Neurons, Blood Vessels and the Surface of the Brain

3.1.1 Astrocytes are Star-shaped Cells Characterized by the Presence of Glial Filaments in Their Cytoplasm

Astrocytes are small star-shaped cells with numerous fine, tortuous, ramified processes covered with varicosities (Figure 3.1). The cell body is typically 9–10 μm in diameter and the processes extend radially over 40–50 μm. These often have enlarged terminals in contact with neurons or non-neuronal tissue (like the walls of blood vessels).

Two kinds of astrocytes are recognized. Some astrocytes contain in their cytoplasm numerous glial filaments: these are fibrillary astrocytes, principally located in the white matter (Figure 3.1). They have numerous, radial processes which are infrequently branched and covered with ('expansions en brindilles'). Other astrocytes contain few, if any, glial filaments: these are protoplasmic astrocytes, found normally in the gray matter. They have more delicate processes, some of which are velate (veil-like). Both types of astrocytes send out processes that end on the walls of blood vessels or beneath the pial surface of the brain and spinal cord.

Figure 3.1 Fibrillary astrocyte. Micrograph of a fibrillary astrocyte stained with a Golgi stain observed through an optical microscope. The processes of this astrocyte make contact with a blood vessel: these are the terminal end feet. (Photo: Olivier Robain.)

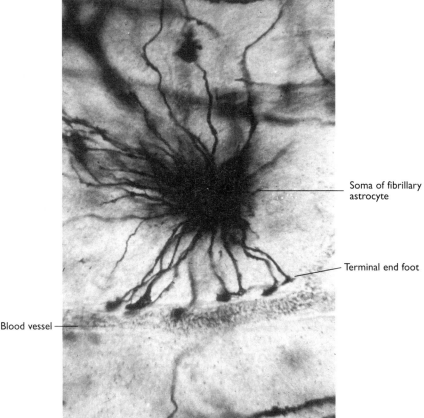

Soma of fibrillary astrocyte

Terminal end foot

Blood vessel

The principal ultrastructural characteristics of astrocytes are the glial filaments and glycogen granules present in the cytoplasm of their somata and processes. The filaments are 'intermediate filaments' with an average diameter of 8–10 μm. They are composed of a protein specific to astrocytes, glial fibrillary acidic protein (GFAP), consisting of a single type of subunit with a molecular weight of 50 kD, different from that of neurofilaments. This characteristic has been exploited as a method of identifying astrocytes. By using an antiserum to glial fibrillary acidic protein (anti-GFAP) linked to fluorescein, one can stain astrocytes, *in situ* or in culture, without marking either neurons or other types of glial cells.

Astrocytes, like all glial cells, do not form chemical synapses. They do, however, mutually form junctional complexes. Two types of junctions have been demonstrated: communicating junctions (or gap junctions, see Section 5.4.4) and desmosomes (puncta adhaerentia). Coupled to each other by numerous junctional complexes, astrocytes therefore constitute a vast cellular network, or syncytium, extending from neurons to blood vessels and the external surface of the brain.

3.1.2 The Processes of Astrocytes Form End Feet on the Walls of Blood Vessels

The essential characteristic of astrocytic processes is their termination on the walls of blood vessels in astrocytic end feet (Figure 3.2). Here the end feet are joined, forming a 'palisade' between neurons and vascular endothelial cells. The space between the layer of astrocyte end feet and the endothelial cells is about 40–100 nm and is occupied by a basal lamina. Astrocytes also send processes to the external surface of the central nervous system where the astrocyte end feet, together with the basal lamina that they produce, form the 'glia limitans externa', which separates the pia mater from the nervous tissue. Astrocytes therefore constitute a barrier between neurons and the external medium (blood), preventing access of substances foreign to the central nervous system. They can thus be thought of as protecting neurons. This barrier is not, however, totally impermeable and astrocytes are involved in selective exchange processes.

Astrocyte end feet are not the blood–brain barrier. This is formed, in most regions of the central nervous system, by vascular endothelial cells joined together by tight junctions. Even though the astrocyte end feet do not form the blood–brain barrier, they have an important role in its development and maintenance. Thus, if the layer of astrocyte end feet in the adult is destroyed, by a tumor or by allergic illnesses, for example, the capillary endothelial cells immediately take on the characteristics normally observed in capillaries outside the central nervous system: they are no longer bound by tight junctions and become 'fenestrated'. In such capillaries the blood–brain barrier disappears (see Section 4.2).

Figure 3.2   Diagram of the covering formed by astrocyte end feet around a capillary in the central nervous system (CNS). (From Goldstein G and Betz L, 1986. La barrière qui protège le cerveau, *Pour la Science*, November, 84–94, with permission.)

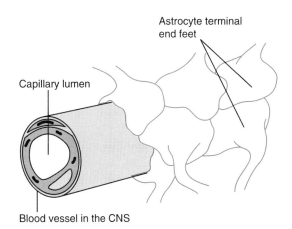

Astrocyte terminal end feet

Capillary lumen

Blood vessel in the CNS

3.1.3 Astrocytes Regulate the Composition of the Extracellular Fluid

We have seen that astrocyte end feet are involved in the formation and maintenance of the blood–brain barrier, and that astrocytes thus contribute to regulation of the brain extracellular fluid. However, astrocytes have other important roles in controlling the composition of the extracellular fluid. We shall give as examples the regulation of the extracellular potassium concentration and the reuptake of neurotransmitters following their release at chemical synapses.

The extracellular potassium concentration needs to be tightly regulated: if potassium increased it would depolarize neurons, first increasing neuronal excitability and then inactivating action potential propagation. Regulation of the extracellular potassium concentration must occur in the face of large fluxes of potassium ions into the extracellular space during neuronal activity, when potassium ions leave neurons through voltage-activated potassium channels (see Chapter 7). Astrocytes are thought to regulate extracellular potassium by the mechanism of 'spatial buffering'. This means that astrocytes take up potassium ions in regions where the concentration rises and eventually release through their end feet an equivalent amount of potassium ions into the vicinity of blood vessels or across the glia limitans externa. The details of the process are complicated, but potassium ions are thought to enter astrocytes via channels or the sodium pump and to exit at the end feet through channels. This potassium buffering role of astrocytes is likely to be of particular importance at the nodes of Ranvier, where marked accumulation of potassium ions in the restricted extracellular space can occur, due to the conduction of action potentials.

After neurotransmitters are released during synaptic transmission, they need to be removed from the extracellular space to prevent the extracellular neurotransmitter concentration from rising. Steady high concentrations of transmitter would interfere with synaptic transmission, and tonic activation of receptors (particularly glutamate receptors) can damage neurons. Most transmitters are removed from the extracellular space by reuptake into cells (but acetylcholine is hydrolyzed, see Chapter 2). Transmitters are taken up by specialized carrier molecules in the cell membrane (Section 5.5.2). Although both neurons and glia express such carrier proteins, it seems that uptake into astrocytes is of particular importance. This is especially clear for the case of glutamate: astrocytes have an enormous capacity to take up this transmitter, presumably reflecting the abundance of this transmitter and the toxicity to neurons of high glutamate concentrations.

3.2 Oligodendrocytes Form the Myelin Sheaths of Myelinated Axons in the Central Nervous System

Two types of oligodendrocyte are recognized: interfascicular or myelinating oligodendrocytes, found in the white matter where they make the sheaths of myelinated axons; and satellite oligodendrocytes which surround neuronal somata in the gray matter. We will deal with the former type in detail.

3.2.1 The Cell Bodies of Interfascicular Oligodendrocytes are Situated Between Bundles of Axons

Interfascicular, or myelinating, oligodendrocytes have small spherical or polyhedral cell bodies of diameter 6–8 μm and few processes. They are called interfascicular because their cell bodies are aligned between bundles (fascicles) of axons. They are distinguished from astrocytes by the sites of termination of their processes: oligodendrocyte processes enwrap axons and make no contact with blood vessels. They are responsible for the formation of the myelin sheath of central axons.

Observed by electron microscopy, the nucleus and perikaryon of oligodendrocytes appear dark (Figure 3.3), there are no glial filaments, and there are many microtubules in the somatic and dendritic cytoplasm. Because of this, oligodendrocyte processes may be

Figure 3.3 Myelinating oligodendrocyte. Electron micrograph of an oligodendrocyte. The cell body and one of its processes enwrapping several axons can be seen. Section taken through the spinal cord. (Photo: Olivier Robain.)

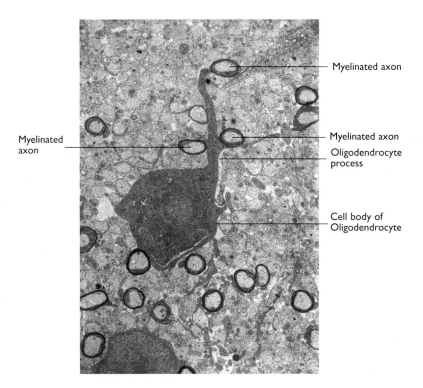

confused with fine dendrites, and it is by the absence of chemical synapses that the glial processes are identified.

Oligodendrocytes can be demonstrated by immunohistochemistry. This is done using an anti-galactoceramide immune serum (anti-gal-C), galactoceramide being a glycolipid found exclusively in the membrane of processes of myelinizing oligodendrocytes.

3.2.2 The Myelin Sheath is Formed by a Compact Roll of the Plasmalemma of an Oligodendrocyte Process: This Glial Membrane is Rich in Lipids

Myelinated axons are surrounded by a succession of myelin segments, each about 1 mm in length. The covered regions of axons alternate with short exposed lengths where the axonal membrane (axolemma) is not covered. These unmyelinated regions (of the order of a micron) are called nodes of Ranvier (Figures 3.4 and 3.5a).

A myelinated segment comprises the length of axon covered by an oligodendrocyte. One oligodendrocyte can form 20 to 70 myelin segments around different axons (Figure 3.4). Thus the degeneration or dysfunction of a single oligodendrocyte leads to the disappearance of myelin segments on several different axons.

Formation and ultrastructure of a myelin segment

Myelinization represents a crucial stage in the ontogenesis of the nervous system. In the human at birth, myelinization is only just beginning, and in some regions is not complete even by the end of the second year of life. The first step in the process is migration of oligodendrocytes into the bundles of axons, then the myelinization of some, but not all, axons. Once contact has been made between the oligodendrocyte and axon, the initial turn of myelin around the axon is rapidly formed. Myelin is then slowly deposited over a period which in humans can reach several months. Myelinization is responsible for a large part of the increase in weight of the central nervous system following the end of neurogenesis.

In order to form the compact spiral of myelin mem-

Figure 3.4 Diagram of a myelinating oligodendrocyte and its numerous processes which each form a segment of myelin around a different axon in the central nervous system. Two myelin segments are represented, one partially, and the other completely, unrolled. (Drawing: Tom Prentiss. In Morell P and Norton W, 1980. La myéline et la sclerose en plaques, *Pour la Science* **33**, with permission.)

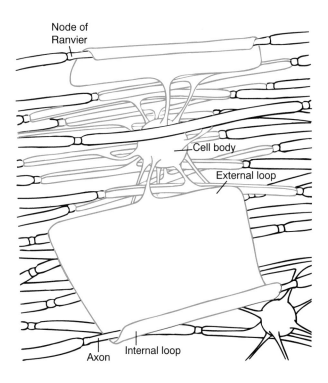

brane, the oligodendrocyte process must roll itself around the axon many times (up to 40 turns) (Figure 3.5). It is the terminal portion of the process, called the inner loop, situated at the interior of the roll, which progressively spirals around the axon. This movement necessitates the sliding of myelin sheets which are not firmly attached. During this period, the oligodendrocyte synthesizes several times its own weight of myelin membrane each day.

Within the spiral the cytoplasm disappears entirely (except at the internal and external loops). The internal leaflets of the plasma membranes can thus adhere to each other. This adhesion is so intimate that the internal leaflets virtually fuse, forming the period, or major, dense line of thickness of 3 nm (Figure 3.5b). The extracellular space between the different turns of membrane also disappears, and the external leaflets

Figure 3.5   Myelin sheath of central axons. (a) Three-dimensional diagram of the myelin sheath of an axon in the central nervous system (CNS). The sheath is formed by a succession of compact rolls of glial processes from different oligodendrocytes. (b) Cross-section through a myelin sheath. The dark lines, or major dense lines, and clear bands (in the middle of which are found the interperiod lines) visible with electron microscopy are accounted for by the manner in which the myelin membrane surrounds the axon, and by the composition of the membrane. The dark lines represent the adhesion of the internal leaflets of the myelin membrane while the interperiod lines represent the adhesion of the external leaflets. The lines are formed by membrane proteins while the clear bands are formed by the lipid bilayer. (a: From Bunge MB, Bunge RP and Ris H, 1961. Ultrastructural study of remyelination in an experimental lesion in adult cat spinal cord, *J. Biophys. Biochem. Cytol.*, **10**, 67–94, with permission of The Rockerfeller University Press. b: Drawing: Tom Prentiss. In Morell P and Norton W, 1980. La myéline et la sclérose en plaques, *Pour la Science* **33**, with permission.)

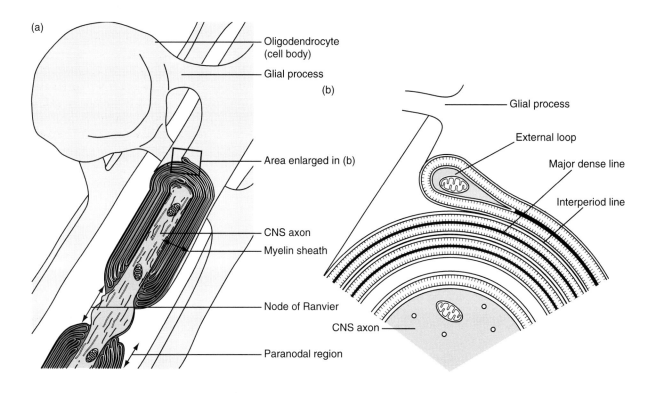

also stick to each other. This apposition is, however, less close and a small space remains between the external leaflets. The apposed external leaflets form the minor, or interperiod, dense line (Figure 3.5b).

Thus, a cross-section of a myelinated axon observed by electron microscopy shows alternating dark and light lines forming a spiral around the axon. The major dense line terminates where the internal leaflets separate to enclose the cytoplasm within the external loop. The interperiod dense line disappears at the surface of the sheath at the end of the spiral (Figure 3.5b).

In the central nervous system there is no basal lamina around myelin segments, so myelin segments of adjacent axons may adhere to each other forming an interperiod dense line.

Nodes of Ranvier

In the central nervous system the nodes of Ranvier, regions between myelin segments, are relatively long (several microns) compared with those in the peripheral nervous system. Here the axolemma is exposed and an accumulation of dense material is seen on the cytoplasmic side. The myelin sheath does not terminate abruptly. Successive layers of myelin membrane terminate at regularly spaced intervals along the axon, the internal layers (close to the axon) terminating first. This staggered termination of the different layers of myelin constitutes the paranodal region (Figure 3.5a).

Myelin

Myelin consists of a compact spiral (without intracellular or extracellular space) of glial plasma membrane of a very particular composition. Lipids make up about 70% of the dry weight of myelin and proteins only 30%. Compared with the membranes of other cells, this represents an inversion of the lipid:protein ratio (Figure 3.6).

The lipids of myelin are divided into three groups: cholesterol, phospholipids and glycolipids. It is the high proportion of the last group, and of galactoceramide (gal-C) in particular, that characterizes the lipid composition of myelin. This glycolipid, being specific to oligodendrocytes and also very immunogenic, is, as we have already seen, often used as a marker of oligodendrocytes. Another glycolipid, sulfogalactosyl ceramide, is also present in myelin at high concentrations, but is a little less specific since it is found in other cells of the central nervous system.

We have seen that myelin has an inverted lipid:protein ratio, while the cell body membrane of the oligodendrocyte has a ratio comparable to that of other cell membranes. As the myelin of the oligodendrocyte process is in continuity with the plasma membrane of the cell body, it is necessary to postulate gradients in the composition of lipids and proteins (in opposite directions to each other) between the cell body and the various processes.

The proteins of myelin are not only less abundant than in other plasma membranes, but also less varied. Two types of protein characteristic of central myelin predominate: myelin basic proteins (MBPs), so named because they are highly charged proteins soluble in acidic solutions, and proteolipid proteins (PLP/DM20, two splicing derivatives). These, like lipids, are soluble in organic solvents. Myelin basic proteins are found on the cytoplasmic side and play a role in the adhesion of the internal leaflets of the specialized oligodendroglial plasma membrane. Proteolipid proteins are integral membrane proteins. Though they are in high abundance (they represent around 50% of the total myelin protein in the central nervous system) their exact biological role has not yet been elucidated.

3.2.3 Myelination Enables Rapid Conduction of Action Potentials

The high lipid content and compact structure of the myelin sheath help make it impermeable to hydrophilic substances such as ions. It prevents transmembrane ion fluxes and acts as a good electrical insulator between the intracellular (i.e. intra-axonal) and extracellular media. Between the nodes of Ranvier the axon therefore behaves as an insulated cable. This permits rapid, saltatory conduction of action potentials along the axon (see Section 7.4.4).

Figure 3.6 Comparison of the lipid content of plasma membrane (left) and myelin (right). The protein/lipid ratio is inverted between the two membranes. The proportions of the three groups of lipids are also different.

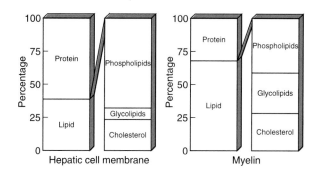

3.3 Microglia: Ramified Microglial Cells Represent the Quiescent Form of Microglial Cells in the Central Nervous System

Ramified microglial cells (Figure 3.7b) are small cells present throughout the whole adult central nervous system, and make up about 5–12% of central glial and neuronal cells. They are found in greater numbers in the gray matter.

Microglial cells have an embryological origin different from that of other glial cells in that they derive

Figure 3.7 Microglial cells. (a) Differentiation of monocytes into microglial cells during the development of the central nervous system as studied in the corpus callosum of the rat brain. Circulating monocytes (m) enter the brain parenchyma during the prenatal and early postnatal period. The cells acquire an abundant cytoplasm and become ameboid microglial cells (a.m). They show mitotic activity but many die *in situ* in the first postnatal week. The surviving cells begin to undergo morphological changes between the second and third postnatal week. They then present a branched appearance and are identified as ramified microglial cells (r.m). (b) Photograph taken using optical microscopy of an adult microglial cell (Golgi stain). (Photo: Olivier Robain.) (a: Adapted from Ling EA and Wong WC, 1993. The origin and nature of ramified and amoeboid microglia: a historical review and current concepts, *Glia* 7; 9–18, with permission.)

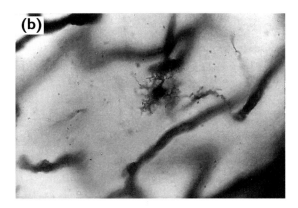

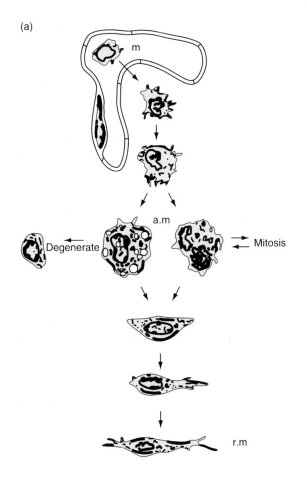

from mesodermal (meningeal) tissue. By using a monoclonal antibody specific for a membrane glycoprotein of mouse macrophages, the mouse IgG Fc receptor, and for the myelomonocytic type 3 complement receptor and with the aid of immunocytochemical techniques (Appendix 2.2), the localization of antibody-positive cells was observed in embryonic brains. This led to the conclusion that during the embryonic development of the central nervous system monocytes cross the brain capillaries to enter central structures and become 'ameboid' microglial cells. These cells are active macrophages phagocytosing degenerating cells and processes resulting from degeneration or remodelling of fibers in developing brain. At that stage they are endowed with a variety of hydrolytic enzymes. They then undergo a series of morphological transformations and differentiate into ramified microglia during the postnatal period, a quiescent form that persists through adulthood (Figure 7a).

Ameboid microglia therefore disappear in the adult, but reappear upon injury of central nervous tissue. These microglial cells are able to move and ingest particles. In contrast, ramified microglial cells are deprived of all hydrolytic enzymes and do not ingest particles. No labeling of ramified microglial cells in young or adult rats was found after systemic injection of ³H-thymidine. These cells do not divide in normal brain. They are probably a 'resting' form of microglia, of which the function is unknown.

3.3.1 Microglial Cells have Long Meandering Processes

Microglial cells have an elongated soma from which fine wavy processes carrying numerous protrusions ramify (Figure 3.7b). The nucleus is small and flattened or angular. It contains chromatin masses at the periphery. The endoplasmic reticulum forms very narrow, long cisternae which meander through the cytoplasm.

3.3.2 Do Adult Microglial Cells Play a Role in Immune Processes?

Are adult microglial cells capable of phagocytosis?

Phagocytosis (the ability to ingest extracellular particles) involves immune processes. It requires the presence of Fc receptors or type 3 complement (C3) receptors. These receptors have indeed been demonstrated on microglial cells, but the phagocytic capability of these cells remains disputed.

Are ramified glia transformed into macrophages following injury to nervous tissue?

Following injury to nervous tissue a proliferation of glial cells around the lesion is observed. Which are the glial cells capable of proliferation and of generating this reaction, called gliosis? According to Rio del Hortega, microglia present in the normal central nervous system could be transformed into reactive glial cells, i.e. divide and become macrophages capable of migration and ingestion of cellular debris. For example, in several human neurological disorders, a microglial activation characterized by proliferation, increased expression of surface antigens, migration and changes into a macrophage-like morphology and immunophenotype is observed. However, the studies to date have been unable to provide a clear answer to this question and the problem is still not resolved. In fact, if the blood–brain barrier is damaged during injury to nervous tissue, circulating monocytes are recruited in large numbers and it becomes technically difficult to distinguish macrophages derived from monocytes from any macrophages resulting from division of 'resident' microglia.

3.4 Ependymal Cells Form an Epithelium at the Surface of the Ventricles of the Central Nervous System

Ependymal cells cover the walls of the cerebral ventricles (the lateral ventricles, third ventricle, cerebral aqueduct (of Sylvius) and the fourth ventricle) as well as the walls of the central canal of the spinal cord (see Figure 4.2). In these cavities they form a continuous epithelium which is heterogeneous, because there are several types of ependymal cell.

All ependymal cells have a well-defined polarity: an apical, or luminal, side (in contact with the cerebrospinal fluid), site of cilia or microvilli, depending on the cell type, and a basal, or subependymal, side which rests on a basal lamina. Ependymal cells are joined to each other by junctional complexes at the edge of the apical pole. These junctions ensure the cohesion of the entire ependyma.

Ependymal cells are grouped into two main classes: ependymal cells of the choroid plexus and extrachoroidal ependymal cells which include ciliated ependymal cells and tanycytes. The distinction between these two classes is based on cytological and positional criteria. The differences used to classify ependymal cells indicate differences of function, but these remain obscure.

3.4.1 Ependymal Cells of the Choroid Plexus Form a Barrier Between Blood Capillaries and the Cerebrospinal Fluid

The choroid plexuses are situated in the lateral ventricles, where they stretch from the interventricular foramen (of Monro), to the tips of the inferior cornua, in the third ventricle where they cover the superior wall of the third ventricle, and on the roof of the fourth ventricle.

Ependymal cells of the choroidal plexus are characterized by a cuboidal shape. Observed in the scanning electron microscope, the luminal face has the form of a dome (Figure 3.8). The apical pole presents numerous microvilli, 2–3 μm long, and occasional cilia. The spherical nucleus occupies the centre of the cell and contains relatively homogeneous chromatin. The numerous mitochondria and vesicles (30–40 nm in diameter) are largely situated towards the apical pole.

Figure 3.8 Ependymal cells. (a) Junction between choroidal and extrachoroidal ependyma: choroidal ependymal cells with their villous surface are directly adjacent to ciliated extrachoroidal ependymal cells. (b) Diagram of a choroidal ependymal cell. Numerous villi and a few cilia are found at the apical pole. The lateral membranes of adjacent cells are attached near the apical pole by junctional complexes. Lower down there are numerous interdigitations between neighboring cells. The basal pole rests on a basal lamina. (Adapted from Peters A and Swan RC, 1979. Choroidal epithelium, *Anat. Rec.* **194**, 325–353, with permission.)

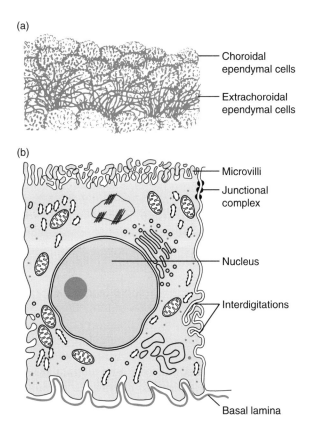

The other characteristic feature of ependymal cells of the choroidal plexus is that they are joined to each other by tight junctions (zonula occludens). These junctions, situated at the apical end of the lateral plasma membrane, form a continuous circumferential ring around each ependymal cell. At the level of the junction there is no extracellular space between the cells. This means that exchange between blood vessels (on the basal side) and the cerebrospinal fluid (apical side) can only occur via the ependymal cells. This is of considerable importance, because the capillaries in the choroidal plexuses, being fenestrated, do not form a blood–brain barrier. Instead, the barrier here consists of the ependymal cells joined by tight junctions (see Section 4.2.4).

Below the tight junctions, the plasma membranes of the choroidal cells have numerous and complex interdigitations. The many (apical) microvilli, as well as the interdigitations of the basolateral region, are structures that greatly increase the area available for exchange between the cells and their environment (cerebrospinal fluid and extracellular fluid). These are, along with the presence of numerous vesicles in their cytoplasm, indicators of a large exchange of substances via secretion and absorption. Indeed, if a marker such as horseradish peroxidase (HPR) is injected into the circulation, the marker remains trapped in the region of the interdigitations and within

Figure 3.9 Tanycytes. Drawing of the ultrastructure of a beta tanycyte of the rat. (I) perikaryon; (II) process; (III) termination of process. (Adapted from Akmayev IG and Popov AP, 1977. Morphological aspects of the hypothalamic hypophyseal system, *Cell Tiss. Res.* **180**, 263–282, with permission.)

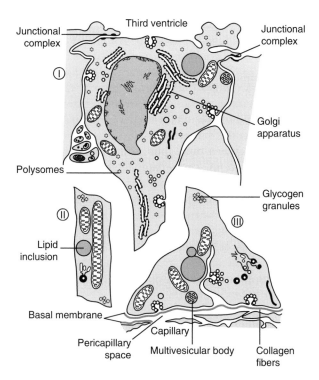

the choroidal cells. This block of the entry of certain substances into the cerebrospinal fluid may be an important element of the active barrier between blood and cerebrospinal fluid. Conversely, tracers injected into the cerebrospinal fluid are later found in the lysosomal apparatus of the ependymal cells.

3.4.2 Extrachoroidal Ependymal Cells Line the Walls of the Cavities of the Central Nervous System

Outside the choroid plexus, the ventricles are lined by ciliated ependymal cells and by non-ciliated tanycytes. The transition between choroidal and extrachoroidal ependyma is abrupt.

Ciliated ependymal cells have numerous cilia projecting into the cavity (Figure 3.8). Their movements presumably aid the circulation of the cerebrospinal fluid. These cells are not joined by tight junctions.

Tanycytes are covered on their apical surface by microvilli and have characteristic long basal processes which make contact with blood capillaries, neurons or other glial cells (Figure 3.9). They contain numerous secretory vesicles.

3.4.3 Roles of Ependymal Cells

Choroidal ependymal cells occupy a special position, interposed between fenestrated blood capillaries of the choroid plexus and the cerebrospinal fluid. They constitute an active barrier between these two media (blood and cerebrospinal fluid), but also play a role in the production of cerebrospinal fluid (see Section 4.1.1).

The function of extrachoroidal ependymal cells seems not to be restricted solely to moving the cerebrospinal fluid with their cilia. They may also play a role in the regulation of the activity of the cells situated at their basal pole. This regulation would be controlled by signals in the cerebrospinal fluid. The discovery of the presence of various hormones and neurotransmitters in the cerebrospinal fluid suggested that ependymal cells may absorb such substances (apically) and then secrete them (basally). Such a process would permit regulation of neurons in the region of the third ventricle.

3.5 Schwann Cells Are the Glial Cells of the Peripheral Nervous System

There are three types of Schwann cell:

- those forming the myelin sheath of peripheral myelinated axons (myelinating Schwann cells);
- those encapsulating non-myelinated peripheral axons (non-myelinating Schwann cells);
- those that encapsulate the bodies of ganglion cells (non-myelinating Schwann cells or satellite cells).

3.5.1 Myelinating Schwann Cells Make the Myelin Sheath of Peripheral Myelinated Axons

Along an axon, several Schwann cells form successive segments of the myelin sheath. In contrast to oligo-dendrocytes, it is not a process that enwraps the peripheral axon to form the segment of myelin, but the whole Schwann cell (Figure 3.10). Each Schwann cell therefore only forms one myelin segment.

The composition of peripheral myelin differs from that of central myelin only in the proteins it contains. The principal protein constituents of peripheral myelin are: peripheral myelin protein 22 (PMP 22), protein zero (P0) and myelin basic proteins (MBPs). The first two proteins are specific to peripheral myelin. Peripheral myelin protein 22 is a small, hydrophobic integral membrane glycoprotein. Protein zero is a glycoprotein that has adhesive properties and is located in the interperiod line. It functions, in part, as a homotypic adhesion molecule throughout the full thickness of the myelin sheath. It is a good marker for myelinating Schwann cells.

3.5.2 Non-myelinating Schwann Cells Encapsulate the Axons and Cell Bodies of Peripheral Neurons

Non-myelinated axons are not uncovered in the peripheral nervous system as they are in the central nervous system; they are encapsulated. A single non-myelinating Schwann cell surrounds several axons (about 5–20) for a distance of 200–500 μm in man.

In addition, spinal and cranial ganglia contain a large number of Schwann cells that do not produce myelin.

Figure 3.10   Myelin sheath of a peripheral axon. (a) Three-dimensional diagram of the myelin sheath of an axon of the peripheral nervous system. The sheath is formed by successive rolled Schwann cells. (Adapted from Maillet M, 1977. Le tissue nerveux, Vigot, Paris, with permission.) (b) Process of myelinization. The internal loop wraps around the axon several times. During this process the axon grows and the myelin becomes compact. Contact between the Schwann cell and axon occurs only at the paranodal and nodal regions. Elsewhere an extracellular, or periaxonal, space always remains. (Drawing: Tom Prentiss. In Morell P and Norton W, 1980. La myéline et la sclerose en plaques, *Pour la Science* 33, with permission.)

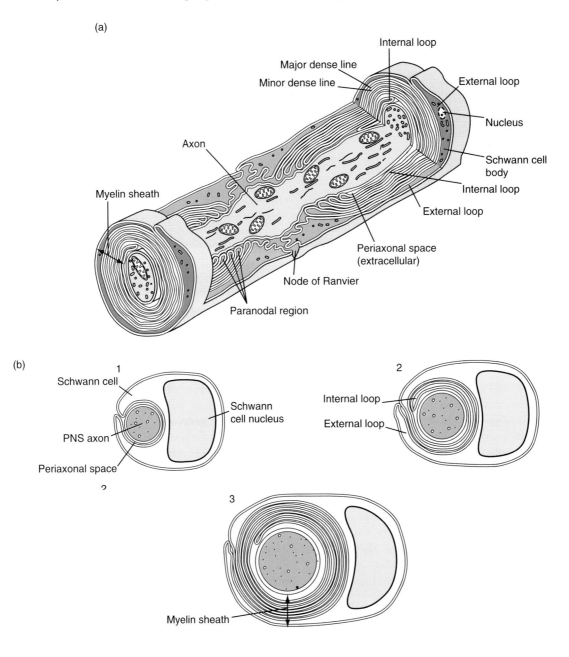

These Schwann cells cover the somata of the ganglionic cells, leaving an extracellular space of about 20 nm between themselves and the surface of the covered neuron (see Figure 4.6a).

The lipid and protein composition of the plasma membrane of non-myelinating Schwann cells is the same as that of other eukaryotic cells (30% lipid, 70% protein).

3.5.3 Roles of Schwann Cells

Apart from their role in the saltatory conduction of action potentials (myelinating Schwann cells), Schwann cells also play a role in the regeneration of peripheral nerve cells. It has long been known that cut peripheral nerves can, within certain limits, regrow and reinnervate deafferented regions while central axons are not capable of this. This property of regeneration is due in large part to an enabling effect of Schwann cells on axon regrowth (see Section 4.3).

Further Reading

Del Rio Hortega, P. (1932) Microglia. In: Penfield, W. (Ed) *Cytology and Cellular Pathology of the Nervous System*, vol. 2, pp. 481–534, P.B. Hoeber, New York.

Eddleston, M. and Mucke, L. (1993) Molecular profile of reactive astrocytes – implications for their role in neurologic disease. *Neuroscience*, **54**, 15–36.

Filbin, M.T. (1995) Myelin-associated glycoprotein: a role in myelination and in the inhibition of axonal regeneration? *Curr. Opin. Neurobiol.* 5; 588–595.

Giulian, D. (1987) Ameboid micoglia as effectors of inflammation in the central nervous system. *J. Neurosci.* **18**, 155–171.

Kettenmann, H. and Ranson, B.R. (Eds) (1995) *Neuroglia*, Oxford University Press, New York.

Morell, P. (1984) *Myelin*, 2nd edn, Plenum Press, New York.

Palay, S.L. and Chan-Palay, V. (1977) General morphology of neurons and neuroglia. In: Brookhart, J.M., Mountcastle, V.B., Kandel, E.R. and Geiger, S.R. (Eds), *Handbook of Physiology*, vol. 1, part 1, pp. 5–37, American Physiological Society, Bethesda, MD.

Perry, V.H. and Brown, M.C. (1992) Role of macrophages in peripheral nerve degeneration. *BioEssays* **14**, 401–410.

Special issue on microglial cells (1993) *Glia* 7 (1).

Streit, W.I., Graeber, M.B. and Kreutzberg, G.W. (1988) Functional plasticity of microglia: a review. *Glia* **1**, 301–307.

4

The Nervous Tissue

The nervous tissue is composed of nerve cells and non-neuronal elements (glial cells, extracellular matrix and blood vessels). The neuronal and non-neuronal elements are organized as subcortical nuclei, brain cortex, bundles, commissures, ganglions, nerves, brain and spinal cord, terms that will be defined in this chapter.

4.1 The Central and Peripheral Nervous Tissues Are Different at the Level of Their Non-neuronal Elements

4.1.1 The Central Nervous System is Comprised of the Brain and Spinal Cord

The brain and spinal cord

Protected by the meningeal coverings, skull and spinal column, the central nervous system occupies a central position in vertebrates (Figure 4.1a). The brain (encephalon) consists of the telencephalon (brain hemispheres), diencephalon and brainstem, which includes the mesencephalon (midbrain), pons, cerebellum and medulla oblongata. The spinal cord is the prolongation of the medulla oblongata. The diencephalon and the brainstem are in greater part covered by the telencephalon and are visible only from the base of the brain (Figure 4.1b) or by sectioning the brain (Figure 4.3). The brain and the spinal cord give rise to the cranial and spinal nerves, respectively (see Section 4.1.3).

The meningeal coverings

The central nervous system is covered by three layers of meninges of mesodermic origin. They are, from the outside to the inside, the dura mater, arachnoid mater and pia mater. The meninges are innervated and their lesions are painful. At the brain level, the dura mater covers the inside surface of the skull, and constitutes

Figure 4.1   The central nervous system. (a) Human central nervous system (posterior and lateral views). The brain is lodged in the skull, and the spinal cord in the spinal column. At the first lumbar vertebra level the spinal cord terminates as conus medullaris. Below this level the vertebral canal only contains spinal nerves. (b) Lateral view of the encephalon.

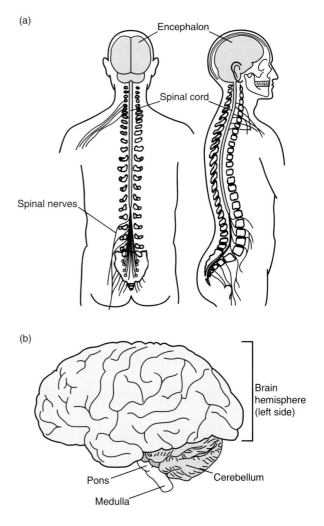

the periosteum. It also contains the venous sinuses which transport blood to the cervical veins.

The arachnoid mater adheres to the inside surface of the dura mater, and constitutes the outer layer of the subarachnoid spaces, where the cerebrospinal fluid circulates. The villous expansions or the arachnoid granulations of the arachnoid are responsible for the absorption of the cerebrospinal fluid (CSF).

The pia mater contains the blood vessels and directly covers the brain and the spinal cord, and for some short distance follows the blood vessels that penetrate the central nervous system tissue. It also constitutes, with the marginal layer of the glial cells, the glia limitans externa (see Section 3.1.2).

In the spinal cord, the dura mater is not attached to the vertebrae. The space left between the two is called the epidural space; this contains the veins, lymphatic vessels and fatty tissues, which facilitate the head and vertebral column movements.

The dura mater and arachnoid mater follow the spinal nerve roots, cover the spinal ganglions and mix with the other coverings of the spinal nerves.

Different fluid compartments

In the central nervous system, the fluid compartments are: the blood, the cerebrospinal fluid, and the extracellular and intracellular fluids.

Blood is distributed throughout the central nervous tissue by a capillary network. These capillaries are devoid of smooth muscles, except for those capillaries located near the surface. The endothelial cell lining of the wall of these small vessels is tightly related and so most substances present in the blood cannot pass through this blood–brain barrier (see Section 4.2). These capillaries are surrounded from the outside by a basal membrane (see Section 4.1.4) and by astrocyte endings (glial perivascular feet) (see Figures 3.1 and 3.2).

The *cerebrospinal fluid* (CSF) is a clear liquid deprived of protein and cells. It circulates inside the central nervous system through a cavity network formed by the ventricles and canals. This fluid also circulates around the central nervous system in the subarachnoid space (Figure 4.2a). It is secreted by the choroid plexus, a group of capillary villosities, lined with choroid ependymal cells and protruding inside the ventricles (Figures 4.2 and 4.10) (see also Section 3.4.1).

At the level of the choroidal vessels, the blood–brain barrier is absent (see Figure 4.10) and the substances filter freely from the blood toward the ependymal choroidal cells. However, the CSF is not simply a plasma filtrate. Its formation is achieved by a secretion process of ependymal choroidal cells which demands energy. The CSF thus formed in the ventricles circulates through openings in the fourth ventricle (Figure 4.2a), reaching the subarachnoid space, where it is absorbed through arachnoid granulations into the venous system (Figure 4.2b).

The *extracellular fluid* is found in the extracellular space all around the nerve and glial cells. Its composition is very similar to that of the CSF (Figure 4.10b). The *intracellular fluid* is located inside the nerve cells and is called cytosol. The extracellular and intracellular fluids are totally different in their ionic composition (see Figure 5.2) and remain stable by active transport through the plasma membrane of neuronal and glial cells.

4.1.2 The Central Nervous System is Composed of Nerve and Glial Cells That are Organized in Cortex, Nuclei, Horns, Funiculi, Commissures and Tracts: These Central Cells are Protected From the Blood Elements by the Blood–Brain Barrier

Gray matter and white matter

A cross-section of the nervous tissue seen in optic microscopy shows two distinct regions: the white and gray matters (Figure 4.3). The gray matter contains the cell bodies, the dendrites, the beginning of the axons, the axonal endings and the synapses. The white matter contains mainly the axons. Its white color in freshly cut tissue is due to the presence of myelin. Myelin is absent in the gray matter though glial cells and blood vessels are encountered in both regions.

Cortex, nuclei and horns (gray matter)

The cortex envelops the surface of the encephalon (cerebral, cerebellar), whereas the nuclei are situated deep in the brain (thalamic nuclei, inferior olive, etc.) (Figure 4.3a,b). Inside the cortex, the cell bodies are arranged in layers (Figure 4.4), whereas in the nuclei, the cell bodies are more or less organized in a

Figure 4.2   Meninges and cerebrospinal fluid. (a) Sagittal cross-section of the central nervous system demonstrating the circulation of the cerebrospinal fluid, which is secreted by the choroid plexus and circulates through the ventricles and subarachnoid space: 1, lateral ventricle; 2, third ventricle; 3, cerebral (Sylvius) aqueduct; 4, fourth ventricle; 5, central canal. (b) Frontal cross-section of cranial bone showing the relation of meninges with the cerebrospinal fluid (CSF), venous sinuses and blood vessels (see text). (After Kahle W, Leonhardt H and Platzer W, 1981. *Anatomie, Système Nerveux*, Tome 3, p. 269, Flammarion Médecine-Sciences, Paris, with permission.)

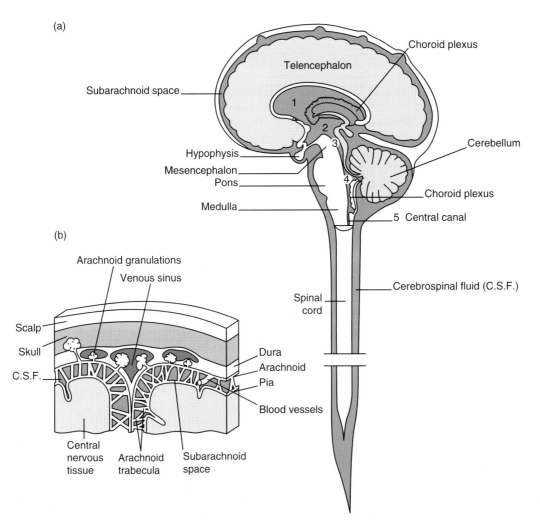

particular pattern. In the spinal cord, the gray matter is shaped like a butterfly. It is centrally located and has anterior, lateral and posterior horns (Figure 4.3c).

Tracts, bundles, commissures and fasciculi

These terms represent a group of axons that leave or reach target structures such as the cortex, nuclei or spinal horns. The terms tracts and bundles are the same whereas the term commissures refers to bundles of fibers that cross the midline and reach the opposite side of the brain. The term fasciculi is used to describe different regions of the white substance in the spinal cord.

An afferent pathway to a neuronal population is a pathway composed of axons that conduct the impulses toward the neurons of this neuronal popula-

Figure 4.3 White and gray substances. Frontal cross-section of the brain at the hippocampus level (a), cerebellum level (b) and horizontal cross-section of the spinal cord at the sacrum level (c).

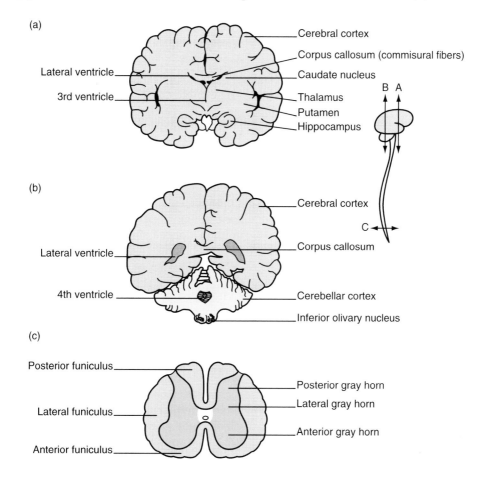

tion (for example, the climbing fibers and parallel fibers are afferent pathways to the cerebellar cortex, see Figures 2.6 and 2.7). An efferent pathway of a neuronal population is composed of axons that conduct impulses from this neuronal population to a target cell (e.g. the thalamo-cortical pathway, see Figure 1.14).

The central nervous tissue observed under the electron microscope

In the gray matter, the following elements can be observed under the electron microscope: dendrites, dendritic spines, axonal endings, glial cell extensions and sometimes the soma of the neurons or glial cells and blood vessels (see Figures 1.7 and 2.3). These different elements are recognized by their ultrastructures and the presence of pre- and post-synaptic specializations, which permit the localization of the synapses.

In an ultra-thin cross-section it is possible for an axonal ending and a dendrite to be seen in contact with one another over many microns. Yet the synapse sometimes cannot be observed, since it can be located in the preceding or the following sections of the same tissue.

The extracellular space between cells is very narrow: the membranes of the neurons and the glial cells are spaced from each other as far as 10 nm. In this space, the fluid (extracellular fluid) has a composition very similar to that of CSF.

Finally, central neurons are not in direct contact

Figure 4.4 Laminar organization of the hippocampus. (a) Transverse cross-section of the hippocampus demonstrating pyramidal cells in the CA1 (3) and CA3 regions (2) and the cells of the dentate gyrus (1). (b) Microphotograph of the area outlined in (a) under the optic microscope (Golgi stain). (Microphotograph: Paul Derer.)

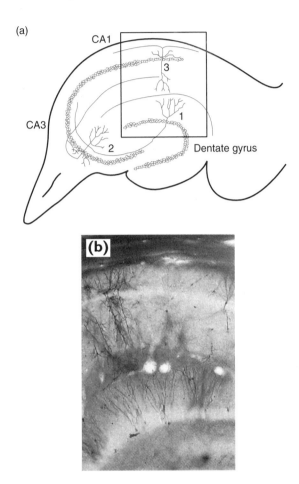

with the blood vessels since glial cells are intercalated between the central neurons and the blood vessels (see Section 3.1).

4.1.3 The Peripheral Nervous System is Comprised of Somatic and Autonomic (Visceral) Nervous Systems

The peripheral nervous system is composed of axons and neurons that are *not* located in the central nervous system. The somatic system innervates the skin, skeletal joints, muscles and sensory organs, whereas the autonomic nervous system innervates the smooth muscles of the internal organs, the blood vessels, the meninges and the glandular tissues.

The somatic system

The somatic system consists of motoneuron axons that innervate the skeletal muscles and the primary sensory neurons that bring sensory information to the central nervous system.

The motoneuron cell bodies are located in the motor nuclei of the cranial nerves or in the ventral horn of the spinal cord, and their axons follow the trajectory of the cranial or spinal nerves (Figures 4.5, see also Figures 1.13a and 4.1a).

The cell bodies of sensory neurons are located in the cranial ganglia (except for the olfactory and optic nerves) and in the dorsal root ganglia of the spinal nerves. Their axons follow the cranial or spinal nerve trajectories from the receptors situated in the skin, muscles and skeletal joints (Figures 1.13a and 1.14). There are 12 cranial nerves, of which the first two pairs (the olfactory and optic nerves) are not real peripheral nerves since they belong to the central nervous system. There are 31 pairs of spinal nerves, of which eight pairs are cervical, 12 pairs are thoracic, five pairs are lumbar, five other pairs are sacral and one last pair is coccygeal.

The autonomic nervous system

From an anatomical and functional point of view, the autonomic nervous system is divided into two groups: sympathetic and parasympathetic systems. Both systems are composed of efferent and afferent components to the central nervous system. The efferent component is composed of the axons of the pre-ganglionic neurons and the post-ganglionic viscero-motor and viscero-secretory neurons. The pre-ganglionic neurons have their cell bodies located in the central nervous system, more specifically in the vegetative nuclei of the cranial nerves or in the intermedio-lateral horn of the spinal cord (Figures 4.3c and 4.5b, c). The pre-ganglionic neurons control the activity of the post-ganglionic neurons. The cell bodies of the post-

Figure 4.5 Peripheral nervous system (only efferent neurons are represented). (a) Somatic system. The efferent side is formed by motoneuron axons that innervate skeletal muscles. The axons form the cranial motor nerves (III, IV, V, VI, VII, IX, XII, which are not represented) and the spinal motor nerves. (b) Sympathetic system. The efferent side is formed by the axon of the pre-ganglionic neurons (Pre) which have their cell bodies situated in the thoraco-lumbar section of the spinal cord, and by the post-ganglionic neurons (Post) which have their cell bodies situated in ganglia. The synapses between pre- and post-ganglionic neurons are therefore located in ganglions that lie in a long interconnected chain called the sympathetic ganglionic chain or are situated along the abdominal aorta. The post-ganglionic neurons directly innervate internal organs and glands. The adrenal glands are innervated directly by the pre-ganglionic neurons that form the splanchnic nerve. (c) Parasympathetic nervous system. The efferent side is formed of axons from the pre-ganglionic neurons (Pre) which have their cell bodies located in the brain stem (nerves III, VII, IX and X) or in the sacral part of the spinal cord (S2, S3, S4), and by post-ganglionic neurons which have their cell bodies located in ganglia that lie near their targets. The post-ganglionic nerves innervate internal organs and glands. In the upper drawings only one or a few neurons of each system are represented. The neurotransmitters of efferent neurons are shown in the lower drawings. ACh, acetylcholine; NA, noradrenaline.

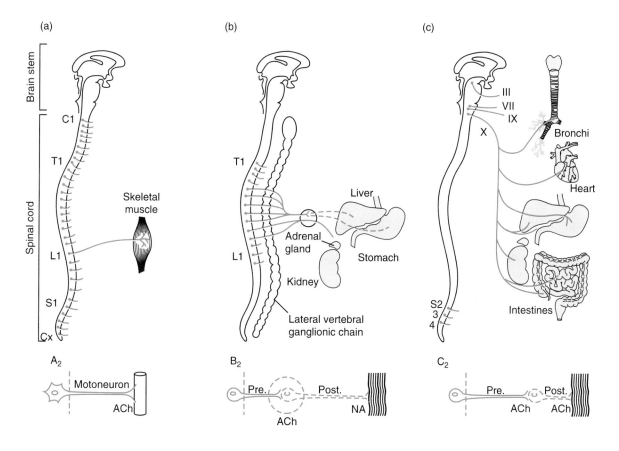

ganglionic viscero-motor and viscero-secretory neurons are situated in ganglia (Figure 4.5b, c). For this reason, they are called post-ganglionic neurons. The cell bodies of the viscero-sensory neurons are located in the spinal or cranial sensory ganglia. These afferent neurons transport the sensory information that comes from the body's internal organs and their peripheral coverings to the central nervous system.

Figure 4.6 Cross-sections of a spinal ganglion (a) and a peripheral nerve (b). See text for details. (After Kahle W, Leonhardt H, and Platzer W, 1981. *Anatomie Système Nerveux*, Tome 3, p. 57(a), p. 37(b), Flammarion Medecine-Sciences, Paris, with permission.)

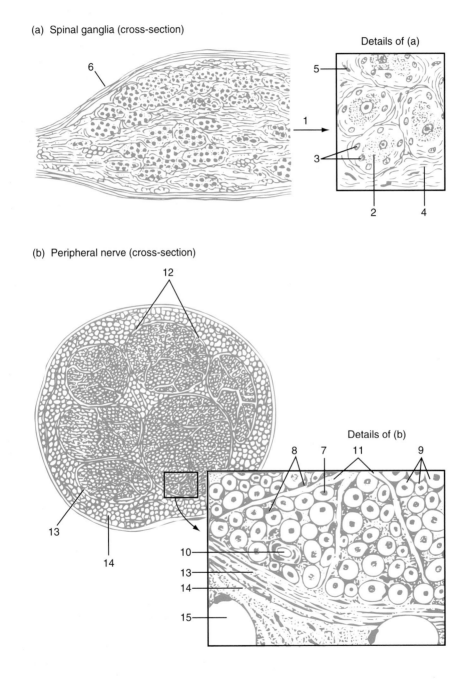

(a) Spinal ganglia (cross-section)

Details of (a)

(b) Peripheral nerve (cross-section)

Details of (b)

4.1.4 The Peripheral Nervous Tissue Consists of Nerve Cells, Glial Cells and Elements of the Extracellular Matrix, which Form Nerves and Ganglia

The ganglia

The ganglia contain the cell bodies of the peripheral nerves, Schwann cells that do not produce myelin (satellite cells, see Section 3.5.2) and the elements of the extracellular matrix. For example, the spinal ganglion, which contains the cell bodies of somato-sensitive and viscero-sensitive neurons, is spindle-shaped and is located on the dorsal root of the spinal nerves (see Figure 1.13a and 1.14). The somato-sensitive and viscero-sensitive neurons lack dendrites and have a T-shaped axon in which one branch comes from the periphery and the other leads to the central nervous system. Their cell bodies gather in groups surrounded by axons (Figure 4.6a, (1)). These cell bodies (2) are covered by satellite Schwann cells (3) and a basal membrane. Surrounding the whole is connective tissue, called the endoganglional tissue (4), which comprises endoganglionic fibroblasts (5). The spinal ganglion is protected by a capsule (6) which is the continuation of the perinerve tissue of the spinal nerve (Figure 4.6b, (13)).

The nerves

Nerves are made of many peripheral axons, embedded in many layers of connective tissue (Figure 4.6b). Each axon (7) is covered by Schwann cells (capable or not of producing myelin) (8) (see Section 3.5) and a basal membrane that securely separates each axonal fiber. Each axon with its envelope is called a nerve fiber (9). These fibers are surrounded by capillaries (10) and collagen fibers, which together form a very loose connective tissue called endonerve (11). Nerve fibers and the endonerve are grouped in bundles (12) that are surrounded by the perinerve (13). The perinerve is composed of: (i) several internal layers of epithelial cells connected to each other by junctions (zonulae occludentes). These constitute a barrier between the nerve fibers and the surrounding tissue, and (ii) an external layer of fibroblasts. The perinerve is enveloped by the epinerve (14), a connective tissue that contains fibroblasts, blood vessels, lymphatic vessels and fatty tissue (15).

The extracellular matrix

This macromolecular network is present in the peripheral nerve tissue and is practically absent in the central nervous system. One of the components of this network is the basal membrane that envelops the axons and the cell bodies in the peripheral nerve tissue. Other components are the connective tissue of nerves and ganglia, and the basal membrane that covers the small blood vessels and central canal cells.

The extracellular matrix mainly serves as supporting tissue, but it also plays an active role, for example, in the nerve regeneration of the peripheral nervous tissue. The cells that synthesize the macromolecules of the matrix are the Schwann cells, the endothelial cells of the blood vessels, the fibroblasts and the epithelial cells. The matrix is made of proteins and glycosaminoglycans that are covalently linked to other proteins to form proteoglycans. The glycosaminoglycans form a gel in which hormones, nutrients, metabolites, etc., diffuse. The proteins form the skeletal part of the matrix.

The principal proteins found in the matrix are: collagen, laminin and fibronectin (Figure 4.7).

A collagen molecule is made of three polypeptides rolled up into a triple spiral. Several collagen molecules have been described and the most prominent types have been numbered I to V. Collagen molecules are linked together to form collagen fibers. Fibronectin is a glycoprotein that adheres the cells, and laminin stimulates the growth and regeneration of peripheral axons. Laminin is made of three polypeptides connected together to make a cross-shaped molecule. The use of an anti-laminin antibody has localized the connection site of the protein to nerve and non-nerve cells. It has also identified the membrane receptors implicated in the recognition of laminin.

The glycosaminoglycans are or are not associated with proteins. Also called mucopolysaccharides, the glycosaminoglycans are formed by repeated sequences of disaccharides that are either *N*-acetyl-glycosamine or *N*-acetyl-galactosamine. Heparan sulfate and hyaluronic acid are two types of glycosaminoglycans. Some glycosaminoglycans are associated with proteins and are called proteoglycans. Their carbohydrate content is approximately 90%. All these materials form a hydrated gel that permits the rapid diffusion of hydrated molecules and the migration of nerve cells or their extensions.

Figure 4.7 The macromolecules of the extracellular matrix. (a) The collagen molecule is a triple α-helix. (b) Laminin is formed by three polypeptide chains, and is a cross-shaped molecule. In the area outlined are fragments that adhere to neuronal and/or non-neuronal elements. (c) A proteoglycan. (a and c: After Alberts B *et al*, 1986. *Biologie Moléculaire de la Cellule*, pp. 294, 705, Flammarion Médecine-Sciences, Paris, with permission. b: After Edgard D, 1989. Neuronal laminin receptors, *TINS* **12**, 248–251, with permission.)

(a) Collagen molecule

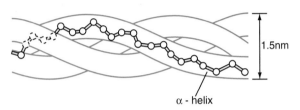

1.5nm

α - helix

(b) Laminin

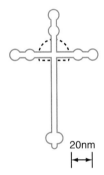

20nm

(c) Proteoglycan

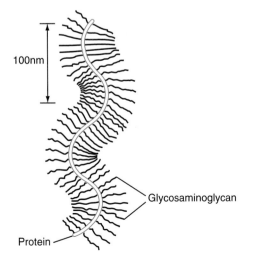

100nm

Glycosaminoglycan

Protein

The basal membrane is a specialized form of the extracellular matrix. The basal membrane is a fine layer of specialized extracellular matrix that is found in all kinds of epithelium. It also surrounds the central and peripheral vessels, the peripheral axon–Schwann cell complex, the skeletal muscle fibers, etc. The basal membrane separates these cells from the surrounding tissue. It represents the only form of extracellular matrix present in the central nervous system where it is located around the blood vessels and under the epithelium that borders the cavities of the brain and the spinal cord. Under the electron microscope, this basal layer is composed of a very dense zone (lamina densa), surrounded by two pale regions. The lamina densa contains type IV collagen, and the pale regions are glycoproteins (laminin and fibronectin) and glycosaminoglycans. The basal membrane not only is a selective filter but also plays an important role in nerve cell migration, the induction of differentiation and the organization of proteins in the adjacent membranes. For example, the basal membrane that surrounds the muscles presents special antigenic properties at the neuromuscular junction level. During development, this allows the formation of the synapse and the differentiation of the pre- and post-synaptic elements.

4.1.5 The Differences Between the Central and Peripheral Nervous Systems are Seen at the Non-neuronal Element Level

The central and peripheral nervous tissues are both made of neurons that are very similar. The ultrastructural differences between these two tissues are related to the nature of the glial cells, the presence or absence of the extracellular matrix and of the junctions between endothelial cells of the blood vessels. As explained in Section 4.2, the endothelial cells that form the capillary walls in the central nervous system protect the nervous tissue from blood. In the peripheral nervous tissue this protection does not exist. On the other hand, each peripheral neuron is covered by a basal membrane and other elements of the extracellular matrix, whereas central neurons do not have this covering. In Section 4.3, the role of this microsurrounding in the peripheral nervous systems is analyzed.

4.2 The Blood–Brain Barrier Protects the Central Neurons From Blood Content and Maintains the Composition of the Extracellular Medium

In all organs, the substances freely move from blood capillaries to the surrounding tissue by passively crossing the blood vessel walls. In the central nervous system the situation is different. The concept of a barrier between the blood and the central nervous system (blood–brain barrier) comes from the work of Paul Ehrlich. This researcher observed that the injection of a colored solution into the blood circulation stains all organs except the brain and spinal cord. On the other hand, injections of staining material into the CSF stains the central nervous system tissue, but does not stain the blood or any of the other organs. This indicates the presence of a 'barrier' between the central nervous system and the blood.

4.2.1 The Tight Junctions That Link the Endothelial Cells Together in the Blood Vessel Walls of the Central Nervous System Represent the Main Element of the Blood–Brain Barrier

Studies performed by electron microscopy have proven that the endothelial cells that comprise the capillary walls present in the central nervous system are linked together by tight junctions. This provides a very strong barrier for many substances, preventing them from passing between endothelial cells (Figure 4.8a). At the tight junction level, the external layers of the membranes of two endothelial cells fuse together, thus suppressing the extracellular space in that region (Figure 4.8b). Blood substances therefore cannot diffuse in between the endothelial cells and so have to pass through the plasma membrane of these cells to reach the central extracellular space. In humans

Figure 4.8 Capillary vessels in the central nervous system. (a) Transverse cross-section of a capillary vessel indicating an endothelial cell with a tight junction forming the capillary wall. Blood vessels with a large diameter have many endothelial cells connected to each other by tight junctions and forming the perimeter of the vessel. These cells are surrounded by pericytes, a basal membrane and astrocyte foot extensions (glial perivascular feet). (b) Diagram of a tight junction. Neighboring membranes are tightly coupled along their entire length, and in some places by protein chains. The cytoplasmic layer of one of the plasma membranes is elevated to show the protein chain. (a: After Goldstein G and Betz L, 1986, La barrière qui protège le cerveau, *Pour la Science*, **Nov**: 84–94, with permission. b: After Alberts B *et al*, 1986, *Biologie Moléculaire de la Cellule*, p. 686, Flammarion Mèdicine-Sciences, Paris, with permission.)

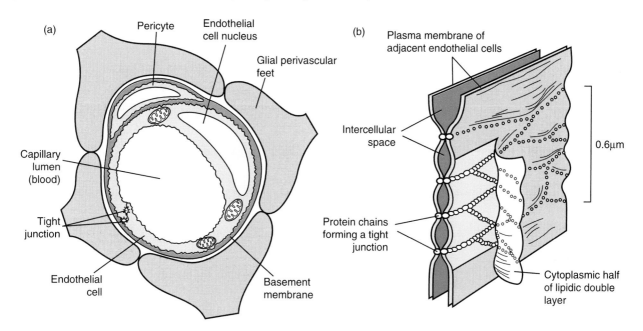

this isolating layer is formed in the third month of embryonic life, and is the principal element of the blood–brain barrier. It prevents the passage of macromolecules, especially proteins, and limits the passage of smaller molecules. It also protects the central nervous system cells from foreign elements.

The blood vessel walls outside the central nervous system present different characteristics compared with the blood vessels that irrigate the central nervous system. Outside the central nervous system, the endothelial cells are not connected to each other by tight junctions. Therefore, there exists an interstitial space where the plasma substances circulate freely from blood vessels to adjacent tissues. For this reason, the blood vessels outside the central nervous system are said to be 'fenestrated'.

However, in the central nervous system, in a few places, fenestrated blood vessels are observed. They are mostly encountered in structures of the nervous system where activity is modulated by the hormonal system such as the pineal gland, some nuclei of the hypothalamus and the postrema area of the medulla oblongata.

Many experiments have been performed in order to determine the role played by the surrounding medium in the acquisition of the special properties observed in the central capillaries. In these experiments, cerebral and muscle tissues were transplanted in a bird embryo at different locations. After the transplantation of cerebral tissue in the embryonic intestines, the micro-blood vessels of the intestines that colonized the cerebral tissue comprised endothelial cells connected to each other by tight junctions. Conversely, when muscle tissue was transplanted into the brain tissue, the endothelial cells of the blood vessels that irrigated the graft lose their barrier capabilities, and become fenestrated. Thus it would seem that the development of the blood–brain barrier is stimulated by the central nervous tissue, and has nothing to do with genetic programming.

4.2.2 Liposoluble Substances and Actively Transported Substances are Capable of Passing Through the Central Blood Vessel Walls

If the central nervous system tissue was totally isolated from circulating blood, the neuronal and non-

neuronal elements of the central nervous system would be deprived of any source of energy and would degenerate. Many essential molecules and other materials pass the blood–brain barrier, by active transport or because they are liposoluble. This transport is achieved through the membrane of endothelial cells. For this reason the term 'barrier' is not adequate as it refers to a physical obstacle being present between the plasma and the extracellular medium. The blood–brain barrier more likely represents a dynamic interface between the blood and the central nervous system.

To study the characteristics of the substances that can traverse the blood–brain barrier, different radioactively labeled molecules have been used. The probability of the studied radioactive molecule crossing the barrier is compared with the probability of a molecule that is known to traverse easily or not cross it at all. This is achieved by comparing the concentration of the two molecules in the cerebral tissue and in the blood that flows back from the brain. We can then establish the 'coefficient of penetration' of the substances that have been the subject of the study by comparison with the reference molecules. The liposolubility of the substances is one of the characteristics that facilitates their passage through the blood–brain barrier. Oxygen, carbon dioxide and other liposoluble molecules such as alcohol, nicotine, different types of anesthetics and heroïn traverse the endothelial cell membranes by simple diffusion. Hydrosoluble molecules that are essential to the proper function of the central nervous system are actively transported by specific transport mechanisms. For example, D-glucose is recognized by a protein situated in the membrane of the endothelial cells which allows its passage from the blood to the nervous system. The same procedure is used for neutral amino acids that in some cases are essential in the synthesis of some of the neurotransmitters released by central neurons. The proteins implicated in the transport of different substances are present in the luminal and anti-luminal membranes of the endothelial cells. The luminal membrane is in contact with the blood, whereas the anti-luminal membrane is directly in contact with the extracellular medium of the central nervous system. Other molecules that are mostly brought in by a nutritional diet are also transported: the precursors of the nucleic acids, cetonic bodies and choline (precursor of acetylcholine).

4.2.3 The K⁺ Ions and Amino Acids used as Neurotransmitters are Transported Through the Endothelial Cell Membrane from the Extracellular Space to Enter the Bloodstream

The blood–brain barrier does not act as a simple semi-permeable barrier functioning in one direction, from blood to central nervous system. For example, the K^+ ion concentration has to be kept at low levels in the extracellular fluid to maintain the excitability properties of the neurons. This regulation is achieved by the glial cells (see Section 3.1.3) and the endothelial cells of the blood vessels. Likewise, the amino acids glutamate, aspartate and glycine, which are also neurotransmitters, are recaptured not only by neurons and glial cells but also by endothelial cells. This is assured by several systems that actively transport these substances from the extracellular space toward the blood and are localized in the endothelial cells at the anti-luminal membrane level (Figure 4.9).

In conclusion, the blood–brain barrier maintains the strict composition of the extracellular fluid by permitting the passage of essential molecules, but also by

Figure 4.9 Examples of a local transport system in the luminal (in contact with blood) and antiluminal (in contact with extracellular fluid) membranes of endothelial cells. The proposed model depicts only some receptors and carrier systems. D-glucose and small neutral amino acids enter the central nervous tissue by localized transport mechanisms (GT and AS, respectively). I, insulin receptor; LDL, low density lipoprotein receptor; T, transferrin receptor. (From Schlosshauer B, 1993. The blood–brain barrier: morphology, molecules and neurothelin, *Bioessays*, **15**, 341–346, with permission.)

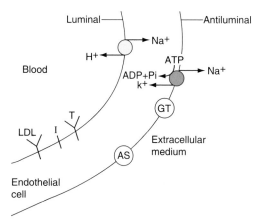

preventing the entry or by supplying a system of recapture of molecules, ions and toxic substances that could change the excitability of the neurons.

4.2.4 Summary of Exchanges Between the CSF and the Central Nervous System

In a cross-section drawing of the central nervous tissue (Figure 4.10) we represent the endothelial cells of the capillaries situated in the central nervous tissue. The endothelial cells are bound together by tight junctions and form the blood–brain barrier. These blood vessels are surrounded by the basal membrane and astrocyte endings (glial perivascular feet) coupling up with each other and separating the perivascular space from the nervous system.

At the level of the choroid plexus, the blood vessels of the plexus are fenestrated. However, the choroid ependymal glial cells of this choroid plexus that are coupled together by tight junctions (see Section 3.4.1) form a physical barrier that prevents the passage of many choroidian blood molecules toward the CSF. Thus, different systems exist to isolate the central nervous system from the circulating blood.

The molecules that can avoid these obstacles, namely the blood–brain barrier or the layers of the choroid ependymal cells (by being liposoluble or by being transported actively), diffuse freely into the CSF and the extracellular space, where the neurons are located. Neurons are joined together by synaptic contacts, and the glial cells communicate with each other via gap junctions. In fact, the CSF and the extracellular fluid are in continuity, each penetrating freely through the layers of the ependymal choroid cells.

4.3 In Adult Mammals, Non-neuronal Peripheral Elements Favor the Regrowth of Injured Axons Though in the Central Nervous System Non-neuronal Elements do not Allow this Regrowth

When a nerve is cut or damaged, the axon segment and its myelin sheath which are distal to the lesion site will degenerate. The proximal part of the axon, which is nourished by the neuron's cell body, remains alive and grows to replace the degenerated distal part. It

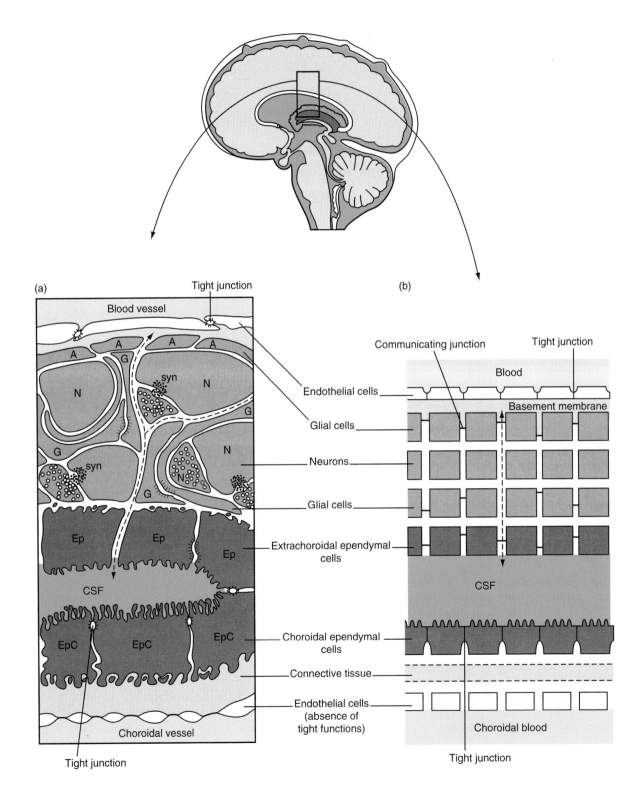

will also restore its function. The regrowth of axons in the central nervous system is very short and the axon never re-establishes synaptic contacts with the target neurons.

4.3.1 The Glial Cells of the Central and Peripheral Systems Have Opposite Effects on the Regrowth of Axons

Schwann cells favor regrowth and guide the peripheral axons

Studies showing the evolution of an injured peripheral nerve demonstrate that first the distal section of the axon degenerates, then the myelin sheath is absorbed, and finally there is a proliferation of the Schwann cells that are present in the empty nervous canals (these canals are lined by a basal membrane, and an axon passes through each one of them). These Schwann cells excrete trophic factors that stimulate the growth of the proximal sections of the neurons. Nerve growth factor (NGF), discovered by Levi-Montalcini, Cohen and Hamburger, is the prototype for trophic factors.

NGF is a protein produced by the target tissues of NGF-responsive neurons and acts as a retrograde neurotrophic messenger (see Section 1.3.5). In this role NGF regulates the extent of the survival and differentiation of sympathetic neurons, for example, during development and maintenance of their specific function in adulthood. NGF is not expressed to a significant extent in non-neuronal cells of adult peripheral nerves. However, this situation changes dramatically after nerve lesion (e.g. sciatic nerve lesion). A rapid, transient and massive increase in NGF mRNA occurs in the nerve region immediately proximal to the lesion (Figure 4.11a, b). Simultaneously with the enhanced synthesis of NGF, the lesion

of the sciatic nerve leads to re-expression of NGF receptor mRNA by Schwann cells, receptors normally expressed only in early stages of development (Figure 4.11b). Then, regenerating nerve fibers reverse the increases in both mRNAs produced by injury.

Contact of the peripheral axons with the white matter of the central nervous system inhibits axonal regrowth

Even though growth factors such as NGF are necessary for lengthening of the peripheral axons, their presence alone is not sufficient for the growth of axons when the neurons are co-cultured with the central nervous system tissue. This has been demonstrated in a study where peripheral nerve cells were taken from the sensory or sympathetic ganglia of newborn rats and cultured on different types of tissues: either central nervous system tissue of the adult rat (spinal cord, cerebellum and optic nerve) or peripheral nerve tissue (sciatic nerve). After 2 weeks of culture, the neurons were stained and the cross-sections were observed under the microscope (Figure 4.12).

The peripheral neurons grew extensions over the whole surface of the peripheral nerve tissue, whereas the peripheral neurons that were cultured over the optic nerve (white substance) did not develop any extensions and disappeared. The cells cultured over tissue extracted from the spinal cord or cerebellum grew extensions only over the gray matter. This suggests that the white matter of the adult central nervous system has a non-permissive effect on the growth of the cultured neurons and their axon extensions.

Moreover, the destruction of a great portion of the oligodendrocytes of the central nervous system tissue by the use of an antimitotic agent (5-azacytidine) greatly diminishes the non-permissive ability of the

Figure 4.10 Relationship between the central nervous system cells, cerebrospinal fluid (CSF) and blood. (a) Cross-section of the central nervous tissue including the choroid plexus. (b) Simplified version of the drawing in (a). Spaces between endothelial cells of the blood vessels are closed by tight junctions. Spaces between choroid ependymal cells (EpC) are also closed by tight junctions which prevent the direct passage of substances in choroidian blood toward the CSF. On the other hand, the substances diffuse freely from the CSF toward the extracellular fluid, and vice versa (arrows). The communicating junctions between glial cells (G and Ep) are not obstacles to this diffusion. A, Astrocytes; Ep, extrachoroid ependymal cells; N, neurons; Syn, synapse. (a: After Brightman MW and Reese TS, 1969. The junctions between intimately apposed cell membranes in the vertebrate brain, *J. Cell. Biol.* **40**, 648–677, with permission. b: After Cohen MW, Gerschenfeld HM and Kuffler SW, 1968. Ionic environment of neurons and glial cells in the brain of an amphibian, *J. Physiol.* **197**, 363–380, with permission.)

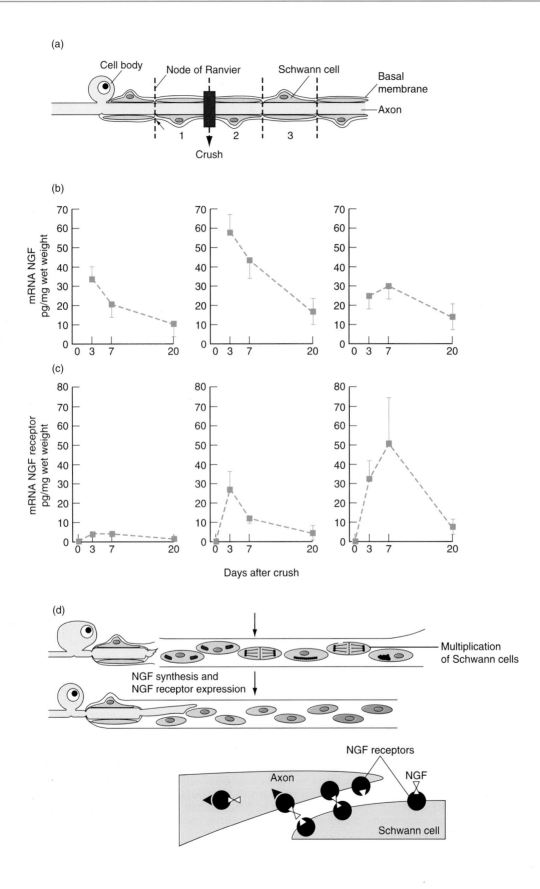

white matter in the central nervous system. This indicates that the oligodendrocytes may be implicated in prevention of the growth of the neurons and their extensions in the central nervous system. However, the glial cells would not be the only elements at the nervous system level that inhibit or induce the growth of the axons.

The following hypothesis is proposed: other factors besides the growth factors are present in the peripheral nerve tissue and allow elongation of the axons (permissive factors), and there are other factors present in the central nervous system of the adult mammals that do not favor, and even inhibit, the growth of the axons (non-permissive factors). The non-permissive factors are absent from the central nervous system of immature mammals and are also absent from the central nervous system of the inferior vertebrates such as fish and amphibians for which elongation of the central axons is normally observed.

4.3.2 Grafting of a Peripheral Nerve into the Central Nervous System Induces Regrowth of Central Axons and Functional Reinnervation of their Target Cells: Bridging Experiments

The hypothesis was that peripheral non-neuronal elements favor the growth and lengthening of axons. In an experiment, the central microenvironment was substituted by the peripheral environment and thus central neurons were exposed to permissive peripheral factors for axonal growth. The experiment consisted more specifically of implanting fragments of peripheral nerves between neurons of the central nervous system that were previously denervated or deafferented (Figures 4.13 and 4.14a, left). Later, after the grafting operation, the peripheral axons inside the nerve fragments degenerate and only the glial and extracellular matrix remained inside the 'empty nerve conduct'. The question was: is there any possibility that this empty tube made of non-neuronal elements could guide and permit the regrowth of cut axons of central neurons?

We will present two types of experiments demonstrating this procedure: (i) reinnervation of central target neurons by central neurons; and (ii) reinnervation of peripheral target cells by central neurons. Reinnervation is studied at different levels (Figure 4.14, left):

- Identification and localization of the neurons where axons have grown inside the graft and have reached the target cells: these neurons are marked by retrograde tracers injected either at the level of the target structures or at the level of the peripheral graft. Their morphology and location are studied under the optic microscope.
- Identification and localization of new synapses formed in the target structures: the newly grown

Figure 4.11   Synthesis of the mRNA of NGF and re-expression of the mRNA of NGF receptors during axonal regrowth. (a) Drawing of a peripheral neuron and its myelin sheath formed by Schwann cells (many of these form a peripheral nerve). In this experiment, the sciatic nerve was crushed with forceps cooled in liquid nitrogen and the crush site was marked with a thread. At various times (3 to 20 days) after the nerve was crushed, the rats were killed and the nerve was cut into three segments: 1 (proximal), 2 and 3 (distal), each 4 mm long. (b) Changes in sciatic mRNA NGF levels proximal (segment 1) and distal (segments 2 and 3) to the crush. Values represent means ± SEM of three or four experiments. Level of mRNA NGF for intact sciatic nerve is 3.4 ± 0.6 fg/mg wet weight. (c) Changes in mRNA NGF receptor levels proximal (segment 1) and distal (segments 2 and 3) to the crush. Level of mRNA NGF receptor in intact sciatic nerve is 240 ± 100 fg/mg wet weight. (d) Hypothesis concerning the regulation of NGF synthesis and NGF receptor expression during axonal regrowth. After crushing, the distal part of axons degenerates and the myelin sheath disappears. Schwann cells proliferate. The loss of contact between the Schwann cell membranes and the axonal membrane would induce the expression of NGF and its receptor by Schwann cells. During axonal regrowth, the Schwann cells resume contact with the axonal membrane, remake the myelin sheath, and cease the expression of NGF and its receptor. Enlarged diagram shows the transfer of NGF between the Schwann cell and the regenerating axon. (After Johnson EM, Taniuchi M Jr, and Di Stefano PS, 1988. The expression and possible function of nerve growth factor receptors on Schwann cells, *TINS* **11**, 299–304, with permission, and Heumann R, Lindholm D, Bandtlow C, *et al*, 1987. Differential regulation of mRNA encoding nerve growth factor and its receptor in rat sciatic nerve during development, degeneration and regeneration: role of macrophages, *Proc. Natl. Acad. Sci. USA*, **84**, 8735–8739, with permission.)

Figure 4.12   Non-permissive role of the central white substance. Neurons cultured for 2 days on sections of adult sciatic nerve (peripherial nerve, a) grow and multiply and their extensions become longer, whereas when cultured on sections of spinal cord (central gray and white substances, b), they show a strong preference for gray matter. Growth inhibition is observed on the funiculus part of the spinal cord (white substance, B). Cresyl violet stain, original magnifications: a ×36, b ×17. (After Savio T and Schwab ME, 1989. Rat CNS white matter but not gray matter is non-permissive for neuronal cell adhesion and fiber outgrowth, *J. Neurosci.* 9, 1126–1133, with permission.

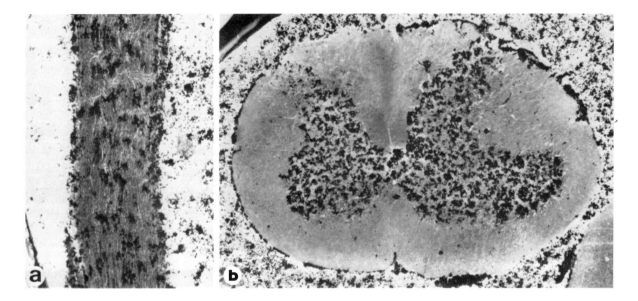

axons are marked anterogradely by injecting anterograde tracers at the level of the cell bodies. The synapses formed between the marked axonal endings and the dendrites or the soma of the target cells are studied under the electron microscope.

- Study of the electrophysiological properties of the newly formed synapses.

Formation of new and functional central synapses between the ganglion cell axons of the retina and the superior colliculus neurons in peripheral nerve graft experiments

The axons of the ganglion cells of the retina form the optic nerve. These axons take visual information to the visual structures of the brain, among them the superior colliculus. In the adult rat, any damage to the optic nerve causes degeneration of the ganglion cells, and deafferentation of the target neurons, such as the neurons of the superior colliculus.

To study the prevention of the degenerating process of the axons of ganglion cells and the stimulating factors that cause their regrowth, the optic nerve is severed as close as possible to the eye. An autogenous nerve graft (peroneal nerve of the same animal) is then applied between the severed optic nerve and the superior colliculus neurons (Figure 4.13): the tip of the nerve graft is sutured to the tip of the severed optic nerve, the rest of the graft is left under the scalp inside a groove that leads to the occipital region and the nerve graft's end is left near the superior colliculus. This extracranial approach is used because normally the optic nerve is in contact only with the superficial cells of the superior colliculus. This approach allows the regenerating axons to establish connections directly with the target neurons.

The results of these experiments indicated that the ganglion cells which showed axonal regrowth were situated only in the retina. The damaged ganglion cell axons were capable of growing inside the grafted nerve, for a distance of twice the length that normally they have to grow inside the brain. This indicates the remarkable plasticity of the central axons when placed

Figure 4.13 Sagittal section of an adult rat that has been grafted with a portion of the peripheral nerve, between the sectioned optic nerve and the superior colliculus. (After Vidal-Sanz M, Bray GM, Villegas-Perez MP, Thanos S and Aguayo AJ, 1987. Axonal regeneration and synapse formation in the superior colliculus by retinal ganglion cells in the adult rat, *J. Neurosci.* 7, 2894–2909, with permission.)

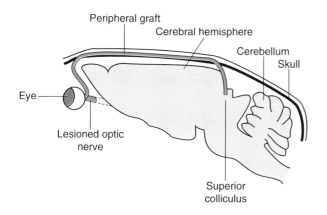

in favorable conditions. However, once the target structures were reached, very few axons penetrated the superior colliculus and coursed over only a short distance (500 µm maximum). The non-neuronal peripheral elements were then capable of stimulating the growth of the axons, but were not capable of permitting the deep penetration of the axons inside the central nervous system. Those axons that did penetrate the superior colliculus formed terminal branches and synapses that under the electron microscope presented pre- and post-synaptic specialization. The synapses were functional and visual stimulations of the retina evoked the response of the collicular cells.

Formation of new functional neuromuscular junctions

New junctions are observed between the motoneurons that have grown axons inside a peripheral nerve graft and the muscle cells that were previously denervated. Experiments carried out on rats consisted of: (i) sectioning and tying a nerve that innervates a neck muscle. The cell bodies of this nerve are situated in the cervical spine (C1); and (ii) grafting a fragment of the peripheral nerve (peroneal) between the spinal cord at the C5 level and a denervated muscle (Figure 4.14A, left). One end of the graft is sutured to C5 near the dorsal horn of the spinal cord, and the other end is sutured to the denervated muscle. The central motor axons that previously innervated this neck muscle and the axons located in the nerve graft all degenerate. The nerve graft then becomes an empty tube. What is peculiar in this type of experiment is that the new axons that penetrated and grew into the hollow graft are not issued from the same neurons that were innervating the muscle before (since those have degenerated). In fact, one of the purposes of this experiment was to understand if the collateral axons of intact motoneurons were able to grow inside the graft and could innervate the denervated muscle.

The end results were analyzed after 6 weeks to 5 months after applying the nerve graft. They showed that the neurons that grew axons and reached the muscle cells were essentially motoneurons (Figure 4.14b). In fact, many types of neurons were present near the graft and could grow collaterals to innervate the denervated muscle fibers: motoneurons and medular neurons inside local circuits, medular neurons that have principal axons that project to other central structures, and finally visceral neurons that innervate the meninges and blood vessels of the spinal cord (Figure 4.14c). If all of them sent a collateral axon to enter the nerve graft, only the motoneurons could really establish synaptic contacts with the muscle cells. The contact site (the new neuromuscular junction) could be at the former site or even another nearby location, away from the primary site (ectopic junctions) (Figure 4.14A, left). These new junctions were perfectly functional since stimulating the new axons in the graft produced muscle contractions (Figure 4.14A, right). Finally, all pharmaceutical substances that normally block synaptic transmission at the neuromuscular junction by preventing acetylcholine fixation were effective at the newly formed junction. This again proved that the neurons that reinnervated the denervated muscle were effectively motoneurons using acetylcholine as a neurotransmitter.

In conclusion, some central neurons have kept their capacity to regenerate their axons over long distances and express this capacity in permissive microenvironments. They can also establish new synaptic contacts, which are perfectly selective and functional, with target cells. However, it must be noted that not all the central neurons are able to regenerate axons inside peripheral nerve grafts (for example, the Purkinje cells).

Figure 4.14   Innervation of a neck muscle by collateral axons of motor neurons, growing through a periph-eral nerve graft. (a) This graft is lodged between the dorsal horn of the spinal cord and a neck muscle (rat). Once axonal growth is achieved, the newly formed neuromuscular junctions are localized by a colored acetyl-cholinesterase reaction (left). The junctions are located at the same level as the older junctions (**a** and **b**) but also in a central ectopic region. Stimulation of axons present in the graft evokes a response in muscle cells (right). This response is monitored in the ectopic junction (left, extracellular electrode). (b) An HRP injection into the muscle labels the neurons with axons that have grown and reached the muscle cells (left). The cell bod-ies of these labeled neurons are mainly localized in the ventral ipsilateral and contralateral horns of the spinal cord (right) where the cell bodies of motoneurons are normally located. (c) When HRP is injected at the proximal end of the severed graft (left) many more spinal neurons are labeled with cell bodies located in the ventral, dorsal and intermediate horn (right). After Horvat JC, Pecot-Dechavasisne M, Mira JS and Davapanach Y, 1989. Formation of functional endplates by spinal axons regenerating through a peripheral nerve graft. A study in the adult rat, *Brain Res. Bull.* **22**, 103–114, with permission, and Horvat JC, Pecot-Dechavassine M and Mira JC, 1988. Functional reinnervation of a denervated skeletal muscle of the adult rat by axons regen-erating from the spinal cord through a peripheral nervous graft, *Prog. Brain Res.*, **78**, 219–224, with permis-sion.)

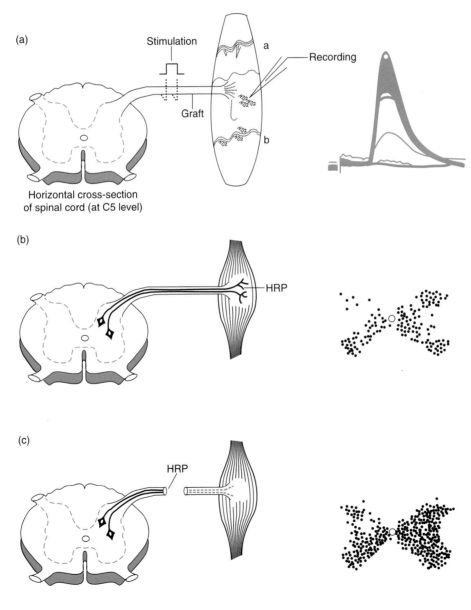

Further Reading

Allan, V.J., Vale, R.D. and Navone, F. (1992) Microtubule-based organelle transport in neurons. In: Burgoyne, R.D. (Ed), *The Neuronal Cytoskeleton*, pp. 257–282, Wiley-Liss, New York.

Aubert, I., Ridet, J.L. and Gage, F.H. (1995) Regeneration in the adult mammalian CNS: guided by development. *Curr. Opin. Neurobiol.*, **5**, 625–635.

Begley, D.J. (1994) Peptides and blood brain barrier. The status of our understanding. *Ann. NY Acad. Sci.*, **739**, 89–100.

Bonate, P.L. (1995) Animal models for studying transport across the blood brain barrier. *J. Neurosci. Methods*, **56**, 1–15.

Nixon, R.A. (1992) Axonal transport of cytoskeletal proteins. In: Burgoyne, R.D. (Ed), *The Neuronal Cytoskeleton*, pp. 283–308, Wiley-Liss, New York.

Shaw, G. (1992) Neurofilament proteins. In: Burgoyne, R.D. (Ed), *The Neuronal Cytoskeleton*, pp. 185–214, Wiley-Liss, New York.

Part II

Neurons and Excitable and Secretory Cells

The Neuronal Plasma Membrane

The neuronal plasma membrane delimits the whole neuron, from the dendritic spines to the axon terminals. It is a barrier between the intracellular and extracellular environments. The general structure of the neuronal plasma membrane is similar to that of other plasma membranes. It is made up of proteins inserted in a lipid bilayer forming as a whole a 'fluid mosaic' (Figure 5.1). However, insofar as there are functions that are exclusively neuronal, the neuronal membrane differs from other plasma membranes by the nature, density and spatial distribution of the proteins of which it is composed.

5.1 The Intracellular and Extracellular Environments Have Different Ionic Compositions

All cells have an unequal distribution of ions across the plasma membrane: regardless of the animal's environment (seawater, freshwater or air) potassium (K^+) ions are the predominant cations in the intracellular fluid and sodium (Na^+) ions are the predominant cations in the extracellular fluid. The main anions of the intracellular fluid are organic molecules (P^-): negatively charged amino acids (glutamate and aspartate), proteins, nucleic acids, etc. In the extracellular fluid the predominant anions are chloride (Cl^-) ions. A marked difference between the cytosolic and extracellular Ca^{2+} concentration (Figure 5.2) is also observed. This difference in concentration between two compartments is called a concentration gradient.

Spatial distribution of Ca^{2+} ions inside the cell deserves a more detailed description. Ca^{2+} ions are present in the cytosol as 'free' Ca^{2+} ions at a very low concentration ($10^{-8} - 10^{-7}$ M) and as bound Ca^{2+} ions (bound to Ca^{2+}-binding proteins). They are also distributed in organelles able to sequester calcium, which include endoplasmic reticulum, calciosome and mito-

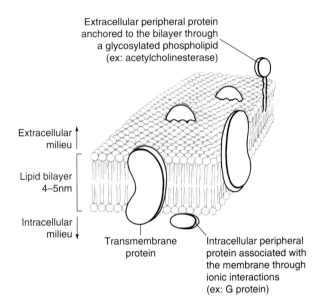

Figure 5.1 Fluid mosaic: transmembrane proteins and lipids are kept together by non-covalent interactions (ionic and hydrophobic).

Extracellular peripheral protein anchored to the bilayer through a glycosylated phospholipid (ex: acetylcholinesterase)

Extracellular milieu

Lipid bilayer 4–5nm

Intracellular milieu

Transmembrane protein

Intracellular peripheral protein associated with the membrane through ionic interactions (ex: G protein)

chondria, where they constitute the intracellular Ca^{2+} stores. Free intracellular Ca^{2+} ions act as second messengers and transduce electrical activity in neurons into biochemical events such as exocytosis. Ca^{2+} ions bound to cytosolic proteins or present in organelle stores are not active Ca^{2+} ions. Exchanges of Ca^{2+} ions occur between these compartments (extracellular, cytosolic, intraorganelles) in response to specific signals, but, as for Na^+ and K^+ ions, the intracellular concentration of free Ca^{2+} ions is precisely controlled (see below and Chapter 8).

Inorganic ions such as Na^+, K^+, Ca^{2+} and Cl^- can cross the membrane and the membrane is said to be permeable to these ions. Organic ions (such as proteins) cannot diffuse through the membrane: the

Figure 5.2   Asymmetric distribution of ions across the plasma membrane (terrestrian vertebrates).

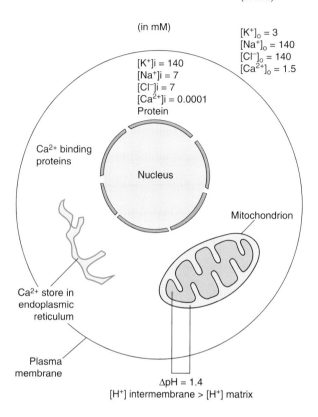

(in mM)

(in mM)

$[K^+]_o = 3$
$[Na^+]_o = 140$
$[Cl^-]_o = 140$
$[Ca^{2+}]_o = 1.5$

$[K^+]i = 140$
$[Na^+]i = 7$
$[Cl^-]i = 7$
$[Ca^{2+}]i = 0.0001$
Protein

Ca²⁺ binding proteins

Nucleus

Mitochondrion

Ca²⁺ store in endoplasmic reticulum

Plasma membrane

ΔpH = 1.4
$[H^+]$ intermembrane > $[H^+]$ matrix

membrane is impermeable to them. Passive ion movements occur only through specialized transmembrane transport proteins, called protein channels, since the lipid bilayer is impermeable to ions as well as to most polar molecules.

Passive ion movements across the membrane would cause concentration changes in the extracellular and intracellular compartments if the concentrations were not constantly regulated during the entire life of the neuron. This regulation is carried out by proteins that continually re-establish the ionic concentration difference by active transport (see Section 5.5 and Chapter 6). These proteins are known as pumps and transporters.

Thus, the plasma membrane is not a passive barrier between the intracellular and extracellular environments. Proteins that are part of the membrane allow a strict regulation of the passage of ions and molecules between these two environments.

5.2 The Lipid Bilayer is the Solvent for Membrane Proteins and a Barrier for Diffusion

5.2.1 Membrane Lipids Organize Themselves into a Bilayer

Membrane lipids belong to three main classes: phospholipids, cholesterol and glycolipids. They have a polar head which is hydrophilic and a non-polar tail which is hydrophobic. This defines them all as amphiphilic molecules (Appendix 5.1).

Phospholipids

The most commonly found phospholipids in the neuronal plasma membrane are phosphoglycerides. They are made up of two chains of fatty acids and a phosphorylated alcohol attached to glycerol-3-phosphate. Fatty acids form the hydrophobic tail and the phosphodiester forms the hydrophilic head (Figure 5.3a). Fatty acid chains are formed by 14 to 24 carbon atoms: palmitic acid (a saturated fatty acid of 16 carbon atoms) and oleic acid (unsaturated fatty acid of 18 carbon atoms). Depending on the phosphodiester that forms the head group, one can identify phosphatidylserine, phosphatidylethanolamine, phosphatidylcholine and phosphatidylinositol (Figure 5.3).

When phosphoglycerides are placed in an aqueous solution, they spontaneously orient themselves, their hydrophilic heads in contact with water and their hydrophobic tails oriented towards each other in order to exclude water. Within the membrane, they form two parallel monolayers facing each other, called a lipid bilayer. In this bilayer the heads are in contact with the intracellular and the extracellular environments and the tails form the interior of the bilayer (see Figure 5.1). Such a structure, where the polar heads, but not the hydrophobic tails, are in contact with the surrounding aqueous environments, is thermodynamically stable and has the tendency to reform spontaneously if it is perturbed.

Cholesterol

Cholesterol molecules insert themselves between, and parallel to, membrane phospholipids. They orient themselves in such a way that their polar hydroxyl

Figure 5.3   Membrane lipids: structural characteristics of phospholipids (a) and cholesterol (b) Schematic representation of a cholesterol molecule inserted between two phospholipid molecules in the membrane (c) The table illustrates the polar heads (H) and the most common bonds (B). PC, phosphatidylcholine; PE, phosphatidylethanolamine; PG, phosphatidylglycerol; PI, PIP or PIP$_2$, phosphatidylinositol, phosphatidylinositol phosphate or phosphatidylinositol biphosphate; PS, phosphatidylserine. (a: From Béréziat G, Chambaz J, Colard O and Wolf C, 1988. The various functions of cellular phospholipids, *Med. Sci.*; **1**, 8–15, with permission). b, c: From Alberts B, Bray D, Lewis J, Raff M, Roberts K and Watson JD, 1986. *Biologie moléculaire de la Cellule*, p. 259: Flammation Médecine-Science, Paris, with permission.)

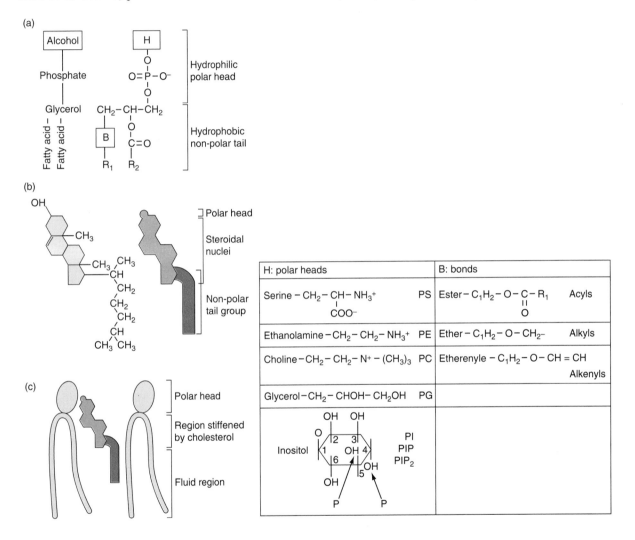

group is close to the phospholipid polar groups (Figure 5.3b, c). Cholesterol represents approximately 10% of the plasma membrane lipids. This molecule plays an important role in determining the fluidity of the membrane. It consists of a flat and rigid portion made of steroid nuclei (Figure 5.3b), renders the plasma membrane less fluid and, consequently, ensures a certain mechanical stability.

Glycolipids

Glycolipids are molecules whose polar head group comprises one or several sugar residues and whose hydrophobic portion is made of ceramide. The most common glycolipids in the neuronal plasma membrane are cerebrosides and gangliosides (Figure 5.4). The latter are characterized by the presence of one or several sialic acid residues (*N*-acetyl neuraminic acid or NANA) in their polar head group. This confers the gangliosides with a net negative charge. Glycolipids appear to be localized exclusively in the external sheath of the membrane with their sugar residues oriented towards the extracellular environment. This suggests that they may play a role in the process of intercellular communication and recognition.

5.2.2 The Lipid Bilayer is Asymmetric and Fluid

The lipid bilayer is asymmetric: the preferential localization of certain lipids in one of the two sheaths of the bilayer provides it with an asymmetry of both

Figure 5.4 Glycolipids. (left) A cerebroside, galactocerebroside; (right) a ganglioside, GM_1. Gangliosides contain in their polar group one or more residues of *N*-acetyl neuraminic acid (NANA). They are called GM_1 when they contain one, GM_2 when they contain two and GM_3 when they contain three NANA residues. (Lower right) Symbolic representation of glycolipids. Glu, glucose; Gal, galactose; Gal/NAc, *N*-acetylgalactosamine.

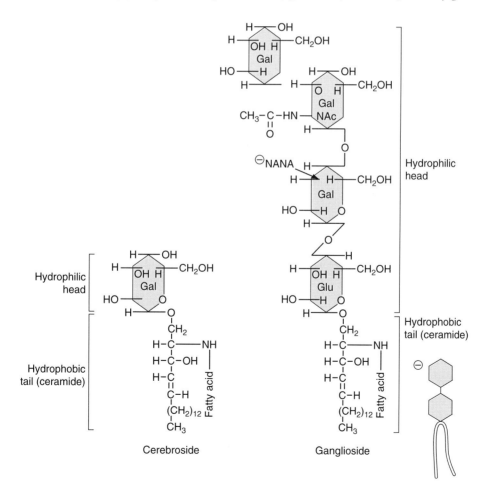

Figure 5.5   Voltage sensitive channels. (a) This channel opens as a result of changes in transmembrane potential (ΔV). (b) Model of the transmembrane organization of a voltage dependent Na^+ channel. This model has been developed from a hydrophobicity profile of the protein (see Appendix 5.2). The channel is made up of only one subunit. (Left) Linear representation of the subunit in the lipid bilayer. (Right) Representation of the subunit as it would be seen from the top of the membrane. One can distinguish four homologous domains (labeled I to IV) each one containing six transmembrane α-helices (labeled 1 to 6). The model assumes that the four domains are arranged symmetrically around a central aqueous pore. From Salkoff L, Butter A, Wei A, *et al*, 1987. Molecular biology of the voltage-gated sodium channel, *TINS* **10**, 522–527, with permission.)

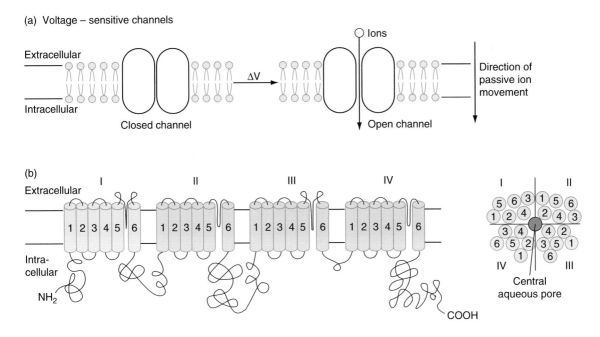

5.2.3 The Lipid Bilayer is a Barrier for the Diffusion of Ions and Most Polar Molecules

Owing to its central hydrophobic region, the lipid bilayer has a low permeability to hydrophilic substances such as ions, water and polar molecules (Appendix 5.1). Therefore, ions can only cross the membrane *passively* through specialized transport molecules known as channel proteins. Likewise, they only cross the membrane *actively* through specialized proteins known as pumps or transporters. This passage of ions through the membrane is then regulated and the flow of ions is not a simple and anarchic diffusion through the lipid bilayer. Instead, it is restricted to proteins whose opening (channel proteins) or activation (pumps or transporters) is tightly controlled by different factors.

structure and function. Thus, for example, phosphatidylinositol biphosphate is localized preferentially in the internal sheath while glycolipids are localized in the external sheath of the membrane.

The lipidic phase of the membrane is fluid. It means that phospholipids are mobile and can move laterally (lateral diffusion) or rotate (rotational diffusion). This fluidity, which depends on temperature and on cholesterol content, allows proteins to move laterally within the membrane (lateral diffusion) or new proteins to enter a given area as a result of the fusion of two membranes. This represents the basic mechanism for the continued renewal of membrane content.

5.3 Proteins Are Responsible for Most of the Functions of the Plasma Membrane

While the lipid bilayer represents a diffusion barrier and separates the intracellular and extracellular compartments, proteins ensure all the dynamic functions

Figure 5.6   Receptor channels. (a) Ligand dependent channels open when a ligand is bound to the receptor site or sites located on the extracellular domain of the protein. A neurotransmitter is an example of such a ligand. (b) Model of the transmembrane organization of receptor channels: example of the nicotinic acetylcholine receptor (nAChR). This receptor is made up of two α, one β, one γ, and one δ subunit, all of which present sequence homologies and a similar transmembrane organization. The α subunit is illustrated here in a linear representation in the membrane. This model has been developed from hydrophobicity profiles of the protein subunit (Appendix 5.2). Both acetylcholine receptor sites are located in the extracellular domains of each α subunit. All five subunits are assembled into an $\alpha_2\beta\gamma\delta$ pentamer which forms a rosette and delimits a central aqueous pore (see also Chapter 9).

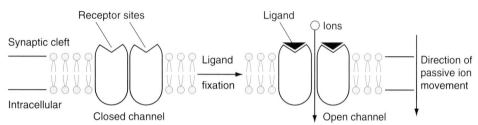

(a) Channel receptors

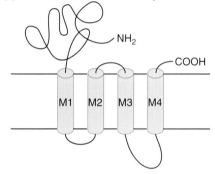

(b) Structure of the nicotinic acetylcholine receptor α subunit

of the membrane (permeability, enzymatic functions, etc.). Among these proteins we shall study those that participate in the transport of ions across the membrane. They are the basis of the electrical properties of a neuron.

5.3.1 Transmembrane and Peripheral Membrane Proteins

Transmembrane proteins

These proteins span the entire width of the lipid bilayer (see Figure 5.1). They have hydrophobic regions containing a high fraction of non-polar amino acids and hydrophilic regions containing a high frac-

tion of polar amino acids (Appendix 5.2). Certain hydrophobic regions organize themselves inside the bilayer as transmembrane α-helices while more hydrophilic regions are in contact with the aqueous intracellular and extracellular environments. In the following paragraphs we shall analyze two examples of this type of protein: channel proteins and G-protein coupled receptors (Figures 5.5–5.7).

Interaction energies are very high between hydrophobic regions of the protein and hydrophobic regions of the lipid bilayer, as well as between hydrophilic regions of the protein and the extracellular and intracellular environments. These interactions strongly stabilize transmembrane proteins within the bilayer, thus preventing their extracellular and cytoplasmic regions from flipping back and forth.

Figure 5.7 G-protein coupled receptors (neurotransmitter and sensory receptors). (a) When a ligand or a sensory signal activate the receptor (R*), the receptor activates in turn several G-proteins (G*) which then modify directly or indirectly --->) the ionic channel properties. (b) Model of the receptor transmembrane organization: example of rhodopsin. The ligand receptor site would be located in the central region of the protein. (b, left: From Peralta EG, Winslow JW, Peterson GL *et al*, 1987. Primary structure and biochemical properties of an M_2 muscarinic receptor, *Science*, **236**, 600–650, with permission. b, right: From Dratz EA and Hargrave PA, 1983. The structure of rhodopsin and the rod outer segment disk membrane, *Trends Biochem. Sci.*, **8**, 128–131, with permission.)

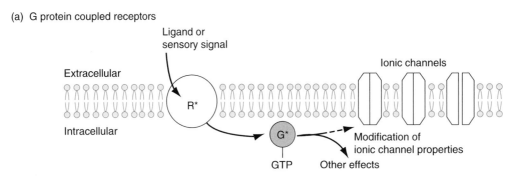

(a) G protein coupled receptors

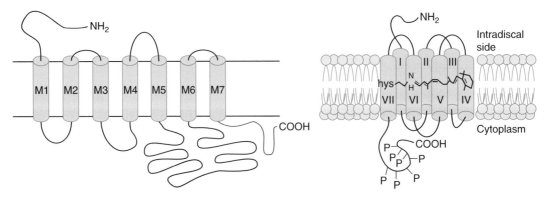

(b) Ex: the light sensitive pigment: rhodopsin

Peripheral proteins

Peripheral proteins are those proteins present on the cytoplasmic or extracellular side of the membrane which do not span the lipid bilayer (see Figure 5.1). They are either 'attached' to the membrane or anchored to it. Proteins that are *attached* to the membrane probably interact with polar regions of transmembrane proteins through ionic interactions. We call them 'attached' because they can be solubilized without detergents. This is the case, for example, of G-proteins (Figure 5.7). Peripheral proteins *anchored* to the membrane contain in their structure a lipid chain that is covalently bound to one of their amino acids. Those proteins that anchor themselves to the cytoplasmic side do so through a myristic acid bound to a glycine residue or through palmitic acid bound to a cysteine residue. This is the case, for example, of the catalytic subunit of protein kinase A. Other proteins are anchored to the extracellular side, in this case through a complex glycosylated phospholipid or through a hydrophobic peptide. An example of the former case is acetylcholinesterase (AChE) the enzyme that hydrolyses acetylcholine (see Figure 2.10b), whereas an example of the latter case is aminopeptidases.

5.3.2 Proteins That Allow or Modulate the Transport of Ions Across the Membrane

Proteins that play a role in the transport of ions belong to two broad categories: those that participate in the *passive* transport of ions (Table 5.1) and those that participate in the *active* transport of ions. Proteins that *participate in* the passive transport of ions are ionic channels. Proteins *that modulate* the passive transport of ions are G-protein-coupled receptors (Table 5.1)

Ionic channels have a three-dimensional structure that delimits an aqueous pore through which certain ions can pass. They provide the ions with a passage through the membrane, and are called ionic channels (Table 5.2). These proteins exist in different states: closed and open. Their opening (the switch from the closed to the open state) is tightly controlled, for example, by: (i) a change in the membrane potential: voltage sensitive channels (see Section 5.4.1); (ii) by the binding of an extracellular ligand, e.g. a neurotransmitter: receptor channels or ionotropic receptors (see Section 5.4.2); or (iii) by the binding of intracellular Ca^{2+}.

Table 5.1 Examples of proteins controlling passive ion transport (ionotropic and metabotropic receptors)

Protein type	Activated by	Examples
Ionic channels		
Voltage sensitive channels	Membrane depolarization	Na^+ channel of action potential K^+ channel of action potential Ca^{2+} channels type L, N, P and T
	Membrane hyperpolarization	K^+ channel of I_f current Cationic channel of I_Q current
Ca^{2+} sensitive channels	Intracellular Ca^{2+} ions (and/or not depolarization)	Ca^{2+} dependent K^+ channels Ca^{2+} dependent cationic channels Ca^{2+} dependent Cl^- channels
Receptor channels or ionotropic receptors	Neurotransmitters: acetylcholine glutamate GABA Glycine	nAChR (permeable to cations) GluR: NMDA and non-NMDA channels (permeable to cations) $GABA_A$ (permeable to Cl^-) GlyR (permeable to Cl^-)
Mechanoreceptors	Sensory stimulus: pressure, stretch movement of stereociliae	Receptors located in Pacini corpuscle (permeable to cations) or in Auditory and vestibular ciliated cells (permeable to cations)
G-protein coupled receptor or metabotropic receptors	Neurotransmitters: ACh glutamate GABA adrenalin	mAChR mGluR $GABA_B$ αAd and βAd
	Sensory stimulus: light	Rhodopsin modulates a nucleotide-activated cation channel via a G_T protein and cGMP
	olfactory molecules	Odorant receptor modulates a nucleotide-activated cation channel via a G_s protein and cAMP

NMDA, *N*-methyl-D-aspartate; nAChR, nicotinic acetylcholine receptor (ionotropic receptor); mAChR, muscarinic acetylcholine receptor (metabotropic receptor); $GABA_A$, γ-aminobutyric acid receptor type A (ionotropic receptor); $GABA_B$, γ-aminobutyric acid receptor type B (metabotropic receptor); mGluR, metabotropic glutamatergic receptors; αAd and βAd, α and β adrenoceptors (metabotropic receptors). I_f K^t inward retifyer; I_Q, cationic inward rectifyer; G_T, tranuducin; G_s, G protein type S.

Table 5.2   Examples of ionic channels

Channels	Voltage-gated	Ligand-gated			Stretch activated
Open by	Depolarization caused by synaptic or pacemaker current	Extracellular ligand	Intracellular ligand		Stretch
Membrane	Plasma	Plasma	Plasma	Organelle	Plasma
Examples	Na$^+$ channel Ca^{2+} channels K$^+$ channels	nAChR iGluR 5-HT$_3$ GABA$_A$ GlyR	G-protein gated Ca^{2+} gated cAMP gated cGMP gated IP$_3$ gated	IP$_3$ gated Ca^{2+} gated	Cationic (mechano-receptors)
Roles	action potentials ↑[Ca^{2+}]$_i$	EPSP IPSP ↑[Ca^{2+}]$_i$	EPSP IPSP ↑[Ca^{2+}]$_i$	↑[Ca^{2+}]$_i$	Transduce stretch into depolarization
Closed by	Inactivation Repolarization	Desensitization Ligand recapture or degradation			

EPSP, excitatory post-synaptic potential; IPSP, inhibitory post-synaptic potential; iAChR, nGluR, 5-HT$_3$, cationic channels; GABA$_A$, GlyR, anionic channels (Cl$^-$); G-protein gated, Ca^{2+} or K$^+$ channels; Ca^{2+} gated, K$^+$, Cl$^-$ or Ca^{2+} channels; ATP gated, K$^+$ channel; cAMP gated and cGMP gated, cationic channels; IP$_3$ gated: Ca^{2+} channel.

G-protein-coupled receptor proteins have a structure that does not encompass an aqueous pore. Their role is to modulate the opening of totally separate ionic channels in response to the binding of an extracellular ligand (e.g. neurotransmitters, photons, olfactory molecules). The receptor (activated by its ligand) is coupled to its effectors via a GTP-binding protein (and therefore called G-protein, see Section 5.4.2). G-proteins couple this type of receptor to various effectors: ionic channels, enzymes that produce second messengers. They are also called metabotropic receptors (Table 5.1).

Proteins participating in the active transport of ions: pumps and transporters

These proteins require energy to operate. Pumps obtain energy from the hydrolysis of ATP, whereas transporters use the energy of an ionic gradient, for example, the sodium driving force (see Section 5.5).

In the following section we shall present the characteristics of these different proteins according to their function in the neuronal membrane.

5.4 Proteins That Carry or Modulate Ion Passage Through the Membrane Underlie the Electric Properties of Neurons

5.4.1 Depolarization-Activated Membrane Channels Determine the Excitability Properties of Neurons (Table 5.2)

Channels opened by voltage changes are transmembrane proteins. They have a three-dimensional structure which contains an aqueous pore and a voltage 'sensitive' region. Depending on the membrane potential these channels may be in an open state (ions can pass through the aqueous pore) or in a closed state (ions cannot pass through the aqueous pore). Conformational changes (switch from one state to the other) depend on membrane potential changes. Most of these channels open transiently in response to membrane depolarization (Figure 5.5a).

The aqueous pore of voltage sensitive channels is essentially permeable to one ionic species. Such is the case of voltage dependent Na$^+$ channels, voltage dependent K$^+$ channels and voltage dependent Ca^{2+} channels (Tables 5.1 and 5.2). The voltage sensitive Na$^+$ channel is responsible for the initial inward current of Na$^+$ ions during the depolarizing phase of action potentials. It thus underlies the generation and propagation of action potentials (Chapter 7). The multiple types of voltage sensitive Ca^{2+} channels control the entry of Ca^{2+} ions into the cell. These ions then participate in membrane potential depolarization and in the regulation of several intracellular processes including the release of neurotransmitters from presynaptic terminals (Chapter 8). The multiple types of voltage sensitive K^+ channels do not have a single function that can be assigned to them as a group. In general, they participate in action potential repolarization or in the duration of the interval between two consecutive action potentials (Chapters 7 and 17).

The voltage dependent Na^+ channel consists of a single protein subunit (α subunit) which contains four structurally homologous domains (denoted I to IV) each one approximately 300 amino acids long and containing six putative membrane-spanning α-helical regions. These four domains are said to be homologous because they share a high percentage of identical amino acid residues. They are separated from each other by non-homologous regions of variable lengths. The α subunit comprises the pore of the ion channel which is believed to be formed by the four homologous domains organized in a rosette (Figures 5.5b and A5.1). This structure is similar to the predicted structure of voltage dependent Ca^{2+} channels and the functional tetrameric form of K^+ channels.

5.4.2 Neurotransmitter Receptors (Receptor Channels and G-protein-Coupled Receptors) are the Basis of Synaptic Transmission and its Modulation (Table 5.1)

Receptor channels are channels that open as a result of the binding of an extracellular ligand (e.g. a neurotransmitter). Their common characteristic is that the receptor sites for the ligand and the ionic channel that they control are part of the *same protein*. Receptor channels are made up of several subunits (linked together by non-covalent bonds) which form the central aqueous pore. In general, the receptor sites of the neurotransmitter are present in the extracellular domains of two identical subunits. When the neurotransmitter binds to its receptor sites, the receptor channel changes conformation and transiently switches to a state in which the aqueous pore is open (Figure 5.6a). Thus, receptor channels ensure fast

synaptic transmission by triggering a rapid increase of ionic permeability in response to the binding of a neurotransmitter. It should be noted that these channels may also present receptor sites for other endogenous molecules such as allosteric agonists which modulate their activity.

The best-known members of this group open in response to neurotransmitters (Tables 5.1 and 5.2): acetylcholine (nicotinic receptors), γ-aminobutyric acid ($GABA_A$ receptors) and glutamate (NMDA and non-NMDA receptors). Nicotinic receptors (nAChR, Chapter 9) and glutamate receptor channels (Chapter 11) are permeable to cations (Na^+, K^+ and Ca^{2+}). Conversely, $GABA_A$ receptors (Chapter 10) are mainly permeable to Cl^- ions.

The primary structures of the nAChR, $GABA_A$ and glutamate receptor channels show many similarities (Figures 5.6b and A5.2). The nAChR, for example, is a pentamer of stoichiometry $\alpha_2\beta\gamma\delta$. Its different subunits show very high levels of sequence and hydrophobicity profile homologies. The neurotransmitter receptor sites have been localized in the large extracellular domain of two identical subunits (the two α subunits of the nAChR receptor and the two β subunits of the $GABA_A$ receptor). On the other hand, the ionic walls of the channel are assumed to be formed by the same putative transmembrane segment (M2 segment) of each subunit.

G-protein-coupled neurotransmitter receptors modulate the properties of different ionic channels in response to the binding of a neurotransmitter (Table 5.1). These receptors are entirely separate from the ionic channels that they modulate, and exert their influence through a peripheral protein located on the cytoplasmic side of the membrane. This peripheral protein is capable of binding GTP and is thus called G-protein (Figure 5.7a).

An activated G-protein-coupled receptor (bound to a neurotransmitter) can in turn activate several G-proteins because of the fluidity of the membrane. These directly (or indirectly via a second messenger) modulate the opening of ionic channels and the metabolic activity of the neuron (see Chapters 13–15). Thus, G-proteins convert and amplify the signal corresponding to the binding of neurotransmitter to the receptor. Examples of such receptors are the muscarinic acetylcholine receptors (mAChR), the metabotropic glutamate receptors (mGluR) and the α- and β- adrenergic receptors (αAd and βAd).

Primary structures of muscarinic, metabotropic glutamate and β-adrenergic receptors, for example, show great similarities (see Section 5.4.3 and Figures 5.7b and A5.3). These receptors are formed by a single subunit presenting seven hydrophobic segments and a large cytoplasmic hydrophilic domain. The seven segments are believed to form seven transmembrane α-helices, while the hydrophilic cytoplasmic domain is believed to contain phosphorylation sites that regulate receptor activation.

5.4.3 Certain Sensory Receptors are Ionic Channels Directly Opened by Sensory Stimuli: Others are G-protein-Coupled Receptors (Tables 5.1 and 5.2)

Sensory receptors underlying the transduction of pressure, stretching, taste, auditory and vestibular stimuli are ionic channels directly opened by the corresponding sensory stimulus. Consequently, transduction in these cases is very rapid. On the other hand, the sensory receptors coupled to G-proteins are found, for instance, in photoreceptor membranes (rods and cones of the retina) and in membranes of olfactory epithelium cells where they transduce visual and olfactory stimuli, respectively.

We shall take rhodopsin as an example of a G-protein-coupled sensory receptor. This light-sensitive pigment (or light receptor) located in the rod membranes of the retina has a very similar structure to that of other G-protein-coupled receptors such as the muscarinic acetylcholine receptors (Figures 5.7 and A5.3).

5.4.4 Other Ionic Channels of the Neuronal Plasma Membrane

Channels sensitive to intracellular Ca^{2+}

K^+, Cl^- and cation permeable channels belong to this class of channels. An intracellular increase in Ca^{2+} concentration favors the probability of Ca^{2+} binding to Ca^{2+} receptor site(s) located on the cytoplasmic side of these channels. This in turn triggers the opening of channels and the passage of ions through them. Some of these channels are also voltage dependent (see Chapter 7).

Junctional channels or gap junctions

These channels are different from all the channels mentioned so far because they are built with transmembrane proteins from two apposed plasma membranes (Figure 5.8a). At the point of apposition the extracellular space is very narrow. These structures are called gap junctions because they connect the cytoplasms of two adjacent cells. These are poorly selective channels but are more permeable to cations than to anions. They are also permeable to small molecules, i.e. molecules with molecular weights lower than 1200 D.

Junctional channels have a hexameric structure with a central aqueous pore 15 nm long, 2 nm wide at the ends and approximately 1.5 nm wide at its center. Each hexamer belongs to the membrane of one of the coupled cells and constitutes a connexon formed by six connexins. A junctional channel is formed by the apposition of two connexons and its axis is perpendicular to the plane of the plasma membranes. Genes coding for connexins were first sequenced from rat and human heart and liver cells and the amino acid sequences deduced. Hydrophobicity profiles and specific antibody binding to certain regions of the protein have led to a transmembrane model of the connexins. Each connexin has four putative transmembrane α-helices and both NH_2 and COOH terminals are oriented to the cytoplasmic side, accessible to intracellular regulatory elements (Figure 5.8b).

Junctional channels are usually open at the resting membrane potential. Their opening can be modulated by either the transjunctional potential (the voltage difference between the two internal sides of the coupled membranes), by intracellular or extracellular factors or by second messengers. Thus, depending on the cell type they may open or close as a function of membrane potential, intracellular pH, intracellular concentration of Ca^{2+} ions and the presence of cyclic nucleotides.

There is a high density of gap junctions at electrical synapses. The function of these gap junctions is electrical and metabolic coupling as well as transfer of second messengers between the associated cells. Electrical coupling allows the rapid propagation of action

Figure 5.8 Junction channels. (a) These channels allow ions and molecules of low molecular weight (less than 1200 D) to cross them. The flow is generally bidirectional. The opening of these channels is regulated, among other factors, by intracellular Ca^{2+} ions and pH. (b) Diagram of the structure of gap junctions in a lipid bilayer. These junctions are made up of 12 connexins molecules organized into two hexamers, called connexons. Each connexon has two domains, a transmembrane and a cytoplasmic domain. The aqueous pore situated at the center of the connexon spans both plasma membranes. (From Makowski L, Caspar DLD, Phillips WC, Baker TS and Goodenough DA, 1984. Gap junction structures. VI. Variation and conservation in connexon conformation and packing, *Biophys. J.*, **45**, 208–218, with permission.)

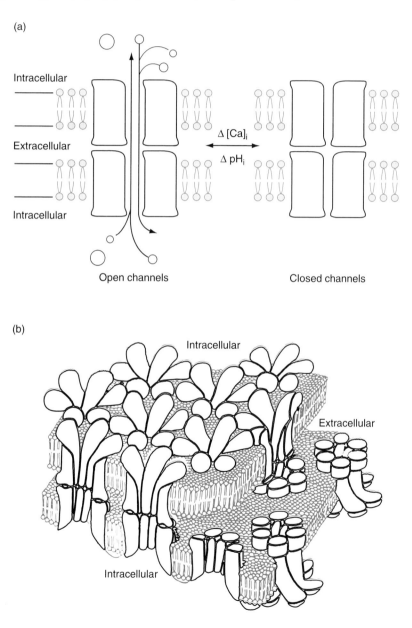

potentials between neurons. This would give synchrony among a population of active neurons for the purpose of escape behaviors, for example (electrical coupling of crayfish cord neurons). In the heart the primary function of gap junctions is to allow current flow from the pacemaker cells to ventricular muscle cells leading to their synchronized rhythmic contraction. Metabolic coupling is particularly important in the case of non-vascularized cells such as those of the eye lens. The exchange of second messengers (cyclic AMP, cyclic GMP, inositol triphosphate, Ca^{2+}, etc.) allows the transfer of information between coupled cells.

5.5 Pumps Are Proteins That Actively Transport Ions to Maintain Ionic Concentration Differences Between the Intracellular and Extracellular Environments: These Transmembrane Ion Gradients Provide the Energy for Other Active Transports

In order to keep intracellular and extracellular ionic concentrations constant, certain proteins actively transport ions against their electrochemical gradients. Active transport requires energy in order to oppose the electrochemical potential gradient of the transported ions (see Chapter 6).

5.5.1 Ionic Pumps are Ion Transport Proteins That Use the Energy Obtained From the Hydrolysis of ATP

Pumps have ATPase activity (they hydrolyze ATP). This ATPase activity is generally the easiest way of identifying them. Pumps are membrane-embedded enzymes that couple the hydrolysis of ATP to active translocation of ions across the membrane. The central issue of ion motive ATPases is to couple the hydrolysis of ATP (and their auto-phosphorylation) to the translocation of ions.

The Na/K/ATPase pump

Na/K/ATPases maintain the unequal distribution of Na^+ and K^+ ions across the membrane (Figures 5.2).

Na^+ and K^+ ions cross the membrane through different Na^+ and K^+ permeable channels (voltage sensitive Na^+ and K^+ channels plus receptor channels). This pump operates continuously at a rhythm of 10^2 ions s^{-1} (compared with 10^6 ions for a channel), adjusting its activity to the electrical activity of the neuron. It actively transports 3 Na^+ ions towards the extracellular space for each 2 K^+ ions that it carries into the cell. It catalyses the following reaction:

$$3\,Na^+_i + 2\,K^+_o + Mg^-ATP + H_2O \quad \rightleftharpoons$$

$$3\,Na^+_o + 2\,K^+_i + ADP + \text{inorganic P} + Mg^{2+}$$

The energy of ATP hydrolysis is needed for the conformational changes that allow the pump to change its affinity for the ion transported whether the binding sites are accessible from the cytoplasmic or the extracellular sides. For example, when the Na^+ binding sites are accessible from the cytoplasm, the protein is in a conformation with a high affinity for Na^+ ions and thus 3 Na^+ bind to their sites. On the contrary, when the 3 Na^+ have been translocated to the extracellular side, the protein is in a conformation with a low affinity for Na^+ ions so that the 3 Na^+ are released in the extracellular space. These conformational changes are energy dependent. The Na/K/ATPase has a catalytic α-subunit comprising about 1000 amino acids with a molecular weight of approximately 100 kD. A second β-subunit, whose function is unknown, is closely associated with it.

The steady unequal distribution of Na^+ and K^+ ions constitutes a reserve of energy for a cell. The neuron uses this energy to produce electric signals (action potentials, synaptic potentials) as well as to actively transport other molecules (see Section 5.5.2).

The Ca/ATPase pump

The function of Ca/ATPases is to maintain the intracellular Ca^{2+} concentration at very low levels. In fact, the intracellular Ca^{2+} concentration is 10 000 times lower than the extracellular concentration despite the inflow of Ca^{2+} (through receptor channels and voltage sensitive Ca^{2+} channels) and the intracellular release of Ca^{2+} from intracellular stores. This unequal distribution of Ca^{2+} ions is maintained in part by the operation of Ca/ATPases, which remove intracellular

Figure 5.9 Comparison of the structures of proteins involved in neuronal functions. Schematic diagrams showing the transmembrane putative topology of the entire proteins (Na$^+$ and Ca^{2+} channels, G-protein coupled receptors, neurotransmitter transporters) and of a subunit of the proteins (K$^+$ channels, neurotransmitter-gated channels). (From Jessel TM and Kandel ER, 1993. Synaptic transmission: a bidirectional and self-modifiable form of cell–cell communication, *Cell* **72**/*Neuron* **10**, 1–30, with permission.)

Na$^+$ channel

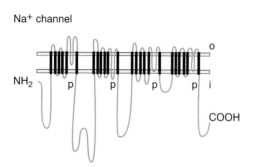

Transmitter-gated channel subunit

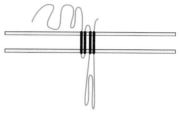

Ca^{2+} channel

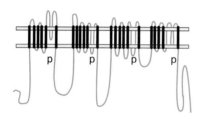

G – protein-coupled receptor

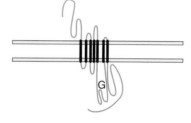

K$^+$ channel subunit

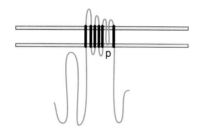

Neurotransmitter uptake carrier

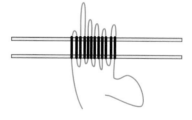

Synaptic vesicle transporter

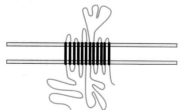
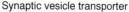

Ca^{2+} ions by active transport (see also Section 5.5.2). Maintaining a low intracellular Ca^{2+} concentration is critical since Ca^{2+} ions control several intracellular reactions and are toxic at a high concentration.

Ca/ATPases have been isolated from the sarcoplasmic reticulum of rabbit muscle cells. They have only one subunit, called α, which presents a transmembrane organization similar to that of the α subunit of the Na/K/ATPase. There are several sequence homologies between these two subunits. Most homologous regions are located in the large cytoplasmic domain implicated in ATP recognition and hydrolysis.

5.5.2 Transporters Are Proteins That Use the Energy Stored in the Transmembrane Electrochemical Gradient of Na$^+$ or H$^+$ to Drive the Active Transport of Ions or Molecules

When transporters carry Na$^+$ or H$^+$ ions (along their electrochemical gradient) in the same direction as the transported ion or molecule (against its electrochemical gradient), the process is called symport. When the movements occur in opposite directions the process is called antiport. We shall only study transporters implicated in the electrical or secretory activity of neurons.

Na/neurotransmitter co-transporters (Figure 5.9)

Inactivation of most neurotransmitters present in the synaptic cleft is achieved by rapid reuptake into the pre-synaptic neural element and astrocytic glial cells. This is performed by specific neurotransmitter transporters, transmembrane proteins that couple neurotransmitter transport to the movement of Na$^+$ down its concentration gradient (maintained by the activity of the Na/K/ATPase). Certain neurotransmitter precursors are also taken up by this type of active transport (glutamine and choline, for instance). Once in the cytoplasm, neurotransmitters are concentrated inside synaptic vesicles by distinct transport systems driven by the H$^+$ concentration gradient (maintained by the vesicular H$^+$/ATPase).

The Na/Ca exchanger

This transporter uses the energy of the Na$^+$ gradient to actively carry Ca^{2+} ions towards the extracellular environment. It is situated in the neuronal plasma membrane and operates in synergy with the Ca/ATPase and with transport mechanisms of the smooth sarcoplasmic reticulum to maintain the intracellular Ca^{2+} concentration at a very low level.

5.6 Distribution of Different Ionic Channels in the Neuronal Plasma Membrane (Figure 5.10)

Voltage sensitive channels

Voltage sensitive Na$^+$ channels underlie the generation and propagation of sodium and sodium–calcium action potentials. They are localized at high densities at the initial segment and nodes of Ranvier of the axon (in the case of myelinated axons) or all along the axon (in the case of non-myelinated axons). Na$^+$ channels are also found in the membrane of the cell body, but they are generally absent or present at a very low density in dendritic membranes. In fact, dendrites rarely generate or propagate sodium action potentials. The distribution of voltage dependent K$^+$ channels will not be analyzed here because of the large diversity of these channels.

Voltage dependent Ca^{2+} channels are located at high density at pre-synaptic terminals: axon terminal membranes, pre-synaptic dendrites or somatic pre-synaptic regions where they ensure the Ca^{2+} inflow essential for the release of neurotransmitters. They can also be present in the dendritic or somatic membranes where they are the basis of the generation and propagation of calcium (dendrites) or sodium–calcium (soma) action potentials.

Neurotransmitter receptors

Neurotransmitter receptors are localized at post-synaptic regions: post-synaptic membrane of the dendritic spines, the dendritic branches, the soma or the axon (the latter in the case of axo-axonic synapses). They underlie synaptic transmission. They can also be

Figure 5.10   Ionic channel localization in the neuronal plasma membrane. The diagram illustrates a moto-neuron innervating a striated muscle cell (nicotinic cholinergic post-synaptic receptor) and receiving excitatory (glutamate) and inhibitory (GABAergic) afferences originating in local circuit neurons from the spinal cord. General localization of voltage dependent Na^+ and Ca^{2+} channels (Vdep channels) and receptor channels (nAChR, Glu and $GABA_A$ receptors). Voltage sensitive K^+ channels and $GABA_B$ channels have been omitted. One channel symbolizes a population of channels of the illustrated type. nAChR, nicotinic acetylcholine receptor; $GABA_A$, type A GABA receptor; Glu, glutamate.

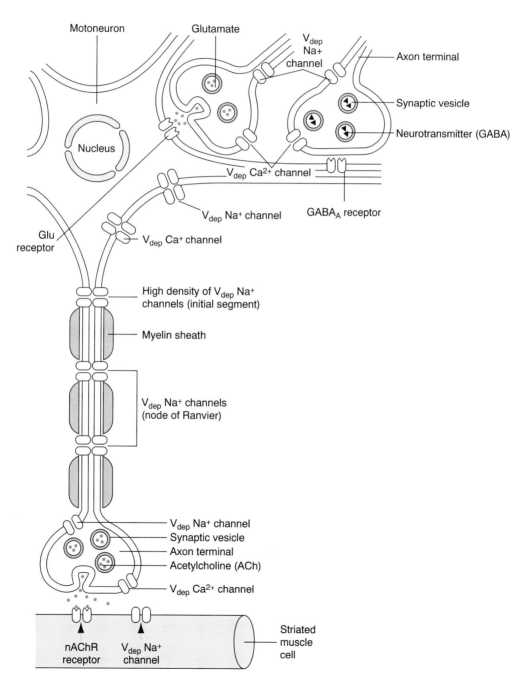

found in pre-synaptic regions where they play a role in the control of neurotransmitter release.

Sensory receptors

They are localized exclusively in membranes of sensory receptor cells where they underlie sensory signal transduction.

5.7 Processes of Exocytosis and Endocytosis at Pre-synaptic Active Zones

5.7.1 Exocytosis of Synaptic Vesicles is Responsible for Neurotransmitter Release into the Synaptic Cleft

Neurotransmitter secretion from pre-synaptic elements into the synaptic cleft takes place by exocytosis of synaptic vesicles. Exocytosis is the process by which vesicles containing the secretion product (synaptic vesicles) fuse with the plasma membrane (pre-synaptic membrane) in response to a triggering signal (the inflow of Ca^{2+} into the pre-synaptic element). Their content is thus released into the extracellular space (synaptic cleft). Once the membranes have fused, they become continuous in such a way that the internal side of the vesicular membrane faces the extracellular space (Figure 5.11a).

Membrane fusion takes place in several phases (Figure 5.11a):

- First, synaptic vesicles are docked at the plasma membrane (targeting and docking). This seems to be the result of the particular organization of the cytoskeleton at this region.
- A stable adhesion of the two membranes then occurs. This attraction between the lipid bilayers is mediated by Van Der Waals forces.
- Finally, water molecules bound to polar groups of the membranes have to be removed to enable the close contact and fusion of the membranes. This requires energy, because phospholipid polar heads are extremely hydrated. This energy requirement explains why vesicles rarely fuse with the plasma membrane without a triggering signal.

The mechanisms underlying the process of vesicular exocytosis are not well understood. Two hypotheses have been suggested. One of them proposes that osmotic pressure would cause vesicles to swell, thus exposing the hydrophobic fatty acid chains and favoring membrane fusion. The second hypothesis proposes that, prior to vesicle swelling, a pore traverses both apposed membranes constituting the first connection between the extracellular and the intravesicular environment (Figure $5.11a_3$). This pore could later either dilate to allow the release of the vesicular content or close again. This hypothesis is based on studies of mastocytes, cells that enclose large secretory granules. A protein, synaptophysine, present in the vesicular membrane could participate in the formation of the putative pore. In fact, its transmembrane organization shows homologies with the connexon of gap junctions (compare Figures 5.8 and 8.10). According to this hypothesis, the junction of two proteins of this type, one in the vesicular membrane and the other in the plasma membrane, would form the transmembrane pore.

5.7.2 Pre-synaptic Membrane Endocytosis Allows the Recycling of Vesicular Membranes

Endocytosis is the process by which the plasma membrane invaginates and then closes on itself to form a cytoplasmic vesicle. In this process some extracellular fluid is trapped inside the vesicle (Figure 5.11b). This has been shown by adding a marker such as horseradish peroxidase to the extracellular environment. In this way the process can be demonstrated and quantified (the product of the reaction between peroxidase and its substrate becomes electron dense after fixation with osmium tetroxide).

The endocytotic vesicles are frequently covered by a fuzzy substance that appears under the electron microscope as an ensemble of fibrous structures on their cytoplasmic surface (see Figure 2.4). This coating comprises a fibrous protein called clathrine (molecular weight 18 kD) which is associated with a smaller polypeptide. This results in vesicles covered by a characteristic polyedric envelope: the coated vesicles.

Figure 5.11   Synaptic vesicle exocytosis and endocytosis. (a) Exocytosis. Vesicular and plasma membranes first appose tightly to each other (bilayer adhesion, a_1) giving a temporary five-layered image. The dense central line corresponds to the apposition of the vesicular external sheath and plasma internal sheath (a_2). Later the bilayers reorganize and fuse forming a continuous membrane and the vesicle opens towards the extracellular space. a_3, Schematic representation of the formation of a transmembrane pore during exocytosis. (b) Endocytosis. In this case one observes two regions of the external sheath of the membrane approaching each other and sticking together. (a_1, a_2 and b: From B. Alberts *et al.*, 1986, *Biologie Moléculaire de la Cellule*, Flammarion Médecine-Science, Paris, with permission. a_3: From Lindstedt AD and Kelly RB, 1987. Overcoming barriers to exocytosis, *TINS* **10**, 446–448, with permission.)

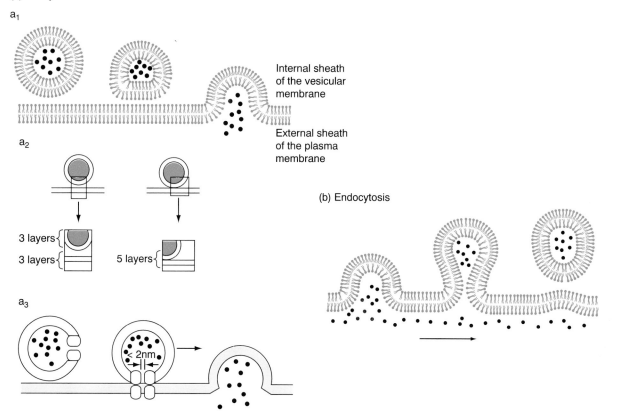

(a) Exocytosis

a_1

Internal sheath
of the vesicular
membrane

External sheath
of the plasma
membrane

a_2

3 layers
3 layers

5 layers

a_3

< 2nm

(b) Endocytosis

Appendix 5.1
Influence of Water on the Behavior of Biological Molecules

A5.1.1 Water is a Polar Molecule

The total charge of a water molecule (H_2O) is zero (because it has the same number of protons and electrons). However, its electrons are distributed unevenly between the oxygen atom and the two hydrogen atoms. Oxygen and hydrogen atoms carry partial charges denoted δ^- or δ^+. The orbitals of the unbound electrons of the oxygen are therefore oriented in specific directions in space. The oxygen atom has four external electronic orbitals which are oriented towards the vertices of a tetrahedron centered on the atom. Each orbital contains two electrons. The electrons of two of those orbitals are paired with two hydrogen atoms and the other two contain the remaining two electron pairs. Since the two hydrogen atoms are both located on the same side of the oxygen atom, a partially positive charge is localized on that side of the water molecule, whereas the other side has a partially negative charge. Thus, a water molecule can be compared to an electrical dipole. Water is a polar molecule.

The oxygen atom (charge δ^-) of a water molecule is pulled by the hydrogen atoms (charged δ^+) of a neighboring water molecule. This creates bonds between the oxygen atom of one water molecule and the hydrogen atoms of neighboring water molecules, called hydrogen bonds. These bonds can also be formed with other molecules, such as proteins, nucleic acids, etc.

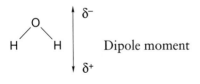

Dipole moment

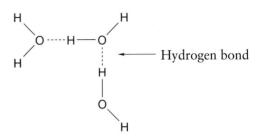

Hydrogen bond

A5.1.2 Other Polar Molecules

Polar molecules are all the molecules presenting one or more polar radicals such as hydroxyl (–OH), carboxyl (–COOH) and phosphate ($-PO_4$) radicals. Membrane lipids have a polar head owing to the presence of polar groups in that region. These polar groups vary according to the lipid:

Lipids	Polar group
Phosphoglycerides	Phosphodiester
Glycolipids	Sugar residues
Cholesterol	–OH radical

Amino acids of a protein, bound to each other by peptide bonds, are more or less polar depending on the nature of their lateral chain R:

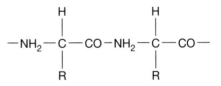

Amino acids	Polar lateral chain R
Arginine	$-CH_2-CH_2-CH_2-NH-C\begin{smallmatrix}NH_2+\\ \\NH_2\end{smallmatrix}$
Lysine	$-CH_2-CH_2-CH_2-CH_2-NH_3+$
Asparagine	$-CH_2-C\begin{smallmatrix}O\\ \\NH_2\end{smallmatrix}$
Aspartate	$-CH_2-C\begin{smallmatrix}O^-\\ \\O\end{smallmatrix}$
Glutamate	$-CH_2-CH_2-C\begin{smallmatrix}O^-\\ \\O\end{smallmatrix}$

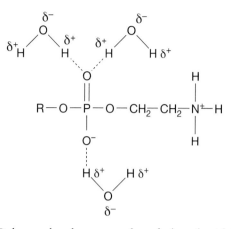

Polar molecules: examples of phosphatidyl ethanolamine

A5.1.3 Hydrophilic Properties

Substances that interact with water molecules by forming dipole–dipole bonds, such as hydrogen bonds, are hydrophilic substances. These are charged substances, i.e. a non-zero charge (ions, amino acid residues that interact with water molecules through Van Der Waals bonds) or polar substances that interact with water through dipole bonds (phospholipids, some amino acids). These substances are soluble or relatively soluble in water. For ions, we have:

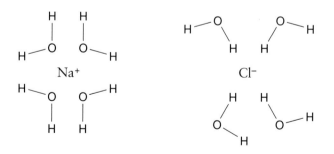

A hydration ring is formed around ions in aqueous solution. For a given charge (mono- or divalent ions), an ion is increasingly hydrated the smaller its ionic radius. Thus, the heaviest ions are the least hydrated ones.

A5.1.4 Hydrophobicity

All uncharged substances that do not form dipole bonds with water molecules are hydrophobic. In contact with those substances, water molecules form a kind of cage by establishing hydrogen bonds between each other and therefore limiting their mobility. This is the reason why hydrophobic molecules stick together and are not soluble in water. 'Hydrophobic interactions', which bring hydrophobic molecules together, are an expression of the tendency of water molecules to limit their interactions with those molecules. Such an organization of water molecules imposed by the presence of hydrophobic molecules is thermodynamically unfavorable because it increases the entropy of the system.

A5.1.5 Amphiphilicity

This is the name given to molecules that contain hydrophilic and hydrophobic regions within the same molecule (from the Greek *amphis* meaning two sides), such as phospholipids and transmembrane proteins. In the case of proteins, this term is used particularly if a hydrophilic and a hydrophobic domain can be distinguished and eventually separated.

Figure A5.1   Hydrophobicity profile of two voltage sensitive channels, the voltage activated Na$^+$ channel underlying the sodium action potential, and the voltage activated dihydropyridine sensitive Ca^{2+} channel. One can distinguish four hydrophobic domains (I to IV) in each protein, each composed of six segments (1 to 6). The hydrophilic COOH terminal domain of the Na$^+$ channel is approximately twice as long as that of the Ca^{2+} channel. The transmembrane organization model of these two channels is given in Figure 5.5b. (From Alsobrook JP II and Stevens CF, 1988. Cloning the calcium channel, *TINS* 11, 1–2, with permission.)

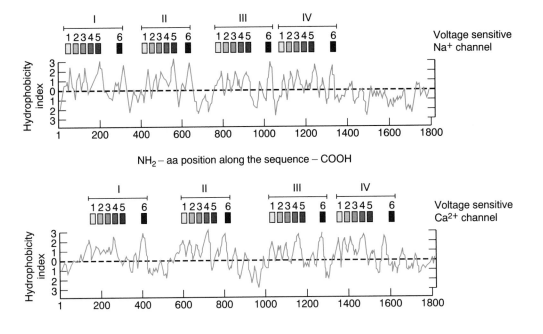

Appendix 5.2
Hydrophobicity Profile of a Transmembrane Protein

The hydrophobicity profile of a protein represents the degree of attraction to water of different regions of the molecule. By convention, the more hydrophilic regions are denoted – and the more hydrophobic ones are denoted +. Hydrophilicity and hydrophobicity are the two extremes of the hydrophobicity scale.

A5.2.1 Determination of the Hydrophilic and Hydrophobic Characters of a Protein

This determination is possible when the primary structure of the protein is known. Each one of the 20 amino acids has been given a value for its hydropathic character that approximately reflects the hydrophilic or hydrophobic nature of its side chain, i.e. its tendency to remain in contact with water (hydrophilicity) or its tendency to repel it (hydrophobicity) (Table A5.1).

Figure A5.2   Hydrophobicity profile of subunits of receptor channels: the glycine receptor (GlyR), the β subunit of the GABA$_A$ receptor, the α$_3$ subunit of the nicotinic acetylcholine receptor (nAChR) and of the GluR-1 subunit of the glutamatergic AMPA receptor. One can distinguish four hydrophobic segments (M1 to M4) in each subunit and a large hydrophilic NH$_2$ terminal domain. For the GluR-1 subunit two models are presented. The GluR subunits have almost twice as many amino acid residues as the other three receptor channel subunits and what appears to be a large extracellular domain spanning approximately the amino-terminal half. The transmembrane organization model of receptor channel subunits is given in Figure 5.6b. (From Gasic GP and Heinemann S, 1991. Receptors coupled to ion channels: the glutamate receptor family, *Curr. Opin. Neurobiol.* 1, 20–26, with permission.)

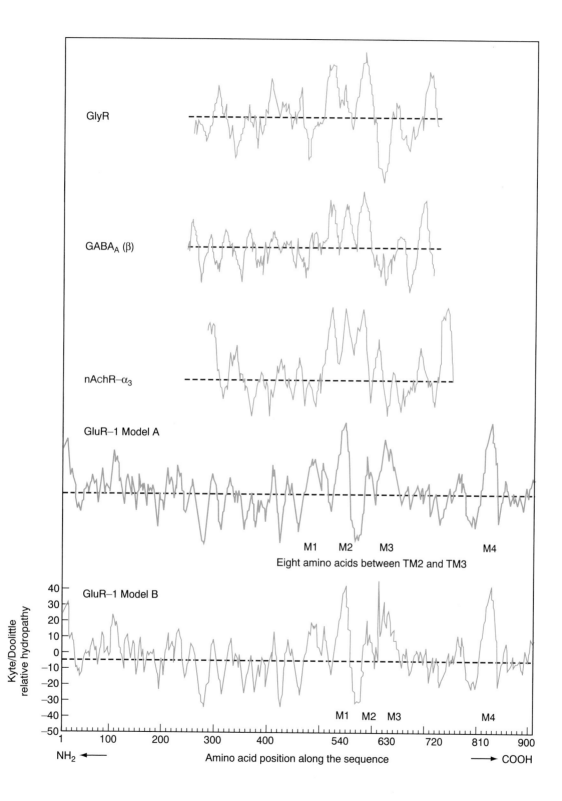

GlyR

GABA_A (β)

nAchR–α_3

GluR–1 Model A

M1 M2 M3 M4

Eight amino acids between TM2 and TM3

GluR–1 Model B

M1 M2 M3 M4

Kyte/Doolittle relative hydropathy

NH_2 ← Amino acid position along the sequence → COOH

Figure A5.3   Hydrophobicity profile of the β adrenergic receptor (βAd), the muscarinic acetylcholine receptor (mAChR) and of rhodopsin. In each receptor one can distinguish seven hydrophobic segments (I to VII) and one hydrophilic domain of variable length, located between segments V and VI. The transmembrane organization model of rhodopsin is illustrated in Figure 5.7b. (From (top to bottom). Dixon RAF *et al.*, 1986. Cloning of the gene and cDNA for mammalian β-adrenergic receptor and homology with rhodopsin, *Nature* **321**, 75–79, with permission. Kubo T *et al.*, 1986. Cloning, sequencing and expression of complementary DNA encoding the muscarinic acetylcholine receptor, *Nature* **323**, 411–416, with permission. Nathans J, Thomas D and Hogness DS, 1986. Molecular genetics of human color vision: the genes encoding blue, green and red pigments, *Science* **232**, 193–202, with permission.)

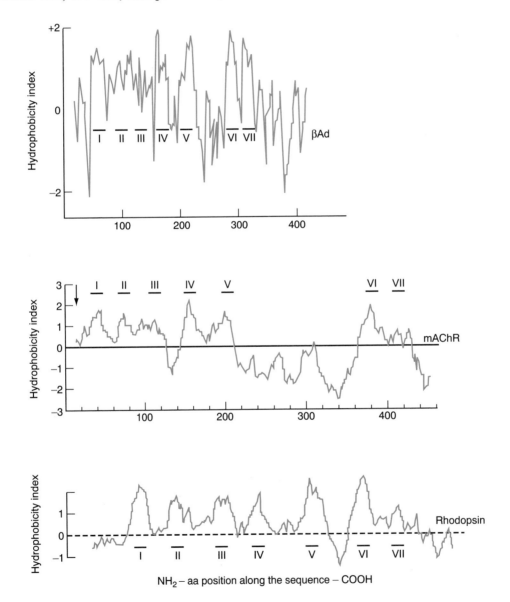

Table A5.1   Hydrophobicity index of the side chains of each of the 20 amino acids (From Kyte J and Doolittle RF, 1982. A simple method for displaying the hydropathic character of a protein, *J. Mol. Biol.* **157**, 105–132, with permission.)

Lateral chain	Hydropathy index
Isoleucine	4.5
Valine	4.2
Leucine	3.8
Phenylalanine	2.8
Cysteine/cystine	2.5
Methionine	1.9
Alanine	1.8
Glycine	−0.4
Threonine	−0.7
Tryptophane	−0.9
Serine	−0.8
Tyrosine	−1.3
Proline	−1.6
Histidine	−3.2
Glutamic acid	−3.5
Glutamine	−3.5
Aspartic acid	−3.5
Asparagine	−3.5
Lysine	−3.9
Arginine	−4.5

Protein segments containing a high percentage of polar or charged amino acids are hydrophilic, whereas segments containing a high percentage of non-polar amino acids (isoleucine or valine) are hydrophobic.

Computer programs exist that are capable of evaluating the hydrophilic or hydrophobic character all along a peptide sequence. By convention this analysis is performed from the NH_2 towards the COOH terminal. The length of each segment analyzed is chosen by the experimenter, usually between 7 and 20 amino acids. The results can be expressed graphically: the hydrophobicity index of each segment is plotted against the position of the segment in the protein. Thus, one obtains the hydrophobicity profile (Figures A5.1–A5.3).

A5.2.2 Determination of the Transmembrane Organization of the Protein

In the case of transmembrane proteins one assumes that the more hydrophobic regions, usually characterized by stretches of approximately 20 amino acids with positive values, are localized in the interior of the lipid bilayer, in the form of transmembrane α-helices. On the other hand, the more hydrophilic regions, characterized by uninterrupted negative values, are in contact with aqueous environments, thus constituting the hydrophilic extracellular or intracellular domains of the protein (see Figures 5.5–5.7).

Further Reading

Conklin, B.R. and Bourne, H. R. (1993) Structural elements of Gα subunits that interact with Gβγ, receptors and effectors. *Cell* **73**, 631–641.

Gilman, A.G. (1995) G proteins and regulation of adenylate cyclase (Nobel Lecture). *Angew. Chem. Int. Ed. Engl.* **34**, 1406–1419.

Güdermann, T., Nürnberg, B. and Schultz, G. (1995) Receptors and G proteins as primary components of transmembrane signal transduction. Part 1. G-protein-coupled receptors: structure and function. *J. Mol. Med.* **73**, 51–63.

Marshall, J. Molloy, R. Moss, G.W.J., Howe, J.R. and Hughes, T.E. (1995) The jelly fish fluorescent protein: a new tool for studying ion channel expression and function. *Neuron* **14**, 211–215.

Nürnberg, B., Gudermann, T. and Schultz, G. (1995) Receptors and G proteins as primary components of transmembrane signal transduction. Part 2. G proteins: structure and function. *J. Mol. Med.* **73**, 123–132.

Schertler, G.F.X., Villa, C. and Henderson, R. (1993) Projection structure of rhodopsin. *Nature* **362**, 770–772. See also references in Chapters 9–15.

6

Basic Properties of Excitable Cells at Rest

If a fine-tipped glass pipette (usually called a micro-electrode), connected via a suitable amplifier to a recording system such as an oscilloscope, is pushed through the membrane of a living nerve cell to reach its cytoplasm, a potential difference is recorded between the cytoplasm and the extracellular compart-ment (Figure 6.1a). In fact, the cell interior shows a negative potential (typically between −60 and −80 mV) with respect to the outside, which is taken as the zero reference potential. In the absence of ongoing electrical activity, this negative potential remains stable and is therefore termed the resting membrane potential (V_{rest}). Since nerve cells communicate through rapid (ms) or slow (s) changes in their mem-brane potential, it becomes important to understand first how V_{rest} is maintained and the various mecha-nisms responsible for this phenomenon. It was Julius Bernstein (1902) who pioneered the theory of V_{rest} as due to selective permeability of the membrane to one ionic species only and that nerve excitation developed when such a selectivity was transiently lost. This con-cept leads us to consider various ways in which ions can cross a biological membrane and how these prin-ciples are applicable to the understanding of V_{rest}.

6.1 Ionic Channels Open at Rest Determine the Resting Membrane Potential

Basically, membranes can use the following processes to shift ions across:

- *Passive movement*: if the membrane contains permeable pores for a particular ionic species, such ions will move because of two physical causes, namely down their concentration gradient (obeying to Fick's law) and according to the membrane elec-tric field. Both processes are established by the transmembrane electrochemical (i.e. dependent on concentration and potential) gradient. The electro-chemical gradient determines the direction of move-ment for a particular ion while the amount of ionic current generated by the passage of these ions through a permeable pore depends not only on this gradient but also on the conductance (a measure of how easily ions can pass through a pore) of the pore itself. A classical theory to account for pore con-ductance is discussed later.

Figure 6.1   Resting membrane potential and ion con-centrations. (a) Schematic representation of micro-electrode impalement of a nerve cell with a resting membrane potential of −80 mV. (b) Idealized nerve cell (depicted as a sphere) with relative concentrations of intra- and extracellular ions. Direction of arrows indicates the direction of ion movement through open channels. Ion concentrations are expressed in millimoles.

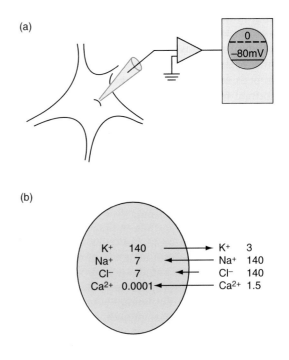

- *Facilitated diffusion*: this process relies on carrier molecules residing in the cell membrane to help the translocation of ions without expenditure of external energy, while the concentration and electrical gradients remain the factors controlling the direction of movement and the final distribution attained.
- *Active transport*: this requires selective transporter molecules plus energy expenditure (for example, obtained from hydrolysis of ATP or from movement of Na⁺ down its electrochemical gradient). In this way, ions can be transported against electrochemical gradients. Often two (or more) ionic species are coupled to a single carrier molecule: if there is no net charge transfer (for example, one positive ion is moved out while a similarly charged ion enters into the cell), then the process is said to be electroneutral. However, the *stoichiometry* (i.e. the relative number of individual ions bound to a carrier molecule) of the carrier-mediated transport is often more complex (for instance three Na⁺ are counter transported with one Ca²⁺) so that there is a net gain or loss of charges in the cell and a resultant change in V_{rest} as discussed in a subsequent section.

Of the three mechanisms considered above, passive diffusion is by far the most important process for the immediate control of the membrane potential of nerve cells and thus their V_{rest}. The chief factor is the permeability of the membrane through specific pores of *ionic channels*, a phenomenon that depends on:

- the conductance of single channels;
- the probability of the channels opening;
- the density of channels in the neuronal membrane.

If the channels are open, then the movement of a particular ionic species will depend on the electrochemical gradient. However, the crucial point is the mechanism that opens (or *gates*) channels: in the case of ligand-gated channels the signal is a chemical substance interacting with a specific receptor site of the channel; in the case of voltage-gated channels a rapid change in membrane potential will open them. Furthermore, some channels appear to be persistently open and are thus important in determining the actual value of V_{rest}. The principal ionic mechanisms of V_{rest} will thus be examined.

6.1.1 The Plasma Membrane Separates Two Media of Different Ionic Composition

The cytoplasm of a nerve cell is rich in K⁺ (approximately 140 mM) while it is relatively poor in Na⁺ (approximately 7 mM). The internal concentration of Cl⁻ is also usually low (assume about 7 mM, though this value differs considerably depending on the cell considered) while the intracellular free Ca²⁺ is only about 0.1 μM. The cell inside is also rich in anions such as proteins and phosphates which have a large molecular weight and do not permeate through membrane channels. The cell membrane (with its lipoprotein composition) can be equated to an insulator separating two electrically conductive media (intracellular and extracellular electrolytes): it thus plays the role of a dielectric in a capacitor and it can be assigned an average capacity (C) value of 1 μF/cm².

The composition of the extracellular solution (in mM) is the opposite of the internal one: for example, Na⁺ is about 140, K⁺ is only about 3, Cl⁻ is about 140 and Ca²⁺ is around 1.5 (Figure 6.1b). The extracellular concentration of large anions is very low. These large asymmetries in ion distribution imply a dynamic state through which cell to cell signalling is made possible.

6.1.2 At Rest Most of the Channels Open are K⁺ Channels

According to the original theory of Bernstein, under resting conditions the cell membrane permeability is minimal to Na⁺, Cl⁻ and Ca²⁺ while it is high to K⁺. This condition can be verified experimentally by measuring ionic fluxes with radioactive tracers or by electrophysiological tests (as explained later). K⁺ will therefore move outwards following its concentration gradient: in doing so it will subtract negative charges from the cell interior and will induce a relatively negative internal potential. Such a negativity will oppose further outward movements of K⁺ until an equilibrium is reached when the concentration gradient for K⁺ cancels the drive exerted by the electrical gradient. In other words, an *equilibrium potential* (E_{rev}) is obtained. Hence, at a membrane potential corresponding to E_{rev}, although K⁺ keeps moving in and out of the cell, there is no net change in its concentration across the membrane (Figure 6.2). E_{rev} is given by the Nernst equation (Eq. 1), which for excitable cells according to Bernstein's theory related to K⁺ is:

$$E_{rev} = \frac{RT}{zF} \ln \frac{[K^+]_o}{[K^+]_i} \qquad (1)$$

where R=gas constant, T=absolute temperature, z=valency, F=Faraday number and $[K^+]_o$ and $[K^+]_i$ indicate extra- and intracellular potassium ion concentrations, respectively. Eq. (1) is a particular case of the Boltzmann Law, relating molecular concentration at some place to potential energy of the molecule in that place. At 20°C RT/zF=25 mV. This value can be multiplied by 2.3 to convert the natural logarithm into base 10 (log), thus giving 58 mV (at 37°C this value is 61 mV). Taking the K⁺ concentration values indicated above means that E_{rev} for K⁺ is –97 mV, i.e. the value at which there is no net transfer of K⁺ across the cell membrane. Of course, this description of the K⁺ potential is entirely based on a physical theory of passive ion movements. Its transmembrane flux, however, involves active transport of ions as well.

Note that, in the case of central neurons with a strongly asymmetrical distribution of Cl⁻ between the extracellular and intracellular compartments, the Nernst equation for Cl⁻ (based on the concentrations stated above) yields an E_{rev} for this anion of –75 mV since E_{rev} = –58 log $[Cl^-]_o/[Cl^-]_i$ (due to the negative value of z in Eq. 1) which transforms into E_{rev} = 58 log $[Cl^-]_i/[Cl^-]_o$. The Nernst equation applied to Na⁺ predicts an E_{rev} value of +75 mV. However, the gradients for Na⁺ and, in particular, for Ca²⁺ are regulated by complex mechanisms relying on transporters and intracellular sequestration so that the possibility of predicting the precise reversal potential of responses mediated by rises in Na⁺ or Ca²⁺ permeability on the basis of their apparent transmembrane concentrations is limited. Figure 6.1b presents a scheme of ion distribution across the cell membrane at rest while Table 6.1 summarizes these values.

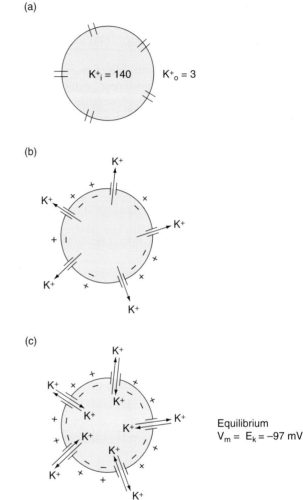

Figure 6.2   The establishment of V_{rest} in a cell where most of the channels open are K⁺ channels.

(a)

(b)

(c)

Equilibrium
$V_m = E_k = -97$ mV

Table 6.1   Examples of ionic concentrations in the extracellular and intracellular media.

Ion	Intracellular concentration (mM)	Extracellular concentration (mM)	Nernst reversal potential (mV)
K⁺	140	3	–97
Na⁺	7	140	+75
Cl⁻	7	140	–75
Ca²⁺	0.0001	1.5	+129

6.1.3 In Muscle Cells, K^+ and Cl^- Ion Movements Equally Participate in Resting Membrane Potential

Some excitable cells, notably skeletal muscle fibres, have a demonstrably high resting permeability not only to K^+ but also to Cl^-. This condition can be equated to that of a semipermeable membrane separating two water solutions containing permeable ions (K^+ and Cl^- in this case) but with an impermeable large ionic species (e.g. proteins) present on one side only. It is also necessary to suppose that the semipermeable membrane can withstand considerable hydrostatic pressure. In this system the non-permeable negatively charged ions will attract K^+ while repelling Cl^-. At equilibrium the following relation is established:

$$\frac{RT}{zF} \ln \frac{[K^+]_o}{[K^+]_i} = -\frac{RT}{zF} \ln \frac{[Cl^-]_o}{[Cl^-]_i} \qquad (2)$$

since $z = 1$ for K^+ and $z = -1$ for Cl^-, respectively. Eq. (2) can be simplified to Eq. (3):

Figure 6.3 Theoretical diagram of E_K versus the external concentration of K^+ ions ($[K^+]_o$). $E_K = (RT/zF) \times 2.3 \log ([K^+]_o/[K^+]_i)$.

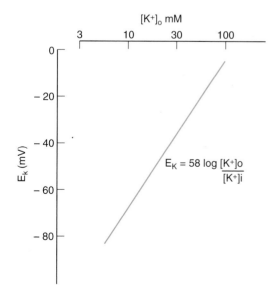

$$[K^+]_o \cdot [Cl^-]_o = [K^+]_i \cdot [Cl^-]_i \qquad (3)$$

which is an example of the *Donnan equilibrium* applied to a cell. Note that one side of the membrane (corresponding to the intracellular compartment) will have a total concentration of ions larger than on the opposite side. This situation will tend to attract water molecules (which are considered to move freely across the membrane) until the larger hydrostatic pressure resulting from water accumulation prevents further movement of water molecules, thus yielding an equilibrium condition. Donnan equilibrium is a process whereby some cells can establish asymmetrical ion gradients at rest without the need of an active transport system.

6.1.4 In Central Neurons, K^+, Cl^- and Na^+ Ion Movements Participate in Resting Membrane Potential: the Goldman–Hodgkin–Katz Equation

Unlike muscle fibres, the value of V_{rest} of central neurons is not as negative as the predicted E_{rev} for K^+, nor can it be adequately accounted for by the Donnan equilibrium for K^+ and Cl^-. Furthermore, inspection of the Nernst equation applied to K^+ indicates that a 10-fold change in the concentration ratio should alter the membrane potential of a neuron by 58 mV (Figure 6.3). This relation can be tested in experiments in which the extracellular (or intracellular) concentration of this ion is altered and the resulting membrane potential measured with a sharp or patch microelectrode. A semilog plot of the extracellular K^+ concentration (abscissa) against the membrane potential (ordinate) should thus have a slope of 58 mV per 10-fold change in K^+: this condition is rarely encountered in neurons but it seems to be more common for glial cells (which sometimes are termed K^+ electrodes because their membrane potential is linearly dependent on K^+). In the case of neurons non-linearity of this plot is frequently seen, particularly at low levels of extracellular K^+.

These observations confirm that K^+ is a very important ion for setting the value of neuronal V_{rest} but that other ionic mechanisms must also play a significant role. Since the intracellular concentration of Na^+ is not negligible, this implies that this ionic species can accumulate inside the cytoplasm, presumably because its rather positive E_{rev} (+75 mV) versus a very negative V_{rest} creates an electrochemical gradient extremely favorable to Na$^+$ entry. Equally, the asymmetric distribution of Cl$^-$ suggests its possible role in determining V_{rest}. In order to take into account various ionic species it was useful to introduce what is commonly called the *Goldman–Hodgkin–Katz equation* (GHK; Eq. 4):

$$V_{rest} = 58 \times \log \frac{p_K[K^+]_o + p_{Na}[Na^+]_o + p_{Cl}[Cl^-]_i}{p_K[K^+]_i + p_{Na}[Na^+]_i + p_{Cl}[Cl^-]_o} \quad (4)$$

where p is the permeability coefficient (cm/s) for each ionic species as explained in 6.1.5.

Note that if the resting permeability to Na$^+$ and Cl$^-$ is very low, the GHK equation closely resembles the Nernst equation for K$^+$.

In applying the GHK equation to nerve cells, the following assumptions must be made:

- The voltage gradient across the membrane is uniform in the sense that it changes linearly within the membrane. This assumption has led to the GHK equation being termed as the *constant field equation*.
- The overall net current flow across the membrane is zero as the currents generated by individual ionic species are balanced out.
- The membrane is at steady state since there is no time-dependent change in ionic flux or channel density. This is obviously not applicable to non-steady state conditions of rapidly changing membrane potential as produced when a nerve cell fires action potentials.
- Any role of active transport mechanisms is ignored. However, as discussed later, there is evidence for this transport of various ionic species.
- The ionic species are monovalent cations or anions which do not interact among themselves or with water molecules. This point does not hold true if there is a measurable permeability to divalent cations such as Ca^{2+}. Furthermore, it has been reported that ions can interact among themselves within the same channel.
- The role of membrane surface charges is ignored. This is a relatively major limitation because the cell membrane contains negative charges on its inner and outer layers (amino acid residues of membrane proteins which are typically negatively charged). The electric field generated by these charges is able

to influence the kinetic properties of ionic channels (gating, activation and inactivation). Adding divalent cations such as Ca^{2+} or Mg^{2+} leads to screening of these charges and consequent changes in channel properties.

- The mobility of each ionic species and its diffusion coefficient (D) within the membrane of thickness (δ) is constant.
- The ions do not bind to specific sites in the membrane and their concentration (C) can be expressed by a linear partition coefficient ($\beta = C_{membrane}/C_{solution}$). However, there is evidence that ions can bind to sites inside channels and influence channel kinetics.
- The ionic activities (a) can be replaced by their concentrations.

In summary, according to the GHK equation, the cell membrane potential is considered as a tridimensional space through which ions move, whereas in real terms the membrane contains distinct narrow pores for different ions.

6.1.5 Some Principles Related to the Derivation of the GHK Equation

In spite of the fact that several of these assumptions do not appear to be applicable to nerve cells, the GHK model can be a useful tool to describe the behavior of an excitable membrane. It is of interest to understand the basic principles behind the derivation of this equation because they have important implications for the basic neurophysiological properties of excitable cells. The starting point is the Nernst–Planck diffusion equation which describes the dependence of the ionic flux across the membrane on the electrochemical and concentration gradients of a given ion. This can be represented by:

$$j = u \cdot c \left[RT \frac{d(\ln a)}{dx} + zF \frac{dV}{dx} \right]. \quad (5)$$

where j is the net ionic flux of a given ionic species, u is the absolute mobility of the ion (cm/s per unit force) through the membrane, c is the ion concentration at a point x in the membrane, R and T have the same meaning as in Eq. (1), a is the ionic activity and dV/dx is the potential gradient.

For the GHK equation the permeability coefficient for an ionic species can be calculated as: $p = \beta^* \, D/\delta$ (these terms are explained above). If only one ionic species permeates across the nerve cell membrane the Nernst–Planck flux equation (Eq. 5) can then be rewritten as Eq. (6):

$$j = \frac{pzFV}{RT}\left[\frac{C_o - C_i \exp\left(\dfrac{zFV}{RT}\right)}{1 - \exp\dfrac{zFV}{RT}}\right] \qquad (6)$$

where C_o and C_i are the concentrations of the ion outside and inside the cell, respectively (all the other terms have been described earlier in the text). It is clear that membrane permeability to more than one ionic species will be described by the sum of similar equations for each ion considered. It was mentioned earlier that in order to measure the permeability coefficient (p) of an ion it is possible to perform radioactive tracer experiments although a major limitation of this approach resides in the difficulty to resolve ion fluxes on a timescale of a few seconds or even milliseconds. An alternative approach of high temporal resolution is to use electrophysiological techniques working on the principle that movement of ions through the membrane will generate an ionic current (I). This phenomenon is described by Eq. (7):

$$I = J \cdot F \cdot z \qquad (7)$$

The term (I) is the current density expressed in ampere/cm^2, while F is the Faraday number (coulombs/mole) and J is the net ionic flux density (moles/s)/cm^2. If the terms of Eq. (4) are multiplied by zF, for the case of a single ionic species Eq. (8) is obtained:

$$I = \frac{p(zF)^2 V}{RT} \times \frac{C_o - C_i \exp\left(\dfrac{zFV}{RT}\right)}{1 - \exp\left(\dfrac{zFV}{RT}\right)} \qquad (8)$$

6.2 Membrane Pumps are Responsible for Keeping Constant the Concentration Gradients Across Membranes

Expressions such as the GHK or Nernst equations (Eqs 4 or 1) describe the behavior of ions in purely physical terms and, in doing so, they cannot take into account biological processes influencing ionic gradients. It was already noted at the beginning of this century that heart muscle cells, which fire Na$^+$ and K$^+$ dependent action potentials through the lifetime of the individual, should gradually lose their intracellular concentration of K$^+$ and replace it with Na$^+$; yet, the K$^+$ content of these cells is virtually the same in young and old animals, suggesting that an ion redistribution process is continuously taking place. Later work suggested that skeletal muscle fibres probably use a transport mechanism to restore their ionic gradients after fatigue and proposed the existence of a 'sodium pump', namely a system able to exchange Na$^+$ for K$^+$ across the cell membrane using intracellular ATP. The sodium pump, which appears to be a ubiquitous characteristic of cells, exerts the fundamental role of exchanging intracellularly accumulated Na$^+$ for extracellular K$^+$ in order to preserve the correct ionic gradients.

The pump is a protein with enzymatic function, located in the cell membrane and comprising four subunits (two α and two β, see Chapter 5) of which several isoforms are known. One important feature of the pump activity is its stoichiometry whereby three Na$^+$ are exchanged for two K$^+$: in practice, this means that for each cycle of pump activity one extra positive charge is subtracted from the cell cytoplasm, thus generating a hyperpolarization (i.e. making the intracellular compartment more negative as a result of positive current outflow). This phenomenon is shown in Figure 6.4. Consequently, not only is the sodium pump necessary to re-establish ionic gradients after intense nerve cell activity but it also helps the membrane potential to return to the initial V_{rest} value or to be even more negative, thus providing temporary inhibition against further excitation.

The operation of the pump is thought to be triggered by binding of intracellular Na$^+$ and ATP to internal facing sites of this protein. Transformation of ATP into ADP releases a phospho group which leads to a conformational change in the pump with trapping of three Na$^+$ which are released into the outside compartment. K$^+$ then binds to the pump outer sites and

Figure 6.4 Different states of the sodium–potassium pump to shift Na^+ and K^+ across the cell membrane. P, phospho group.

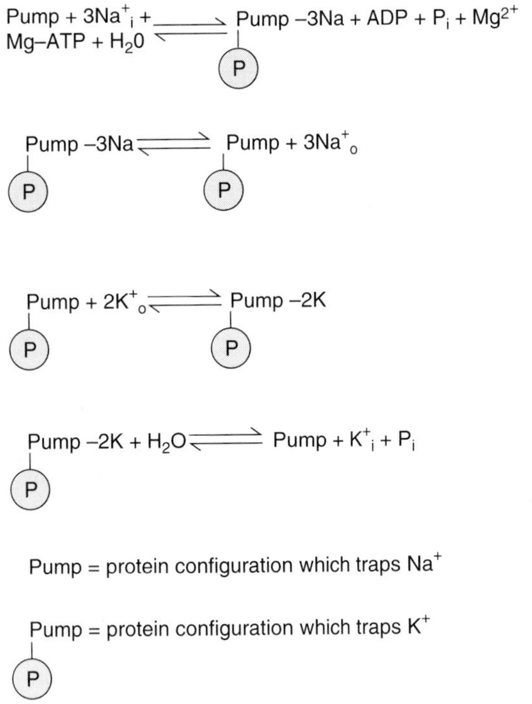

Pump + $3Na^+_i$ + $\longrightarrow$ Pump $-3Na$ + ADP + P_i + Mg^{2+}
Mg–ATP + H_2O $\longleftarrow$ |
                              Ⓟ

Pump $-3Na$ $\rightleftharpoons$ Pump + $3Na^+_o$
| |
Ⓟ   Ⓟ

Pump + $2K^+_o$ $\rightleftharpoons$ Pump $-2K$
| |
Ⓟ   Ⓟ

Pump $-2K$ + H_2O $\rightleftharpoons$ Pump + K^+_i + P_i
|
Ⓟ

Pump = protein configuration which traps Na^+

Pump = protein configuration which traps K^+
|
Ⓟ

Figure 6.5 Schematic drawing of the Na–K–ATPase and Na–Ca pumps.

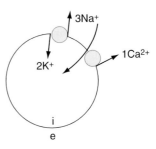

releases the phospho group into the extracellular water: removal of the phospho residues induces a conformational change in the pump with translocation and release of K^+ to the cell inside.

Pharmacological block of the sodium pump is produced by cardiac glycosides (e.g. ouabain) or oligomycin; a K^+-free extracellular solution is a useful experimental tool to block the pump activity of cells *in vitro*. Lowering the ambient temperature will also depress the sodium pump activity.

While the sodium pump is probably the main representative of membrane transporters for ions, other mechanisms also exist. In particular, extracellular Na^+ is exchanged for intracellular Ca^{2+} with a 3:1 stoichiometry; such a mechanism is again electrogenic (because it is based on a net inflow of positive charges) and has the role of keeping the intracellular concentration of Ca^{2+} low (Figure 6.5). Since Na^+ moves according to its gradient, the system does not require energy in the form of ATP hydrolysis. It uses the energy of Na^+ in the extracellular space and it relies on the operation of the sodium pump to maintain a

low intracellular level of Na^+. Intracellular Ca^{2+} at rest is also kept at submicromolar level by sequestration into cell organelles via distinct pump mechanisms (see Figure 8.5). Finally, in mature brain neurons the intracellular concentration of Cl^- is usually found to be very low because various pumps (coupling its transport with that of Na^+, K^+ or bicarbonate) actively extrude this anion. When inhibitory neurotransmitters such as GABA (or glycine) activate Cl^- permeable channels, the gradient caused by pumps allows an influx of Cl^- to hyperpolarize (and thus inhibit) neuronal membranes (see Chapter 10).

6.3 A Simple Equivalent Electrical Circuit for Resting Membrane Properties

6.3.1 Membrane Potential has an Ohmic Behavior at Rest

A convenient description of the electrical behavior of nerve cells is provided by formally applying to them *Ohm's law*, which establishes the relation between current (I) and potential (V): thus, $I = V/R$ where V is the cell membrane potential and R is the cell resistance. Taking $1/R$ as the conductance (g), $I = g \times V$. One can then relate I to V with a simple plot (usually called the I/V curve), the slope of which will be a measure of g (Figure 6.6). If the I/V curve is linear, this is said to display *ohmic* behavior. Conversely, if diffusion is involved in the ionic current flow, the I/V curve becomes non-linear because g becomes a function of membrane potential.

The Nernst equation (Eq. 1) predicts that the net ion flow across the cell membrane ceases when the transmembrane potential (V_m) is the same as the

Figure 6.6   Ohmic behavior of the membrane potential around the resting potential. (a) Time-dependent responses to ± 0.4 nA current injected for 300 ms. Upper traces, current (I); lower traces, membrane potential changes (V_m). (b) Membrane potential at the end of the current pulse (i.e. at 300 ms) plotted against current intensity. (From Adams PR, Brown DA and Constanti A, 1982. M-currents and other potassium currents in bullfrog sympathetic neurones. *J. Physiol. (Lond.)* 330, 537–572, with permission.)

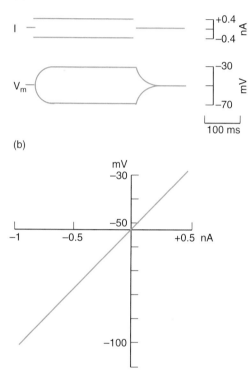

(a)

(b)

or for macroscopic current:

$$I = g(V_m - E_{ion})   \text{knowing that } I = N\, p_o\, i$$

where N is the total number of channels, g is the macroscopic conductance and p_o is the probability of these channels to be in the open state. Note that the microscopic conductance of a single channel (Eq. 10) is often termed γ. Since the present chapter is not concerned with distinct species of single channels responsible for V_{rest}, for sake of simplicity the notation g will be used here for the micro as well as the macroscopic conductance.

By electrophysiological convention, the current leaving the cell has a positive sign while the one entering the cell has a negative one. The same equation may be adopted for a single ionic channel, in spite of the possibility of interaction of ions within the channel itself. Indeed, every channel may be characterized by a potential, E_{ion}, at which the current stops flowing through it. Obviously, one may not *a priori* assume that the value of g for each channel is a constant which does not depend on V, i.e. that $i–V$ is a linear function according to Ohm's law. However, the use of Ohm's law for a description of channel current is an approximation justified by its simplicity and, to a certain extent, by experimental evidence. In fact, the current through the open pore of many types of ionic channel is actually found to be linearly dependent on the membrane potential while g always depends on the concentration of the current-carrying ions (g is an empirical measure of how easily and quickly ions can go through a pore of the membrane). Important functional consequences are that the channel conductance (g) is switched on and off by neurotransmitters or variations in membrane potential (and the speed of such a change) as described elsewhere.

Eq. (9) may be used to describe many electrical events in the nerve cell, including its resting state. One should expect that there must be a V_{rest} value at which the sum of all membrane currents (active pump currents included) is equal to zero. This value represents a condition of electrical equilibrium for the membrane since the current does not change the total charge and hence the potential is also not changing. The equilibrium value of the potential, or resting potential, V_{rest}, is thus given by the following equation (Eq. 10):

Nernst E_{rev} of the ion. One may instead adopt a simple electrical circuit to represent this phenomenon so that the transmembrane gradient for a given ion concentration produces an electromotive force (E) which is equal to the Nernst potential (Table 6.1). In other words, there is an electrochemical current source for each ion. The current source is characterized by its internal conductance, g, in addition to E_{ion}. The current is then described as:

for unitary current

$$i = g(V_m - E_{ion})   \text{(9)}$$

$$g_K (V_{rest} - E_K) + g_{Na}(V_{rest} - E_{Na}) + g_{Ca}(V_{rest} - E_{Ca})$$
$$+ g_{Cl}(V_{rest} - E_{Cl}) + \ldots + i_{Na/K} + i_{Ca} + \ldots = 0   \text{(10)}$$

where i is the current generated by operation of the various ionic pumps and it may depend upon V, ion concentrations, etc. The ellipses indicate possible addition of other channels and pumps. It should also be noted that for each ion there are often several different types of channel with distinct conductance and gating properties but that, in the present simplified scheme, these are all lumped together into a single species.

6.3.2 Stability, Bistability and Instability of Resting Membrane Potential

At this point, it is of utmost importance to discuss the notion of equilibrium stability. V_{rest} is stable whenever any small deviation of it (ΔV_{rest}) elicits a current of same polarity which restores V_{rest} to its normal value. Let us consider, for example, a slight depolarization ($\Delta V_{rest} > 0$). Then, a positive current will be generated to cancel membrane depolarization. Similarly, a hyperpolarization ($\Delta V_{rest} < 0$) will evoke a negative current which restores again V_{rest}. This situation occurs, for example, in ohmic systems. A steady resting potential (Figure 6.7a) is therefore a characteristic of most excitable and all non-excitable cells. Of course, very large signals (depolarizations or hyperpolarizations) will not be cancelled out by currents of the same polarity and regenerative membrane responses may appear (for instance action potentials are triggered when membrane depolarization reaches a certain threshold, as discussed in Chapter 7).

Some nerve cells (e.g. motoneurons) have an additional stable level of electrical equilibrium. This stable point corresponds to a steady depolarization generated by a voltage-activated slow inward current. Such cells are called *bistable* and their steady depolarization level may be considered as a *metastable* point. It only exists until such a time when slow changes in ion concentration, conductance and/or pump current changes make the second stable solution of Eq. (10) impossible. Thus, a short excitatory input is sufficient to shift the cell from the stable state, V_{rest}, to the metastable steady depolarization; *vice versa*, a short inhibitory process is enough to return the cell to V_{rest} (Figure 6.7b).

In pacemaker cells (for example, some cells present in the heart or in certain brainstem or hypothalamic nuclei) V_{rest} is intrinsically *unstable* and, as such, it cannot be reliably measured. Any deviation (ΔV_{rest}) of membrane potential generates membrane currents that further enhance it, i.e. depolarization activates a negative (depolarizing) current, while hyperpolarization activates a positive one. This situation results in membrane potential oscillations around a 'resting' level (Figure 6.7c), which are precisely what a pacemaker cell should spontaneously express to drive the activity of nearby cells.

6.3.3 An Electrical Model of Resting Membrane Potential

Let us simplify Eq. (10) by reducing the currents to the passive movement of K^+, Na^+ and Cl^-, which substantially determine V_{rest}. Figure 6.8a presents an electrical equivalent for such simplification. Pump currents may be neglected since the main current through the Na/K ATPase is a counterflow of K^+ and Na^+. By transforming the simplified Eq. (10), we obtain Eq. (11):

Figure 6.7   Schematic representation of a stable (a), a bistable (b) and an unstable (c) resting membrane potential.

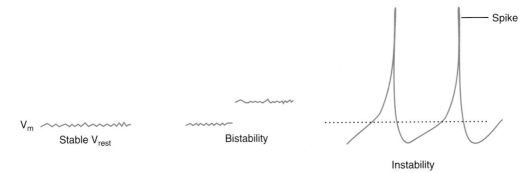

Figure 6.8 Simplified equivalent scheme to account for membrane electrical characteristics near the resting potential. (a) Three main ionic current sources. Note: E_K and E_{Cl} are negative while E_{Na} is positive. (b) An equivalent current source for the resting potential. (c) Electrical scheme for below-threshold potential changes (passive de- and hyperpolarizations) relative to the resting potential. Battery symbols indicate electromotive forces, boxes represent conductances and parallel plates indicate membrane capacitors.

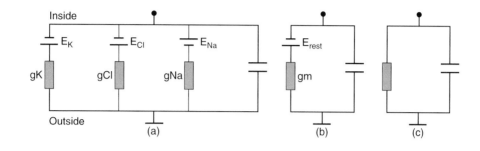

$$V_{rest} = \frac{g_K E_K + g_{Na} E_{Na} + g_{Cl} E_{Cl}}{g_K + g_{Na} + g_{Cl}} \quad (11)$$

The meaning of Eq. (11) is as follows (Figure 6.8b). Instead of three parallel current sources for K⁺, Na⁺ and Cl⁻, we have lumped them together into only one source with electromotive force (E) equal to V_{rest} and an inward conductance gm equal to the sum of the specific ionic (channel) conductances $g_K + g_{Na} + g_{Cl}$. One may consider, instead of the absolute value of membrane potential, only its deviation from V_{rest}. In this case the equivalent electromotive force becomes equal to 0 and the equivalent scheme of the cell membrane simplifies to an RC-circuit (Figure 6.8c). If one includes more channel types in the circuit of Figure 6.8a, then the notion of resting current still holds true. The equivalent scheme of Figure 6.8c is applicable only to depolarizations and hyperpolarizations characterized by linear (ohmic) current–voltage relations.

In standard excitable cells it means that these potential changes from V_{rest} are not activating voltage-gated currents, e.g. they are below the threshold for spike generation. For bistable cells, instead of Ohm's law, one must consider an N-shaped current–voltage relation as shown in Figure 6.9. In pacemaker cells approximately ohmic current–voltage relations with *negative* membrane conductance exist. The direction of the current–voltage relation when crossing the voltage axis determines the stability of the corresponding equilibrium (zero-current) point (Figure 6.9).

From the scheme of Figure 6.1 and Eqs (10) and (11), the resting potential should be very close to the electromotive force for the ion with largest membrane

Figure 6.9 Theoretical current–voltage curves exemplifying the case of a cell with one stable resting potential (line labeled a) or with an unstable resting potential (line labeled b). The example of a bistable cell current–voltage relation is presented by the thin line (labeled c, partly including also the thick lines a and b). The arrows along the horizontal voltage axis indicate the direction of membrane potential change (ΔV_{rest}) which in the case of the stable cell (a) evokes an outward (positive) current (see vertical arrow) which forces the membrane potential to return to resting level. When the signs of potential and current change are the same, as in (a), the conductance (given by the slope of the line) is positive and V_{rest} is stable; if these signs are different, as in the case of (b) (note negative conductance), V_{rest} becomes unstable as an inward (negative) current depolarizes the membrane potential. In bistable cells both extreme zero-current points (V_{rest} and steady depolarization) are stable while the middle one is unstable.

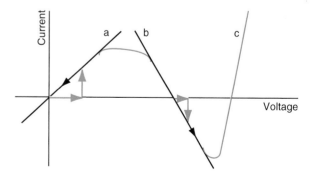

conductance. As a rule, g_K is the largest one. (Note: It may seem that the Eqs (10) and (11) for V_{rest} have little in common with the Donnan equilibrium (see Eq. 3.) Nonetheless, this is not so. The principal small inorganic permeable cation that is screening non-permeable organic anions in the cytoplasm is K^+. Its electromotive force is the closest to the Donnan equilibrium because considerable additional energy would otherwise be needed to maintain the cell potential and the concentration gradients at resting state.) This is why the V_{rest} is so susceptible to E_K changes. The high intracellular K^+ concentration actually does not change much during electrical activity, while the low extracellular concentration can do so markedly. During sustained convulsive activity a considerable amount of K^+ leaves the cell; hence, the extracellular concentration of this ion increases and, consequently, E_K and V_{rest} are shifted toward less negative values.

6.4 Advantages and Disadvantages of Sharp (Intracellular) Versus Patch Electrodes for Measuring the Resting Membrane Potential

In order to measure membrane potential, optical and electrophysiological techniques can be employed. The optical techniques make use of membrane-soluble substances whose light absorption or luminescence is a function of the electric field applied. The transmembrane electric field is strong enough, approximately 20 MV/m, to produce such effects. At the present time optical techniques are in the process of further development and their sensitivity is increasing, although they are used by just a few laboratories. It is still unclear to what extent the molecules used for optical measurements affect cell properties. Furthermore, optical techniques are used to measure potentials, not currents.

Membrane potentials and currents (under voltage clamp) are measured by employing methods of cellular electrophysiology. Nerve cell impalement with a tapered, sharp saline-filled pipette has been used for almost half a century. However, this technique entails some problems. Firstly, in order to provide the pipette with the necessary ability to pass current, the filling salt solution has to be more concentrated (by one order of magnitude) than the cytoplasm. Leakage of ions from the pipette into the cell shifts their physiological concentration in the cytoplasm and might

therefore affect the normal performance of cellular organelles, enzymes, pumps and channels with consequent changes in membrane potential. Secondly, it is possible that the impalement itself (in addition to any alterations in the cytoplasm composition) may introduce considerable artefactual leakage (often termed *shunt*) of the membrane, which corresponds to a parasitic membrane conductance. Thirdly, the pipette might destroy the cytoskeleton and subcellular structures. The cell is not always able to compensate for all these factors. Indeed, some cells, particularly smaller ones, cannot survive the impalement. Major signs of cell deterioration are high membrane conductance and low V_{rest}, which can be present even in those neurons that do survive. Fourthly, the electrode resistance and capacitance are often large and thus difficult to compensate. Finally, a junctional current may arise at the interface between pipette orifice and cytoplasm owing to the differences in electrolyte composition and concentration.

Whole-cell patch clamp is another electrophysiological technique to measure the cell potential and current. In this case negative pressure is applied to a pipette (usually of larger orifice than the ones used for intracellular recording) in order to establish a tight contact (*seal*) with the nerve cell membrane. A small area (*patch*) of the cell is thus forced inside the pipette orifice and eventually ruptured so that the cytoplasm is in direct continuity with the pipette interior (see Appendix 7.3). The tight seal ensures reliable insulation of the inside of the electrode from the extracellular medium, thereby excluding the possibility of membrane shunting. Electrical currents originating from the cell are thus unable to escape at the interface between membrane and electrode tip. When there is a loose contact between membrane and electrode (e.g because of damage to the cell) signals are largely attenuated or even lost (this phenomenon is called shunting). Indeed, in certain cases (e.g. neurons in hippocampal slices), the cell apparent conductance decreases several times compared with that measured with a sharp intracellular microelectrode. The whole cell patch clamp thus enables one to record more reliably potential and current signals from small cells and even from fine processes such as dendrites. Furthermore, the mechanical stability of recording is much improved over conventional intracellular methods.

Nonetheless, the method is not devoid of shortcomings. First of all, the suction effect caused by the initial negative pressure may remove small molecules of biological importance from the cytoplasm. This phenomenon might alter the activity of membrane channels which are controlled by intracellular chemical messengers (e.g. cAMP or cGMP). Gradual replacement of the cell cytoplasm by the pipette internal solution (*intracellular dialysis*) during prolonged recording might compound this effect. Hence, it is feasible that the very low cell conductance observed with whole-cell patch clamping may be, at least in part, artefactual. The negative pressure applied to the cell might disturb the membrane structure and even open stretch-activated channels. Still unresolved are the problems associated with compensation of electrode capacitance and resistance and with the contact between pipette electrolyte and cytoplasm.

In an attempt to reduce the problems caused by intracellular dialysis and washout, a modification of the whole-cell patch clamp technique has been introduced whereby chemical perforation (*perforated patch*) of the membrane patch beneath the pipette is used. This effect is achieved by adding to the pipette solution a *channel-forming* substance, e.g. the antibiotics nystatin or amphotericin. Such substances create artificial pores in the patch of membrane under the electrode tip through which only small monovalent ions can pass. However, one still faces the problem of high and unstable resistance of the clamped membrane patch which, in the case of *in situ* neurons, is not dissimilar to the situation obtained with an intracellular sharp microelectrode. Furthermore, the perforating molecules endow the membrane with a selective ion permeability, thereby affecting the membrane electrical properties and turning on an artefactual electromotive force.

From this discussion it is clear that an ideal electrophysiological method to study membrane potential and current is not yet available. The present techniques are useful but impose several experimental constraints. The shortcomings inherent in electrophysiological measurements are well described by Niels Bohr's famous statement that any biological measurement entails interference with the object's life activities and, hence, a bias in the values obtained. Choosing the method of measurement most appropriate for a given objective is an arduous task for a neuroscientist who must be able to measure not only the resting potential and apparent cell conductance but also to detect the presence of an injury shunt.

6.5 Background Currents Which Flow Through Voltage-Gated Channels Open at Resting Membrane Potential Also Participate in V_{rest}

Under resting conditions many nerve cells normally display a stable V_{rest} as a result of the combined action of the so-called *leak* conductance (measured as the linearity of the I–V curve according to Ohm's law) caused by passive permeability mainly to K^+ (and, to a smaller extent, to other ions), and a variable degree of shunt conductance generated by the presence of the recording electrode itself. In certain neurons this picture is complicated by the overlapping presence of other currents caused by flow of ions through specific membrane channels which are permanently open at or around V_{rest}. In this case such channels are persistently activated by either intracellular (or extracellular) chemicals or the actual level of V_{rest}. A necessary property of these channels is that they do not undergo significant inactivation (i.e. spontaneous closure despite the continuous presence of the gating signal): under these circumstances the current flowing through these channels is termed *background* current.

The interest in background currents stems from the fact that they may be the target for the action of neurotransmitters or drugs which can change the membrane potential and the excitability of neurons by selective up- or down-regulation of channels already open at rest. This situation may be exemplified by the action of some endogenously occurring neuropeptides, of which substance P and TRH are notable representatives. Let us suppose that one is recording from a brain neuron that has an apparently stable V_{rest} which (assuming ideal experimental conditions of minimal conductance shunt by the electrode) is actually due to two mechanisms: passive permeability to various ions (K^+, Na^+, Cl^- and Ca^{2+}) and selective permeability to K^+ through membrane channels that are activated by hyperpolarization. The relatively negative membrane potential ensures constant opening of these channels which will tend to hyperpolarize the cell towards the value of E_K, an action opposed by the leak channel activity (with reversal potential less negative than E_K). Binding of substance P to specific receptors (coupled to G-proteins) will activate a series of intracellular biochemical reactions leading to closure of the hyperpolarization-activated K^+ channels (called *inward rectifier* channels). The result will be a depolarization of the cell with a *decrease* in conductance (because channels have been closed). The depolarization will thus bring the membrane nearer the threshold for action potential generation; at the same time, the conductance decrease will make the membrane more sensitive to signals coming from other cells because (according to Ohm's law) synaptic currents generated by various transmitters now evoke larger variations in membrane potential. In this fashion substance P can produce a sustained up-regulation of the excitability of a neuron. The action of TRH is similar (though not identical) to that of substance P since it also involves suppression of a background K^+ current apparently distinct from the inward rectifier current.

Other background currents that operate at V_{rest} are also known to exist in brain neurons with different degrees of expression depending on the cell type considered: some are selectively mediated by K^+, such as the *M-current* (so-called because it is blocked by acetylcholine acting via muscarinic receptors, see Appendix 17.3); others are generated by channels permeable to Na^+ and K^+ (with a reversal potential positive to V_{rest}, such as I_Q or I_h; see Appendix 17.5); or to Cl^- especially when cells contain a high concentration of this anion owing its efflux from the recording electrode.

Further Reading

Adams, P.R., Brown, D.A. and Constanti, A. (1982) Pharmacological inhibition of the M-current. *J. Physiol.* **332**, 223–262.

Baginskas, A., Gutman A. and Svirskis, G. (1993) Bi-stable dendrite in constant electric field: a model analysis. *Neuroscience* **53**, 595–603.

Glynn, I.M. (1993) All hands to the sodium pump. *J. Physiol.* **462**, 1–30.

Hamill, O.P., Marty, A., Neher, E., Sakmann, B. and Takahashi, T. (1981) Improved patch-clamp techniques for high resolution current recording from cells and cell-free membrane patches. *Pflugers Arch.* **391**, 85–100.

Hultborn, H. and Kiehn, O. (1992) Neuromodulation of vertebrate motor neuron membrane properties. *Curr. Opin. Neurobiol.* **2**, 770–775.

Nistri, A., Fisher, N.D. and Gurnell, M. (1990) Block by the neuropeptide TRH of an apparently novel K^+ conductance of rat motoneurones. *Neurosci. Lett.* **120**, 25–30.

Staley, K. (1994) The role of an inwardly rectifying chloride conductance in postsynaptic inhibition. *J. Neurophysiol.* **72**, 273–284.

Yamaguchi, K., Nakajima, Y., Nakajima, S. and Stanfield, P.R. (1990) Modulation of inwardly rectifying channels by substance P in cholinergic neurones from rat brain in culture. *J. Physiol.* **426**, 499–520.

7

The Voltage-Gated Channels of Action Potentials

The ionic basis for nerve excitation was first elucidated in the squid giant axon by Hodgkin and Huxley (1952) using the voltage clamp technique. They made the key observation that two separate, voltage-dependent currents underlie the action potential: an early transient inward Na^+ current which depolarizes the membrane, and a delayed outward K^+ current largely responsible for repolarization. This led to a series of experiments that resulted in a quantitative description of impulse generation and propagation in the squid axon.

Nearly 30 years later, Sakmann and Neher, using the patch clamp technique, recorded the activity of the voltage-gated Na^+ and K^+ channels responsible for action potential initiation and propagation. Taking history backwards, we will explain action potentials from the single channel level to the membrane level.

7.1 Properties of Action Potentials

7.1.1 The Different Types of Action Potentials

The action potential is a sudden and transient depolarization of the membrane. The cells that initiate action potentials are called excitable cells. Action potentials can have different shapes, i.e. different amplitudes and durations. In neuronal somas and axons, action potentials have a large amplitude and a small duration: these are the Na^+-dependent action potentials (Figures 7.1 and 7.2a). In other neuronal cell bodies, heart ventricular cells and axon terminals, the action potentials have a longer duration with a plateau following the initial peak: these are the Na^+/Ca^{2+}-dependent action potentials (Figure 7.2b–d). Finally, in some neuronal dendrites and some endocrine cells, action potentials have a small amplitude and a long duration: these are the Ca^{2+}-dependent action potentials.

Action potentials have common properties, for example they are all initiated in response to a mem-

brane depolarization. They also have differences, for example in the type of ions involved, their amplitude, duration, etc. We will first explain the Na^+-dependent action potential.

Figure 7.1 The action potential of the giant axon of the squid. Action potential recorded intracellularly recorded in the giant axon of the squid at resting membrane potential in response to a depolarizing current pulse (the extracellular solution is sea-water). The different phases of the action potential are indicated. (Adapted from Hodgkin AL and Katz B, 1949. The effect of sodium ions on the electrical activity of the giant axon of the squid, *J. Physiol.* **108**, 37–77, with permission.)

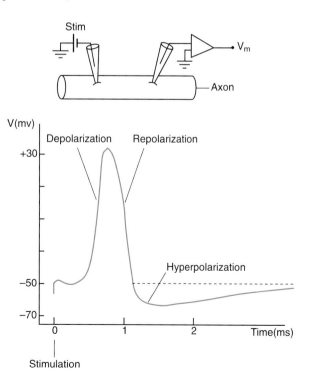

Figure 7.2   Different types of action potentials recorded in excitable cells. (a) Sodium-dependent action potential recorded intracellularly in a node of Ranvier of a rat nerve fiber. Note the absence of a hyperpolarization phase. (b–d) Sodium–calcium-dependent action potentials. Intracellular recording of the complex spike in a cerebellar Purkinje cell in response to climbing fiber stimulation: an initial Na$^+$-dependent action potential and a later larger slow potential on which are superimposed several small Ca^{2+}-dependent action potentials. The total duration of this complex spike is 5–7 ms (b). Action potential recorded from axon terminals of *Xenopus* hypothalamic neurons (these axon terminals are located in the neurohypophysis) in control conditions (top) and after adding blockers of Na$^+$ and K$^+$ channels (TTX and TEA, bottom) in order to unmask the Ca^{2+} component of the spike (this component has a larger duration due to the blockade of some of the K$^+$ channels) (c). Intracellular recording of an action potential from an acutely dissociated dog heart cell (Purkinje fiber). Trace **a** is recorded when the electrode is outside the cell and represents the trace 0 mV. Trace **b** is recorded when the electrode is inside the cell. The peak amplitude of the action potential is 75 mV and the total duration 400 ms (d). All these action potentials are recorded in response to an intracellular depolarizing pulse or to the stimulation of afferents. Note the differences in their durations. (Adapted from: a: Brismar T, 1980. Potential clamp analysis of membrane currents in rat myelinated nerve fibres, *J. Physiol.* **298**, 171–184, with permission. b–d: Coraboeuf E and Weidmann S, 1949. Potentiel de repos et potentiels d'action du muscle cardiaque, mesurés à l'aide d'électrodes internes. C. R. Soc. Biol. **143**, 1329–1331; Eccles JC, Llinas R and Sasaki K, 1966. The excitatory synaptic action of climbing fibres on the Purkinje cells of the cerebellum, *J. Physiol.* **182**, 268–296; Obaid AL, Flores R and Salzberg BM, 1989. Calcium channels that are required for secretion from intact nerve terminals of vertebrates are sensitive to ω-conotoxin and relatively insensitive to dihydropyridines, *J. Gen. Physiol.* **93**; 715–730; with permission.)

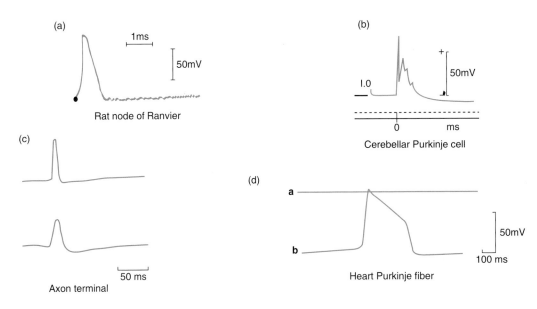

7.1.2 Na$^+$ and K$^+$ Ions Participate in the Action Potential of Nerve Fibers

The activity of the giant axon of the squid is recorded with an intracellular electrode (in current clamp, Appendix 7.1) in the presence of sea water as the external solution.

Na$^+$ ions participate in the depolarization phase of the axon potential

When the extracellular solution is changed from sea water to an Na$^+$-free solution, the amplitude and rise time of the depolarization phase of the action potential gradually and rapidly decreases until after 8 s the current pulse can no longer evoke an action potential (Figure 7.3). Moreover, tetrodotoxin (TTX), a specific blocker of voltage-gated Na$^+$ channels, completely blocks action potential initiation (Figure 7.4a, c), thus confirming a major role of Na$^+$ ions.

Figure 7.3 The action potential of the squid giant axon is abolished in an Na$^+$-free external solution. **1** Control action potential recorded in sea water; **2–8**, recordings taken at the following times after the application of a dextrose solution (Na-free solution): 2.30, 4.62, 5.86, 6.10, 7.10 and 8.11 s; **9**, recording taken 9 s after reapplication of sea water; **10**, recording taken at 90 and 150 s after reapplication of sea water; traces are superimposed. (From Hodgkin AL and Katz B, 1949. The effect of sodium ions on the electrical activity of the giant axon of the squid, *J. Physiol.* **108**, 37–77, with permission.)

Figure 7.4 Effects of tetrodotoxin (TTX) and tetraethylammonium chloride (TEA) on the action potential of the squid giant axon. (a) Control action potential. TEA application lengthens the action potential (b, left), which then has to be observed on a different time scale (b, right). TTX totally abolishes the initiation of the action potential (c). (Adapted from Tasaki I and Hagiwara S, 1957. Demonstration of two stable potential states in the squid giant axon under tetraethylammonium chloride, *J. Gen. Physiol.* **40**, 859–885, with permission.)

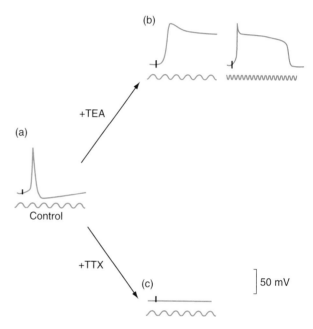

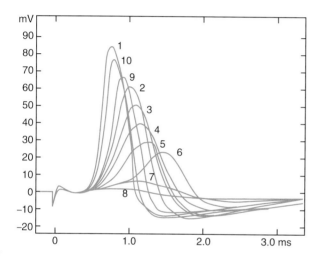

K$^+$ ions participate in the repolarization phase of the action potential

Application of tetraethylammonium chloride (TEA), a blocker of K$^+$ channels, greatly prolongs the duration of the action potential of the squid giant axon without changing the resting membrane potential. The action potential treated with TEA has an initial peak followed by a plateau (Figure 7.4a, b) and the prolongation is sometimes 100-fold or more.

7.1.3 Na$^+$-Dependent Action Potentials Are All or None and Propagate Along the Axon with the Same Amplitude

Depolarizing current pulses are applied through the intracellular recording electrode, at the level of a neuronal soma or axon. We observe that (i) to a certain level of membrane depolarization called the threshold potential, only an ohmic passive response is recorded (Figure 7.5a, right); (ii) when the membrane is depolarized just above threshold, an action potential is recorded. Then, increasing the intensity of the stimulating current pulse does not increase the amplitude of the action potential (Figure 7.5a, left). The action potential is all or none.

Once initiated, the action potential propagates along the axon with a speed varying from 1 to 100 m s^{-1} according to the type of axon. Intracellular recordings at varying distances from the soma show that the amplitude of the action potential does not attenuate: the action potential propagates without decrement (Figure 7.5b).

Figure 7.5   Properties of the Na$^+$-dependent action potential. (a) The response of the membrane to depolarizing current pulses of different amplitudes is recorded with an intracellular electrode. Upper traces are the voltage traces, bottom traces are the current traces. Above 0.2 nA an axon potential is initiated. Increasing the current pulse amplitude does not increase the action potential amplitude (left). With current pulses of smaller amplitudes, no action potential is initiated. (b) An action potential is initiated in the soma–initial segment by a depolarizing current pulse (stim). Intracellular recording electrodes inserted along the axon record the action potential at successive nodes at successive times. See text for further explanations.

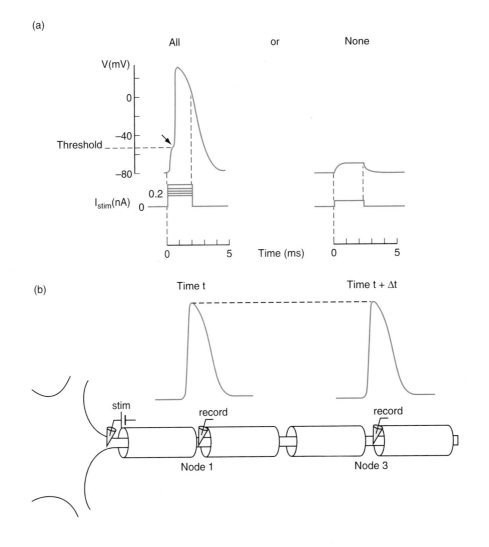

7.1.4 Questions About the Na$^+$-Dependent Action Potential

- What are the structural and functional properties of the Na$^+$ and K$^+$ channels of the action potential (Sections 7.2 and 7.3)?
- What represents the threshold potential for action potential initiation (Section 7.4)?
- Why is the action potential all or none (Section 7.4)?
- What are the mechanisms of action potential propagation (Section 7.4)?

7.2 The Depolarization Phase of Na⁺-Dependent Action Potentials Results from the Transient Entry of Na⁺ Ions Through Voltage-Gated Na⁺ Channels

7.2.1 The Na⁺ Channel Consists of a Principal Large α-Subunit with Four Internal Homologous Repeats and Auxiliary β-Subunits

The primary structures of the *Electrophorus* electroplax Na⁺ channel, the three distinct Na⁺ channels from rat brain (designated types I, II and III) and the Na⁺ channel from skeletal and heart muscle cells have been elucidated by cloning and sequence analysis of the complementary DNAs. The Na⁺ channel in all these structures is composed of a large polypeptide consisting of about 2000 amino acid residues, the principal α-subunit. It exhibits four homologous internal repeats (I to IV) each of which has six putative membrane-spanning segments (S1 to S6) (Figures 5.9 and 7.6). The four homologous domains are presumably oriented in a pseudosymmetric fashion across the membrane in order to form a central pore (see Figure 5.5).

Each homology unit contains a unique segment, the S4 segment, with positively charged residues: an arginine or a lysine residue at every third position with mostly non-polar residues intervening between the basic residues (see Figure 7.15a). The structure of the S4 segment is strikingly well conserved in all the types of Na⁺ channels analysed so far. It has been proposed that the positive charges in this segment represent the voltage sensor (see Section 7.2.7).

The brain Na⁺ channels have two auxiliary subunits designated β1 and β2. They are small proteins of about 200 amino acid residues, with a substantial N-terminal extracellular domain, a single putative membrane-spanning segment and a small C-terminal intracellular domain (Figure 7.6). The β2-subunit is covalently attached to the α-subunit by disulfide linkage, whereas the β1-subunit is non-covalently associated. The Na⁺ channel from skeletal muscle sarcolemma contains a non-covalently associated β-subunit similar to brain β1.

The α-subunit mRNA isolated from rat brain or the α-subunit RNAs transcribed from cloned cDNAs from rat brain are sufficient to direct the synthesis of functional Na⁺ channels when injected into oocytes. These results establish that the protein structures necessary for voltage gating and ion conductance are contained within the α-subunit itself. However, the properties of these channels are not identical to native Na⁺ channels and it has been shown that the auxiliary β-subunits play a role in the targeting and stabilization of the α-subunit in the plasma membrane, its sensitivity to voltage and rate of inactivation.

7.2.2 Membrane Depolarization Favors Conformational Change of the Na⁺ Channel Towards the Open State: Then the Na⁺ Channel Quickly Inactivates

The function of the Na⁺ channel is to transduce *rapidly* membrane depolarization into an entry of Na⁺ ions.

The activity of a single Na⁺ channel was first recorded by Sigworth and Neher in 1980 from rat muscle cells with the patch clamp technique (cell-attached patch, Appendix 7.3). It must be first explained that the experimenter does not know before recording it, which type of channel(s) is in the patch of membrane isolated under the tip of the pipette. He or she can only increase the chance of recording a Na⁺ channel, for example, by studying a membrane where this type of channel is frequently expressed and by pharmacologically blocking the other types of channels that could be activated together with the Na⁺ channels (voltage-gated K⁺ channels are blocked by TEA). The recorded channel is then identified by its voltage dependence, reversal potential, unitary conductance, ionic permeability, mean open time, etc. Finally, the number of Na⁺ channels in the patch of membrane cannot be predicted. Even when pipettes with small tips are used, the probability of recording more than one channel can be high because of the type of membrane patched. For this reason, very few recordings of single native Na⁺ channels have been performed (the number of Na⁺ channels in a patch is known from recordings where the membrane is strongly depolarized in order to increase to a maximum the probability of opening the voltage-gated channels present in the patch) (see Appendix 7.3).

Voltage-gated Na⁺ channels of the skeletal muscle fiber

A series of recordings obtained from a single Na⁺ channel in response to a 40 mV depolarizing step

Figure 7.6 Putative transmembrane organization of the α and β subunits of the voltage-gated Na⁺ channel. (a) Cylinders represent putative membrane-spanning segments, ψ sites of probable N-linked glycosylation and P sites of demonstrated protein phosphorylation. (b) Each of the four domains has a region linking segments S5 and S6 that forms a pore loop (upper trace). Diagram of a voltage-activated channel arranged to form a central pore (lower trace). Pore loops enter into the pore to form an active site where ion selectivity occurs (one quarter of the channel is omitted). (a: From Isom LL, De Jongh KS and Caterall WA, 1994. Auxiliary subunits of voltage-gated ion channels, *Neuron* **12**, 1183–1194, with permission. b: Adapted from MacKinnon R, 1995. Pore loops: an emerging theme in ion channel structure, *Neuron* **14**, 889–892, with permission.)

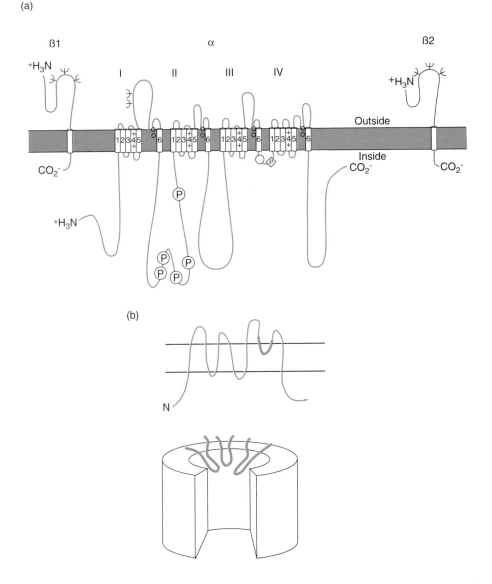

given every second is shown in Figure 7.7a, c. The holding potential is around −70 mV (remember that in the cell-attached patch, the membrane potential can only be estimated). A physiological extracellular concentration of Na⁺ ions is present in the pipette.

At holding potential, no variations in the current traces are recorded. After the onset of the depolarizing step, current pulses of varying durations but of the

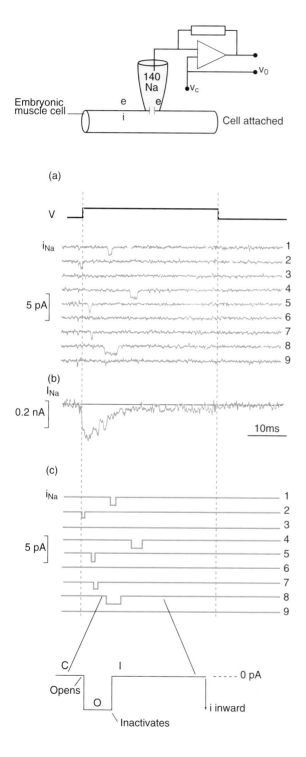

(a)

(b)

(c)

Figure 7.7 Single Na+ channel openings in response to a depolarizing step (muscle cell). The activity of the Na+ channel is recorded in patch clamp (cell-attached patch) from an embryonic muscle cell. (a) Nine successive recordings of single channel openings (i_{Na}) in response to a 40 mV depolarizing pulse (V trace) given at 1 s intervals from a holding potential 10 mV more hyperpolarized than the resting membrane potential. (b): Averaged inward Na+ current from 300 elementary Na+ currents as in (a). (c) The same recordings as in (a) are redrawn in order to explain more clearly the different states of the channel. On the bottom line one opening is enlarged. C, closed state; O, open state; I, inactivated state. The solution bathing the extracellular side of the patch or intrapipette solution contains (in mM): 140 NaCl, 1.4 KCl, 2.0 MgCl$_2$, 1 CaCl$_2$ and 20 HEPES at pH 7.4. TEA 5 mM is added to block K+ channels and bungarotoxin to block acetylcholine receptors. (Adapted from Sigworth FJ and Neher E, 1980. Single Na+ channel currents observed in rat muscle cells, *Nature* **287**, 447–449, with permission.)

same amplitude are recorded (lines 1, 2, 4, 5, 7 and 8) or not recorded (lines 3, 6 and 9). It means that six times out of nine, the Na+ channel has opened in response to the depolarization. The Na+ current has a rectangular shape and is downward. By convention, inward currents of + ions are represented as downward (inward means that + ions enter the cell). The histogram of the Na+ current amplitudes recorded in response to a 40 mV depolarizing step gives a mean amplitude for i_{Na} of around −1.6 pA (Appendix 7.3). It is interesting to note that once the channel has opened, there is a low probability that it will reopen during the depolarization period. Moreover, even when the channel does not open at the beginning of the step, the frequency of appearance of Na+ currents later in the depolarization is very low, i.e. the Na+ channel inactivates.

Rat brain Na+ channels

The rat brain Na+ channel has been described in cerebellar Purkinje cells in culture. Each trace of Figure 7.8a, c shows the unitary Na+ currents (i_{Na}) recorded during a 20 ms membrane depolarization to −40 mV test potential from a holding potential of −90 mV. Rectangular inward currents occur most frequently at the beginning of the depolarizing step but can also be found at later times (Figure 7.8a, line 2). The histogram of the Na⁺ current amplitudes recorded at −40 mV test potential gives a mean amplitude for i_{Na} of around −2 pA (Figure 7.8d). Events near −4 pA correspond to double openings (at least two channels are present in the patch).

The unitary current has a rectangular shape

The rectangular shape of the unitary current means that when the Na⁺ channel opens, the unitary current is nearly immediately maximal. The unitary current then stays constant: the channel stays open for a time

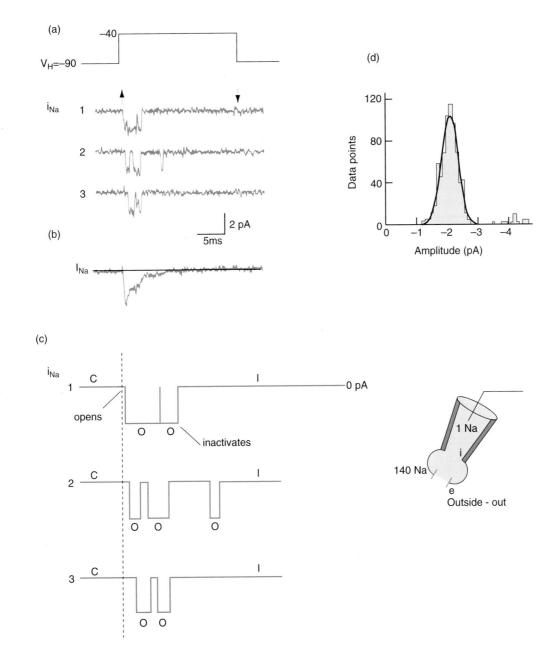

which varies; finally the unitary current goes back to 0 pA though the membrane is still depolarized. The channel may not reopen (Figure 7.7a, c) since it is in an inactivated state (Figure 7.7c, bottom trace). After being opened by a depolarization, the channel does not come back to the closed state but inactivates. In that state, the pore of the channel is closed (no Na^+ ions flow through the pore) as in the closed state but the channel cannot reopen immediately (which differs from the closed state). The inactivated channel is refractory to opening unless the membrane repolarizes to allow it to return to the closed (resting) state.

In other recordings, such as that of Figure 7.8a, c, the Na^+ channel seems to reopen once or twice before inactivating. This may result from the presence of two (as here) or more channels in the patch so that the unitary currents recorded do not correspond to the same channel. It may also result from a slower inactivation rate of the channel recorded, which in fact opens, closes, reopens and then inactivates.

The unitary current is carried by a few Na^+ ions

How many Na^+ ions are entering through a single channel? Knowing that in the preceding example, the unitary Na^+ current has a mean amplitude of -1.6 pA during 1 ms, the number of Na^+ ions flowing through one channel during 1 ms is $1.6 \times 10^{-12}/1.6 \times 10^{-19} \times 10^3 = 10\,000$ Na^+ ions (since 1 pA = 1 pC/s and the elementary charge of one electron is 1.6×10^{-19} C). This number, 10^4 ions, is negligible compared with the number of Na^+ ions in the intracellular medium: if $[Na^+]_i = 14$ mM, knowing that 1 mole represents 6×10^{23} ions, the number of Na^+ ions per liter is $6 \times 10^{23} \times 14 \times 10^{-3} = 10^{22}$ ions/l. In a neuronal cell body or a section of axon, the volume is in the order of $10^{-12} - 10^{-13}$ liter. Then the number of Na^+ ions is around $10^9 - 10^{10}$.

The Na^+ channel fluctuates between the closed, open and inactivated states

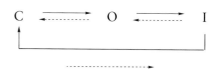

where C is the channel in the closed state, O in the open state and I in the inactivated state. Both C and I states are non-conducting states. The C to O transition is triggered by membrane depolarization. The O to I transition is due to an intrinsic property of the Na^+ channel. The I to C transition occurs when the membrane repolarizes or is already repolarized. In summary, the Na^+ channel opens when the membrane is depolarized, stays open during a mean open time of less than 1 ms and then usually inactivates.

7.2.3 The Time During Which the Na+ Channel Stays Open Varies Around an Average Value, τ_o, Called the Mean Open Time

In Figures 7.7a and 7.8a we can observe that the periods during which the channel stays open, t_o, are variable. The mean open time of the channel, τ_o, at a given potential is obtained from the frequency

Figure 7.8 Single-channel activity of a voltage-gated Na^+ channel from rat brain neurons. The activity of a Na^+ channel of a cerebellar Purkinje cell in culture is recorded in patch clamp (outside-out patch) in response to successive depolarizing steps to -40 mV from a holding potential of -90 mV. (a) The 20 ms step (upper trace) evokes rectangular inward unitary currents (i_{Na}). (b) Average current calculated from all the sweeps which had active Na^+ channels within a set of 25 depolarizations. (c) Interpretative drawing on an enlarged scale of the recordings in (a). (d) Histogram of elementary amplitudes for recordings as in (a). The continuous line corresponds to the best fit of the data to a single Gaussian distribution. C, closed state; O, open state; I, inactivated state. The solution bathing the outside face of the patch contains (in mM): 140 NaCl, 2.5 KCl, 1 $CaCl_2$, 1 $MgCl_2$, 10 HEPES. The solution bathing the inside of the patch or intrapipette solution contains (in mM): 120 CsF, 10 CsCl, 1 NaCl, 10 EGTA-Cs^+, 10 HEPES-Cs^+. Cs^+ ions are in the pipette instead of K^+ ions in order to block K^+ channels. (Adapted from Gähwiler BH and Llano I, 1989. Sodium and potassium conductances in somatic membranes of rat Purkinje cells from organotypic cerebellar cultures, *J. Physiol.* **417**; 105–122, with permission.)

Figure 7.9 The single channel current–voltage (i_{Na}–V) relation is linear. (a) The activity of the rat type II Na$^+$ channel expressed in *Xenopus* oocytes from cDNA is recorded in patch clamp (cell-attached patch). Plot of the unitary current amplitude versus test potential: each point represents the mean of 20–200 unitary current amplitudes measured at one potential (left) as shown at –32 mV (right). The relation is linear between test potentials –50 and 0 mV (holding potential = –90 mV). The slope is γ_{Na} = 19 pS. (b) Drawings of an open voltage-gated Na$^+$ channel to explain the direction and amplitude of the net flux of Na$^+$ ions at two test potentials (–40 and 0 mV). [], force due to the concentration gradient across the membrane; ⤳, force due to the electric gradient; V_m–E_{Na}, driving force. The solution bathing the extracellular side of the patch or intrapipette solution contains (in mM): 115 NaCl, 2.5 KCl, 1.8 CaCl$_2$, 10 HEPES. (a: Adapted from Stühmer W, Methfessel C, Sakmann B, Noda M and Numa S, 1987. Patch clamp characterization of sodium channels expressed from rat brain cDNA, *Eur. Biophys. J.* **14**, 131–138, with permission.)

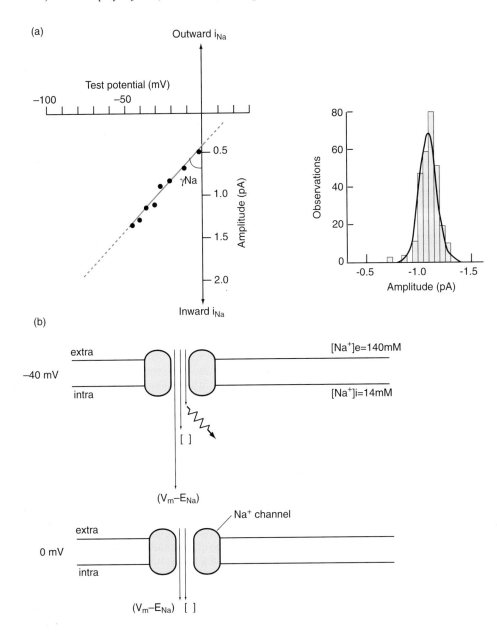

histogram of the different t_o at this potential. When this distribution can be fitted by a single exponential, its time constant provides the value of τ_o (Appendix 7.3). The functional significance of this value is the following: during a time equal to τ_o the channel has a high probability of staying open.

For example, the Na^+ channel of the skeletal muscle fiber stays open during a mean open time $\tau_o = 0.7$ ms. For the rat brain Na^+ channel of cerebellar Purkinje cells, the distribution of the durations of the unitary currents recorded at −32 mV can be fitted with a single exponential with a time constant of 0.43 ms ($\tau_o = 0.43$ ms).

7.2.4 The i_{Na}–V Relation is Linear: the Na^+ Channel has a Constant Unitary Conductance γ_{Na}

When the activity of a single Na^+ channel is now recorded at different test potentials, we observe that the amplitude of the inward unitary current diminishes as the membrane is further and further depolarized (see Figure 7.10a). In other words, the net entry of Na^+ ions through a single channel diminishes as the membrane depolarizes. The i_{Na}–V relation is obtained by plotting the amplitude of the unitary current (i_{Na}) versus membrane potential (V_m). It is linear between −50 mV and 0 mV (Figure 7.9a). For membrane potentials more hyperpolarized than −50 mV, there are no values of i_{Na} since the channel rarely opens or does not open at all. Quantitative data for potentials more depolarized than 0 mV are not available.

The critical point of the current–voltage relation is the membrane potential for which the current = 0 pA, i.e. the reversal potential of the current (E_{rev}). If only Na^+ ions flow through the Na^+ channel, the reversal potential, E_{rev}, is equal to E_{Na}. From −50 mV to E_{rev}, i_{Na} is inward and its amplitude decreases. This results from the decrease of the Na^+ driving force ($V_m - E_{Na}$) as the membrane approaches the reversal potential for Na^+ ions. For membrane potentials more depolarized than E_{rev}, i_{Na} is now outward. Above E_{rev}, the amplitude of the outward Na^+ current increases as the driving force for the exit of Na^+ ions increases.

The linear i_{Na}–V relation is described by the equation $i_{Na} = \gamma_{Na} (V_m - E_{Na})$, where V_m is the test potential, E_{Na} is the reversal potential of the Na^+ current, and γ_{Na} is the conductance of a single Na^+ channel (unitary conductance). The value of γ_{Na} is given by the slope of the linear i_{Na}–V curve. It has a constant value at any given membrane potential. This value varies between 5 and 18 pS depending on the preparation.

7.2.5 The Probability of the Na^+ Channel Being in the Open State Increases with Depolarization to a Maximal Level

An important observation at the single channel level is that the more the membrane is depolarized, the higher is the probability that the Na^+ channel will open. This observation can be made from two types of experiments:

- The activity of a single Na^+ channel is recorded in patch clamp (cell-attached patch). Each depolarizing step is repeated several times and the number of times the Na^+ channel opens is observed (Figure 7.10a). With depolarizing steps to −70 mV from a holding potential of −120 mV, the channel very rarely opens and if it does, the time spent in the open state is very short. In contrast, with depolarizing steps to −40 mV, the Na^+ channels open for each trial.
- The activity of 2–3 Na^+ channels is recorded in patch clamp (cell-attached patch). In response to depolarizing steps of small amplitude, Na^+ channels do not open or only one Na^+ channel opens at a time. With larger depolarizing steps, the overlapping currents of 2–3 Na^+ channels can be observed, meaning that 2–3 Na^+ channels open with close delays in response to the step (not shown).

From the recordings of Figure 7.10a, we can observe that the probability of the Na^+ channel being in the open state varies with the value of the test potential. It also varies with time during the depolarizing step: openings occur more frequently at the beginning of the step. The open probability of Na^+ channels is voltage- and time-dependent. By averaging a large number of records obtained at each test potential, the open probability (p_t) of the Na^+ channel recorded can be obtained at each time t of the step (Figure 7.10b). We observe from these curves that after 4–6 ms the probability of the Na^+ channel being in the open state is very low, even with large depolarizing steps: the Na^+ channel inactivates in 4–6 ms.

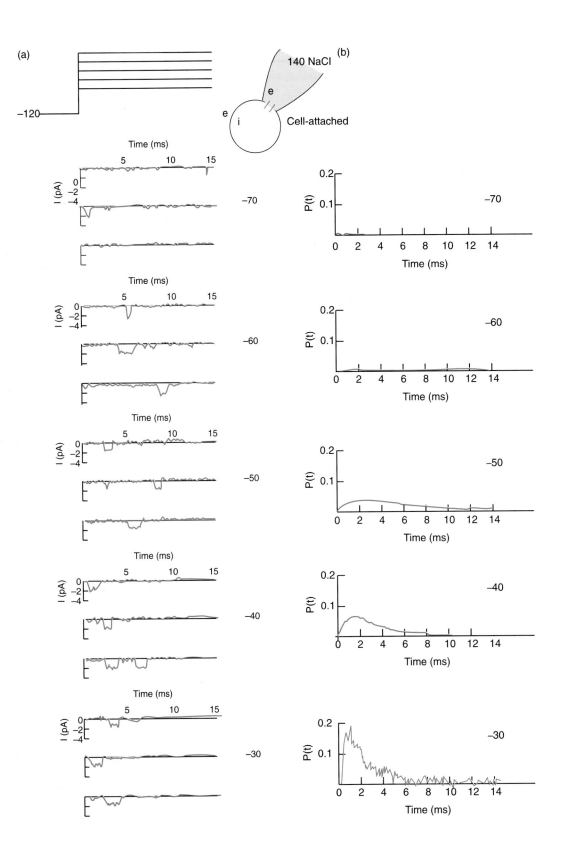

When we compare now the open probabilities at the different test potentials, we observe that the probability of the Na$^+$ channel being in the open state at time $t = 2$ ms increases with the amplitude of the depolarizing step.

7.2.6 The Macroscopic Na$^+$ Current (I_{Na}) has a Steep Voltage Dependence of Activation and Inactivates Within a Few Milliseconds

The macroscopic Na$^+$ current, I_{Na}, is the sum of the unitary currents, i_{Na}, flowing through all the open Na$^+$ channels of the recorded membrane

At the axon initial segment or at nodes of Ranvier, there is a number of N Na$^+$ channels that can be activated. We have seen that the unitary Na$^+$ current flowing through a single Na$^+$ channel has a rectangular shape. What is the time course of the macroscopic Na$^+$ current, I_{Na}?

If we assume that the Na$^+$ channels in one cell are identical and function independently, the sum of many recordings from the same Na$^+$ channel should show the same properties as the macroscopic Na$^+$ current measured from thousands of channels with the voltage clamp technique. In Figure 7.7b, an average of 300 unitary Na$^+$ currents elicited by a 40 mV depolarizing pulse is shown. For a given potential, the 'averaged' inward Na$^+$ current has a fast rising phase and presents a peak at the time $t = 1.5$ ms. The peak corresponds to the time when the Na$^+$ channel more often opens at each trial. Then the averaged current decays with time because the Na$^+$ channel has a low probability of being in the open state later in the step (owing to the inactivation of the Na$^+$ channel). At each trial, the Na$^+$ channel does not inactivate exactly at the

same time which explains the progressive decay of the averaged macroscopic Na$^+$ current. A similar averaged Na$^+$ current is shown in Figure 7.8b. The averaged current does not have a rectangular shape because the Na$^+$ channel does not open with the same delay and does not inactivate at the same time at each trial.

The *averaged* macroscopic Na$^+$ current has a similar time course to the *recorded* macroscopic Na$^+$ current from the same type of cell at the same potential. However, the averaged current from 300 Na$^+$ channels still presents some angles in its time course. In contrast, the macroscopic recorded Na$^+$ current is smooth. The more numerous are the Na$^+$ channels opened by the depolarizing step, the smoother is the Na$^+$ current. The value of I_{Na} at each time t at a given potential is:

$$I_{Ka} = N \times p_{(o)} \times i_{Ka}$$

where N is the number of Na$^+$ channels in the recorded membrane and $p_{(t)}$ is the open probability at time t of the Na$^+$ channel; it depends on the membrane potential and on the channel opening and inactivating rate constants. i_{Na} is the unitary Na$^+$ current and $Np_{(t)}$ is the number of Na$^+$ channels open at time t.

The I_{Na}–V relation has a bell-shape though the i_{Na}–V relation is linear

We have seen that the amplitude of the unitary Na$^+$ current decreases linearly with depolarization (see Figure 7.9a). In contrast, the I_{Na}–V relation is not linear. The macroscopic Na$^+$ current is recorded from a myelinated rabbit nerve with the double electrode

Figure 7.10 The open probability of the voltage-gated Na$^+$ channel is voltage- and time-dependent. Single Na$^+$ channel activity is recorded in a mammalian neuroblastoma cell in patch clamp (cell-attached patch). (a) In response to a depolarizing step to the indicated potentials from a holding potential of −120 mV, unitary inward currents are recorded. (b) Ensemble of averages of single-channel openings at the indicated voltages; 64 to 2000 traces are averaged at each voltage to obtain the time-dependent open probability of a channel ($p_{(t)}$) in response to a depolarization. The open probability at time t is calculated according to the equation: $p_{(t)} = I_{Na(t)} / Ni_{Na}$ where $I_{Na(t)}$ is the average current at time t at a given voltage, N is the number of channels (i.e. the number of averaged recordings of single channel activity) and i_{Na} is the unitary current at a given voltage. At −30 mV the open probability is maximum. The channels inactivate in 4 ms. (Adapted from Aldrich RW and Steven CF, 1987. Voltage-dependent gating of sodium channels from mammalian neuroblastoma cells, *J. Neurosci.* 7, 418–431, with permission.)

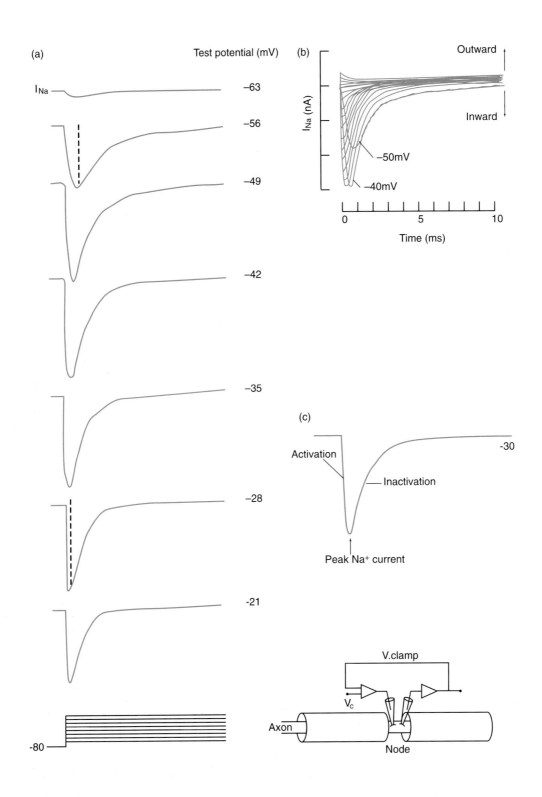

voltage clamp technique. When the amplitude of the peak Na$^+$ current is plotted against membrane potential, it has a clear bell-shape (Figures 7.11 and 7.12a). Analysis of each trace from the smallest depolarizing step to the largest shows that:

- For small steps, the peak current has a small amplitude (0.2 nA) and a slow time to peak (1 ms). At these potentials the Na$^+$ driving force is strong but the Na$^+$ channels have a low probability of opening (Figure 7.11a). Therefore, I_{Na} represents the current through a small number of open Na$^+$ channels. Moreover, the small number of activated Na$^+$ channels open with a delay since the depolarization is just *subliminal*. This explains the slow time to peak.
- As the depolarizing steps increase in amplitude (to −42/−35 mV), the amplitude of I_{Na} increases to a maximum (−3 nA) and the time to peak decreases to a minimum (0.2 ms). Larger depolarizations increase the probability of the Na$^+$ channel being in the open state and shorten the delay of opening (see Figure 7.10). Therefore, though the amplitude of i_{Na} decreases between −63 and −35 mV, the amplitude of I_{Na} increases owing to the large increase of open Na$^+$ channels.
- After this peak, the amplitude of I_{Na} decreases to 0 nA since the open probability does not increase enough to compensate for the decrease of i_{Na}. The reversal potential of I_{Na} is the same as that of i_{Na} since it depends only on the extracellular and intracellular concentrations of Na$^+$ ions.
- I_{Na} changes polarity after E_{rev}: it is now an outward current whose amplitude increases with the depolarization.

It is important to note that membrane potentials more depolarized than +20 mV are non-physiological.

Activation and inactivation curves: the threshold potential

Activation is the rate at which a macroscopic current turns on in response to a depolarizing voltage step. The Na$^+$ current is recorded in voltage clamp from a node of rabbit nerve. Depolarizing steps from −70 mV to +20 mV are applied from a holding potential of −80 mV. When the ratio of the peak current at each test potential to the maximal peak current ($I_{Na}/I_{Na\ max}$) is plotted against test potential, the activation curve of I_{Na} can be visualized. The distribution is fitted by a sigmoidal curve (Figure 7.12b). In this preparation, the threshold of Na$^+$ channel activation is −60 mV. At −40 mV, I_{Na} is already maximal ($I_{Na}/I_{Na\ max}$ = 1). This steepness of activation is a characteristic of the voltage-gated Na$^+$ channels.

Inactivation of a current is the decay of this current during a maintained depolarization. To study inactivation, the membrane is held at varying holding potentials and a depolarizing step to a fixed value is applied where I_{Na} is maximal (0 mV for example). The amplitude of the peak Na$^+$ current is plotted against the holding potential. I_{Na} begins to inactivate at −90 mV and is fully inactivated at −50 mV. Knowing that the resting membrane potential in this preparation is around −80 mV, some of the Na$^+$ channels are already inactivated at rest.

Ionic selectivity of the Na$^+$ channel

To compare the permeability of the Na$^+$ channel to several monovalent cations the macroscopic current is recorded at different membrane potentials in the presence of external Na$^+$ ions and when all the external Na$^+$ are replaced by a test cation. Lithium is as permeant as sodium but K$^+$ ions are weakly permeant

Figure 7.11 Voltage dependence of the macroscopic voltage-gated Na$^+$ current. The macroscopic voltage-gated Na$^+$ current is recorded in a node of a rabbit myelinated nerve in voltage clamp conditions. (a) Depolarizing steps from −70 mV to −21 mV from a holding potential of −80 mV evoke macroscopic Na$^+$ currents (I_{Na}) with different time courses and peak amplitudes. The test potential is on the right. Bottom trace is the voltage trace. (b) The traces in (a) are superimposed and current responses to depolarizing steps from −14 to +55 mV are added. The outward current traces are recorded when the test potential is beyond the reversal potential (+ 30 mV in this preparation). (c) I_{Na} recorded at −30 mV. The rising phase of I_{Na} corresponds to activation of the Na$^+$ channels and the decrease of I_{Na} corresponds to progressive inactivation of the open Na$^+$ channels. The extracellular solution contains (in mM): NaCl 154, CaCl$_2$ 2.2, KCl 5.6, pH 7.4. (Adapted from Chiu SY, Ritchie JM, Bogart RB and Stagg D, 1979. A quantitative description of membrane currents from a rabbit myelinated nerve, *J. Physiol.* **292**, 149–166, with permission.)

Figure 7.12   Activation–inactivation properties of the macroscopic voltage-gated Na$^+$ current. (a) The I_{Na}–V relation has a bell shape with a peak at –40 mV and a reversal potential at +30 mV (the average E_{Na} in the rabbit node is +27 mV). (b) Activation (right curve) and inactivation (left curve) curves obtained from nine different experiments. The voltage protocols used are shown in insets. In the ordinates, I/I_{max} represents the ratio of the peak Na$^+$ current (I) recorded at the tested potential of the abscissae and the maximal peak Na$^+$ current (I_{max}) recorded in this experiment. It corresponds to the peak current recorded at –40 mV in Figure 7.11. (From Chiu SY, Ritchie JM, Bogart RB and Stagg D, 1979. A quantitative description of membrane currents from a rabbit myelinated nerve, J. Physiol. 292, 149–166, with permission.)

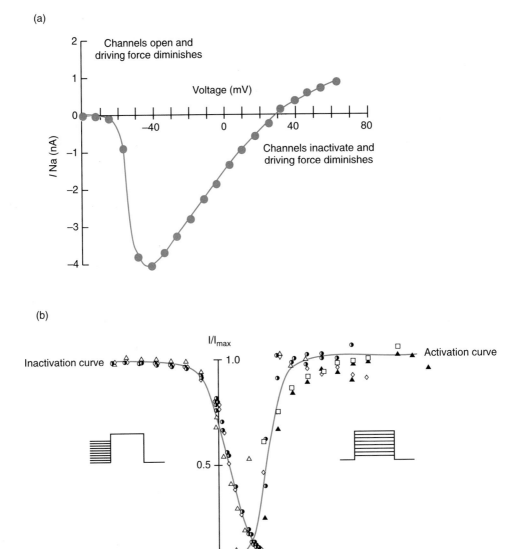

($P_K/P_{Na} = 0.048$). Therefore, Na$^+$ channels are highly selective for Na$^+$ ions and only 4% of the current is carried by K$^+$ ions (Figure 7.13).

Figure 7.13 Ionic selectivity of the Na$^+$ channel. The macroscopic Na$^+$ current is recorded with the double electrode voltage clamp technique in a mammalian skeletal muscle fiber at different test membrane potentials (from −70 to +80 mV) from a holding potential of −80 mV. (a) Inward currents in normal Na$^+$–Ringer (sodium) and in a solution where all Na$^+$ ions are replaced by K$^+$ ions (potassium). The other voltage-gated currents are blocked. (b) I–V relation of the currents recorded in (a). I is the amplitude of the peak current at each tested potential. (Adapted from Pappone PA, 1980. Voltage clamp experiments in normal and denervated mammalian skeletal muscle fibers, *J Physiol.* **306**, 377–410, with permission.)

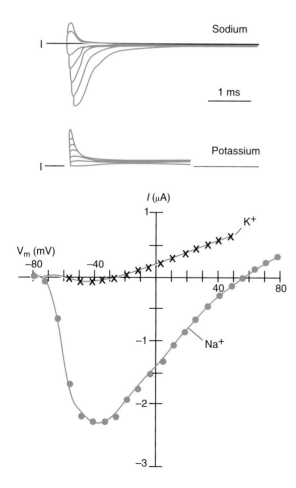

Tetrodotoxin is a selective open Na$^+$ channel blocker

A large number of biological toxins can modify the properties of the Na$^+$ channel. One of these, tetrodotoxin (TTX), which is found in the liver and ovaries of the fish tetrodon, has a binding site supposed to be located near the extracellular mouth of the pore. A single point mutation of the rat brain Na$^+$ channel type II, which changes the glutamic acid residue 387 to glutamine (E387Q) in the repeat I, renders the channel insensitive to concentrations of TTX up to tens of micromolars. *Xenopus* oocytes are injected with the wild-type mRNA or the mutant mRNA and the whole cell Na$^+$ currents are recorded with the double electrode voltage clamp technique. TTX sensitivity is assessed by perfusing TTX-containing external solutions and by measuring the peak of the whole-cell inward Na$^+$ current (the peak means the maximal amplitude of the inward Na$^+$ current measured on the I_{Na}–V relation). The dose–response curves of Figure 7.14 show that 1 μM TTX completely abolishes the wild-type Na$^+$ current, but has no effect on the mutant Na$^+$ current. The other characteristics of the Na$^+$ channel are not significantly affected, except a reduction in the amplitude of the inward current at all potentials tested. All these results suggest that the link between segments S5 and S6 in repeat I of the rat brain Na$^+$ channel is in close proximity to the channel mouth (see Figure 7.6).

7.2.7 Segment S4, the Region Between Segments S5 and S6, and the Region Between Domains III and IV Play a Significant Role in Activation, Ion Permeation and Inactivation, Respectively

The major questions about a voltage-gated ionic channel and particularly the Na$^+$ channel are the following:

- How does the channel open in response to a voltage change?
- How is the permeation pathway designed to define single channel conductance and ion selectivity?
- How does the channel inactivate?

In order to identify regions of the Na$^+$ channels involved in these functions, site-directed mutagenesis

Figure 7.14   A single mutation close to the S6 segment of repeat I completely suppresses the sensitivity of the Na$^+$ channel to TTX. A mutation of the glutamic acid residue 387 to glutamine (E387Q) is introduced in the rat Na$^+$ channel type II. *Xenopus* oocytes are injected with either the wild-type mRNA or the mutant mRNA. The macroscopic Na$^+$ currents are recorded 4–7 days later with the double electrode voltage clamp technique. Dose–response curves for the wild-type (open circles) and the mutant E387Q (filled circles) to tetrodotoxin (TTX). TTX sensitivity is determined by perfusing TTX-containing external solutions and by measuring the macroscopic peak inward current. The TTX concentration that reduces the wild-type Na$^+$ current by 50% (IC$_{50}$) is 18 nM. Data are averaged from 7–8 experiments. (From Noda M, Suzuki H, Numa S and Stühmer W, 1989. A single point mutation confers tetrodotoxin and saxitoxin insensitivity on the sodium channel II, *FEBS Lett.* 259, 213–216, with permission.)

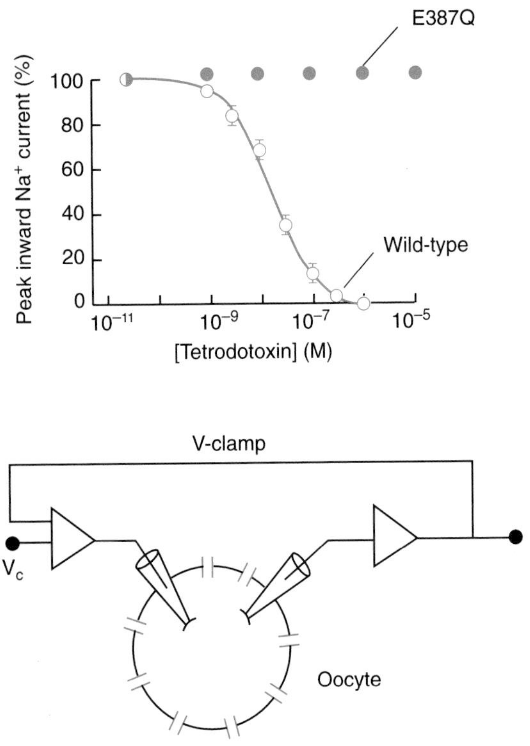

experiments were performed. The activity of each type of mutated Na$^+$ channel is analysed with patch clamp recording techniques.

The short segments between putative membrane-spanning segments S5 and S6 are membrane associated and contribute to pore formation

The Na$^+$ channels are highly selective for Na$^+$ ions. This selectivity presumably results from negatively charged amino acid residues located in the channel pore. Moreover, these amino acids must be specific to Na$^+$ channels (i.e. different from the other members of voltage-gated cationic channels such as K$^+$ and Ca^{2+} channels) to explain their weak permeability to K$^+$ or Ca^{2+} ions.

Studies using mutagenesis to alter ion channel function have shown that the region connecting the S5 and S6 segments forms part of the channel lining (see Figure 7.6). A single amino acid substitution in these regions, in repeats III and IV, alters the ion selectivity of the Na$^+$ channel to resemble that of Ca^{2+} channels. These residues would constitute part of the selectivity filter of the channel. There is now a general agreement that the selectivity filter is formed by pore loops, i.e. relatively short polypeptide segments that extend into the aqueous pore from the extracellular side of the membrane. Rather than extending completely across the lipid bilayer, a large portion of the pore loop is near the extracellular face of the channel. Only a short region extends into the membrane to form the selectivity filter. In the case of the voltage-gated Na$^+$ channel each of the four homologous domains contributes a loop to the ion conducting pore (Figure 7.6b).

The S4 segment is the voltage sensor

The S4 segments are positively charged and hydrophobic (Figure 7.15a). Moreover, the typical amino acid sequence of S4 is conserved among the different voltage-gated channels. These observations led to the suggestion that S4 segments have a transmembrane orientation and are voltage sensors. To test this proposed role, positively charged amino acid residues are replaced by neutral or negatively charged residues in the S4 segment of a rat brain Na$^+$ channel type II. The mutated channels are expressed in *Xenopus* oocytes. When more than three positive residues are mutated in the S4 segments of repeat I or II, no appreciable expression of the mutated channel is obtained. The replacement of only one arginine or lysine residue in

Figure 7.15   Effect of mutations in the S4 segment on Na⁺ current activation. Oocytes are implanted with the wild-type rat brain Na⁺ channel or with Na⁺ channels mutated on the S4 segment. The activity of a population of Na⁺ channels is recorded in patch clamp (cell-attached macropatches). (a) Amino acid sequences of segment S4 of the internal repeats I (I S4) and II (II S4) of the wild-type rat Na⁺ channel. Positively charged amino acids are boxed with solid lines and the numbers of the relevant residues are given. In the mutated channel studied here the lysine residue in position 226 is replaced by a glutamine residue (K226Q). (b) In response to step depolarizations ranging from −60 to +70 mV from a holding potential of −120 mV, a family of macroscopic Na⁺ currents is recorded for each type of Na⁺ channel. The arrow indicates the reponse to the test potential −20 mV. Note that at −20 mV the amplitude of the Na⁺ current is at its maximum for the wild-type and less than half maximum for the mutated channel. (c) Steady-state activation (right) and inactivation (left) curves for the wild-type (circles) and the mutant (diamonds) Na⁺ channels. (Adapted from Stühmer W, Conti F, Suzuki H *et al*, 1989. Structural parts involved in activation and inactivation of the sodium channel, *Nature* 339, 597–603, with permission.)

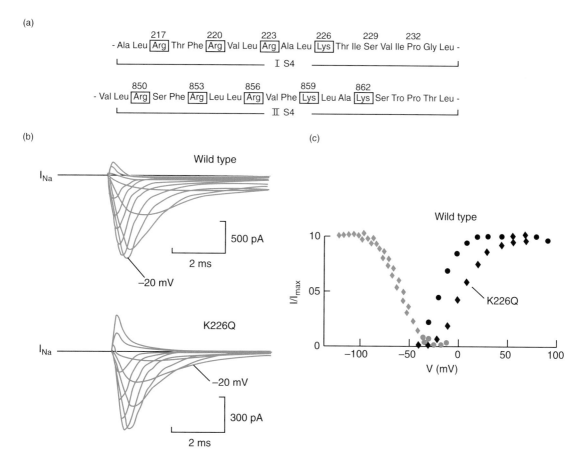

segment S4 of repeat I by a glutamine residue shifts the activation curve to more positive potentials (Figure 7.15b, c).

It is hypothesized that the positive charges in S4 form ion pairs with negative charges in other transmembrane regions, thereby stabilizing the channel in the non-conducting closed conformation. With a change in the electric field across the membrane, these ion pairs would break as the S4 charges move and new ion pairs would form to stabilize the conducting, open conformation of the channel.

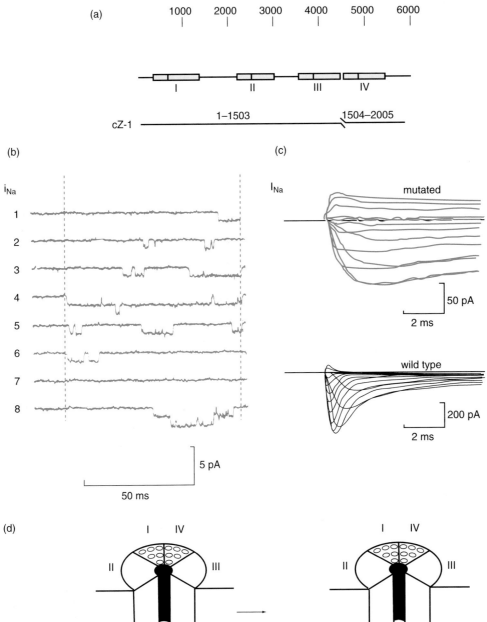

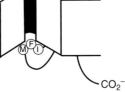

The cytoplasmic loop between domains III and IV contains the inactivation particle which, in a voltage-dependent manner, enters the mouth of the Na⁺ channel pore and inactivates the channel

The results obtained from three different types of experiments strongly suggest that the short cytoplasmic loop connecting homologous domains III and IV, L_{III-IV} loop (see Figures 7.6a and 7.16a), is involved in inactivation: (i) cytoplasmic application of endopeptidases; (ii) cytoplasmic injection of antibodies directed against a peptide sequence in the region between repeats III and IV; and (iii) cleavage of the region between repeats III and IV (Figure 7.16a, b, c); all strongly reduce or block inactivation. Moreover, in some human pathology where the Na⁺ channels poorly inactivate (as shown with single channel recordings from biopsies), this region is mutated.

Positively charged amino acid residues of this L_{III-IV} loop are not required for inactivation since only the mutation of a hydrophobic sequence, isoleucine-phenylalanine-methionine (IFM), to glutamine completely blocks inactivation. The critical residue of the IFM motif is phenylalanine since its mutation to glutamine slows inactivation 5000-fold. It is proposed that this IFM sequence is directly involved in the conformational change leading to inactivation. It would enter the mouth of the pore, thus occluding it during the process of inactivation. In order to test this hypothesis, the ability of synthetic peptides containing the IFM motif to restore fast inactivation to non-inactivating rat brain Na⁺ channels expressed in kidney carcinoma cells is examined. The intrinsic inactivation of Na⁺ channels is first made non-functional by a mutation of the IFM motif. When the recording is now performed with a patch pipette containing the synthetic peptide with an IFM motif, the non-inactivating whole cell Na⁺ current now inactivates. Since the restored inactivation has the rapid, voltage dependent time course characteristic of inactivation of the wild-type Na⁺ channels, it is proposed that the IFM motif serves as an inactivation particle (Figure 7.16d).

7.2.8 Conclusion: The Consequence of the Opening of a Population of N Na⁺ channels is a Transient Entry of Na⁺ Ions Which Depolarizes the Membrane above 0 mV

The function of the population of N Na⁺ channels at the axon initial segment or at nodes of Ranvier is to ensure a *sudden* and *brief* depolarization of the membrane above 0 mV.

Rapid activation of Na⁺ channels makes the depolarization phase sudden

In response to a depolarization to the threshold potential, the closed Na⁺ channels (Figure 7.17a) of the axon initial segment begin to open (b). The flux of Na⁺ ions through the few open Na⁺ channels depolarizes the membrane more and thus triggers the opening of other Na⁺ channels (c). In consequence, the flux of Na⁺ ions increases, depolarizes the membrane more and opens other Na⁺ channels until all the N Na⁺ channels of the segment of membrane are opened (d). In (d) the depolarization phase is at its peak. Na⁺ channels are opened by depolarization and once opened they contribute to the membrane depolarization and therefore to their activation: it is a self-maintained process.

Figure 7.16 Effects of mutations in the region between repeats III and IV on Na⁺ current inactivation. (a) Linear representation of the wild-type Na⁺ channel (upper trace) and the mutated Na⁺ channel (bottom trace). The mutation consists of a cut with an addition of four to eight residues at each end of the cut. An equimolar mixture of the two mRNAs encoding the adjacent fragments of the Na⁺ channel protein separated with a cut is injected in oocytes. (b) Single-channel recordings of the activity of the mutated Na⁺ channel in response to a depolarizing step to –20 mV from a holding potential of –100 mV. Note that late single or double openings (line 8) are often recorded. The mean open time τ_o is 5.8 ms and the elementary conductance γ_{Na} is 17.3 pS. (c) Macroscopic Na⁺ currents recorded from the mutated (upper trace) and the wild-type (bottom trace) Na⁺ channels. (d) Model for inactivation of the voltage-gated Na⁺ channels. The region linking repeats III and IV is depicted as a hinged lid that occludes the transmembrane pore of the Na⁺ channel during inactivation. (a–c: From Pappone PA, 1980. Voltage clamp experiments in normal and denervated mammalian skeletal muscle fibers, *J Physiol*, **306**, 377–410, with permission. d: From West JW, Patton DE, Scheuer T *et al*, 1992. A cluster of hydrophobic amino acid residues required for fast sodium channel inactivation, *Proc. Natl. Acad. Sci. USA* **89**, 10910–10914, with permission.)

Rapid inactivation of Na⁺ channels makes the depolarization phase brief

Once the Na⁺ channels have opened, they begin to inactivate (e). Therefore, though the membrane is depolarized, the influx of Na⁺ ions diminishes quickly. Therefore the Na⁺-dependent action potential is a spike and does not present a plateau phase. Inactivation is a very important protective mechanism since it prevents potentially toxic persistent depolarization.

Figure 7.17 Different states of voltage-gated Na⁺ channels in relation to the different phases of the Na⁺-dependent action potential. C, closed state; O, open state; I, inactivated state; →, driving force for Na⁺ ions.

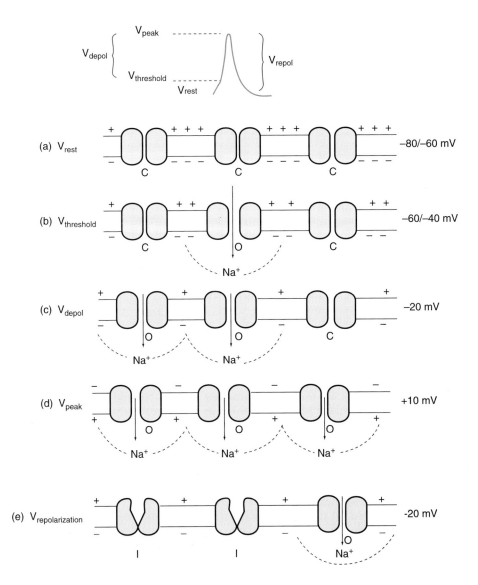

7.3 The Repolarization Phase of the Sodium-Dependent Action Potential Results from Na⁺ Channel Inactivation and Partly from K⁺ Channel Activation

The participation of a voltage-gated K⁺ current in action potential repolarization differs from one preparation to another. For example, in the squid axon the voltage-gated K⁺ current plays an important role in spike repolarization, though in mammalian peripheral nerves, this current is almost absent. However, the action potentials of the squid axon or in non-mammalian nerves have the same duration. This is because the Na⁺ current in mammalian axons inactivates two to three times faster than that of the frog axon. Moreover, the leaked K⁺ currents are important in mammalian axons (see below).

We will explain in this section the structure and activity of the voltage-gated, delayed rectifier K⁺ channels responsible for action potential repolarization in the squid or frog nerves. Then, in Section 7.4, we will explain the other mode of repolarization observed in mammalian nerves, in which the delayed rectifier current does not play a significant role.

7.3.1 The K⁺ Channel Consists of an α-Subunit with a Single Repeat and Auxiliary β-Subunits

K⁺ channels represent an extremely diverse ion channel type. They all consist of an α-subunit with a single repeat made of six putative membrane-spanning segments (S1 to S6) and a typical sequence between S5 and S6 probably tucked into the membrane (Figure 7.18). The hydropathy profile of this single repeat is similar to each of the internal repeats of the Na⁺ channel (see Figures 5.9 and 7.6), suggesting similar transmembrane topologies for these voltage-gated channels. K⁺ channels are therefore generally believed to form homotetramers in the cell membrane. As for the Na⁺ channel, the region linking segments S5 and S6 contributes substantially to the formation of the pore. In this example of a probably homotetrameric channel, four identical loops, one from each subunit, would extend into the pore to form the selectivity filter (see Figure 7.6b).

Purified neuronal K⁺ channels from mammalian

Figure 7.18 Putative transmembrane organization of the α-subunit of the delayed rectifier, voltage-gated K⁺ channel and its associated cytoplasmic β-subunit. Cylinders represent putative α-helical segments, ψ sites of probable N-linked glycosylation and P sites of demonstrated protein phosphorylation. (Adapted from Isom LL, De Jongh KS and Caterall WA, 1994. Auxiliary subunits of voltage-gated ion channels, *Neuron* **12**, 1183–1194, with permission.)

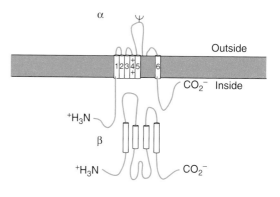

brain have auxiliary small β-subunits considered intracellularly located and associated with the α-subunit. As for Na⁺ channels, these auxiliary subunits play an important role in the inactivation properties of the K⁺ channels.

Voltage-gated K⁺ channels can be classified into two major groups based on physiological properties:

- delayed rectifiers which activate after a delay following membrane depolarization and inactivate slowly;
- A-type channels which are fast activating and fast inactivating.

The first type, the delayed rectifier K⁺ channels, plays a role in action potential repolarization. The A-types inactivate too quickly to do so. Delayed rectifiers form a family of channels with similar properties.

7.3.2 Membrane Depolarization Favors the Conformational Change of the Delayed Rectifier Channel Towards the Open State

The function of the delayed rectifier channel is to transduce, *with a delay*, membrane depolarization into an exit of K⁺ ions.

Figure 7.19 Single K$^+$ channel openings in response to a depolarizing step. The activity of a single delayed rectifier channel expressed from rat brain cDNA in a *Xenopus* oocyte is recorded in patch clamp (inside-out patch). A depolarizing step to 0 mV from a holding potential of –60 mV evokes the opening of the channel. The elementary current is outward. The channel then closes briefly and reopens several times during the depolarization, as shown in the drawing (bottom line) that interprets the current trace. Bathing solution or intracellular solution (in mM): KCl 100, EGTA 10, HEPES 10. Pipette solution or extracellular solution (in mM): NaCl 115, KCl 2, CaCl$_2$ 1.8, HEPES 10. (Adapted from Stühmer W, Stocker M, Sakman B *et al*, 1988. Potassium channels expressed from rat brain cDNA have delayed rectifier properties, *FEBS Lett.* **242**, 199–206, with permission.)

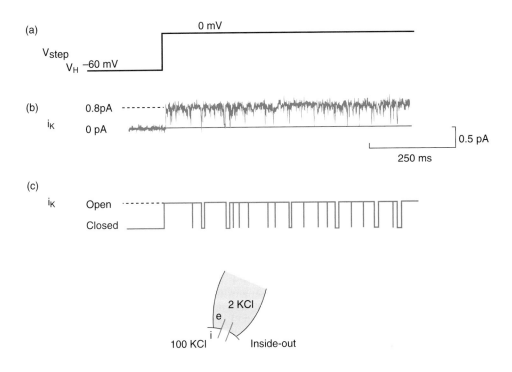

Single channel recordings were obtained by Conti and Neher in 1980 from the squid axon. We shall, however, present recordings obtained from K$^+$ channels expressed in oocytes or in mammalian cell lines from cDNA encoding a delayed rectifier channel of rat brain. Since the macroscopic currents mediated by these channels have time courses and ionic selectivity resembling those of the classical delayed outward currents described in nerve and muscle, these single channel recordings are good examples for describing the properties of a delayed rectifier current.

Figure 7.19 shows a current trace obtained from patch clamp recordings (inside-out patch) of a rat brain K$^+$ channel (RCK1) expressed in a *Xenopus* oocyte. In the presence of physiological extracellular and intracellular K$^+$ concentrations, a depolarizing voltage step to 0 mV from a holding potential of –60 mV is applied.

After the onset of the step, a rectangular pulse of elementary current, upwardly directed, appears. It means that the current is outward; K$^+$ ions leave the cell. In fact, the driving force for K$^+$ ions is outward at 0 mV.

It is immediately striking that the gating behavior of the delayed rectifier channel is different from that of the Na$^+$ channel (compare Figures 7.7a or 7.8a and 7.19). Here, the rectangular pulse of current lasts the whole depolarizing step with short interruptions during which the current goes back to 0 pA. It indicates that the delayed rectifier channel opens, closes briefly and reopens many times during the depolarizing pulse: the delayed rectifier channel does not inactivate within seconds. Another difference, is that the delay of opening of the delayed rectifier is much longer than that of the Na$^+$ channel, even for large membrane depolarizations (mean delay 4 ms in Figure 7.20a).

Figure 7.20   Characteristics of the elementary delayed rectifier current. Same experimental design as in Figure 7.19. The patch of membrane contains a single delayed rectifier channel. (a) Successive sweeps of outward current reponses to depolarizing steps from –60 mV to 0 mV (C for closed state, O for open state of the channel). (b) Averaged current from 70 elementary currents as in (a). (c) Amplitude histogram of the elementary outward currents recorded at test potential 0 mV. The mean elementary current amplitude observed most frequently is 0.8 pA. (d) Single channel current–voltage relation (i_K–V). Each point represents the mean amplitude of at least 20 determinations. The slope is γ_K = 9.3 pS. The reversal potential E_{rev} = –89 mV. (From Stühmer W, Stocker M, Sakman B *et al*, 1988. Potassium channels expressed from rat brain cDNA have delayed rectifier properties, *FEBS Lett.* **242**, 199–206, with permission.)

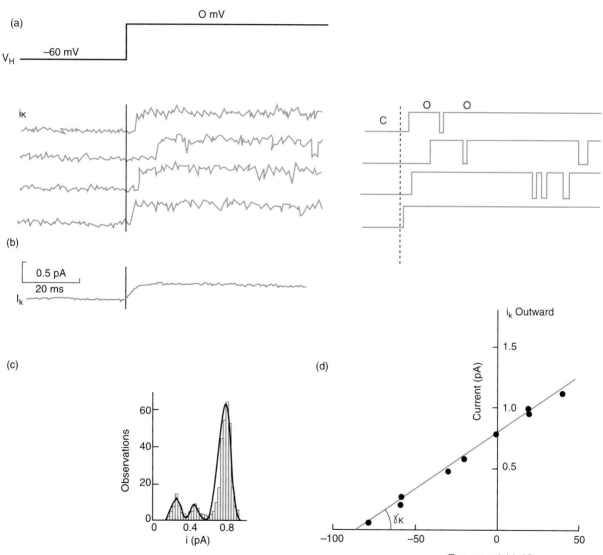

When the same depolarizing pulse is now applied every 1–2 s, we observe that the delay of channel opening is variable (1–10 ms) but gating properties are the same in all recordings: the channel opens, closes briefly and reopens during the entire depolarizing step (Figure 7.20a). Amplitude histograms collected at 0 mV membrane potential from current recordings, such as those shown in Figure 7.20a, give a mean amplitude of the unitary currents of +0.8 pA (Figure 7.20c). It means that the most frequently occurring main amplitude is +0.8 pA.

7.3.3 The Open Probability of the Delayed Rectifier Channel is Stable During a Depolarization in the Second Range

The average open time τ_o measured in the patch illustrated in Figure 7.19 is 4.6 ms. The mean closed time is 1.5 ms. As seen in Figures 7.19 and 7.20a, during a depolarizing pulse to 0 mV, the delayed rectifier channel spends much more time in the open state than in the closed state: at 0 mV its average open probability is high ($p_o = 0.76$).

In order to test if the delayed rectifier channels show some inactivation, long-lasting recordings are performed. Though no significant inactivation is apparent during test pulses in the range of seconds, during long test depolarizations (in the range of minutes), the channel shows steady-state inactivation at positive holding potentials (not shown). Therefore, in the range of seconds, the inactivation of the delayed rectifier channel can be omitted: the channel fluctuates between the closed and open states:

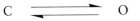

$$C \rightleftharpoons O$$

The transition from the closed (C) state to the open (O) state is triggered by membrane depolarization with a delay. The delayed rectifier channel activates in the range of milliseconds. In comparison, the Na$^+$ channel activates in the range of submilliseconds. The O to C transitions frequently happen though the membrane is still depolarized. It results also from membrane repolarization.

7.3.4 The K$^+$ Channel has a Constant Unitary Conductance γ_K

In Figure 7.21a, unitary currents are shown in response to increasing depolarizing steps from –50 to +20 mV from a holding potential of –80 mV. We observe that both the amplitude of the unitary current and the time spent by the channel in the open state increase with depolarization.

When the mean amplitude of the unitary K$^+$ current is plotted versus membrane test potential, a linear i_K–V relation is obtained (Figures 7.20d and 7.21b). This linear i_K/V relation (between –50 and +20 mV) is described by the equation $i_K = \gamma_K (V_m - E_K)$, where V_m is the membrane potential, E_K is the reversal potential of the K$^+$ current, and γ_K is the conductance of the single delayed rectifier K$^+$ channel, or unitary conductance. Linear back-extrapolation gives a reversal potential value around –90/–80 mV, a value close to E_K calculated from the Nernst equation. It means that from –80 mV to more depolarized potentials, which correspond to the physiological conditions, the K$^+$ current is outward. For more hyperpolarized potentials, the K$^+$ current is inward.

The value of γ_K is given by the slope of the linear i_K/V curve. It has a constant value at any given membrane potential. This value varies between 10 and 15 pS depending on the preparation (Figures 7.20d and 7.21b).

7.3.5 The Macroscopic Delayed Rectifier K$^+$ Current (I$_K$) has a Delayed Voltage Dependence of Activation and Inactivates Within Tens of Seconds

Whole cell currents in *Xenopus* oocytes expressing delayed rectifier channels start to activate at potentials positive to –30 mV and their amplitude is clearly voltage dependent. When unitary currents recorded from 70 successive depolarizing steps to 0 mV are average (Figure 7.20b), the macroscopic outward current obtained has a slow time to peak (4 ms) and lasts the entire depolarizing step. It closely resembles the whole cell current recorded with two electrodes voltage clamp in the same preparation (rat brain delayed rectifier channels expressed in oocytes, Figure 7.22a). The whole cell current amplitude (I_K) at steady state (once it has reached its maximal amplitude) for a given potential is:

Figure 7.21   The single channel current–voltage (i_K–V) relation is linear. Delayed rectifier K⁺ channels from rat brain are expressed in a myoblast cell line. (a) The activity of a single channel is recorded in patch clamp (cell-attached patch). Unitary currents are recorded at different test potentials (from −50 mV to +20 mV) from a holding potential at −80 mV. Bottom trace is the voltage trace. (b) i_K–V relation obtained by plotting the mean amplitude of i_K at the different test potentials tested. i_K reverses at V = −75 mV and γ_K = 14 pS. Intrapipette solution (in mM): 145 NaCl, 5.5 KCl, 2 CaCl₂, 2 MgCl₂, 10 HEPES. (Adapted from Koren G, Liman ER, Logothetis DE, Nadal-Ginard B and Hess P, 1990. Gating mechanism of a cloned potassium channel expressed in frog oocytes and mammalian cells, *Neuron* **2**, 39–51, with permission.)

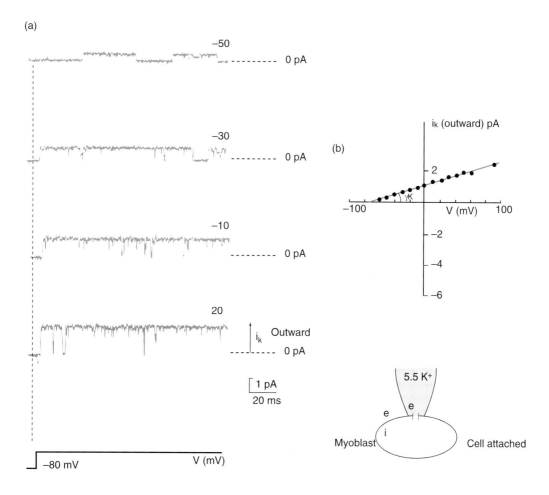

$$I_{Ka} = N \times p_{(o)} \times i_{Ka}$$

where N is the number of delayed rectifier channels in the membrane recorded, p_o the open probability at steady state and i_K the elementary current. The number of open channels Np_o increases with depolarization (to a maximal value) and so does I_K.

The I_K–V relation shows that the whole cell current varies linearly with voltage from a threshold potential which in this preparation is around −40 mV (Figure 7.22b). When the membrane is more hyperpolarized than the threshold potential, very few channels are open and I_K, is equal to 0. For membrane potentials more depolarized than the threshold potential, I_K depends on p_o and the driving force state ($V_m − E_K$) which augments with depolarization. Once p_o is maximal, I_K augments linearly with depolarization since it depends only on the driving force.

Figure 7.22   Characteristics of the macroscopic delayed rectifier K+ current. The activity of N delayed rectifier channels expressed from rat brain cDNA in oocytes is recorded in double electrode voltage clamp. (a) In
response to depolarizing steps of increasing amplitude (given every 2 s) from a holding potential of −80 mV
(upper traces), a non-inactivating outward current of increasing amplitude is recorded (lower traces). (b) The
amplitude of the current at steady state is plotted against test potential. The potential threshold for its activation is −40 mV. (c) The value of the reversal potentials of the macroscopic current is plotted against the extracellular concentration of K+ ions on a semi-logarithmic scale. The slope is −55 mV. (From Stühmer W, Stocker
M, Sakman B *et al*, 1988. Potassium channels expressed from rat brain cDNA have delayed rectifier properties, *FEBS Lett.* **242**, 199–206, with permission.)

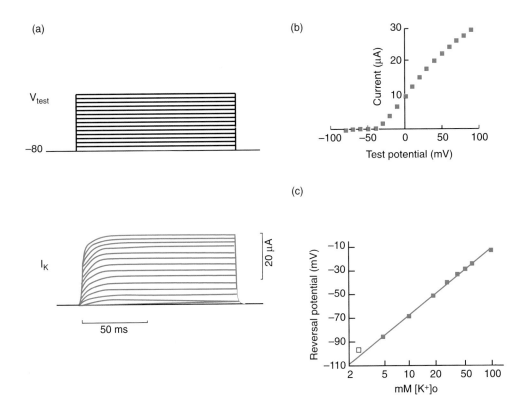

*The delayed rectifier channels are selective to
K+ ions*

Ion substitution experiments indicate that the reversal
potential of I_K depends on the external K+ ions concentration as expected for a selective K+ channel. The
reversal potential of the whole cell current is measured
as in Figure 7.22b in the presence of different external
concentrations of K+ ions. These experimental values
are plotted against the external K+ concentration,
$[K^+]_o$, on a semi-logarithmic scale. For concentrations
ranging from 2.5 (normal frog Ringer) to 100 mM, a
linear relation with a slope of 55 mV for a 10-fold

change in $[K^+]_o$ is obtained (Figure 7.22c). These data
are well fitted by the Nernst equation. It indicates that
the channel has a higher selectivity for K+ ions over
Na+ and Cl− ions.

*The delayed rectifier channels are blocked by
millimolar concentrations of tetraethylammonium
(TEA) and by Cs+ ions*

Ammonium ions can pass through most K+ channels,
whereas its quaternary derivative TEA cannot, resulting in the blockade of most of the voltage-gated K+

Figure 7.23   States of the delayed rectifier K⁺ channels in relation to the different phases of the Na⁺-dependent action potential. C, closed state; O, open state; -------, driving force for K⁺ ions.

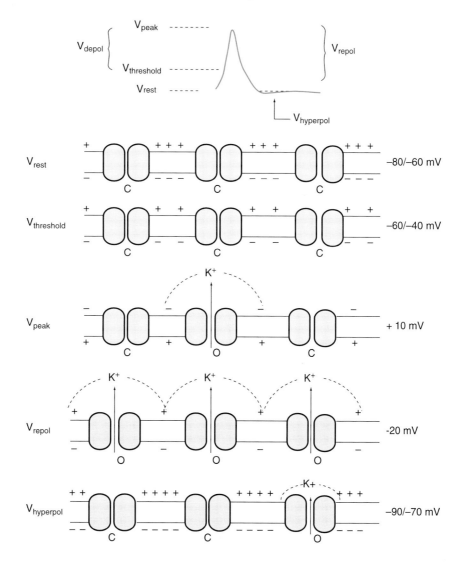

channels: TEA is a small open channel blocker. Amino acids in the carboxyl half of the region linking segments S5 and S6 (i.e. adjacent to S6) influence the sensitivity to pore blockers such as TEA.

7.3.6 Conclusion: During an Action Potential the Consequence of the Delayed Opening of K⁺ Channels is an Exit of K⁺ Ions Which Repolarizes the Membrane to Resting Potential

Owing to their delay of opening, delayed rectifier channels open when the membrane is already depolarized by the entry of Na⁺ ions through open voltage-gated Na⁺ channels (Figure 7.23). Therefore, the exit of K⁺ ions does not occur at the same time as the entry

Figure 7.24   Gating of Na⁺ and K⁺ channels during the Na⁺-dependent action potential. (a) Interpretation of the manner in which the conductances to Na⁺ (g_{Na}) and K⁺ (g_K) contribute to the action potential. (b) State of the Na⁺ and K⁺ voltage-gated channels during the course of the action potential. O, channels open; I, channels inactivate; C, channels close or are closed. (a: Adapted from Hodgkin AL and Huxley AF, 1952. A quantitative description of membrane current and its application to conduction and excitation in nerve, *J. Physiol.* **117**, 500–544, with permission.)

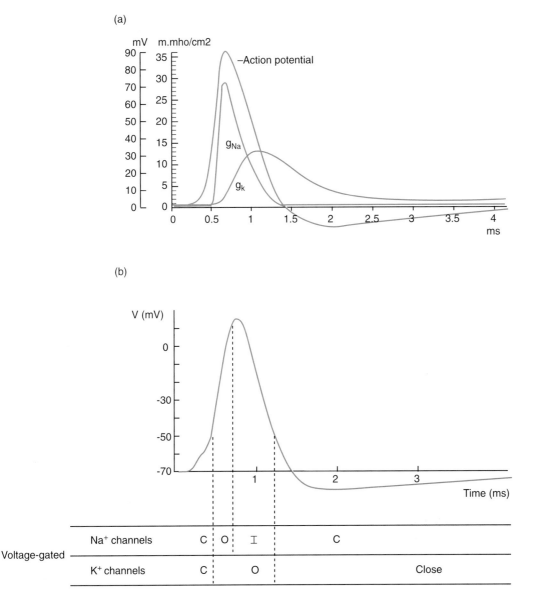

of Na⁺ ions (see also Figure 7.24). This allows the membrane to first depolarize in response to the entry of Na⁺ ions and then to repolarize as a consequence of the exit of K⁺ ions.

7.4 Sodium-Dependent Action Potentials are Initiated at the Axon Initial Segment in Response to a Membrane Depolarization and then Actively Propagate Along the Axon

Na⁺-dependent action potentials, because of their short duration (1–5 ms), are also named spikes. Na⁺ spikes, for a given cell, have a stable amplitude and duration; they all look alike, and are binary, all-or-none. The pattern of discharge (which is often different from the frequency of discharge, see Chapter 18) and not individual spikes carries significant information.

7.4.1 Summary of the Na⁺-Dependent Action Potential

The depolarization phase of Na⁺ spikes is due to the rapid time to peak inward Na⁺ current which flows into the axon initial segment or node. This depolarization is brief because the inward Na⁺ current inactivates in milliseconds (Figure 7.24b).

In the squid giant axon or frog axon, spike repolarization is associated with an outward K⁺ current (Figures 7.24 and 7.25) through delayed rectifier channels since TEA application dramatically prolongs the action potential (see Figure 7.4b). As pointed out by Hodgkin and Huxley: 'The rapid rise is due almost entirely to Na⁺ conductance, but after the peak the K⁺ conductance takes a progressively larger share until, by the beginning of the hyperpolarized phase, the Na⁺ conductance has become negligible. The tail of raised conductance that falls away gradually during the positive phase is due solely to K⁺ conductance, the small constant leak conductance being of course present throughout.'

In contrast, in rat or rabbit myelinated axons the action potential is very little affected by the application of TEA. The repolarization phase in these preparations is largely associated with a leak K⁺ current. Voltage clamp studies confirm this observation. When

Figure 7.25 The currents underlying the action potentials of the rabbit and frog nerves. (a) The action potentials are recorded intracellularly at 14°C. Bottom trace is the current of stimulation injected in order to depolarize the membrane to initiate an action potential. (b) The currents flowing through the membrane at different voltages are recorded in voltage clamp. In the rabbit node, very little outward current is recorded after the large inward Na⁺ current. In the frog nerve, a large outward K⁺ current is recorded after the large inward Na⁺ current. Leak current is subtracted from each trace and does not appear in these recordings. (Adapted from Chiu SY, Ritchie JM, Bogart RB and Stagg D, 1979. A quantitative description of membrane currents in rabbit myelinated nerve, *J. Physiol.* **292**, 149–166, with permission.)

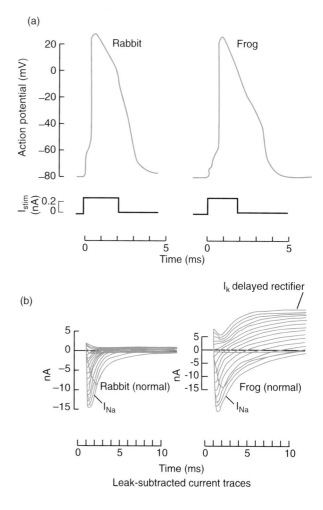

the leak current is subtracted, almost no outward current is recorded in rabbit node (Figure 7.25b).

However, squid and rabbit nerve action potentials have the same duration (Figure 7.25a). In this prepa-

Figure 7.26 TEA-resistant outward current in a mammalian nerve. The currents evoked by depolarizing steps from –60 to +60 mV from a holding potential of –80 mV are recorded in voltage clamp in a node of Ranvier of an isolated rat nerve fiber. Control inward and outward currents (a) after TTX 25 nM (b) and after TTX 25 nM and TEA 5 mM (c) are added to the extracellular solution. The outward current recorded in (c) is the leak K+ current. The delayed outward K+ current is taken as the difference between the steady state outward current in (b) and the leak current in (c). (Adapted from Brismar T, 1980. Potential clamp analysis of membrane currents in rat myelinated nerve fibres, *J. Physiol.* **298**, 171–184, with permission.)

(a) Control

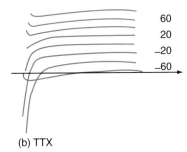

(b) TTX

(c) TTX + TEA

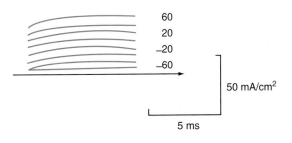

ration, the normal resting membrane potential is around –80 mV which suggests the presence of a large leak K+ current. Moreover, test depolarizations evoke large outward K+ currents insensitive to TEA (Figure 7.26). How does the action potential repolarize in such preparations? First the Na+ currents in the rabbit node inactivate two to three times faster than those in the frog node. Second, the large leak K+ current present at depolarized membrane potentials repolarizes the membrane. The amplitude of the leak K+ current augments linearly with depolarization, depending only on the K+ driving force.

7.4.2 Depolarization of the Membrane to the Threshold for Voltage-Gated Na+ Channel Activation has Two Origins

The inward current which depolarizes the membrane of the initial segment to the threshold potential for voltage-gated Na+ channel opening is either:

- a depolarizing current resulting from the activity of excitatory afferent synapses (see Chapters 9 and 11) or afferent sensory stimuli (see Chapters 12 and 15). In the first case, the synaptic currents generated at post-synaptic sites in response to synaptic activity summate, and when the resulting current is inward it can depolarize the membrane to the threshold for spike initiation (see Chapters 16, 17 and 18); in the second case, sensory stimuli are transduced in inward currents that can depolarize the membrane to the threshold for spike initiation; or
- an intrinsic regenerative depolarizing current such as, for example, in heart cells or invertebrate neurons.

7.4.3 The Site of Initiation of Na+-Dependent Action Potentials is the Axon Initial Segment

The site of initiation was suggested long ago to occur in the axon initial segment since the threshold for spike initiation was the lowest at this level. However, this has only recently been directly demonstrated with the double patch clamp technique. First the dendrites and soma belonging to the same Purkinje neuron of the cerebellum are visualized in a rat brain slice. Then the activity is recorded simultaneously at both these sites with two patch electrodes (whole-cell patches). To verify that somatic and dendritic recordings are made from the same cell, the Purkinje cell is filled with two differently colored fluorescent dyes: Cascade blue at the soma and Lucifer yellow at the dendrite. To determine the site of action potential initiation during synaptic activation of Purkinje cells, action potentials are evoked by stimulation of afferent parallel fibers which make synapses on distal dendrites of Purkinje cells (see Figures 2.6 and 2.7).

In all Purkinje cells tested, the evoked action potential recorded from the soma has a shorter delay and a greater amplitude than that recorded from a dendrite (Figure 7.27a). Moreover, the delay and the difference in amplitude between the somatic spike and the dendritic spike both augment when the distance between the two patch electrodes is increased. This suggests that the site of initiation is proximal to the soma.

Simultaneous whole cell recordings from the soma and the axon initial segment were performed to establish whether action potential initiation is somatic or axonal in origin. The action potential clearly occurs first in the axon initial segment (Figure 7.27b). These results suggest that the actual site of Na⁺-dependent action potential initiation is in the axon initial segment of Purkinje cells. Experiments carried out by Sakmann *et al* in other brain regions give the same conclusion for all the neurons tested. This may be due to a higher density of sodium channels in the membrane of the axon initial segment.

The action potential, once initiated, spreads passively back into the dendritic tree of Purkinje cells (passively means that it propagates with attenuation since it is not reinitiated in dendrites). Simultaneously it actively propagates into the axon (not shown here, see below). In some neurons, for example the pyramidal cells of the neocortex, the action potential actively propagates back into the dendrites, but this is not a general rule.

7.4.4 The Na⁺-Dependent Action Potential Actively Propagates Along the Axon to Axon Terminals

Voltage-gated Na⁺ channels are present all along the axon at a sufficient density to allow firing of axon potentials.

Figure 7.27 The Na⁺-dependent action potential is initiated in the axon initial segment in Purkinje cells of the cerebellum. The activity of a Purkinje cell is recorded simultaneously at the level of the soma and 117 µm away from the soma at the level of a dendrite (a) or 7 µm away from the soma at the level of the axon initial segment (b) with the double patch clamp technique (whole-cell patches). Afferent parallel fibers are stimulated by applying brief voltage pulses to an extracellular patch pipette. In response to the synaptic excitation an action potential is evoked in the Purkinje cell and recorded at the two different neuronal sites: soma and dendrite (a) or soma and axon (b). (Adapted from Stuart G and Hauser M, 1994. Initiation and spread of sodium action potentials in cerebellar Purkinje cells, *Neuron* **13**, 703–712, with permission.)

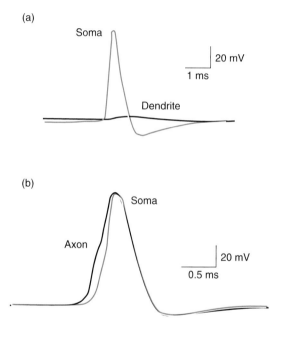

The propagation is active

Active means that the action potential is reinitiated at each node of Ranvier for a myelinated axon or at each point for a non-myelinated axon. The flow of Na⁺ ions through the open Na⁺ voltage-gated channels of the axon initial segment creates a current that spreads passively along the length of the axon to the first node of Ranvier (Figure 7.28). It depolarizes the membrane of the first node to the threshold for action potential initiation. The action potential is now at the level of the first node. The entry of Na⁺ ions at this level will depolarize the membrane of the second node and open

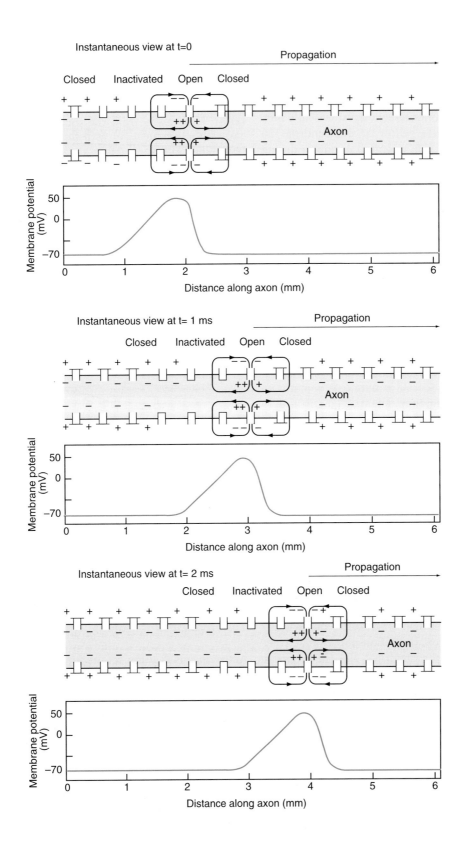

the closed Na⁺ channels. The action potential is now at the level of the second node.

The propagation is unidirectional due to Na⁺ channel inactivation

When the axon potential is, for example, at the level of the second node, the voltage-gated Na⁺ channels of the first node are in the inactivated state since they have just been activated or are still in the open state (Figure 7.28). These Na⁺ channels cannot be activated. The current lines flowing from the second node will therefore activate only the voltage-gated Na⁺ channels of the third node towards axon terminals, where the voltage-gated Na⁺ channels are in the closed state (Figure 7.28). In the axon, under physiological conditions, the action potential cannot back-propagate.

The refractory periods between two action potentials

After one action potential has been initiated, there is a period of time during which a second action potential cannot be initiated or is initiated but has a smaller amplitude (Figure 7.29): this period is called the refractory period of the membrane. It results from Na⁺ channel inactivation. Since the Na⁺ channels do not immediately recover from inactivation, they cannot reopen immediately. It means that once the preceding action potential has reached its maximum amplitude, Na⁺ channels will not reopen before a certain period of time needed for their de-inactivation (Figure 7.24b). This represents the absolute refractory period which lasts in the order of milliseconds.

Then, progressively, the Na⁺ channels will recover from inactivation and some will reopen in response to a second depolarization: this is the relative refractory period. This period finishes when all the Na⁺ channel at the initial axonal segment or at a node are de-inactivated. This actually protects the membrane from being depolarized all the time and enables the initiation of separate action potentials.

Figure 7.29 The refractory periods. A first action potential is recorded intracellularly in the squid axon *in vitro* in response to a small depolarizing stimulus (a). Then a second stimulus with an intensity six times greater than that of the first is applied 4, 5, 6 or 9 ms after. The evoked spike is either absent (b and c, only the stimulation artifact is recorded) or has a smaller amplitude (d to f). Finally, when the membrane is back in the resting state, the evoked action potential has the control amplitude (g). (Adapted from Hodgkin AL and Huxley AF, 1952. A quantitative description of membrane current and its application to conduction and excitation in nerve, *J. Physiol.* **117**, 500–544, with permission.)

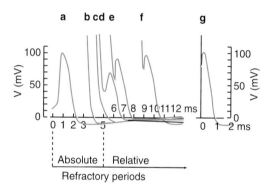

7.4.5 Are the Na⁺ and K⁺ Concentrations Changing in the Extracellular or Intracellular Media During Firing?

Over a small time scale, the external or internal Na⁺ or K⁺ concentrations are not changing during the emission of action potentials. A small number of ions are in fact flowing through the channels during an action potential and the Na–K pump re-establishes continuously the extracellular and intracellular Na⁺ and K⁺ concentrations at the expense of ATP hydrolysis.

Over a longer time scale, during high frequency trains of action potentials, the K⁺ concentration can significantly increase in the external medium. This is due to the very small volume of the extracellular medium surrounding neurons and the limited speed of the Na–K pump. This excess of K⁺ ions is buffered by glial cells which are highly permeable to K⁺ ions (see Section 3.1.3).

Figure 7.28 Active propagation of the Na⁺-dependent action potential in the axon and axon collaterals. (Scheme provided by Alberts B, Bray D, Lewis J, Roff M, Roberts K, Watson JD (1983). Molecular biology of the cell, pp. 1031. New York: Garland Publishing.

7.4.6 The Role of the Na$^+$-Dependent Action Potential is to Evoke Neurotransmitter Release

The role of the Na$^+$-dependent action potential is to propagate, without attenuation, a strong depolarization to the membrane of the axon terminals. There, this depolarization opens the high threshold voltage-gated Ca^{2+} channels. The resulting entry of Ca^{2+} ions into axon terminals triggers exocytosis and neurotransmitter release. The probability value of all these phenomena is not 1. It means that the action potential can fail to invade an axon terminal, the Ca^{2+} entry can fail to trigger exocytosis, etc. Neurotransmitter release is explained in Chapter 8.

7.4.7 Characteristics of the Na$^+$-Dependent Action Potential are Explained by the Properties of the Voltage-Gated Na$^+$ Channel

The *threshold* for Na$^+$-dependent action potential initiation results from the fact that voltage-gated Na$^+$ channels open in response to a depolarization positive to $-50/-40$ mV. The Na$^+$-dependent action potential is *all-or-none* because voltage-gated Na$^+$ channels self-activate (see Figure 7.17). It propagates *without attenuation* since the density of voltage-gated Na$^+$ channels is constant along the axon or at nodes of Ranvier. It propagates *unidirectionally* because of the rapid inactivation of voltage-gated Na$^+$ channels. The instantaneous frequency of Na$^+$-dependent action potentials is limited by the *refractory periods*, which also results from voltage-gated Na$^+$ channel inactivation.

7.5 Other Types of Action Potentials: Generalization

We first explained the Na$^+$-dependent action potential propagated by axons (Sections 7.2 to 7.4) There are two other types of action potentials (Figure 7.2): (i) the Na$^+$/Ca^{2+}-dependent action potential present in axon terminals or heart muscle cells, for example, where it is responsible for Ca^{2+} entry and an increase of intracellular Ca^{2+} concentration, a necessary prerequisite for neurotransmitter release (secretion) or muscle fibre contraction; and (ii) the Ca^{2+}-dependent action potential present in, for example, the dendrites of cerebellar Purkinje cells and in endocrine cells. In Purkinje cell dendrites, it depolarizes the membrane and thus modulates neuronal integration; in endocrine cells it provides a Ca^{2+} entry to trigger hormone secretion.

The voltage-gated Ca^{2+} channels involved in these action potentials are the high threshold Ca^{2+} channels named types L (L for long lasting), N (neither L nor transient (T)) and P (P for Purkinje cells where they have been first described). Since N and P channels show some similarities in their gating behavior, the best way to characterize these three types of channels is their selective sensitivity to toxins or dihydropyridine derivatives. L-type channels are, for example, selectively opened by Bay K 8644 and blocked by nimodipine, both 1,4-dihydropyridine compounds; N-type channels are blocked by a toxin from the marine snail *Conus geographus*, the ω-conotoxin; and P-type channels are selectively blocked by a purified polyamine fraction of the funnel-web spider (*Agelenopsis aperta*) venom (FTX) and a peptide component of the same venom, ω-agatoxin IVA (ω-Aga-IVA).

Structure of Ca^{2+} channels

The voltage-gated Ca^{2+} channels are a diverse group of multisubunit proteins. They are composed of a typical central, channel-forming α-subunit (named α_1) with four internal homologous repeats (I to IV) and different auxiliary subunits which include a β-subunit, the disulfide-linked α_2-δ-subunit. Depending on the tissue of origin, a fifth subunit may also form part of the channel complex (Figure 7.30). At present, at least six isoforms of the α_1-subunit have been cloned. Their identification as forming an L, N or P channel is still under study.

How to record the activity of Ca^{2+} channels in isolation?

To block other voltage-gated channels, different strategies can be used. In whole cell or intracellular recordings, TTX and TEA are added to the extracellular solution and K$^+$ ions are replaced by Cs$^+$ in the intra-pipette solution, in order to block voltage-gated Na$^+$ and K$^+$ channels. In cell-attached recordings the patch pipette is filled with a solution containing Ca^{2+} or Ba^{2+} ions as the charge carrier. When Ba^{2+} substi-

Figure 7.30   Putative transmembrane organization of the α_1 and auxiliary subunits of the voltage-gated Ca^{2+} channels. Cylinders represents putative membrane-spanning segments, ψ sites of probable N-linked glycosylation. (From Figure 7.6a)

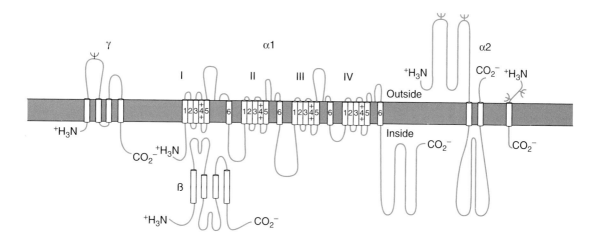

tutes for Ca^{2+} in the extracellular solution, the inward currents recorded in response to a depolarizing step are Ba^{2+} currents. Ba^{2+} is often preferred to Ca^{2+} since it carries current twice as effectively as Ca^{2+} and poorly inactivates Ca^{2+} channels (see Section 7.5.2). As a consequence, unitary Ba^{2+} currents are larger than Ca^{2+} ones and can be studied more easily.

Another challenge is to separate the various types of Ca^{2+} channels in order to record the activity of only one type (since in most of the cells they are co-expressed). These different Ca^{2+} channels are the high threshold L, N and P channels (this chapter) and the low threshold T channel (Section 17.3.2 and Appendix 17.4). By applying different holding potentials and selective agonists or antagonists, these different Ca^{2+} channels can be recorded in isolation.

7.5.1 The L, N and P-type Ca^{2+} Channels Open at Membrane Potentials Positive to −20 mV: They are High Threshold Ca^{2+} Channels

The L-type Ca^{2+} channel has a large conductance and inactivates very slowly with depolarization

The activity of single L-type Ca^{2+} channels is recorded in sensory neurons of the chick dorsal root ganglion in patch clamp (cell-attached patch with Ba^{2+} as the charge carrier). In response to a test depolarization to +20 mV from a *depolarized* holding potential (−40 to 0 mV), unitary inward Ba^{2+} currents are evoked and recorded throughout the duration of the depolarizing step (Figure 7.31a).

The voltage-dependence of activation is studied with depolarizations to various test potentials from a holding potential of −40 mV (Figure 7.32). With test depolarizations up to +10 mV, openings are rare and of short duration. Activation of the channel becomes significant at +10 mV: openings are more frequent and of longer duration. At all potentials tested, openings are distributed relatively evenly throughout the duration of the depolarizing step (Figures 7.31a and 7.32a). At −20 mV, the mean single channel amplitude of the L current (i_{CaL}) is around −2 pA. i_{CaL} amplitude diminishes linearly with depolarization: the i_{CaL}–V relation is linear between −20 and +20 mV. Between these membrane potentials, the unitary conductance, γ_{CaL}, is constant and equal to 20–25 pS in 110 mM Ba^{2+} (Figure 7.32c).

The main characteristics of L-type channels are (i) their very slow inactivation during a depolarizing step; (ii) their sensitivity to dihydropyridines; and (iii) their loss of activity in excised patches.

Bay K 8644 is a dihydropyridine compound that increases dramatically the mean open time of an L-type channel without changing its unitary conductance (Figure 7.33). It has no effect on the other Ca^{2+} channel types (see Figure 7.37). Bay K 8644 binds to a specific site on the α_1 subunit of L channels and changes the gating mode from brief openings to long-lasting openings even at weakly depolarized potentials (V_{step} = −30 mV). Other dihydropyridine derivatives such as nifedipine, nimodipine and nitrendipine selectively block L channels (see Figure 7.44).

The loss of activity of an L channel in excised patch can be observed in outside-out patches. In response to a test depolarization to +10 mV the activity of an L channel rapidly disappears (Figure 7.34). To determine the nature of the cytoplasmic constituent(s) necessary to restore the activity of the L channel, inside-out patches are performed, a configuration that allows a change of the medium bathing the intracellular side of the membrane. The activity of a single L channel is first recorded in cell-attached configuration in response to a test depolarization to 0 mV (Figure 7.35). Then the membrane is pulled out in order to obtain an inside-out patch. The L-type activity rapidly disappears and is not restored by adding ATP-Mg to the intracellular solution. In contrast, when the catalytic subunit of the cAMP-dependent protein kinase (PKA) is added, the L channel activity reappears (the catalytic subunit of PKA does not need the presence of cAMP to be active). This suggests that PKA directly phosphorylates the L channel thus allowing its activation by the depolarization. It means that, in physiological conditions, the activity of L channels requires the activation of the following cascade: the activation of adenylate cyclase by the α_s-subunit of the G_s protein, the formation of cAMP and the subsequent activation of protein kinase A. Other kinases might also play a role.

The N-type Ca^{2+} channel inactivates with depolarization in the tens of milliseconds range and has a smaller unitary conductance than the L-type channel

The activity of single N-type channels is recorded in the same preparation in patch clamp (cell-attached patch, with Ba^{2+} as the charge carrier). In contrast, to the L channels, N channels inactivate with depolarization. Therefore their activity has to be recorded in response to a test depolarization from a *hyperpolarized* holding potential (−80/−60 mV) (Figure 7.31b). At holding potentials positive to −40 mV (e.g. −20 mV, Figure 7.31a), the N channel(s) are inactivated and their activity is absent on the recordings.

N channel activity differs from that of the L channel in several aspects: (i) N channels often open in bursts and inactivate with time and voltage (see Section 7.5.2); (ii) measured at the same test potential, the mean amplitude of the N unitary current is smaller than that of L (e.g. i_{CaN} = −1.22 ± 0.03 pA and i_{CaL} = 2.07 ± 0.09 at −20 mV, Figure 7.31a, b) which makes its mean unitary conductance also smaller (γ_{CaN} = 13 pS in 110 mM Ba^{2+}, Figure 7.36b); (iii) N channels are insensitive to dihydropyridines but are selectively blocked by ω-conotoxin; and (iv) they do not need to be phosphorylated to open (Figure 7.34).

The P-type Ca^{2+} channel differs from the N channel by its pharmacology

The activity of a single P-type channel is recorded

Figure 7.31 Single channel recordings of the high threshold Ca^{2+} channels: the L, N and P channels. The activity of single L (a) and N (b) Ca^{2+} channels is recorded in patch clamp (cell-attached patches) from dorsal root ganglion cells and that of a single P channel (c) is recorded from a lipid bilayer in which a P channel isolated from cerebellum has been incorporated. All recordings are performed with Ba^{2+} (110 or 80 mM) as the charge carrier. In response to a test depolarizing step to +20 mV (a, b) or at a depolarized holding potential of −15 mV (c), unitary inward currents are recorded. Voltage traces are upper traces and the corresponding unitary current traces are the bottom traces (5–10 trials). V_H = −20 mV in (a), −80 mV in (b) and −15 mV in (c). In (a) and (b) the intrapipette solution contains (in mM): 110 $BaCl_2$, 10 HEPES and 200 µM TTX. The extracellular solution bathing the membrane outside the patch contains (in mM): 140 K aspartate, 10 K-EGTA, 10 HEPES, 1 $MgCl_2$ in order to zero the cell resting membrane potential. In (c) the solution bathing the extracellular side of the bilayer contains (in mM): 80 $BaCl_2$, 10 HEPES. The solution bathing the intracellular side of the bilayer in (c) contains (in mM): 120 CsCl, 1 $MgCl_2$, 10 HEPES. (a, b: Adapted from Nowycky MC, Fox AP and Tsien RW, 1985. Three types of neuronal calcium channel with different calcium agonist sensitivity. *Nature* **316**, 440–443, with permission. c: Adapted from Llinas R, Sugimori M, Lin JW and Cherksey B, 1989. Blocking and isolation of a calcium channel from neurons in mammals and cephalopods utilizing a toxin fraction (FTX) from funnel-web spider poison, *Proc. Natl. Acad. Sci. USA.*, **86**, 1689–1693, with permission.)

from lipid bilayers in which purified P channels from cerebellar Purkinje cells have been incorporated. Ba^{2+} ions are used as the charge carrier. The activity of the P channel is recorded at different steady holding potentials. At −15 mV, the channel opens, closes and reopens during the entire depolarization, showing little time-dependent inactivation (Figure 7.31c). The mean unitary conductance, γ_{CaP}, is 10–15 pS in

80 mM Ba^{2+}. Recordings performed in dendrites or the soma of cerebellar Purkinje cells with patch clamp techniques (cell-attached patches) gave similar values of the unitary conductance (γ_p = 9–19 pS in 110 mM Ba^{2+}), but for undetermined reasons the threshold for activation is at a more depolarized potential (−15 mV) than for isolated P channels inserted in lipid bilayers (−45 mV). When the funnel web toxin fraction (FTX)

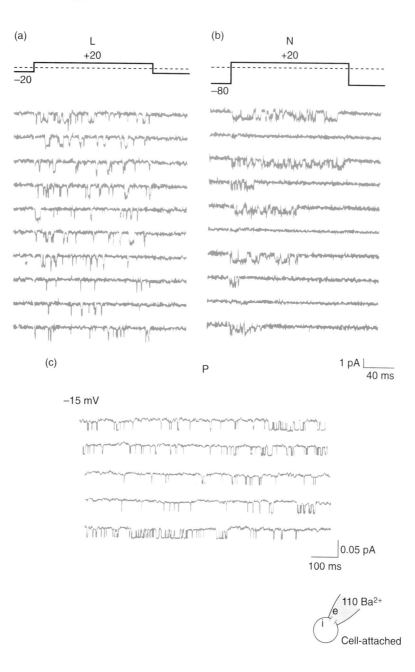

Figure 7.32   Voltage-dependence of the unitary L-type Ca²⁺ current. (a) The activity of L channels (the patch of membrane contains more than one L channel) is recorded in patch clamp (cell-attached patch) in a sensory dorsal root ganglion neuron. The patch is depolarized to −30, −10, 0, +10 and +20 mV from a holding potential of −40 mV. (b) Macroscopic current traces obtained by averaging at least 80 corresponding unitary current recordings such as those in (a). The probability of the L channels being in the open state increases with the test depolarization so that at +20 mV, openings of the 4–5 channels present in the patch overlap, leading to a sudden increase in the corresponding macroscopic current. (c) The unitary L current amplitude (i_{CaL}) is plotted against membrane potential (from −20 to +20 mV) in the absence (+, □) or presence (Δ, ◇) of Bay K8644 in the patch pipette. The amplitude of i_{CaL} decreases linearly with depolarization between −20 and +20 mV with a slope $\gamma_L = 25$ pS. The intrapipette solution contains (in mM): BaCl₂ 110, HEPES 10. The extracellular solution bathing the extracellular side of the membrane outside of the recording pipette contains (in mM): K-aspartate 140, K-EGTA 10, MgCl₂ 1, HEPES 10. A symmetric K⁺ solution is applied in order to zero the cell resting potential. (Adapted from Fox AF, Nowycky MC and Tsien RW, 1987. Single-channel recordings of three types of calcium channels in chick sensory neurons, *J. Physiol.* **394**, 173–200, with permission.)

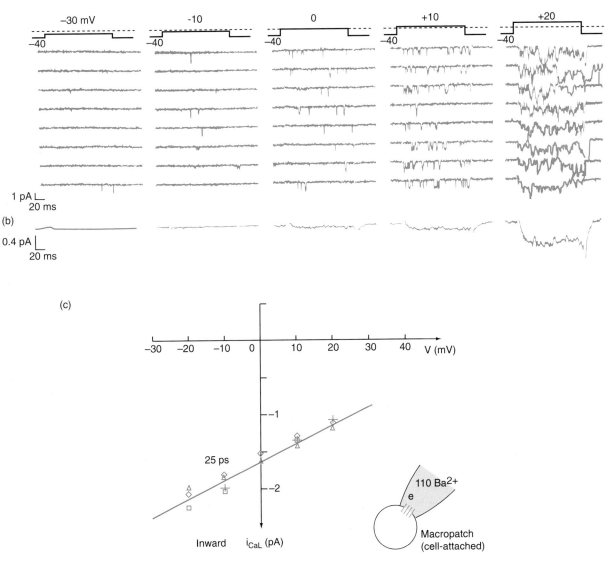

Figure 7.33 Bay K8644 promotes long-lasting openings of L-type Ca^{2+} channels. The activity of three L channels is recorded in patch clamp (cell-attached patch). Top traces: a depolarizing step to +10 mV from a holding potential of –40 mV is applied at a low frequency. Middle traces (1 to 5): five consecutive unitary current traces recorded in the absence (left) and presence (right) of 5 μM Bay K8644 in the bathing solution. Recordings are obtained from the same cell. Dashed line indicates the mean amplitude of the unitary current (–1.28 pA) which is unchanged in the presence of Bay K. Bottom traces: macroscopic current traces obtained by averaging at least 80 corresponding unitary current recordings. (a: Adapted from Fox AP, Nowycky MC and Tsien RW, 1987. Single channel recordings of three types of calcium channels in chick sensory neurones, *J. Physiol.* **394**, 173–200, with permission.)

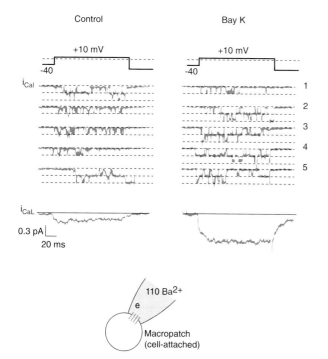

7.5.2 Macroscopic L, N and P-type Ca^{2+} Currents Activate at a High Threshold and Inactivate with Different Time Courses

The macroscopic L, N and P-type Ca^{2+} currents (I_{Ca}), at time t during a depolarizing voltage step, are equal to: $I_{Ca} = Np_t i_{Ca}$ where N is number of L, N or P channels in the membrane, p_t is their probability of being open at time t during the depolarizing step, Np_t is the number of open channels at time t during the depolarizing step and i_{Ca} is the unitary L, N or P current. At steady state, $I_{Ca} = Np_o i_{Ca}$, where p_o is the probability of the channel being open at steady state.

The I–V relations for L, N and P-type Ca^{2+} currents have a bell shape with a peak amplitude at positive potentials

The *I–V* relation of the different types of high threshold Ca^{2+} currents is studied in whole cell recordings in the presence of external Ca^{2+} as the charge carrier. To separate the L, N and P currents, specific blockers are added to the external medium or the membrane potential is clamped at different holding potentials. With this last procedure, the L current can be separated from other Ca^{2+} currents since it can be evoked from depolarized holding potentials. As shown in Figures 7.32b and 7.37, the L and N currents averaged from the corresponding unitary currents recorded in 110 mM Ba^{2+} clearly differ in their time course. The averaged N current decays to zero level in 40 ms while the averaged L current remains constant during the 120 ms depolarizing step to +10 mV. As already observed (Figure 7.31a, b), by holding the membrane at a depolarized potential, the N current inactivates and the L current can be studied in isolation.

The macroscopic N- and L-type Ca^{2+} currents are studied in spinal motoneurons of the chick in patch clamp (whole cell patch) in the presence of Na$^+$ and K$^+$ channel blockers and in the presence of a T-type Ca^{2+} channel blocker (see Appendix 17.4, P channels are almost absent). In response to a depolarizing voltage step to +20 mV from a holding potential of –80 mV, a mixed N and L whole cell current is recorded (Figure 7.38a). When the holding potential is depolarized to 0 mV, a voltage step to +20 mV now only evokes the L current (Figure 7.38b). The difference current obtained by subtracting the L current

is added to the recording patch pipette (the intra-pipette solution bathes the extracellular side of the patch), only rare high threshold unitary currents are recorded from Purkinje cell dendrites or soma at all potentials tested (Bay K 8644 or ω-conotoxin have no effect). These results suggest that the P channel is the predominant high threshold Ca^{2+} channel expressed by Purkinje cells. They also show that the use of selective toxins allows the differentiation between P, N and L channels.

Figure 7.34 In excised patches, the activity of L channels disappears within minutes. The activity of an L and N channel is recorded in patch clamp (outside-out patches from a pituitary cell line in culture) in response to a depolarizing pulse to +10 mV from a holding potential of –80 mV. (Left) One minute after forming the excised patch, the two types of channels open one at a time or their openings overlap (line 3, *). Five minutes after, only the activity of the N-type is still present. The activity of the L-type will not reappear spontaneously. The extracellular solution contains (in mM): BaCl, 90, TEACl 15, TTX 2 × 10⁻³, HEPES 10. The intrapipette solution contains (in mM): CsCl 120, HEPES 40. (Adapted from Armstrong D and Eckert R, 1987. Voltage-activated calcium channels that must be phosphorylated to respond to membrane depolarization, *Proc. Natl. Acad. Sci. USA.* **84**, 2518–2522, with permission.)

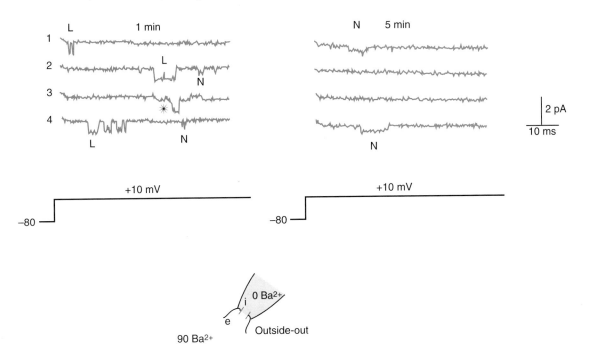

from the mixed N and L current gives the N current (Figure 7.38c). The I–V relations of these two Ca^{2+} currents have a bell-shape with a peak around +20 mV (Figure 7.38d, e). For comparison the peak amplitude of the macroscopic Na^+ current is around –40 mV (see Figure 7.12a).

The macroscopic P-type Ca^{2+} current is studied in cerebellar Purkinje cells. These neurons express T, P and few L-type Ca^{2+} channels. In presence of Na^+ and K^+ channel blockers and by choosing a holding potential where the low threshold T current is inactivated, the macroscopic P current can be studied. The I_{CaP}–V relation has a bell-shape. The maximal amplitude is recorded around –10 mV (Figure 7.39).

The bell-shape of all the I_{Ca}–V relations is explained by the gating properties of the Ca^{2+} channels and the

driving force for Ca^{2+} ions. The peak amplitude of I_{Ca} increases from the threshold potential to a maximal amplitude (Figures 7.38d, e, 7.39b and 7.40a) as a result of two opposite factors: the probability of opening which strongly increases with depolarization (Figure 7.40b) and the driving force for Ca^{2+} which linearly decreases with depolarization (i_{Ca} linearly diminishes, see Figure 7.32c). After a maximum, the peak amplitude of I_{Ca} decreases owing to the progressive decrease of the driving force for Ca^{2+} ions and the increase of the number of inactivated channels. Above +30/+40 mV, the probability of opening (p_o) no longer plays a role since it is maximal (Figure 7.40b). I_{Ca} reverses polarity between +50 mV and +100 mV, depending on the preparation studied. This value is well below the theoretical E_{Ca}.

Figure 7.35 Phosphorylation reverses the loss of activity of the L channels in an inside-out patch. The activity of an L-type channel is recorded in patch clamp (inside-out patch from a pituitary cell line in culture) in response to a depolarizing pulse to 0 mV from a holding potential of −40 mV. The horizontal traces are the unitary current traces and the vertical histogram represents the average number of channel openings per trace, determined over 30 s intervals and plotted versus time of the experiment (0–40 min). After 5 min of recording in the cell-attached configuration, the activity of the channel is recorded in the inside-out configuration. See text for further explanations. The intra-pipette solution contains (in mM): BaCl, 90, TEACl 15, TTX 2×10^{-3}, HEPES 10. The solution bathing the intracellular side of the patch contains (in mM): CsCl 120, HEPES 40. (From Armstrong D and Eckert R, 1987. Voltage-activated calcium channels that must be phosphorylated to respond to membrane depolarization, *Proc. Natl Acad. Sci. USA* **84**, 2518–2522, with permission.)

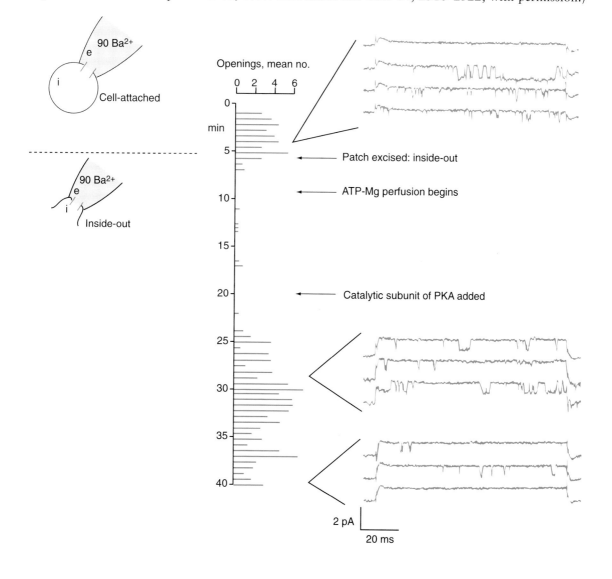

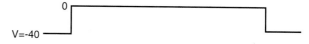

Figure 7.36 Voltage-dependence of the unitary N current, i_{CaN}. (a) The activity of an N channel is recorded in patch clamp (cell-attached patch) in a granule cell of the hippocampus. The patch is depolarized to –25, –20 and –10 mV from a holding potential of –80 mV. The amplitude of the unitary current at these voltages is indicated at the end of each recording. (b) The unitary N current amplitude (i_{CaN}) is plotted against membrane potential (from –60 to +20 mV). The amplitude of i_{CaN} decreases linearly with depolarization between –60 and +20 mV with a slope γ_N = 14 pS (n = 14 patches). (Adapted from Fisher RE, Gray R and Johnston D, 1990. Properties and distribution of single voltage-gated calcium channels in adult hippocampal neurons, *J. Neurophysiol.* **64**, 91–104, with permission.)

Figure 7.37 Averaged N and L-type Ca^{2+} currents. Single channel N current averages (top traces) and L current averages (bottom traces) from cell-attached recordings of dorsal root ganglion cells with Ba^{2+} as the charge carrier (see Figure 7.31a, b). Currents are averaged before (left) and after (right) exposure to 5 µM Bay K8644. Voltage steps from –80 mV to +10 mV (top traces) and from –40 to +10 mV (bottom traces). (From Nowycky MC, Fox AP and Tsien RW, 1985. Three types of neuronal calcium channel with different calcium agonist sensitivity, *Nature* **316**, 440–443, with permission.)

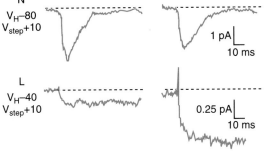

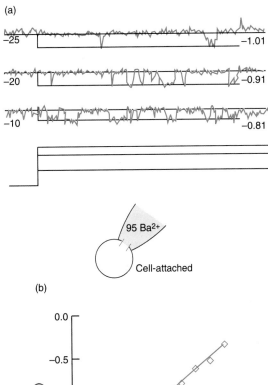

This discrepancy is partly due to the strong asymmetrical concentrations of Ca^{2+} ions. To measure the reversal potential of I_{Ca}, the outward current through Ca^{2+} channels must be measured. This outward current, caused by the extremely small intracellular concentration of Ca^{2+} ions, is carried by Ca^{2+} ions but also by internal K^+ ions, which are around 10^6 times more concentrated than internal Ca^{2+} ions. This permeability of Ca^{2+} channels to K^+ ions 'pulls down' the reversal potential of I_{Ca} towards E_K.

Activation–inactivation properties

Activation properties are analyzed by recording the macroscopic L, N or P currents in response to increasing test depolarizations from a fixed hyperpolarized holding potential (–80 mV, Figures 7.41b, 7.42b and 7.43b). In dorsal ganglion neurons, the L and N currents are half activated around 0 mV (Figures 7.41c and 7.42c) while in Purkinje cells the P current is half activated around –20 mV (Figure 7.43c).

Voltage-gated Ca^{2+} channels show varying degrees of

Figure 7.38 N- and L-type macroscopic Ca²⁺ currents. (a) The mixed N and L macroscopic current is recorded with Ca²⁺ as the charge carrier (whole-cell patch) from chick limb motoneurons in culture in response to a voltage step from −80 to +20 mV. (b) The macroscopic L current is recorded in isolation by changing the holding potential to 0 mV. (c) The difference current obtained by subtracting the L current (b) from the N and L current (a) is the N current. (d) I–V relation for the L current recorded as in b. (e) I–V relation for the N current obtained as the difference current. The intrapipette solution contains (in mM): 140 Cs aspartate, 5 MgCl₂, 10 Cs EGTA, 10 HEPES, 0.1 Li₂GTP, 1 MgATP. The bathing solution contains (in mM): 146 NaCl, 2 CaCl₂, 5 KCl, 1 MgCl₂, 10 HEPES. (Adapted from McCobb DP, Best PM and Beam KG, 1989, Development alters the expression of calcium currents in chick limb motoneurons, *Neuron* 2, 1633–1643, with permission.)

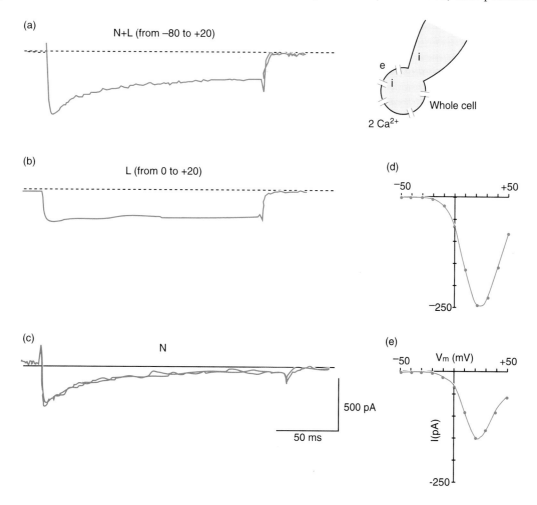

inactivation. Inactivation properties are analyzed by recording the macroscopic L, N or P-type Ca²⁺ currents evoked by a voltage step to a fixed potential from various holding potentials (with Ca²⁺ as the charge carrier). The L current is half inactivated around −40 mV (Figure 7.41a, c), the N current around −60 mV (Figure 7.42a, c) and the P current around −45 mV (Figure 7.43a, c).

In summary, L channels generate a large Ca²⁺ current that is activated by large depolarizations to 0/+10 mV and inactivates with a very slow time course during a step. N and P channels generate smaller Ca²⁺ currents that are activated with depolarization to −30/0 mV and inactivate or not during a depolarizing step.

The inactivation process of Ca²⁺ channels can be voltage-dependent, time-dependent *and* calcium-dependent. Voltage-dependent inactivation is observed

Figure 7.39 P-type macroscopic Ca^{2+} current. The whole-cell P current recorded from acutely dissociated Purkinje cells (whole-cell patch) with Ca^{2+} as the charge carrier. (a) Whole-cell P current recorded in response to a depolarizing pulse to −20 mV from a holding potential of −80 mV. (b) I–V relation of the P current. In the recordings the low threshold T-type Ca^{2+} current was either absent, inactivated or subtracted. The intrapipette solution contains (in mM): 120 TEA glutamate, 9 EGTA, 4.5 $MgCl_2$, 9 HEPES. The bathing solution contains (in mM): 5 $CaCl_2$, 154 TEACl, 0.2 $MgCl_2$, 10 glucose, 10 HEPES. (Adapted from Reagan LJ, 1991. Voltage-dependent calcium currents in Purkinje cells from rat cerebellar vermis, *J. Neurosci.* 7, 2259–2269, with permission.)

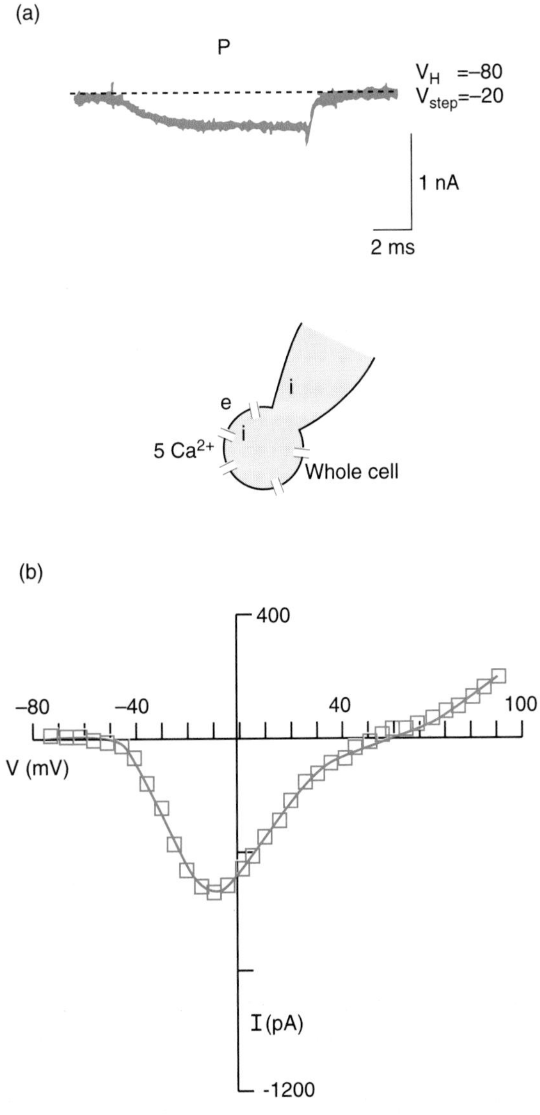

(a)

(b)

by changing the holding potential (see Figures 7.41a, 7.42a and 7.43a). Time-dependent inactivation is observed during a long depolarizing step, in presence of Ba^{2+} as the change carrier (Figure 7.44). Ca^{2+}-dependent inactivation depends on the amount of Ca^{2+} influx through open Ca^{2+} channels. It can be considered as a negative feedback control of Ca^{2+} channels by Ca^{2+} channels.

Calcium-dependent inactivation

Several lines of evidence point to the existence of a Ca^{2+}-induced inactivation of Ca^{2+} currents: (i) the degree of inactivation is proportional to the amplitude and frequency of the Ca^{2+} current; (ii) intracellular injection of Ca^{2+} ions into neurons produces inactivation; (iii) intracellular injection of Ca^{2+} chelators such as EGTA or BAPTA reduces inactivation (Figure 7.45); (iv) substitution of Ca^{2+} ions with Sr^{2+} or Ba^{2+} reduces inactivation; and (v) very large depolarizations to near E_{Ca}, where the entry of Ca^{2+} ions is small, produce little inactivation.

Recordings of L and N channels in Figures 7.41 and 7.42 are obtained with Ca^{2+} as the charge carrier and that of P channels in Figure 7.43 with Ba^{2+} as the charge carrier. Therefore, the inactivation seen in Figures 7.41 and 7.42 result from voltage, time and the increase of intracellular Ca^{2+} ions. In contrast, the inactivation of the P current observed in Figure 7.43 is a voltage- and time-dependent process.

The macroscopic Ca^{2+} current of *Aplysia* neurons is recorded in voltage clamp. During depolarizing voltage steps, the Ca^{2+} current increases to a peak and then declines to a steady state Ca^{2+} current (a noninactivating component of current). The buffering of cytoplasmic free Ca^{2+} ions with EGTA increases the amplitude of the peak current and that of the steady state current (Figure 7.45). This shows that the increase of intracellular Ca^{2+} ions resulting from Ca^{2+} entry through Ca^{2+} channels causes Ca^{2+} current inactivation. It also shows that the peak current is probably contaminated by some early development of inactivation.

In L-type Ca^{2+} channels of cardiac muscle cells, a Ca^{2+}-binding motif located in the COOH terminus of the α_{1C} subunit provides the Ca^{2+} binding site that initiates Ca^{2+}-sensitive inactivation. L channels are transiently expressed in HEK 293 cells from cDNA

Figure 7.40   The peak opening probability of the N current. The macroscopic N current is recorded in a dorsal root ganglion neuron from a cell-attached patch containing hundreds of N channels (macropatch). (a) Current recordings (bottom traces) in response to test potentials (t.p.) ranging from −30 mV to +20 mV from a holding potential (h.p.) of −80 mV (upper traces). (b) Voltage-dependence of the peak opening probability (p_o) from data obtained in (a). Values of p_o are obtained by dividing the peak current I by the unitary current i_{CaN} obtained at each test potential and by an estimate of the number of channels in the patch (599): $p_o = I/Ni_{CaN}$. N was determined by comparison with the single channel experiment in Figure 7.31b which shows that in response to a depolarization to +20 mV from a holding potential of −80 mV, $p_o = 0.32$ and $i_{CaN} = 0.76$ pA. I, the peak current evoked by the same voltage protocol, is 145 pA. $N = I/p_o \, i_{CaN} = 145/(0.32 \times 0.76) = 599$ channels. The intrapipette solution contains (in mM): 100 CsCl, 10 Cs-EGTA, 5 MgCl$_2$, 40 HEPES, 2 ATP, 0.25 cAMP, pH = 7.3. The extracellular solution contains (in mM): 10 CaCl$_2$, 135 TEACl, 10 HEPES, 0.2 TTX, pH = 7.3. (From Nowycky MC, Fox AP and Tsien RW, 1985. Three types of neuronal calcium channel with different calcium agonist sensitivity, *Nature* **316**, 440–443, with permission.)

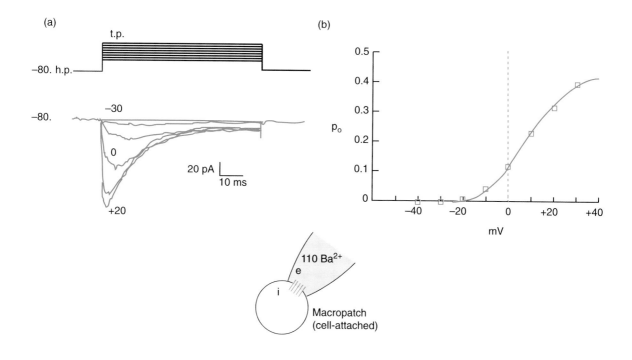

encoding the native α_{1C} or α_{1E} subunits or from a chimeric cDNA encoding an α subunit where the entire COOH terminus of α_{1E} is substituted into α_{1C} (α_{1E} forms a neuronal Ca^{2+} channel lacking Ca^{2+} inactivation). All these α subunits are co-expressed with a β subunit (β_{2a}) in order to ensure robust expression. Ca^{2+} and Ba^{2+} currents are recorded from the chimeric Ca^{2+} channel. Since no Ca^{2+}-dependent inactivation is recorded from the chimeric Ca^{2+} channel, the α_{1C} COOH terminus appears essential for the initiation of Ca^{2+} inactivation in this α subunit.

7.5.3 The Calcium-Dependent Action Potentials

Depolarization of the membrane to the threshold for the activation of L-, N- and P-type Ca$^+$ channels has two origins

L-, N- and P-type Ca^{2+} channels are high threshold Ca^{2+} channels. It means that they are activated in response to a relatively large membrane depolarization. In cells (e.g. neurons, heart muscle cells) where

Figure 7.41   Voltage-dependence of activation and inactivation of the L-type Ca^{2+} current. The macroscopic L current is recorded in a cell with very little T or N current. (a) Inactivation of the L current with holding potential: a test depolarization to +10 mV is applied from holding potentials (h.p.) varying from −70 to −10 mV. (b) Activation of the L current with depolarization: test depolarizations (t.p.) to −30, −20, −10, 0, +10 and +20 mV are applied from a holding potential of −40 mV. (c) Activation–inactivation curves obtained from the data in (b) and (a), respectively. The peak Ca^{2+} current amplitudes (I) are normalized to the maximal current ($I_{max} = 1$) obtained in each set of experiments and plotted against the holding (inactivation curve, □) or test potential (activation curve, ■). For the activation curve, data are plotted as $I = I_{max} [1 + \exp ((V_{1/2} − V)/k)]^{-1}$ and for the inactivation curve as $I = I_{max} [1 + \exp ((V − V_{1/2})/k)]^{-1}$. $V_{1/2}$ is the voltage at which the current I is half-activated ($I = I_{max}/2$ when $V_{1/2} = 2$ mV) or half-inactivated ($I = I_{max}/2$ when $V_{1/2} = −40$ mV). All the recordings are performed in the presence of 10 mM Ca^{2+} in the recording pipette solution which bathes the extracellular side of the channels. (Adapted from Fox AP, Nowycky M and Tsien RW, 1987. Kinetic and pharmacological properties distinguishing three types of calcium currents in chick sensory neurones, *J. Physiol.* **394**, 149–172, with permission.)

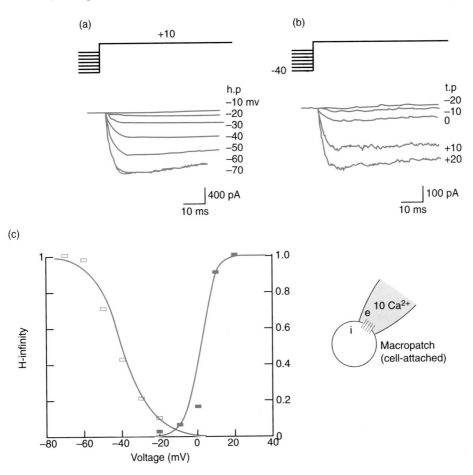

the resting membrane potential is around −80/−60 mV, a 40–60 mV depolarization is therefore needed to activate the high threshold Ca^{2+} channels. Such a membrane depolarization is too large to result directly from the summation of excitatory post-synaptic potentials (EPSPs). This depolarization usually results from the Na$^+$ spike. In heart muscle cells, Na$^+$ entry during the sudden depolarization phase of the action potential depolarizes the membrane to the threshold for L-type Ca^{2+} channel activation: the Na$^+$-dependent depolarization phase is immediately followed by a Ca^{2+}-dependent plateau (Figure 7.2). In axon termi-

Figure 7.42   Voltage-dependence of activation and inactivation of the N-type Ca^{2+} current. The macroscopic N current is recorded in cell-attached patches containing hundreds of channels (macropatch). (a) Inactivation of the N current with holding potential: test depolarization to +10 mV is applied from holding potentials (h.p.) varying from −70 to −10 mV. (b) Activation of the N current with depolarization: test depolarizations (t.p.) to −30, −20, −10, 0, +10 and +20 mV are applied from a holding potential of −80 mV. (c) Activation–inactivation curves obtained from the data in (b) and (a), respectively. The peak Ca^{2+} current amplitudes (I) are normalized to the maximal current ($I_{max} = 1$) obtained in each set of experiments and plotted against the holding (inactivation curve, □) or test potential (activation curve, ●). For the activation curve, data are plotted as $I = I_{max} [1 + \exp ((V_{1/2} − V)/k)]^{-1}$ and for the inactivation curve as $I = I_{max} [1 + \exp ((V − V_{1/2}/k)]^{-1}$. $V_{1/2}$ is the voltage at which the current I is half-activated ($I = I_{max}/2$ when $V_{1/2} = 1.5$ mV) or half-inactivated ($I = I_{max}/2$ when $V_{1/2} = −61.5$ mV). The number of channels is estimated as in Figure 7.40. (Adapted from Fox AP, Nowycky MC and Tsien RW, 1987. Single-channel recordings of three types of calcium channels in chick sensory neurones, *J. Physiol.* **394**, 173–200, with permission.)

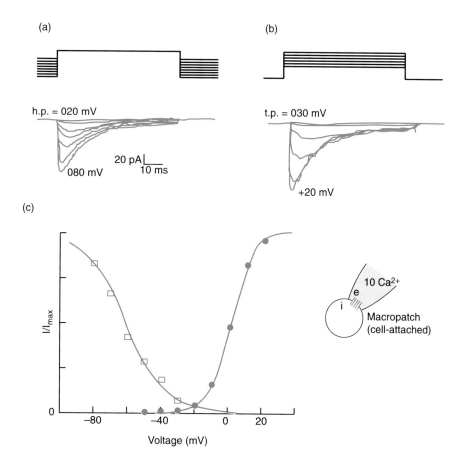

nals, the situation is similar: the Na^+-dependent action potential actively propagates to axon terminals where it depolarizes the membrane to the threshold potential for N- or P-type Ca^{2+} channel activation: an Na^+/Ca^{2+}-dependent action potential is initiated (Figure 7.2c). In Purkinje cells the situation is somehow different. The somatic Na^+-dependent action potential passively

back-propagates to the dendritic membrane where it opens the P-type Ca^{2+} channels: Ca^{2+}-dependent action potentials are initiated and actively propagate in dendrites (Figure 7.2b).

The cells that do not express voltage-gated Na^+ channels and initiate Ca^{2+}-dependent action potentials usually present a depolarized resting membrane

Figure 7.43   Voltage-dependence of activation and inactivation of the P-type Ca^{2+} current. The macroscopic P current is recorded in Purkinje cells (whole-cell patch). The T-type Ca^{2+} current present in these cells is either absent or subtracted. (a) Inactivation of the P current with holding potential: a test depolarization to +20 mV is applied from holding potentials varying from –80 to 0 mV. (b) Activation of the P current with depolarization: test depolarizations (V_{step}) to –40 and –20 mV are applied from a holding potential of –110 mV. (c) Activation–inactivation curves obtained from the data obtained in (b) and (a), respectively. The peak Ca^{2+} current amplitudes (I) are normalized to the maximal current ($I_{max} = 1$) obtained in each set of experiments and plotted against the holding (inactivation curve, O) or test potential (activation curve, ●). For the activation curve, data are plotted as $I = I_{max} [1 + \exp((V_{1/2} – V)/k)]^{-1}$ and for the inactivation curve as $I = I_{max} [1 + \exp((V – V_{1/2})/k)]^{-1}$. $V_{1/2}$ is the voltage at which the current I is half-activated ($I = I_{max}/2$ when $V_{1/2} = –22$ mV) or half-inactivated ($I = I_{max}/2$ when $V_{1/2} = –34$ mV). In all recordings, the extracellular solution contains 5 mM Ba^{2+}. (Adapted from Regan L, 1991. Voltage-dependent calcium currents in Purkinje cells from rat cerebellar vermis, *J. Neurosci.* **11**, 2259–2269, with permission.)

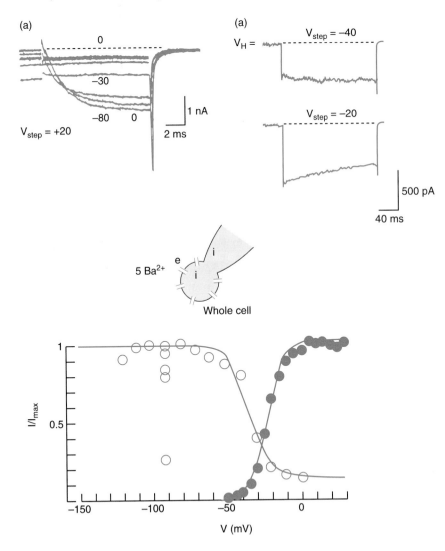

Figure 7.44 Pharmacology of L, N- and P-type Ca^{2+} channels. The macroscopic mixed Ca^{2+} currents are recorded in different neurons with Ba^{2+} as the charge carrier (whole-cell patch). High threshold Ca^{2+} currents are evoked by depolarizations to -30 or -10 mV from a holding potential of -90 or -80 mV. Various blockers or toxins are applied in order to block selectively one type of high threshold Ca^{2+} current at a time: ω-conotoxin (CgTx, 3 μM) selectively blocks N current, nitrendipine or nimodipine (nitr., nimod., 2–4 μM) selectively blocks L current and ω-agatoxin (ω-Aga-IVA, 50–200 nM) selectively blocks P current. In hippocampal cells of the CA1 region and in spinal cord interneurons, the high threshold Ca^{2+} current is a mixed N, L and P current. In sympathetic neurons it is almost exclusively N and in Purkinje cells almost exclusively P. The intrapipette solution contains (in mM): 108 Cs methanesulfonate, 4 MgCl$_2$, 9 EGTA, 9 HEPES, 4 MgATP, 14 creatine phosphate, 1 GTP, pH = 7.4. The extracellular solution contains (in mM): 5 BaCl$_2$, 160 TEACl, 0.1 EGTA, 10 HEPES, pH = 7.4. (Adapted from Mintz IM, Adams ME and Bean B, 1992. P-type calcium channels in rat central and peripheral neurons, *Neuron* **9**, 85–95, with permission.)

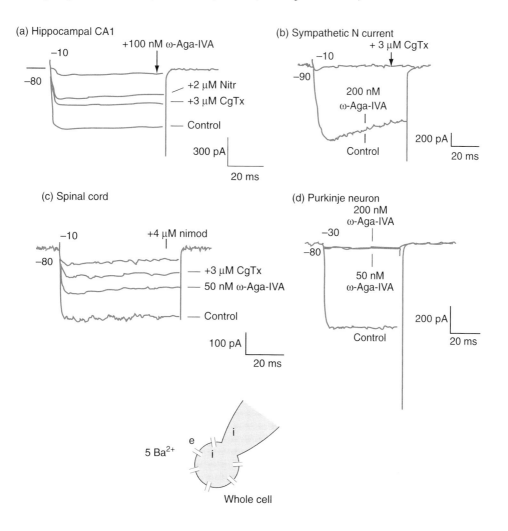

potential ($-50/-40$ mV) close to the threshold for L-type Ca^{2+} channel activation (like some endocrine cells). In such cells, the activation of high threshold Ca^{2+} channels results from a depolarizing current generated by receptor activation or from an intrinsic pacemaker current (for example, activation of the T-type Ca^{2+} current, see Appendix 17.4, or the turning off of a K$^+$ current).

Figure 7.45 Intracellular EGTA slows Ca^{2+}-dependent inactivation of Ca^{2+} channels. The macroscopic Ca^{2+} current is recorded in axotomized *Aplysia* neurons in double electrode voltage clamp (axotomy is performed in order to improve space clamp). Control Ca^{2+} currents are recorded in response to step depolarizations to –20, –10 and 0 mV from a holding potential of –40 mV (control traces). Iontophoretic ejection of EGTA (300–500 nA for 4–8 min) increases the peak amplitude of the Ca^{2+} current and slows its inactivation at all potentials tested (EGTA traces). The amplitude of the non-inactivating component of the current is measured at the end of the steps (▼). (Adapted from Chad J, Eckert R and Ewald D, 1984. Kinetics of calcium-dependent inactivation of calcium current in voltage-clamped neurones in *Aplysia californica*, *J. Physiol. (Lond.)* **347**, 279–300, with permission.)

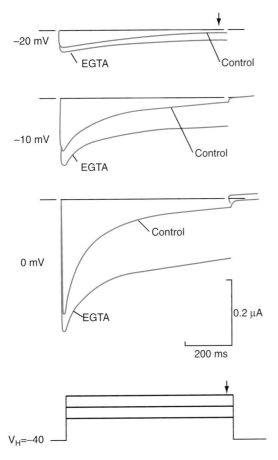

The repolarization of Ca^{2+}-dependent action potentials results from the activation of K$^+$ currents: I$_K$ and I$_{K(Ca)}$

The K$^+$ currents involved in calcium spike repolarization are the delayed rectifier (I_K) studied above and the Ca^{2+}-activated K$^+$ currents ($I_{K(Ca)}$). Meech and Strumwasser in 1970 were the first to describe that a microinjection of Ca^{2+} ions into *Aplysia* neurons activates a K$^+$ conductance and hyperpolarizes the membrane. On the basis of these results, the authors postulated the existence of a Ca^{2+}-activated K$^+$ conductance. The amount of participation of Ca^{2+}-activated K$^+$ currents in spike repolarization depends on the cell type.

The Ca^{2+}-activated K$^+$ currents are classified as maxi-K (or big K) channels and small-K (SK) channels. Maxi-K channels have a high conductance (100–250 pS depending on K$^+$ concentrations) and are sensitive to both voltage *and* Ca^{2+} ions so that their apparent sensitivity to Ca^{2+} ions is increased when the membrane is depolarized. Their activity is blocked by TEA and charybdotoxin, a toxin from scorpion venom. Small-K channels have a smaller conductance (10–80 pS depending on K$^+$ concentrations) and are insensitive to TEA and charybdotoxin but sensitive to apamin, a toxin from bee venom. It is a heterogeneous class containing both voltage-dependent and voltage-independent channels. Maxi-K and small-K channels are very selective for K$^+$ ions over Na$^+$ ions and are acti-

Figure 7.46 Two types of rat brain Ca^{2+}-activated K$^+$ channels incorporated into lipid bilayers. (a, b) (Left) Single channel recordings in symmetrical K$^+$ (the extracellular and intracellular solutions contain 150 mM KCl) at V_H = 40 mV. For all traces channel openings correspond to upward deflections. The recording length of upper traces is 6.4 s and each lower trace is expanded to show a 640 ms recording. (Right) *I–V* relations for the maxi-K channel and the small-K channel in symmetrical K$^+$ (150 mM, circles) and 150 mM KCl inside, 50 mM KCl outside (triangles). The slope conductance for each of these channels in symmetrical 150 mM KCl is 232 pS (maxi-K channel) and 77 pS (small K channel). All the recordings are performed in the presence of 1.05 mM CaCl$_2$ in the intracellular solution. (Adapted from Reinhart PH, Chung S and Levitan IB, 1989. A family of calcium-dependent potassium channels from rat brain, *Neuron* **2**, 1031–1041, with permission.)

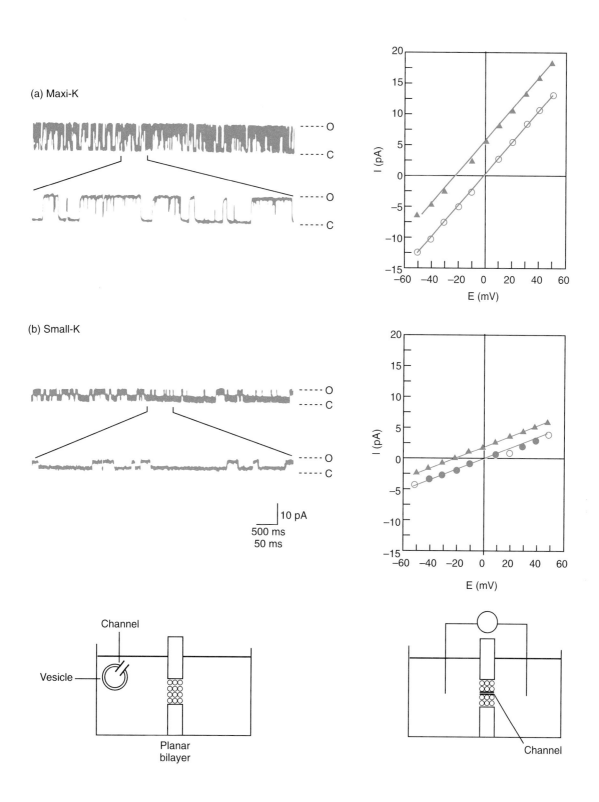

(a) Maxi-K

(b) Small-K

Channel

Vesicle

Planar
bilayer

Channel

10 pA
500 ms
50 ms

Figure 7.47   Ca^{2+}-dependence of Ca^{2+}-activated K$^+$ channels. (a) Single channel activity of Ca^{2+}-activated channels from the rat brain. The activity of the 232 pS maxi-K channel and that of the 77 pS small-K channel is recorded in the presence of 0.1 µM Ca^{2+} (upper traces) and 0.4 µM Ca^{2+} (lower traces) in symmetrical 150 mM KCl (V_H = +20 mV). (b) Single-channel activity of a maxi-K channel from rat skeletal muscle recorded at three different Ca^{2+} concentrations in symmetrical 140 mM KCl (V_H = +30 mV). O, open state; C, closed state. (From Chad J, Eckert R and Ewald D, 1984. Kinetics of calcium-dependent inactivation of calcium current in voltage-clamped neurones in *Aplysia californica*, *J. Physiol. (Lond.)* 347, 279–300, with permission. b: Adapted from McManus OB and Magleby KL, 1991. Accounting for the calcium-dependent kinetics of single large-conductance Ca^{2+}-activated K$^+$ channels in rat skeletal muscle. *J. Physiol.* **443**: 739–777.

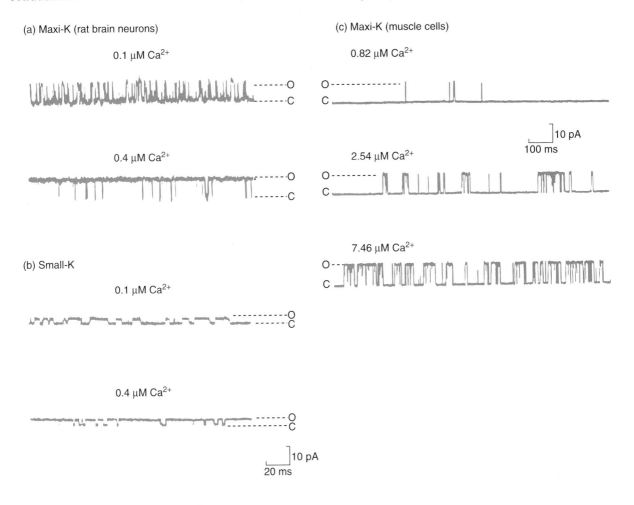

vated by increases in the concentration of cytoplasmic Ca^{2+} ions.

Biochemical purification of maxi-K channels from mammalian smooth muscle shows that they are composed of two structurally distinct subunits, α and β. The β subunits are encoded by a single gene that undergoes alternative splicing. The primary structure of the α-subunits of maxi-K channels reveals a core domain similar to that of other voltage-gated channels that has six putative transmembrane segments (S1 to S6), a string of regularly spaced positive charges in S4 and a highly conserved region between S5 and S6 defining the pore. The primary sequence is approximately twice the length of that of other voltage-gated K$^+$ channels. This additional length is due to an appended sequence on the carboxyl side of the core domain. This raises the possibility that the additional C-terminal sequence may participate in functions particular to maxi-K channels such as Ca²⁺-dependent gating. The smaller β subunit shows no homology with other ion channel subunits.

Although expression of the α subunit alone in *Xenopus* oocytes is sufficient to generate K⁺ channels that are gated by voltage and Ca²⁺, these properties are quantitatively different from the native ones. Currents from cells expressing α/β heteromultimers more closely resemble those of native channels. Immunoprecipitation experiments indicate that the two subunits are tightly associated since antibodies directed against one subunit can precipitate both subunits. These data suggest that both α and β subunits contribute to the functional properties of maxi-K channels and that the α subunit forms part of the transduction machinery of the channels.

To study Ca²⁺-activated K⁺ channels from rat brain neurons, plasma membrane vesicle preparation is incorporated into planar lipid bilayers. In such conditions, the activity of four distinct types of Ca²⁺-activated K⁺ channels is recorded. We will present one example of a maxi-K and one example of a small-K channel. This preparation allows the recording of single channel activity (Figure 7.46). The current–voltage relations obtained in the presence of two different extracellular K⁺ concentrations show that the current reverses at E_K, the theoretical reversal potential for K⁺ ions (Figure 7.46) as expected for a purely K⁺-selective channel. The Ca²⁺-dependence is studied by raising the intracellular Ca²⁺ concentration in the range of 0.1–10 μM. Channels are activated by micromolar concentrations of Ca²⁺. The open probabilities of the maxi-K and small-K channels are largely increased when the medium bathing the intracellular side of the membrane contains 0.4 μM Ca²⁺ instead of 0.1 μM (Figure 7.47a,b). For comparison the Ca²⁺-sensitivity of maxi-K channels from cultured rat skeletal muscle is shown in Figure 7.47c. The rat brain maxi-K channels are sensitive to nanomolar concentrations of charybdotoxin (CTX) and millimolar concentrations of extracellular TEA ions (Figure 7.48).

The macroscopic Ca²⁺-activated K⁺ currents are recorded from a bullfrog sympathetic neuron in a single-electrode voltage clamp ($V_H = -28$ mV). The iontophoretic injection of Ca²⁺ ions through the intracellular recording electrode triggers an outward current (Figure 7.49a). Its amplitude increases when the iontophoretic current is increased, i.e. the amount of Ca²⁺ ions injected is increased. To study the voltage-

Figure 7.48 Pharmacology of the maxi-K channel. Single channel activity of the maxi-K channel (232 pS channel) in symmetrical 150 mM KCl at two different time bases ($V_H = +40$ mV). Control conditions (a), in the presence of 10 nM charybdotoxin (CTX) (b), 100 nM apamin (c) and 0.2 mM tetraethylammonium chloride (TEA) (d) in the extracellular solution. All the recordings are performed in the presence of 1.05 mM Ca²⁺ in the intracellular solution. (From Chad J, Eckert R and Ewald D, 1984. Kinetics of calcium-dependent inactivation of calcium current in voltage-clamped neurones in *Aplysia californica*, *J. Physiol. (Lond.)* **347**, 279–300, with permission.)

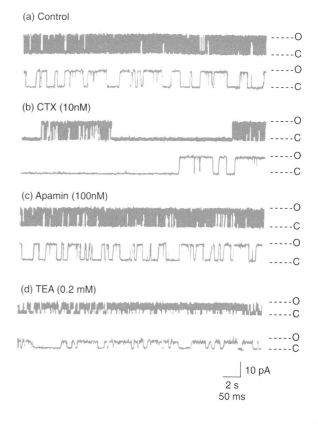

(a) Control

(b) CTX (10nM)

(c) Apamin (100nM)

(d) TEA (0.2 mM)

10 pA
2 s
50 ms

dependence and the kinetics of activation of this Ca²⁺-activated outward current, depolarizing steps from a holding potential of −50 mV are applied in the presence of 2 mM Ca²⁺ in the extracellular medium (Figure 7.49b, 2 Ca). Suppression of Ca²⁺ entry by removal of Ca²⁺ ions from the extracellular medium (0 Ca) eliminates an early Ca²⁺-activated outward current. In the Ca-free medium, only the sigmoidal delayed rectifier K⁺ current I_K is recorded. In the presence of external Ca²⁺ ions, both I_K and a $I_{K(Ca)}$ are

Figure 7.49 The macroscopic Ca²⁺-activated K⁺ current of bullfrog sympathetic neurons. (a) Outward currents recorded in single electrode voltage clamp at a holding potential of −28 mV. In response to increasing 0.4 s intracellular iontophoretic injections of Ca²⁺ from a microelectrode containing 200 mM CaCl₂, increasing outward currents are recorded. (b) Outward currents recorded during voltage steps to −20, −10, 0 and +20 mV from a holding potential of −50 mV in the presence of 2 mM external Ca²⁺ (2 Ca) and a Ca-free external medium (0 Ca). The leak current is subtracted. The two superimposed current traces recorded at the same potential in the presence (+ Ca) or absence (− Ca) of external Ca²⁺ ions show that an early component of the outward current is present ($I_{K(Ca)}$) in the presence of Ca²⁺ ions. (Adapted from Brown DA, Constanti A and Adams PR, 1983. Ca²⁺-activated potassium current in vertebrate sympathetic neurons, *Cell Calcium* **4**, 407–420, with permission.)

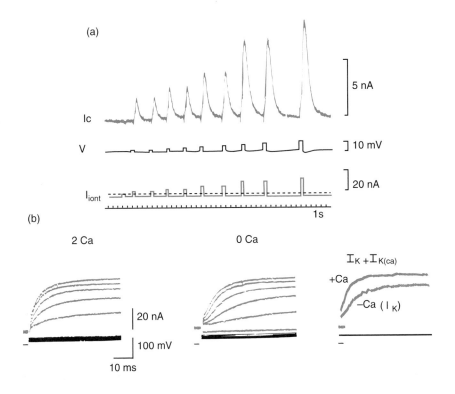

recorded (Figure 7.49b, right). The recorded $I_{K(Ca)}$ corresponds to a maxi-K current also called I_C in some preparations since it is voltage- and Ca²⁺-dependent. It has activation kinetics sufficiently rapid to play a role in spike repolarization (Figure 7.50 and see also Figure 17.5).

In nerve terminals at the motor end plate, maxi-K channels are co-localized with voltage-dependent Ca²⁺ channels. They play an important role in repolarizing the plasma membrane following each action potential. This repolarization resulting from the increased activity of Ca²⁺-activated K⁺ channels closes voltage-dependent Ca²⁺ channels and constitutes an important feedback mechanism for the regulation of voltage-

dependent Ca²⁺ entry. It thereby lowers intracellular Ca²⁺ concentration and dampens neurotransmitter secretion.

7.5.4 The Role of the Calcium-Dependent Action Potentials is to Provide a Local and Transient Increase of [Ca²⁺]ᵢ to Trigger Secretion, Contraction and other Ca²⁺-Gated Processes

The role of Na⁺ action potentials is to propagate information from the cell body to the axon terminals. The general role of Ca²⁺-dependent action potentials

Figure 7.50 Different states of voltage-gated Na⁺, Ca²⁺ and K⁺ channels in relation to the different phases of the Na⁺/Ca²⁺-dependent action potential. Example of the action potential recorded in olivary neurons of the cerebellum.

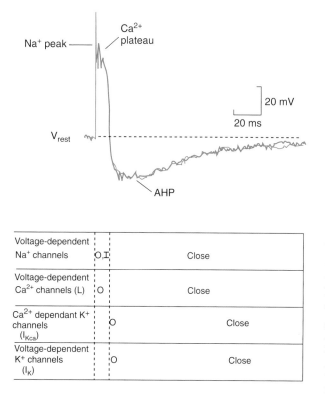

Voltage-dependent Na⁺ channels	O,I		Close	
Voltage-dependent Ca²⁺ channels (L)	O		Close	
Ca²⁺ dependant K⁺ channels (I_{Kca})		O		Close
Voltage-dependent K⁺ channels (I_K)		O		Close

is to provide a local and transient entry of Ca²⁺ ions. A significant entry of Ca²⁺ ions is observed during Ca²⁺-dependent action potentials. Under normal conditions, the intracellular Ca²⁺ concentration is very low, less than 10^{-7} M. The entry of Ca²⁺ ions through Ca²⁺ channels locally and transiently increases the intracellular Ca²⁺ concentration up to 10^{-4} M (see Chapter 8). In some neurons, Ca²⁺ entry through high threshold Ca²⁺ channels participates in the generation of various forms of electrical activity such as dendritic Ca²⁺ spikes (Purkinje cell dendrites) and plays a role in synaptic integration by regulating repetitive firing. Along the same line, Ca²⁺ entry activates Ca²⁺-sensitive channels such as Ca²⁺-activated K⁺ or Cl⁻ channels. However, the more general role of Ca²⁺ entry is to trigger Ca²⁺-dependent intracellular events such as exocytosis of synaptic vesicles or granules and

sliding of the myofilaments actin and myosin. It thus couples action potentials (excitation) to secretion (neurons and other excitable secretory cells, see Chapter 8) or to contraction (heart muscle cells). The influx of Ca²⁺ also couples neuronal activity to metabolic processes and induces long-term changes in neuronal and synaptic activity (see Chapter 19). During development, Ca²⁺ entry regulates outgrowth of axons and dendrites and the retraction of axonal branches during synapse elimination and neuronal cell death.

7.5.5 Generalization on Voltage-Gated Channels and Action Potentials

Voltage-gated Na⁺, K⁺ and Ca²⁺ channels of action potentials share a similar structure (Figure 5.9) and are all activated by membrane depolarization. The Na⁺, Na⁺/Ca²⁺ and Ca²⁺ action potentials have a similar pattern: the depolarization phase results from the influx of cations, Na⁺ and/or Ca²⁺, and the repolarization phase results from the inactivation of Na⁺ or Ca²⁺ channels together with the efflux of K⁺ ions. However, action potentials have at least one important difference. The Na⁺-dependent action potential is all-or-none. In contrast the Ca²⁺-dependent action potential is gradual. This reflects different functions. The Na⁺-dependent action potential propagates on long distances *without attenuation* in order to transmit information from dendrites and soma to axon terminals where they trigger Ca²⁺-dependent action potentials. Ca²⁺-dependent action potentials have the general role of providing a local, *gradual* and transient Ca²⁺ entry.

Appendix 7.1
Current Clamp Recording

The current clamp technique, or intracellular recording in current clamp mode, is the traditional method for recording membrane potential: resting membrane potential and membrane potential changes such as action potentials and post-synaptic potentials. Membrane potential changes result from intrinsic or extrinsic currents. Intrinsic currents are synaptic or autorhythmic currents. Extrinsic currents are currents of known amplitude and duration applied by the experimenter through the intracellular recording electrode, in order to mimic currents produced by synaptic inputs.

Current clamp means that the *current applied* through the intracellular electrode is clamped to a constant value by the experimenter. It does not mean that the *current flowing through the membrane* is clamped to a constant value.

How to record membrane potential

The intracellular electrode (or the patch pipette) is connected to a unity gain amplifier that has an input resistance many orders of magnitude greater than that of the micropipette plus the input resistance of the cell membrane ($R_p + R_m$). The output of the amplifier follows the voltage at the tip of the intracellular electrode (V_p) (Figure A7.1). By definition, membrane potential V_m is equal to $V_i - V_e$ (i for intracellular and e for extracellular). In Figure A7.1, $V_i - V_e = V_p - V_{bath} = V_p - V_{ground} = V_p - 0 = V_p$. When a current I is simultaneously passed through the electrode, this holds true if this current I is very small in order not to cause a

Figure A7.1 A unity gain amplifier A1 and a current source made by adding a second amplifier A2. The micropipette voltage V_p is measured by A1. The command voltage V_{cmd} and V_p are the inputs of A2 (V_p and V_{cmd} are added). The current I applied by the experimenter in order to induce V_m changes flow through R_o and is equal to: $I = V_{cmd} / R_o$ since the voltage across the output resistor R_o is equal to V_{cmd} regardless of V_p. I flows through the micropipette into the cell then out through the cell membrane into the bath grounding electrode. I is here an outward current. Capacitances are ignored. (Adapted from *The Axon Guide*, Axon Instruments Inc, 1993.)

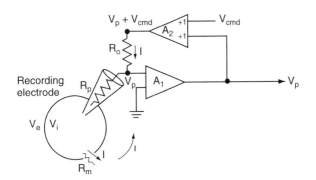

significant voltage drop across R_p (see the last section of this appendix).

How to inject current through the intracellular electrode

If a current injection circuit is connected to the input node, the current injected (I) flows down the electrode into the cell (Figure A7.1). This current source allows a constant (DC) current to be injected, either outward to depolarize the membrane or inward to hyperpolarize the membrane (Figure A7.2). When the recording electrode is filled with KCl, a current that expells K$^+$ ions into the cell interior depolarizes the membrane (V_m becomes less negative) (Figure A7.2a), whereas a current that expells Cl$^-$ ions into the cell interior hyperpolarizes the membrane (V_m becomes more negative) (Figure A7.2b).

Outward means that the current is flowing through the membrane from the inside of the cell to the bath. Inward is the contrary.

The current source can also be used to inject a short duration pulse of current: a depolarizing current pulse above threshold to evoke action potential(s) or a low amplitude depolarizing (Figure A7.3) or hyperpolarizing current pulse to measure the input membrane resistance R_m since $\Delta V_m = R_m \times \Delta I$.

How to measure the membrane potential when a current is passed down the electrode

The injected current (I) causes a corresponding voltage drop (IR_p) across the resistance of the pipette (R_p). It is therefore difficult to separate the potential at the tip of the electrode ($V_p = V_m$) from the total potential ($V_p + IR_p$). For example, if $R_p = 50$ MΩ, and $I = 0.5$ nA, $IR_p = 25$ mV, a value in the V_m range. A special compensation circuitry can be used to eliminate the micropipette voltage drop IR_p.

Appendix 7.2
Voltage Clamp Recording

The voltage clamp technique (or intracellular recording in voltage clamp mode) is a method for recording the current flowing through the cell membrane

Figure A7.2 (a) When the recording electrode is filled with KCl, a current expells K⁺ ions into the cell interior depolarizes the membrane (V_m becomes less negative). (b) A current expells Cl⁻ ions into the cell interior hyperpolarizes the membrane (K_m becomes more negative).

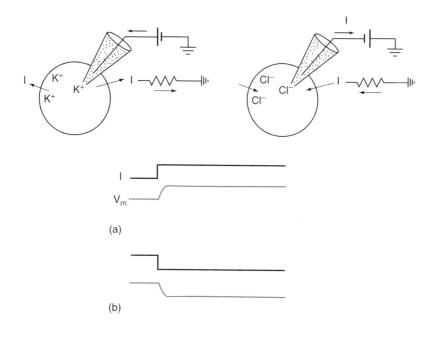

(a)

(b)

while the membrane potential is held (clamped) at a constant value by the experimenter. In contrast to the current clamp technique (Appendix 7.1), voltage clamp does not mimic a process found in nature. However, there are several reasons for performing voltage clamp experiments:

- When studying voltage-gated channels, voltage clamp allows control of a variable (voltage) that determines the opening and closing of these channels.
- By holding the membrane potential constant, the experimenter ensures that the current flowing though the membrane is linearly proportional to the conductance g ($g = 1/R$) being studied. To study, for example, the conductance g_{Na} of the total number (N) of voltage-gated Na⁺ channels present in the membrane, K⁺ and Ca²⁺ voltage-gated channels are blocked by pharmacolgical agents, and the current I_{Na} flowing through the membrane, recorded in voltage clamp, is proportional to g_{Na}:

$$I_{Na} = V_m \, g_{Na} = k \, g_{Na} \text{ since } V_m \text{ is constant.}$$

How to clamp the membrane potential at a known and constant value

The aim of the voltage clamp technique is to adjust continuously the membrane potential V_m to the command potential V_{cmd} fixed by the experimenter. To do so, V_m is continuously measured *and* a current I is passed through the cell membrane to keep V_m at the desired value or command potential (V_{cmd}). Two voltage clamp techniques are commonly used:

Figure A7.3 Injection of a suprathreshold (left) and subthreshold (right) depolarizing pulse.

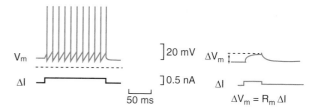

- the two-electrode voltage clamp technique where one electrode is used for membrane potential measurement and the other for passing current (Figure A7. 4);
- the voltage clamp techniques with one electrode:
  (i) the single-electrode voltage clamp technique where the same electrode is used *part time* for membrane potential measurement and part time for current injection (also called discontinuous single-electrode voltage clamp technique, dSEVC). This technique is used for cells that are too small to be impaled with two electrodes; it will not be explained here;
  (ii) the patch clamp technique where the same electrode is used *full time* for simultaneously measuring membrane potential and passing current (see Appendix 7.3).

In the two-electrode voltage clamp technique, the membrane potential is recorded by a unity gain amplifier A1 connected to the voltage-recording electrode E1. The membrane potential measured, V_m (or V_p, see Appendix 7.1) is compared with the command potential V_{cmd} in a high gain differential amplifier A2. It sends a voltage output V_o proportional to the difference between V_m and V_{cmd}. V_o forces a current I to flow through the current passing electrode E2 in order to obtain $V_m - V_{cmd} = 0$. The current I represents the total current that flows through the membrane. It is the same at every point of the circuit.

Figure A7.4 Two-electrode voltage clamp. (Adapted from *The Axon Guide*, Axon Instruments Inc, 1993).

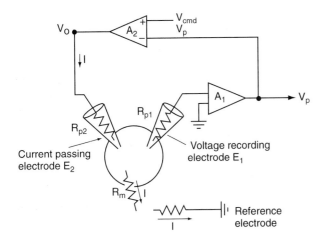

Figure A7.5 The different currents (1 = 1a + 1b + 1c) evoked by a voltage step to −20 mV (V_H = −80 mV) in the presence of K^+ and Ca^{2+} channel blockers.

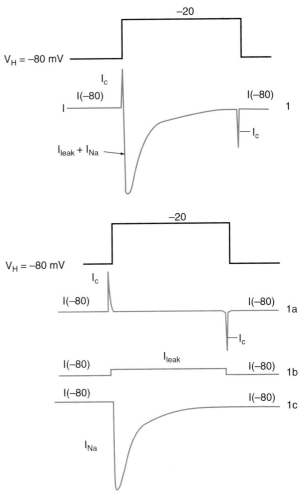

Example of a voltage-clamp recording experiment (Figure. A7.5)

Two electrodes are placed intracellularly into a neuronal soma (an invertebrate neuron for example). The membrane potential is first held at −80 mV. In this condition an outward current flows through the membrane in order to maintain the membrane potential at a value more hyperpolarized than V_{rest}. This stable outward current $I_{(−80)}$ flows through the membrane as long as V_{cmd} = −80 mV.

A voltage step to −20 mV is then applied for

100 ms. This depolarizing step opens voltage-gated channels. In the presence of K+ and Ca2+ channels blockers, only a voltage-gated Na+ current is recorded. To clamp the membrane at the new $V_{cmd} = -20$ mV, a current is sent by the amplifier A2, $I_{(-20)}$. On the rising phase of the step this current $I_{(-20)}$ is equal to the capacitive current I_c necessary to charge the membrane capacitance to its new value plus the leak current I_L flowing through leak channels (lines 1a and 1b). Since the depolarizing step opens Na+ voltage-gated channels, an inward current I_{Na} flowing through open Na+ channels will appear after a small delay (line 1c). Normally, this inward current flowing through the open Na+ channels, I_{Na}, should depolarize the membrane but in voltage clamp experiments it does not: a current constantly equal to I_{Na} but of opposite direction is continuously sent (in the microsecond range) in the circuit to compensate I_{Na} and to clamp the membrane to V_{cmd}. Therefore, once the membrane capacitance is charged, $I_{(-20)} = I_L + I_{Na}$. Usually on recordings, I_C is absent due to the possibility of compensating for it with the voltage clamp amplifier.

Once the membrane capacitance is charged, the total current flowing through the circuit is $I = I_L + I_{Na}$ ($I_c = 0$). Therefore, in all measures of I_{Na}, the leak current I_l must be deduced. To do so, small amplitude hyperpolarizing or depolarizing steps ($\Delta V_m = \pm 5$ to ± 20 mV) are applied at the beginning and at the end of the experiment. These voltage steps are too small to open voltage-gated channels in order to have $I_{Na} = 0$ and $I = I_l$. If we suppose that I_l is linearly proportional to ΔV_m then I_L for a ΔV_m of +80 mV (from −80 to 0 mV), is 8 times the value of I_L for $\Delta V_m = +10$ mV (see Figure 6.6).

Is all the membrane surface clamped?

In small and round cells such as pituitary cells, the membrane potential is clamped on all the surface. In contrast, in neurons, because of their geometry, the voltage clamp is not achieved on all the membrane surface: the distal dendritic and axonal membranes are out of control because of their distance from the soma where the intracellular electrodes are usually placed. Such space clamp problems have to be taken into account by the experimenter in the analysis of the results. In the giant axon of the squid, this problem is overcome by inserting two long axial intracellular electrodes into a segment of axon in order to control the membrane potential all along this segment.

Appendix 7.3
Patch Clamp Recording

The patch clamp technique is a variation of the voltage clamp technique. It allows the recording of current flowing through the membrane: either the current flowing through all the channels open in the whole cell membrane or the current flowing through a single channel in a patch of membrane. In this technique, only one electrode is used full time for both voltage recording and passing current (it is a continuous single-electrode voltage clamp technique, cSEVC). The patch clamp technique was developed by E. Neher and B. Sakmann. By applying very low doses of acetylcholine to a patch of muscle membrane they recorded for the first time, in 1976, the current flowing through a single nicotinic cholinergic receptor channel (nAChR), the unitary nicotinic current.

Some of the advantages of the patch clamp technique are that (i) with all but one configuration (cell-attached configuration) the investigator has access to the intracellular environment (Figure A7.6); (ii) it allows the recording of currents from cells too small to be impaled with intracellular microelectrodes, and (iii) it allows the recording of unitary currents (current through a single channel).

A7.3.1 The Different Patch Clamp Recording Configurations

First a tight seal between the membrane and the tip of the pipette must be obtained. The tip of a micropipette that has been fire polished to a diameter of about 1 μm, is advanced towards a cell until it makes contact with its membrane. Under appropriate conditions, a gentle suction applied to the inside of the pipette causes the formation of a very tight seal between membrane and the tip of the pipette. This is the cell-attached configuration (Figure A7.6). The resistance between the interior of the pipette and the external solution can be very large, of the order of 10 gigaohms (10 GΩ, 1 GΩ = 10^9 Ω) or more. It means that the interior of the pipette is isolated from the extracellular solution by the seal that is formed.

Figure A7.6   The different configurations of patch clamp recording.

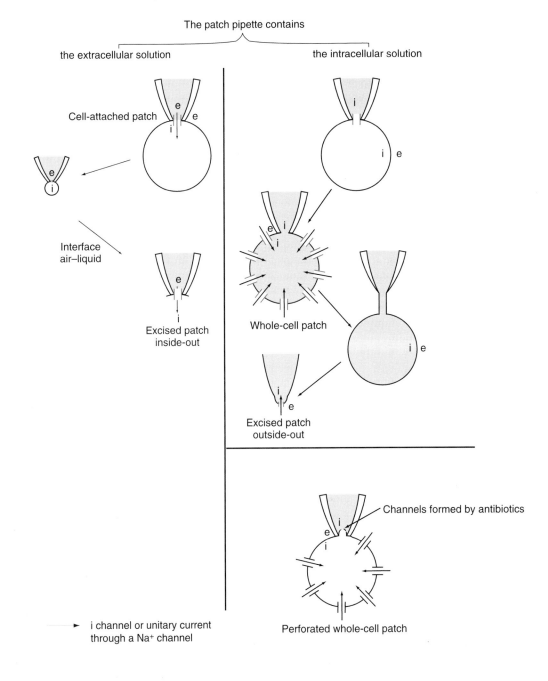

This very large resistance is necessary for two reasons (Figure A7.7):

• It allows the electrical isolation of the membrane patch under the tip of the pipette since practically no current can flow through the seal. This is important because if a fraction of the current passing through the membrane patch leaks out through the seal, it is not measured by the electrode.

Figure A7.7   Good and bad seals. (From *The Axon Guide*, Axon Instruments Inc, 1993.)

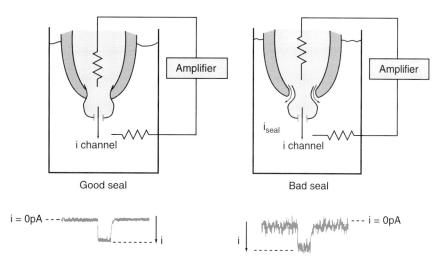

Unitary inward currents

- It augments the signal-to-noise ratio since thermal movement of the charges through a bad seal is a source of additional noise in the recording. A good seal thus enables the measurement of the current flowing through one single channel (unitary current) which is of the order of pA.

From the 'cell-attached' configuration (the last to be explained), one can obtain other recording configurations. In total, three of them are used to record unitary currents, and one (whole-cell) to record the current flowing through all the open channels of the whole cell membrane.

Whole-cell configuration

This configuration is obtained from the cell-attached configuration. If a little suction is applied to the interior of the pipette, it may cause the rupture of the membrane patch under the pipette. Consequently, the patch pipette now records the activity of the whole cell membrane (minus the small ruptured patch of membrane). Rapidly, the intracellular solution equilibrates with that of the pipette, the volume of the latter being many times larger. This is especially true for inorganic ions.

This configuration enables the recording of the current flowing through the N channels open over the entire surface of the cell membrane. Under conditions where all the open channels are of the same type (with the opening of other channels being blocked by pharmacological agents or the voltage conditions), the total current flowing through a population of identical channels can be recorded, such that at steady state:

$$I = N \times p_o \times i$$

where N = number of identical channels, p_o = the probability that these channels are in the open state, Np_o = the number of identical channels in the open state, and i = unitary current.

The advantages of this technique with respect to the two-electrode voltage clamp technique are: (i) the recording under voltage clamp from cell bodies is too small to be impaled with two electrodes and even one; and (ii) a certain control over the composition of the internal environment and a better signal-to-noise ratio. The limitation of this technique is the gradual loss of intracellular components (such as second messengers), which will cause the eventual disappearance of the responses dependent on those components.

Perforated whole-cell configuration

This is a variation of the whole-cell configuration, and also allows the recording of current flowing through the N channels open in the whole membrane but avoids wash-out of the intracellular solution. This configuration is obtained by introducing into the recording pipette a molecule such as nystatin, amphotericin or gramicidin, which will form channels in the patch of membrane under the tip of the electrode. To record in this configuration, first the cell-attached configuration is obtained and then the experimenter waits for the nystatin channels (or amphotericin or gramicidin channels) to form without applying any suction to the electrode. The channels formed by these molecules are mainly permeable to monovalent ions and thus allow electrical access to the cell's interior. Since these channels are not permeant to molecules as large or larger than glucose, whole cell recording can be performed without removing the intracellular environment. This is particularly useful when the modulation of ionic channels by second messengers is studied.

In order to evaluate this problem of 'wash-out', we can calculate the ratio between the cell body volume and the volume of solution at the very end of a pipette. For example for a cell of 20 μm diameter the volume is: $4/3 \, \pi \, (10 \times 10^{-6})^3 = 10^{-15}$ l. If we consider 1 mm of the tip of the pipette, it contains a volume of the solution approximately equal to 10^{-13} l which is 100 times larger than the volume of the cell body.

Excised patch configurations

If one wants to record the unitary current i flowing through a single channel and to control simultaneously the composition of the intracellular environment, the so-called excised or cell-free patch configurations have to be used. The *outside-out configuration* is obtained from the whole-cell configuration by gently pulling the pipette away from the cell. This causes the membrane patch to be torn away from the rest of the cell at the same time that its free ends reseal together. In this case the intracellular environment is that of the pipette, and the extracellular environment is that of the bath. This configuration is used when rapid changes of the extracellular solution are required to test the effects of different ions or pharmacological agents when applied to the extracellular side of the membrane.

The *inside-out configuration* is obtained from the cell-attached configuration by gently pulling the pipette away from the cell, lifting the tip of the pipette from the bath in the air and putting it back into the solution (interface of air–liquid). In this case, the intracellular environment is that of the bath and the extracellular one is that of the pipette (the pipette is filled with a pseudo-extracellular solution). This configuration is used when rapid changes in the composition of the intracellular environment are necessary to test, for example, the effects of different ions, second messengers and pharmacological agents in that environment.

Cell-attached configuration

The intracellular environment is that of the cell itself, and the extracellular environment of the recorded membrane patch is the pipette solution. This configuration enables the recording of current flowing through the channel or channels present in the patch of membrane that is under the pipette and is electrically isolated from the rest of the cell. If one channel opens at a time, then the unitary current i flowing through that channel can be recorded. The recordings in cell-attached mode present two limitations: (i) the composition of the intracellular environment is not controlled; and (ii) the value of the membrane potential is not known and can only be estimated.

Let us assume that the voltage in the interior of the patch pipette is maintained at a known value V_p (p = pipette). Since the voltage across the membrane patch is $V_m = V_i - V_e = V_i - V_p$, it will not be known unless V_i, the voltage at the internal side of the membrane, is also known. V_i cannot be measured directly. One way to estimate this value is to measure the resting potential of several identical cells under similar conditions (with intracellular or whole-cell recordings), and to calculate an average V_i from the individual values. Sometimes, however, V_i can be measured when the cell is large enough to allow a two-electrode voltage clamp recording to be made simultaneously with the patch clamp recording (with a *Xenopus* oocyte, for example). Another method consists of replacing the extracellular medium with isotonic K^+ (120–150 mM). The membrane potential under these conditions will be close to 0 mV.

To leave the intracellular composition intact while recording the activity of a single channel is particularly useful for studies of the modulation of an ionic channel by second messengers.

A7.3.2 The Principles of the Patch Clamp Recording Technique (Figure A7.8)

In the patch clamp technique, as in all voltage clamp techniques, the membrane potential is held constant (i.e. clamped) while the current flowing through a single open channel or many open channels (Np_o) is measured. In the patch clamp technique only one micropipette is used full time for both voltage clamping and current recording. How at the same time via

Figure A7.8 Example of a patch clamp recording in the whole-cell configuration. (a) The amplifier compares V_m to the new $V_{cmd} = -20$ mV. (b) The amplifier sends V_o so that $V_m = V_{cmd} = -20$ mV. Owing to the depolarization to −20 mV, the Na^+ channels open and unitary inward currents i_p flow through the N open channels ($Ni_p = I_p$). (c) The whole cell current I_p flows through the circuit and is measured as a voltage change.

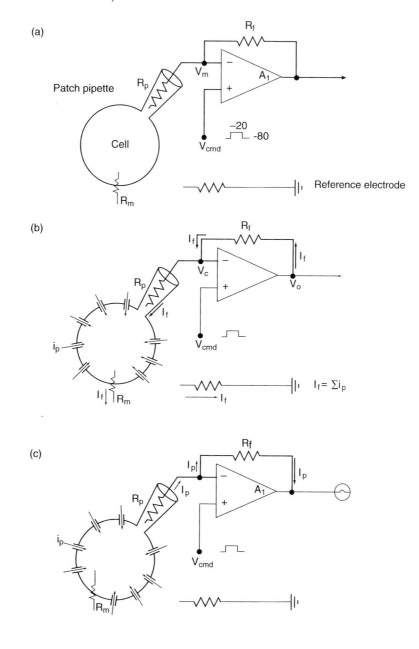

the same pipette can the voltage of the membrane be controlled and the current flowing through the membrane be measured?

When an operational amplifier A1 is connected as shown in Figure A7.8a with a high megohm resistor R_f (f = feedback), a current-to-voltage converter is obtained. The patch pipette is connected to the negative input and the command voltage (V_{cmd}) to the positive one. The resistor R_f can have two values: R_f = 1 GΩ (1 GΩ = 10^9 Ω) in the whole cell configuration and R_f = 10 GΩ in the excised patch configurations.

How the membrane is clamped at a voltage equal to V_{cmd}

R_p represents the electrode resistance and R_m the membrane input resistance (Figure A7.8a). Suppose that the membrane potential is first clamped to –80 mV (V_{cmd} = –80 mV), then a voltage step to –20 mV is applied for 100 ms (V_{cmd} = –20 mV for 100 ms). The membrane potential (V_m) has to be clamped quickly to –20 mV ($V_m = V_{cmd} = -20$ mV) whatever happens to the channels in the membrane (they open or close). The operational amplifier A1 is able to minimize the voltage difference between two inputs to a very small value (0.1 µV or so). A1 compares the value of V_{cmd} (entry +) to that of V_m (entry –). It then sends a voltage output (V_o) in order to obtain $V_m = V_{cmd} = -20$ mV (Figure A7.8b).

What is this value of V_o? Suppose that at the time t of its peak the Na+ current evoked by the voltage step to –20 mV is I_{Na} = 1 nA. V_o will force a current I = –1 nA to flow through $R_f = 10^9$ Ω in order to clamp the membrane potential: $V_o = R_f \times I = 10^9 \times 10^{-9}$ = 1 V. It is said that V_o = 1 V/nA or 1 mV/pA.

The limits of V_o in patch clamp amplifiers are +15 V and –15 V. It means that V_o cannot be bigger than these values, which is largely compatible with biological experiments where currents through the membrane do not exceed 15 nA.

The amplifier A1 compares V_m with V_{cmd} and sends V_o at a very high speed. This speed has to be very high in order to correct V_m according to V_{cmd} very quickly. The ideal clamp is obtained at the output of the circuit via R_f (black dot V_c on the scheme of Figure A7.8b). As in the voltage clamp technique, a capacitive current is present at the beginning and at the end of the voltage step on the current trace and a leak current during the step but they are not re-explained here.

A7.3.3 The Unitary Current i is a Rectangular Step of Current (see Figures 7.8a and c)

We record, for example, in the outside-out patch clamp configuration the activity of a single voltage sensitive Na+ channel. When a positive membrane potential step is applied to depolarize the patch of membrane from –90 mV to –40 mV, an inward current i_{Na} flowing through the open Na+ channel is recorded (inward current means a current that flows across the membrane from the outside to inside). By convention, inward currents are represented as downward deflections and outward currents as upward deflections.

The membrane depolarization causes activation of the voltage-dependent Na+ channel, and induces its transition from the closed (C) state (or conformation) to the open (O) state, a transition symbolized by:

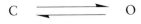

where C is the closed state of the channel (at –90 mV) and O is the open state of the channel (at –40 mV).

While the channel is in the O conformation (at –40 mV), Na+ ions flow through the channel and an inward current caused by the net influx of Na+ ions is recorded. This current reaches its maximum value very rapidly. Thus, the maximal net ion flux is established almost instantaneously given the time scale of the recording (of the order of microseconds). The development of the inward current thus appears as a vertical downward deflection.

A delay between the onset of the voltage step and the onset of the current i is observed. This delay has a duration that varies from one depolarizing test pulse to another and also according to the channel under study. This delay is due to the conformational change or changes of the channel protein. In fact, such changes previous to opening can be multiple:

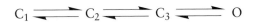

Notice that the opening delay does not correspond to the intrinsic duration of the process of conformational change, which is extremely short. It corresponds to the statistical nature of the equilibrium between the 2, 3, N closed and open conformations.

The opening delay therefore depends on the time spent in each of the different closed states (C_1, C_2, C_3).

The return of the current value to zero corresponds to the closing of the channel. This closure is the result of the transition of the channel protein from the open state (O) to a state in which the channel no longer conducts (state in which the aqueous pore is closed). It can be either a closed state (C), an inactivated state (I) or a desensitized state (D). In the case of the Na^+ channel, the return of the current value to zero is due mainly to the transition of the protein from the open state to the inactivated state ($O \rightarrow I$). Before closing for a long time, the channel can also flicker between the open and closed state ($C \rightleftharpoons O$).

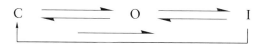

Just as the current reaches its maximum value instantaneously during opening, it also returns instantaneously to its zero value during closing of the pore. Because of this, the unitary current i has a step-like rectangular shape.

A7.3.4 Determination of the Conductance of a Channel

If we repeat several times the experiment shown in Figure 7.8a, we observe that for a given voltage step ΔV, i varies around an average value. The current fluctuations are measured at regular intervals before, during and immediately after the depolarizing voltage pulse. The distribution of the different i values during the voltage pulse describes a gaussian curve in which the peak corresponds to the average i value (Figure 7.8d). There is also a peak around 0 pA (not shown on the figure) which corresponds to the different values of i when the channel is closed. Since the channel is in the closed state most of the time, where i has values around 0 pA, this peak is higher than the one corresponding to $i_{channel}$ (around –2 pA). The width of the peak around 0 pA gives the mean value of the fluctuations resulting from noise. Therefore, the two main reasons for these fluctuations of $i_{channel}$ are: the variations in the noise of the recording system and the changes in the number of ions that cross the channel during a unit of time Δt.

Knowing the average value of i and the reversal potential value of the current (E_{rev}), the average conductance value of the channel under study, γ, can be calculated: $\gamma = i / (V_m - E_{rev})$.

However, there are cases in which the distribution of i for a given membrane potential shows several peaks. Different possibilities should be considered:

- Only one channel is being recorded from but it presents several open conformational states, each one with different conductances. The peaks correspond to the current flowing through these different substates.
- Two or more channels of the *same* type are present in the patch and their activity recorded. The peaks represent the multiple of i (*2i, 3i, . . .*).
- Two or more channels of *different* types are present in the patch and their activity is simultaneously recorded. The peaks correspond to the current through different channel types.

A7.3.5 Mean Open Time of a Channel (Figures A7.9 and A7.10)

An ionic channel fluctuates between a closed state (C) and an open state (O):

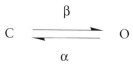

where α is the closing rate constant or, more exactly, the number of channel closures per unit of time spent in the open state O. β is the opening rate constant or the number of openings per unit of time spent in the closed state R (α and β are expressed in s^{-1}).

Once activated, the channel remains in the O state for a time t_o, called open time. When the channel opens, the unitary current i is recorded for a certain time t_o. t_o for a given channel studied under identical conditions varies from one recording to another (Figure A7.9). t_o is an aleatory variable of an aleatory duration. When the number of times a value of t_o (in the order of milli- or microseconds) is plotted against the values of t_o, one obtains the open time histogram, i.e. the distribution of the different values of t_o (Figure A7.10). This distribution declines and the shorter open times are more frequent than the longer ones.

Figure A7.9   Example of the patch clamp recording of a single voltage dependent Ca⁺ channel. In response to a voltage step to +20 mV from a holding potential of −40 mV, the channel opens and closes several times during each of the six trials. (Adapted from Fox AP, Nowyky MC, Tsien RW, 1987. Single-channel recordings of three types of calcium channels in chick sensory neurones, *J. Physiol. (Lond.)* 394, 173–200, with permission.)

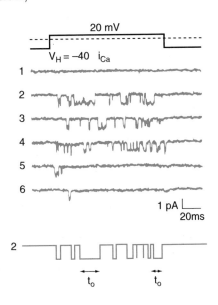

Figure A7.10   Determination of the mean open time of a channel. Trial 2 of Figure A7.9 is selected and all the openings are aligned at time 0. $\tau_o = 1.2$ ms.

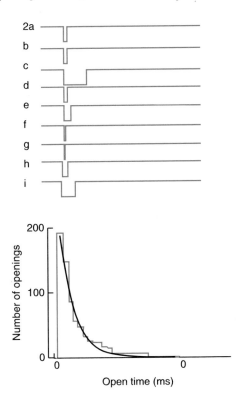

Why does the distribution of t_o *decrease?*

The histogram is constructed as follows: at time $t = 0$, all the channels are open (the delay of opening is ignored, all the openings are aligned at time 0, Figure A7.10). As time t increases, the number of channels that remain open can only decrease since channels progressively close. This can also be expressed as follows: the longer the observation time, the lower the probability that the channel is still in the open state. Or, alternatively, the longer the observation time, the closer the probability will be to 1 that the channel will shut (1 is the maximum value used to express a probability). It is not a Gaussian curve because the delay of opening is ignored and all the openings begin at $t = 0$.

Why is the decrementing distribution of t_o *exponential?*

A channel open at $t = 0$ has a probability of closing at $t + \Delta t$. It has the same probability of closing if it is still open at the beginning of any subsequent observation interval Δt. This type of probability is described mathematically as an exponential function of the observation time. Thus, when the openings of a homogeneous population of channels are studied, the decrease in the number of events is described by a single exponential.

Experimental determination of τ_o, *the mean open time of a channel*

The mean open time τ_o is the time during which a channel has the highest probability of being in the open state: it corresponds to the sum of all the values that t_o may take, weighted by their corresponding probability values. This value is easy to calculate if the distribution is described by a single exponential. In order to verify that the histogram is actually described by a single exponential, one has to first build the histogram by plotting the number of times a value of t_o is observed as a function of t_o, i.e. number of events = $f(t_o)$.

The exponential that describes the histogram has the form $y = y_o e^{-t/\tau_o}$, where y is the number of events observed at each time t. This curve will be linear on semi-logarithmic coordinates if it is described by a single exponential. The slope can be measured with a regression analysis. It corresponds to the mean open time τ_o of the channel. τ_o is the value of t_o for a number of events equal to $1/e$. It is the 'expected value' of t_o. The expected value of t_o is the sum of all the values of t_o weighted by their corresponding probabilities.

In the case of the conformational changes $C \rightleftharpoons O$, the value of τ_o provides an estimate of the closure rate constant α, because at steady state $\tau_o = 1/\alpha$. For example, from the open time histogram of the nicotinic receptor channel, we can determine its mean open time τ_o. Knowing that in conditions where the desensitization of the channel is negligible $\tau_o = 1/\alpha$, we can calculate from τ_o the closing rate constant of the channel. If $\tau_o = 1.1$ ms, $\alpha = 900$ s^{-1}. The channel closes 900 times for each second spent in the open state. In other words there is an average of 900 transitions of the channel to the closed state for each second spent in the open state.

Appendix 7.4
Tail Currents

Tail currents are observed in voltage or patch clamp experiments. 'Tail' means that the voltage-gated current is observed at the end of a depolarizing voltage step, upon sudden removal of the depolarization of the membrane. Tail currents do not exist in physiological conditions; they are 'experimental artifacts'. However, there are several reasons for studying tail currents: they are tools for determining characteristics of currents such as reversal potential and inactivation rate constants. Tail currents were first described by Hodgkin and Huxley (1952) in the squid giant axon.

Single channel tail current

In patch clamp recordings of the activity of a single voltage-gated channel, a unitary current of much larger amplitude is occasionally observed at the end of the voltage step (Figure A7.11). It corresponds to the current flowing through a channel that is not yet closed at the end of the depolarizing step. Therefore tail currents are recorded for voltage-gated channels that do not rapidly close or inactivate during a depolarizing step, such as delayed rectifier K$^+$ or L-type Ca^{2+} channels.

The activity of an L-type Ca^{2+} channel is recorded in patch clamp (cell-attached patch) in the presence of the selective agonist Bay K8644 (see Section 7.5). On stepping back the membrane to the holding potential, the L-type Ca^{2+} channel opened by the preceding depolarization does not immediately close since the transition $O \rightleftharpoons C$ is not immediate. The inward unitary Ca^{2+} current recorded at this moment is larger (Figure A7.11) because of the larger driving force upon removal of depolarization than during the depolarizing step:

during the depolarizing step to 0 mV, i_{Ca}, = γ_{Ca} $(V_m - E_{Ca}) = \gamma_{Ca} (0 - 50) = -50 \gamma_{Ca}$ upon removal of depolarization $i_{Ca} = \gamma_{Ca} (V_m - E_{Ca}) = \gamma_{Ca} (-60 - 50) = -110 \gamma_{Ca}$

Then, after a few milliseconds, due to closing of the channel, the tail current returns to zero (the voltage-gated channel closes in response to the repolarization of the membrane).

Figure A7.11 The activity of an L-type Ca^{2+} channel is recorded in patch clamp (cell-attached patch) in the presence of 110 mM external Ba^{2+}. In response to a depolarizing step from resting potential – 40 mV (RP – 40) to resting potential + 70 mV (RP + 70), in the presence of 5 μM Bay K8644, a current of larger amplitude is recorded on repolarization. It is a single-channel Ca^{2+} tail current.

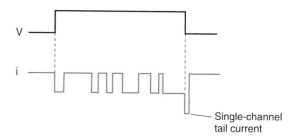

Single-channel
tail current

Whole cell tail current

In voltage or whole cell patch clamp recordings (in the presence of Na^+ and K^+ channel blockers), a voltage step to 0 mV from a holding potential of –40 mV activates a number N of L-type Ca^{2+} channels and an inward Ca^{2+} current is recorded. At the end of the voltage step a Ca^{2+} current of larger amplitude and small duration is always recorded: the tail Ca^{2+} current (Figure A7.12). Then the amplitude of this tail current progressively diminishes. The peak of the whole cell tail current has a larger amplitude than that of the whole cell current recorded during the voltage step since the driving force for Ca^{2+} ions is larger upon removal of depolarization than during the depolarization, as explained above. The tail current diminishes progressively due to the progressive closure of the N open Ca^{2+} channels: the channels do not all close at the same time once the membrane is repolarized. The whole cell tail current of Figure A7.12 represents the summation of hundreds to thousands of recordings of single channel tail currents of Figure A7.11.

In Figures A7.11 and A7.12, the tail currents are inward. The direction of a tail current (as for any type of current) depends on the sign of the driving force, i.e. the value of membrane potential upon repolarization (V_H) and that of the reversal potential of the current (E_{rev}) which depends on the ions flowing through the open channels. By varying the voltage at the end of the depolarizing step the tail current varies in amplitude and direction (inward to outward or the reverse) and it is possible to determine the reversal potential of the tail current under study: when $V_H = E_{rev}$, the tail current is equal to 0 (Figure A7.13). This

Figure A7.12   The activity of a dorsal root ganglion neuron is recorded in single-electrode voltage clamp in the presence of Na^+ and K^+ channel blockers and 2 mM external Ba^{2+}. A depolarization to –10 mV followed by a repolarization to –60 mV is applied to the membrane from a holding potential $V_H = -90$ mV. The depolarizing step evokes an inward whole-cell Ba^{2+} current followed by an inward whole-cell Ba^{2+} tail current (control ○). The presence of 1 μM Bay K 8644 increases the amplitude of the Ba^{2+} current during the step. It also prolongs the Ba^{2+} tail current (●) (Adapted from Carbone E, Formenti A, Pollo A, 1990. Multiple actions of Bay K 8644 on high-threshold Ca channels in adult rat sensory neurons, *Neurosci. Lett.* **111**, 315–320, with permission.)

Figure A7.13   The activity of a chick dorsal root ganglion cell is recorded in single electrode voltage clamp, in the presence of 1 μM TTX and 10 mM Co^{2+} to block, respectively, Ca^{2+} and Na^+ channels. Depolarizations to +10 mV from a holding potential of –50 mV followed by successive repolarizations to –50, –60, –70, –80 and –90 mV are applied (V traces). Bottom I traces show the K^+ tail currents at the corresponding membrane potentials (the outward K^+ current during the step is not shown). The reversal potential of the K^+ tail current is –70 mV. It indicates the value of E_K in these cells. To separate the ionic tail current from the capacitive current, the latter was subtracted from the total current by digital summation of the currents elicited with identical depolarizing and hyperpolarizing test pulses. (Adapted from Dunlap K, Fischbach GD, 1981. Neurotransmitters decrease the calcium conductance activated by depolarization of embryonic chick sensory neurones, *J. Physiol. (Lond.)* **317**, 519–535, with permission.)

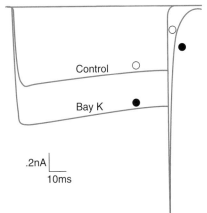

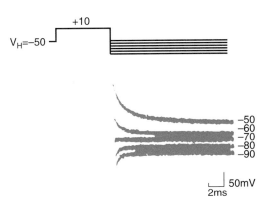

value of E_{rev} is the same for the tail current and the current recorded during the voltage step since it concerns the same channels. The voltage protocol of Figure A7.13, allows the determination of E_{rev} and consequently the identification of the type of ions that carry the current. E_{rev} can also be directly determined by changing the voltage steps value. However, for K^+ channels for example, E_{rev} is near -100 mV, a membrane potential where the open probability of voltage gated channels is very low. By using tail currents, this problem is overcome.

Further Reading

Bertolino, M. and Llinas, R.R. (1992) The central role of voltage-activated and receptor-operated calcium channels in neuronal cells. *Ann. Rev. Pharmacol. Toxicol.* **32**, 399–421.

Eaholtz, G., Scheuer, T. and Catterall, W. A. (1994) Restoration of inactivation and block of open sodium channels by an inactivation gate peptide. *Neuron*; **12**, 1041–1048.

De Leon, M., Wang, Y., Jones, J. *et al.* (1995) Essential Ca^{2+}-binding motif for Ca^{2+}-sensitive inactivation of L-type Ca^{2+} channels. *Science* **270**, 1502–1506.

Hamill, O.P., Marty, A., Neher, E. *et al.* (1981) Improved patch damp technique for high resolution current recording from cells and cell-free membrane patches. *Pflügers Archiv.* **391**, 85–100.

Hofmann, F., Biel, M. and Flockerzi. Molecular basis for Ca^{2+} channel diversity. *Ann. Rev. Neurosci.* **17**, 399–418.

Korn, S.I., Marty, A., Connor, J.A. and Horn R. (1991) Perforated patch recording. *Methods Neurosci.* **4**, 264–373.

Miller, C. (1995) The charybdotoxin family of K^+ channel-blocking peptides. *Neuron* **15**, 5–10.

Neher, E. and Sakmann, B. (1976) Single channel currents recorded from membrane of denervated frog muscle fibres. *Nature* **260**, 779–802.

Noda, M., Ikeda, T., Suzuki, H. *et al.* (1986) Expression of functional sodium channels from cloned cDNA. *Nature* **322**, 826–828.

Numann, K., Caterall, W.A. and Scheuer, T. (1991) Functional modulation of brain sodium channels by protein kinase C phosphorylation. *Science* **254**, 115–118.

Stea, A., Soong, T.W. and Snutch, T.P. (1995) Determinants of PKC-dependent modulation of a family of neuronal calcium channels. *Neuron* **15**, 929–940.

Stuart, G. and Häuser, M. (1994) Initiation and spread of sodium action potentials in cerebellar purkinje cells. *Neuron* **13**, 703–712.

Varadi, G., Mori, Y., Mikala, G. and Schwartz, A. (1995) Molecular determinants of Ca^{2+} channels function and drug action. *Trends Pharmacol. Sci.* **16**, 43–49.

Vassilev, P.M., Scheuer, T. and Catterall, W.A. (1988) Identification of an intracellular peptide segment involved in sodium channel inactivation. *Science* **241**, 1658–1661.

Neurotransmitter Release

The neurotransmitter(s) synthesized by a neuron is (are) stored in the pre-synaptic element, inside the synaptic vesicles. In the absence of pre-synaptic activity, the probability of neurotransmitter release in the synaptic cleft is very low. This probability increases strongly when the pre-synaptic element is excited. The release of neurotransmitter is a discontinuous, 'quantal' phenomenon and, as shown in Figure 2.4, is mediated by the calcium dependent exocytosis of synaptic vesicles, the total content of a single synaptic vesicle being a quantum (Del Castillo and Katz, 1954).

Among the events leading to neurotransmitter release, the local rise of the intracellular Ca^{2+} ion concentration and the need to increase the probability of vesicular exocytosis have been clearly established (Section 8.1). Conversely, only recently have the molecular mechanisms responsible for the coupling between Ca^{2+} ion influx and exocytosis begun to be elucidated. These mechanisms include the identification of the proteins involved in exocytosis, the steps regulating exocytosis and their order of appearance in the phenomenon (Section 8.2).

The exocytosis of a synaptic vesicle is a random phenomenon which can occur in the absence of pre-synaptic activity but with a low probability. Even when all the right conditions come together (depolarization of the pre-synaptic element, opening of Ca^{2+} channels, Ca^{2+} entry), the average probability of the exocytosis of a synaptic vesicle still remains below 1 (Section 8.3).

Many pre-synaptic elements contain small synaptic vesicles as well as large dense-core vesicles (Section 2.1.1). The demonstration at the frog neuromuscular junction that exocytosis of small and large dense-core vesicles (Section 2.3.1) can be dissociated pharmacologically strongly suggests differences in the mechanisms that regulate exocytosis of the two secretory vesicles. However, the two systems share at least some common mechanisms for final fusion since both are sensitive to botulinum toxins. In this chapter we will only consider the mechanisms of transmitter release from small synaptic vesicles.

The vesicle hypothesis of neurotransmitter release, first formulated by Del Castillo and Katz (1954), is one theory attempting to explain neurotransmitter release. The other theory is termed the non-vesicular theory. In this theory, the neurotransmitter molecules released in the synaptic cleft would not be those stored in the vesicles but rather those located in the pre-synaptic cytoplasm (Appendix 8.1). Many recent data demonstrate the existence of vesicular release, such as those obtained with combined capacitance measurements and amperometry or optical analysis of labeled synaptic vesicles. This chapter will focus on data related to the vesicular theory.

In the mammalian central nervous system, the interneuronal synapses, and especially the pre-synaptic elements of those synapses, are too small to be studied with current electrophysiological techniques and *a fortiori* to allow intracellular injection of molecules influencing neurotransmitter release. For this reason, studies have been performed mostly on the neuromuscular junction (Figure 2.10) and for interneuronal synapses on the squid giant synapse (located in the stellate ganglion) (Figure 8.1) or the inhibitory synapses afferent to the Mauthner cell (in teleost fish bulb) (see Figure 8.13a).

8.1 Depolarization of the Pre-synaptic Element Induces a Transient Increase of the Intracellular Ca^{2+} Concentration and Triggers Exocytosis

In a resting pre-synaptic element, Ca^{2+} ions are present at a very low concentration, 10^{-7} to 10^{-8} M. This intracellular Ca^{2+} concentration, $[Ca^{2+}]_i$, is at least 10 000 times smaller than the extracellular Ca^{2+} concentration (see Figure 5.2); it is maintained at this

Figure 8.1   The squid giant synapse. (a) This synapse is located in the stellate ganglion. These neurons are part of a network of giant cells. The primary neurons, whose cell bodies are located in the magnocellular lobe, receive sensory information (from the eyes and tentacles). They transmit this information to secondary neurons located in the palliovisceral ganglion. In this ganglion, the axons of primary neurons make contacts with the axons of secondary neurons. The axons of secondary neurons send projections to the stellate ganglion, where they make giant synaptic contacts with the axons of tertiary neurons. The tertiary neurons are responsible for the contraction of mantle muscles, thus permitting expulsion of water, propelling the animal out of the danger zone. (b) The giant synapse is a synapse between a large size, non-myelinated axon of secondary neurons and a giant axon of tertiary neurons. The contact between the two axons is about 700 μm long and the diameter of the post-synaptic axon is 50 μm. This allows the introduction of many electrodes and the simultaneous recording, in voltage or current clamp, of pre- and post-synaptic activity. The dotted line represents the cutting plane of Figure 8.2. (c) Pre- and post-synaptic spikes recorded simultaneously in current clamp. The post-synaptic action potential arises from an excitatory postsynaptic potential. The synaptic delay is close to 1 ms. $[Ca^{2+}]_o = 10$ mmol/1. AP, Action potential. (From Llinas R, 1982. Calcium in synaptic transmission, *Sci. Am.* **247**, 56–65, with permission.)

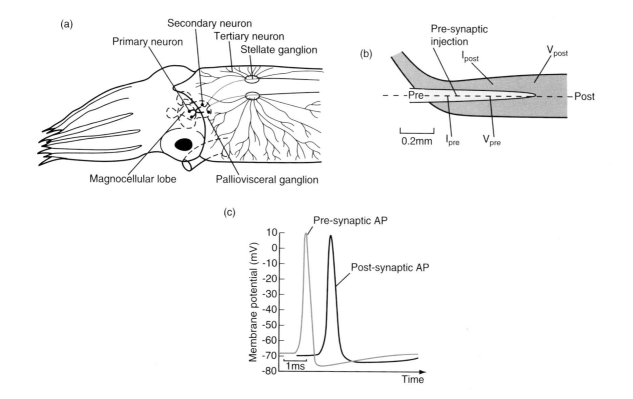

resting level by various Ca^{2+} clearance mechanisms (see Section 8.1.3).

Depolarization of the membrane of a pre-synaptic element by an action potential induces an increase of $[Ca^{2+}]_i$ in the pre-synaptic element and raises the probability of exocytosis of synaptic vesicles and thus transmitter release.

Is the increase of $[Ca^{2+}]_i$ necessary to induce transmitter release? What is the origin of Ca^{2+} ions?

8.1.1 Ca^{2+} Entry in the Pre-synaptic Element Results from the Opening of Voltage-Dependent Ca^{2+} Channels

An extracellular medium deprived of Ca^{2+} ions, or containing Ca^{2+} channel blocking agents (such as Co^{2+} or Cd^{2+} ions), causes the disappearance of post-synaptic potentials although the pre-synaptic potentials are unchanged. The brief membrane depolarization that occurs in the ascending phase of each spike triggers the opening of voltage-dependent Ca^{2+} channels (see Section 7.5) and the subsequent influx of Ca^{2+} ions in the pre-synaptic element. The entry of Ca^{2+} ions through voltage-dependent Ca^{2+} channels is necessary to trigger exocytosis, this being valid for all chemical synapses studied until now.

The type of Ca^{2+} channels present in pre-synaptic terminals and triggering transmitter release is investigated in different preparations. For this purpose pharmacological agents that block relatively selectively a type of Ca^{2+} channel are applied to a preparation and their effects on the amplitude of pre-synaptic Ca^{2+} current and the amplitude of post-synaptic response

are studied. It appears that the Ca^{2+} channels involved differ with the synapse studied and that, at present, no general rule can be given. They are generally of the N and P types.

8.1.2 Strategic Location of Ca^{2+} Channels at Pre-synaptic Active Zones

The short latency, 200–300 µs (see Section 8.1.5), between Ca^{2+} entry and the activation of secretion strongly suggests that the Ca^{2+} channels are close to the release sites in the pre-synaptic terminals.

The localization and the amplitude of the Ca^{2+} rise

Figure 8.2 Ca^{2+} channels are clustered at active zones. (a) In the squid giant synapse, along the region of contact between pre-synaptic (PRE) and post-synaptic (POST) fibers (insert, bottom right), thousands of active zones are present. The $[Ca^{2+}]_i$ variations are seen with the fura-2 technique (see Appendix 11.1) in response to a train of brief pre-synaptic discharges (0.5 s at 80 Hz). The results show that the most prominent increases of $[Ca^{2+}]_i$ are located at active zones (top drawing). (b) In the frog neuromuscular junction, N-type Ca^{2+} channels and nicotinic acetylcholine receptors (nAChR) are labeled with two different selective toxins coupled to different fluorescent dyes. The preparation is viewed with a confocal laser scanning microscope. The diagram below illustrates the structure of the neuromuscular junction on the cylindrical muscle fiber and the box indicates the region scanned by the microscope. The images showing the distribution of pre-synaptic Ca^{2+} channels (top) and post-synaptic nAChR (bottom) are separated for clarity but they are in fact superimposed. The pattern of the two labels is very similar and there is a close registration between them, indicating that each active zone of the pre-synaptic neuron is in almost perfect alignment with each region of the post-synaptic membrane containing a high concentration of nAChR. Bar = 10 µm. (a: From Smith SJ, Augustine GJ, 1988. Calcium ions, active zones and synaptic transmitter release, *TINS* **11**, 458–464, with permission. b: From Robitaille R, Adler EM and Charlton MP, 1990, Strategic location of calcium channels at transmitter release sites of frog neuromuscular synapses, *Neuron* **5**: 773–779, with permission.)

(a)

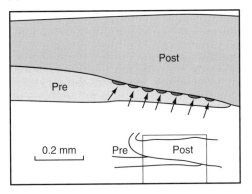

(b)

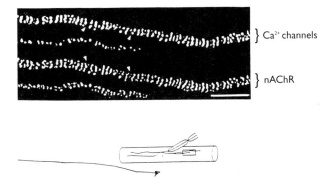

} Ca^{2+} channels

} nAChR

can be studied with imaging techniques. A Ca^{2+} sensitive fluorescent protein with a low affinity for Ca^{2+} ions (in order to visualize only the zones where the Ca^{2+} concentration is high) is injected into the pre-synaptic terminal of the squid giant synapse. When the pre-synaptic element is depolarized, microdomains exhibiting Ca^{2+} concentrations in the range of 200–300 µM are visualized. These microdomains of high Ca^{2+} concentration are localized at active zones of the pre-synaptic plasma membrane. This Ca^{2+} increase is at least 10 times larger than that in other pre-synaptic membrane areas (Figure 8.2a). This observation supports the fact that voltage-dependent Ca^{2+} channels are clustered at active zones.

Other authors investigated the localization of Ca^{2+} channels relative to the position of transmitter release sites in the frog neuromuscular junction using morphological techniques. In this preparation, the pre-synaptic nerve terminal is a long structure (several hundred micrometers) characterized by the presence of neurotransmitter release sites or active zones spaced at regular intervals of 1 µm directly across the synaptic cleft from clusters of nAChR on the edge of the post-junctional folds (see Section 2.3 and Figure 2.10). The preparation is double-labeled to disclose both the nAChR and pre-synaptic N-type Ca^{2+} channels. Ca^{2+} channels are labeled with biotinylated ω-conotoxin, a specific and irreversible blocker of N-type Ca^{2+} channels and of synaptic transmission at the frog neuromuscular junction. To reveal Ca^{2+} channel labeling, preparations are then incubated with streptavidin Texas red (see Figure A2.3) which fluoresces red. nAChRs are labeled with α-bungarotoxin coupled to boron dipyrromethane difluoride which fluoresces green.

Each fluorescent band of nAChR stain is usually matched by a fluorescent band of Ca^{2+} channel stain (Figure 8.2b). Bands of labeled Ca^{2+} channels and labeled nAChRs are thus almost perfectly aligned, suggesting that Ca^{2+} channels are clustered at the similarly spaced active zones opposite the post-junctional folds. When nerve terminals are removed by pulling on branches of the motor nerve, the Ca^{2+} channel labeling totally disappears, indicating that ω-conotoxin binding sites are located on pre-synaptic terminals.

These results exemplify some general principles of rapid Ca^{2+} signaling in neurotransmitter release:

- Ca^{2+} entry into the pre-synaptic element occurs only in close proximity to the exocytotic apparatus.

- Clustering of Ca^{2+} channels close to released sites ensures that a large Ca^{2+} signal (up to hundreds of micromolars) is rapidly available (in the hundreds of microseconds time scale) to the nearby Ca^{2+}-sensitive proteins which initiate transmitter release. The co-precipitation of N-type Ca^{2+} channels (labeled with ω-conotoxin) with a pre-synaptic integral membrane protein (syntaxin, labeled with a specific antibody) and the identification of the syntaxin binding domain on N channels demonstrate the tight physical coupling of N-type Ca^{2+} channels and exocytotic sites, making release as fast as possible (see Section 8.2 and Figure 8.9).

A hypothesis formulated on the basis of these observations is that only high concentrations of cytosolic Ca^{2+} are effective in triggering exocytosis of synaptic vesicles. Thus the cytosolic Ca^{2+} proteins involved in exocytosis would have a low affinity for Ca^{2+} (K_D around 10^{-4} M).

8.1.3 Ca^{2+} Entry Induces a Transient Increase of the Cytosolic Ca^{2+} Concentration

In order to study simultaneously the Ca^{2+} current (I_{Ca}) and the resulting elevation of $[Ca^{2+}]_i$, these two parameters are recorded simultaneously following brief depolarizations of the pre-synaptic terminal (squid giant synapse). The Ca^{2+} current is recorded in voltage clamp in the presence of agents blocking the voltage-dependent Na^+ channels (such as TTX) and the voltage-dependent K^+ channels (TEA, Cs^+ and/or 4-aminopyridine). The $[Ca^{2+}]_i$ variation is measured with arsenazo III, a sensitive probe whose absorbancy properties (at 660 nm) are a function of the intracellular Ca^{2+} concentration (see Appendix 11.1).

When an inward Ca^{2+} current (I_{Ca}) is elicited by a depolarizing pulse, in a pre-synaptic terminal injected with arsenazo III, one can observe that (i) the calcium signal duration, i. e. the length of $[Ca^{2+}]_i$ increase, is larger than the length of I_{Ca} (Figure 8.3a); and (ii) the amplitude of the calcium signal has the same voltage sensitivity as I_{Ca} (Figure 8.3b).

In an attempt to obtain quantitative data on amplitude changes and duration of I_{Ca} and $[Ca^{2+}]_i$ increase, these parameters are recorded following pre-synaptic action potentials instead of pre-synaptic depolarizing pulses. One can observe that (Figure 8.4):

Figure 8.3   Simultaneous recordings of pre-synaptic Ca^{2+} current and intracellular Ca^{2+} ion concentration. (a) Pre-synaptic I_{Ca} is evoked by a 25 ms-long pre-synaptic depolarization (V_{pre}). I_{Ca} (I_{pre}) is recorded in voltage clamp in the presence of agents blocking Na^+ and K^+ currents. The average increase of Ca^{2+} concentration in the pre-synaptic terminal in response to V_{pre} is measured by absorbancy changes of arsenazo III (Ar III). One can see that the calcium signal (increase of $[Ca^{2+}]_i$) lasts much longer than I_{Ca}. In these experimental conditions, an absorbancy variation of 10^{-4} (ΔA) corresponds to a variation of $[Ca^{2+}]_i$ of about 3×10^{-7} mol/l. (b) Voltage dependence of Ca^{2+} current integrals (solid line) and peak $[Ca^{2+}]_i$ elevation ($\square$) elicited by 6 ms-long depolarizations closely correspond when scaled to the same peak value. (a: From Augustine GJ, Charlton MP and Smith SJ, 1985. Calcium entry into voltage clamped presynaptic terminal of squid, *J. Physiol.* 367, 143–162, with permission.)

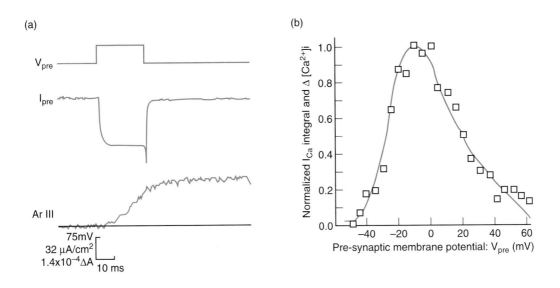

in response to one action potential, $[Ca^{2+}]_i$ increases by 75 nM. The maximal value is obtained in approximately 1 ms, during the repolarizing phase of the action potential (Figure 8.4a);

- in response to two action potentials (at an interval of 12 ms), $[Ca^{2+}]_i$ also increases by 75 nM for each action potential (Figure 8.4b);
- in response to a train of action potentials ($n = 7$ to 74, frequency = 30–40 Hz), $[Ca^{2+}]_i$ increases linearly while the action potentials occur, then slowly decreases with a time constant ranging from 4.5 to 15 s depending on the number of action potentials in the train. The maximal value of $[Ca^{2+}]_i$ elevation corresponds to the theoretical value obtained by multiplying the value of $[Ca^{2+}]_i$ increase for a single action potential by the total number of action potentials in the train (Figure 8.4c).

These results show a clear correlation between I_{Ca} integral and the amplitude of $[Ca^{2+}]_i$ increase.

Moreover, in an active pre-synaptic terminal, the amount of Ca^{2+} ions entering after each action potential is virtually the same. However, as $[Ca^{2+}]_i$ does not decline to its basal level between successive action potentials, there is a cumulative effect of the successive $[Ca^{2+}]_i$ elevations which might account for the residual calcium hypothesis in short-term potentiation (see Section 19.1).

8.1.4 The Amplitude and Time Course of the Increase of $[Ca^{2+}]_i$ in Pre-synaptic Terminals are Determined by the Number of Ca^{2+} Ions Entering the Intracellular Medium and the Efficacy of Ca^{2+} Clearance Mechanisms

The cytosolic free Ca^{2+} concentration ($[Ca^{2+}]_i$) is maintained at a very low level (10^{-7} to 10^{-8} M), the majority of intracellular Ca^{2+} ions being bound to proteins in the cytoplasm, or sequestered in the organelles.

Figure 8.4 Increase of intracellular Ca^{2+} concentration in relation to pre-synaptic activity (squid giant synapse). (a, b) Arsenazo III is injected into the pre-synaptic terminal and its absorbancy changes (see Appendix 11.1) at 660 nm are measured (ΔA, 16 measurements on average) following one (a) or two (b) pre-synaptic spikes (in b, the spikes are at a 12 ms interval). The absorbancy changes correspond to the average of 16 measurements. $[Ca^{2+}]_i$ increase following the second spike is identical to that following the first spike. (c) Absorbancy changes of arsenazo III (ΔA, average of 16 measurements) in repeated activity (33 Hz stimulation for 2 s) of the pre-synaptic axon. $[Ca^{2+}]_o = 11$ mmol/1. (d) The Ca^{2+} cloud is spatially restricted following entry of Ca^{2+} ions through voltage-gated Ca^{2+} channels. The figure shows the distance over which Ca^{2+} ions would diffuse within 2 ms after Ca^{2+} channel opening. During fast neurotransmission, only those synaptic vesicles docked on the pre-synaptic membrane close to Ca^{2+} channels will be able to fuse with the pre-synaptic membrane and release the neurotransmitter. (a–c: Adapted from Charlton MP, Smith SJ and Zucker RS, 1982, Role of presynaptic calcium ions and channels in synaptic facilitation and depression at the squid giant axon synapse, *J. Physiol.* **323**, 173–193, with permission. d: Adapted from Burgoyne RD and Morgan A, 1995. Ca^{2+} and secretory-vesicle dynamics, *Trends Neurosci.* **18**, 191–196, with permission.)

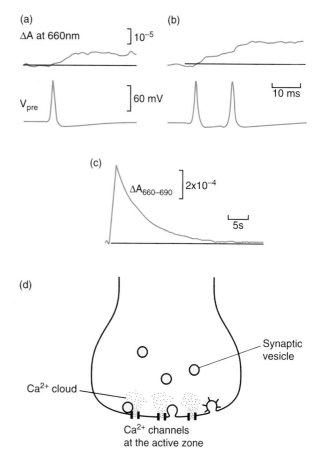

$[Ca^{2+}]_i$ is maintained at this low level by various mechanisms defined here as Ca^{2+} clearance mechanisms.

The Ca^{2+} clearance mechanisms have a very high efficacy, affecting the duration and amplitude of $[Ca^{2+}]_i$ increase. It is estimated that 0.1% to 1% of entering Ca^{2+} ions are actually 'seen' by the intracellular medium as free Ca^{2+} ions, even during the peak of $[Ca^{2+}]_i$ increase.

Thus, the amplitude and duration of the calcium signal are determined by the number of Ca^{2+} ions entering close to the active zones per unit of time and by the efficacy of the Ca^{2+} clearance mechanisms.

The number of Ca^{2+} ions entering in a unit of time through voltage-dependent Ca^{2+} channels *in vivo* depends on the number of opened Ca^{2+} channels, which depends on:

- the pre-synaptic activity (duration, frequency and number of action potentials);
- the number of Ca^{2+} channels that are susceptible to activation;
- the presence of K^+ channels activated by a rise of

$[Ca^{2+}]_i$ (see Section 7.5); the exit of K^+ ions through these channels repolarizes the pre-synaptic membrane and thus reduces the number of Ca^{2+} channels open and the amount of Ca^{2+} ions entering the pre-synaptic terminal. In the pre-synaptic terminals of the neuromuscular junction, the localization of $K_{(Ca)}$ channels labeled with charybdotoxin–biotin matches the localization of N-type Ca^{2+} channels labeled with ω-conotoxin–biotin: a similar banding pattern is observed (as in Figure 8.2b). Other types of K^+ channels can be observed in other preparations.

The neuronal Ca^{2+} clearance mechanisms include Ca^{2+} buffering by cytosolic proteins, Ca^{2+} transport across the neuronal plasma membrane and Ca^{2+} uptake by the plasma membrane of organelles and sequestration in intracellular organelles (Figure 8.5).

Figure 8.5   Schematic representation of components of the Ca^{2+} clearance system in a pre-synaptic terminal. While depolarization occurs, Ca^{2+} ions enter at the level of pre-synaptic active zones through voltage-dependent Ca^{2+} channels and are rapidly buffered by cytoplasmic calcium binding proteins ($Pr\text{-}Ca^{2+}$). Ca^{2+} ions are then cleared from the intracellular medium towards the extracellular medium via the Na–Ca exchanger and the Ca^{2+}–ATPase. Ca^{2+} ions are also actively transported into intracellular Ca^{2+} stores. This clearing has a constant of the order of tens of milliseconds to seconds. Ca^{2+} ions can also be released into the cytosol via Ca^{2+} channels present in the membrane of Ca^{2+}-storing organelles.

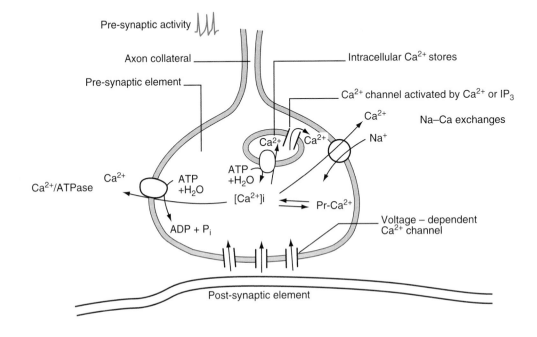

Ca^{2+} buffering by cytosolic proteins. Different cytosolic proteins have the ability to bind Ca^{2+} with a high affinity. These proteins have, in general, a low molecular weight and act primarily as Ca^{2+} buffers (such as parvalbumin and calbindin) or subserve messenger functions (calmodulin).

Parvalbumin is found in large amounts in most GABAergic neurons in the mammalian central nervous system (the co-localization of GABA and parvalbumin has been shown immunohistochemically using highly specific antibodies to GABA and parvalbumin) whereas, in other neurons, the concentration of parvalbumin is much lower. The high concentration of parvalbumin might have a consequence on a neuron's ability to rapidly buffer Ca^{2+}. This is especially important for neurons that are metabolically active (have a tonic activity), such as GABAergic neurons.

Calbindin is a protein that was originally found in the gut, where it binds Ca^{2+} and is vitamin D-dependent. Its presence has been shown in neurons of the mammalian central nervous system, notably the Purkinje cells of the cerebellar cortex and the dopaminergic neurons of the substantia nigra.

Calmodulin has a high affinity for Ca^{2+} and a role of intracellular messenger. When Ca^{2+} binds to these proteins, it triggers intracellular events discussed at the end of Chapter 7.

The buffering of the free intracellular Ca^{2+} ions by cytoplasmic calcium-binding proteins is a very efficient system, responsible for the rapid disappearance of entering Ca^{2+} ions and thus determining the amplitude of the calcium signal.

Extrusion of Ca^{2+} in the extracellular medium. This is achieved by two types of transmembrane proteins, the Ca/ATPase pump and the Na/Ca exchanger. The former uses the hydrolysis of ATP as a source of energy and is independent of the extracellular Na^+ concentration. The latter is driven by the Na^+ electrochemical gradient across the plasma membrane and is thus sensitive to extracellular Na^+ concentration. The Ca/ATPase pump is proposed to be a low capacity, high affinity (K_D = 0.2–0.3 μM) system whereas the Na/Ca exchanger would have a high capacity and a low affinity (K_D = 0.5–1.0 μM). The Ca/ATPase pump would thus be the most efficient system in the presence of a low pre-synaptic activity, and the two systems would act in synergy to regulate the intracellular Ca^{2+} concentration after a train of action potentials.

Sequestration of Ca^{2+} in smooth endoplasmic reticulum and mitochondria. This is achieved by Ca/ATPase pumps present in the membrane of these organelles. The smooth endoplasmic reticulum is a Ca^{2+} storage compartment. In the different cell types studied, the smooth endoplasmic reticulum Ca/ATPase pump has a better affinity for Ca^{2+} than that of a mitochondrion. The latter would function in very rare situations, when there is a massive Ca^{2+} entry. Following an appropriate signal (such as the formation of inositol triphosphate, IP_3), Ca^{2+} can be released in the cytoplasm from these storage compartments.

8.1.5 Correlations Between Increase of Intracellular Ca^{2+} Concentration and Neurotransmitter Release

In order to analyze the relations between the increase of $[Ca^{2+}]_i$ and neurotransmitter release, the following parameters have been recorded simultaneously on the squid giant synapse (see Figure. 8.1b):

- The inward pre-synaptic calcium current, I_{Ca}, taken as a clue to the variation of $[Ca^{2+}]_i$. It was shown previously (Section 8.1.2) that the amplitude of $[Ca^{2+}]_i$ increase varies according to the amplitude of I_{Ca}.
- The excitatory post-synaptic potential (EPSP) taken as a clue to the amount of neurotransmitter released. The post-synaptic response depends largely on the number of excited post-synaptic receptors, which depends on the amount of neurotransmitter released in a unit of time (if one assumes that the efficacy of neurotransmitter inactivation mechanisms does not depend on the amount of neurotransmitter released in the synaptic cleft). The experimental conditions are designed in such a way that desensitization of the post-synaptic receptors can be neglected.

In response to a depolarizing pulse of varying amplitude and stable duration (V_{pre}) (Figure 8.6, bottom traces), the evoked pre-synaptic Ca^{2+} current, I_{Ca} (middle traces), and the EPSP (top traces) are recorded. The pre-synaptic I_{Ca} is recorded in two-electrode voltage clamp mode and the post-synaptic response is recorded in current clamp mode after pharmacological blockade of voltage-dependent Na^+ and K^+ channels (holding potential V_H = –70 mV). Increasing the amplitude of the depolarizing pulse V_{pre} from +30 to +52 mV (Figure 8.6, A to C) produced a larger I_{Ca} with a faster rate of rise. At the end of each pulse, a tail current is recorded during the membrane repolarization, before the repolarization leads to the closing of Ca^{2+} channels (see Appendix 7.4). At the same time (A to C), a larger EPSP is recorded with a faster rate of rise and the EPSP continues to increase after termination of the pulse during the tail current. With a further increase of pre-synaptic depolarization (D and E), I_{Ca} and the EPSP reach a peak. For V_{pre} amplitudes higher than +60 mV (F to H), I_{Ca} decreases but the tail I_{Ca} increases. At the same time, the rate of rise and amplitude of the EPSP during the pulse ('on EPSP') decreases while the part of the EPSP after the break of the voltage clamp pulse ('off EPSP') increases. For V_{pre} = +60 mV I_{Ca} is null because I_{Ca} reverses polarity at a potential less depolarized than the theoretical value calculated from the Nernst equation (see Section 7.5) but the tail I_{Ca} is present. No synaptic transmission was observed during the depolarizing pulse but an 'off EPSP' is generated by the tail I_{Ca}. In conclusion, this experiment shows that the latency and amplitude of the post-synaptic response (EPSP) is a function of the latency and amplitude of pre-synaptic I_{Ca}.

One extremely interesting finding is that the synaptic delay is shorter when the transmitter release is triggered by the tail I_{Ca}. As shown in Figure 8.7, the synaptic delay for the 'on EPSP' is 733 μs. However, in the same synapse, the 'off EPSP' shows a latency of 200 μs. This indicates that the synaptic delay must consist of two parts: one (i) that relates to the time dependence of the Ca^{2+} channels opening and a second (ii) that is determined by the time required for the events that follow the entry of Ca^{2+}. During a voltage clamp pulse, the 1 ms latency of the 'on EPSP' (see Figure. 8.1c) would be composed of both (i) and (ii). The shorter latency of the 'off EPSP' would result from the (ii) events alone. We will now focus on the

Figure 8.6   Amplitude and time course of pre-synaptic calcium current (I_{Ca}) and post-synaptic excitatory potential (EPSP) elicited by 6 ms-long pre-synaptic depolarizing steps (V_{pre}) ranging from 30 to 130 mV (A to I), from a holding potential $V_H = -70$ mV. See text for explanation. (From Llinás R, Steinberg IZ and Walton K, 1981. Relationship between presynaptic calcium current and postsynaptic potential in squid giant synapse, *Biophys. J.* **33**, 323–351, with permission.)

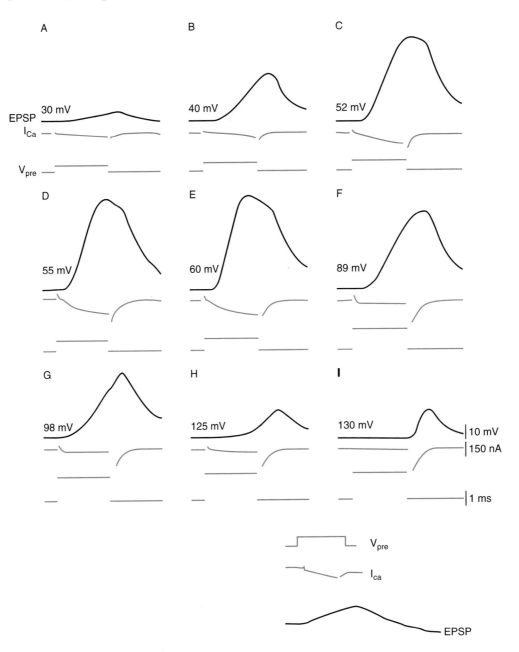

Figure 8.7   The synaptic delay of the 'on EPSP' is longer than that of the 'off EPSP'. (a) The 'on EPSP' is shown for a voltage step to −10 mV. Its latency is 733 µs. The 'off EPSP' is seen following a voltage step to +70 mV. Its latency is 200 µs. (b) Histogram of the variations in the latency (in ms × 10^{-1}) observed for the 'on EPSP' (mean = 0.894 ± 0.168 ms, n = 51) and the 'off EPSP' (mean = 0.192 ± 0.272 ms, n = 25). (From Llinás R, Steinberg IZ and Walton K, 1981. Relationship between presynaptic calcium current and postsynaptic potential in squid giant synapse, *Biophys. J.* **33**, 323–351, with permission.)

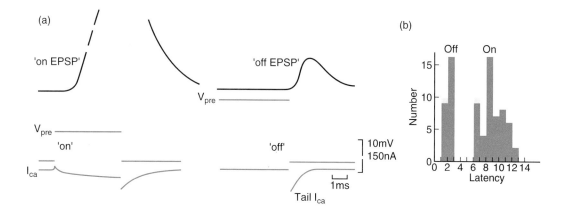

events occurring after the entry of Ca^{2+} into the axon terminal.

8.2 Events Occurring Between the Increase of Intracellular Ca^{2+} Concentration and Neurotransmitter Release

In a resting nerve terminal, synaptic vesicles are loaded with the neurotransmitter. They are localized either in the cytoplasm (linked to filaments) or docked to the active zone at the pre-synaptic plasma membrane. Activation of the nerve terminal by an action potential or a train of action potentials leads to an influx of Ca^{2+} ions triggering fusion (exocytosis) of docked synaptic vesicles and release of neurotransmitter: it is a regulated secretion. We shall explain what is presently known for the different steps between Ca^{2+} entry and release of neurotransmitter.

8.2.1 Synaptic Vesicles are Found in the Active Zones Where They Are Surrounded by a Complex Network of Filaments

The fusion of synaptic vesicles with the pre-synaptic plasma membrane occurs at a restricted, morphologi-

cally distinct domain known as the active zone. An active zone is characterized by: (i) a pre-synaptic membrane area where the density of Ca^{2+} channels is high and specialized in exocytosis of synaptic vesicles; and (ii) a cytoplasmic region where the synaptic vesicles are found close to the pre-synaptic membrane, with a particular cytoskeletal arrangement (Figure 8.8).

However, the active zone is not a characteristic of all synapses. A few monoaminergic synapses and peptidergic synapses do not have discernible active zones. The presence of an active zone would be a clue to focal neurotransmitter release.

In nerve terminals, quick freeze deep-etch electron microscopy demonstrated that a subpopulation of the synaptic vesicles is suspended in a complex network of filaments:

- numerous 40 nm long filaments having globular heads that cross each other, thus enabling the filaments to contract;
- few filaments having a larger diameter, extending from the pre-synaptic membrane to the axoplasm, whose length is about 50 nm. They can be in contact with the vesicles or the smaller filaments.

Moreover, another subpopulation of the synaptic vesicles is docked to the pre-synaptic plasma membrane.

Figure 8.8 Schematic drawing of filaments found in the cytoplasm of pre-synaptic elements. The region close to the active zone is enlarged. One can see the presence of small filaments with a globular head, providing connections with synaptic vesicles and other small filaments. These filaments have the shape and structure of synapsin I (see Figure 8.10). A second type of filament originates from the pre-synaptic membrane and makes contacts with small filaments. The vesicles are sequestered close to the pre-synaptic active zone and others are docked to the pre-synaptic membrane. The exocytosis of a vesicle is shown. (Adapted from Landis DMD, Hall AK, Weinstein LA and Reese TS, 1988. The organization of cytoplasm at the presynaptic active zone of a central nervous system synapse, *Neuron* **1**, 201–209, with permission.)

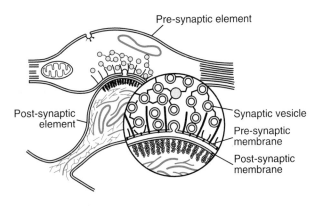

8.2.2 Hypothesis Concerning Vesicle Movement in the Axon Terminals

Intracellular recordings in model synapses such as the squid giant synapse have shown that the latency between Ca^{2+} entry and the release of the transmitter is in the range of 200–300 µs (Section 8.1.4). During this time Ca^{2+} ions diffuse no more than a few vesicle diameters into the cytoplasm (see Figure 8.2a). This suggested that:

- Ca^{2+} channels and release sites are located at a close distance;
- a complex between synaptic vesicles and the plasma membrane is preassembled in the resting state (before intracellular Ca^{2+} levels increase) because the time after Ca^{2+} entry is too short and its diffusion too restricted to allow for vesicle movement before fusion with the plasma membrane.

Studies on freeze-fractured neuromuscular junctions support the first hypothesis since the distance from the

calcium channel to the exocytotic pore is restricted to about 25 nm.

How do synaptic vesicles dock to the target pre-synaptic membrane?

Synaptic vesicle traffic in nerve terminals is considered to involve several hypothetical stages (Figure 8.9). After they fill with neurotransmitter by active transport, synaptic vesicles translocate to the active zone: *mobilization* (i.e transport of vesicles from the reserve pool to the releasable pool); where they dock at morphologically defined sites on the pre-synaptic plasma membrane: *targeting and docking*; the exocytosis of docked vesicles, i.e. the fusion of synaptic vesicle membrane with the plasma membrane (mixing of lipid bilayers of vesicle and target membranes) with the formation of a fusion pore in response to the increase of $[Ca^{2+}]_i$: *fusion*; the empty vesicles form coated pits that undergo endocytosis: *retrieval and recycling*.

The specific targeting of synaptic vesicles to the active zone (Figure 8.9) suggests the specific pairing of protein(s) associated with the membrane vesicle with that associated with the pre-synaptic plasma membrane (docking). The fusion of the synaptic and plasma membranes is triggered in nerve terminals by Ca^{2+} entry: it is a regulated exocytosis. In other secretory systems such as the transport of vesicles between Golgi cisternae, the exocytosis occurs at a constant rate and is Ca^{2+} independent: it is a constitutive exocytosis. Studies on these different systems revealed that both vesicular transports share a common mechanism. The only difference would be the presence of a 'fusion clamp' in regulated exocytosis, a mechanism that prevents a docked vesicle from fusing with the target membrane in the absence of a $[Ca^{2+}]_i$ increase. We shall explain some of the elements involved in the docking and fusion steps on the basis of experiments performed first on the vesicular transport between Golgi cisternae, which led to the discovery and purification of several proteins crucial for membrane docking and fusion processes.

Everything began with the discovery that *N*-ethyl maleimide (NEM), a sulfhydryl reagent, blocks the fusion of Golgi vesicles with Golgi stacks in a cell-free system: the vesicles still bud off from cisternae but the released vesicles no longer fuse with the next stack membrane, and accumulate close to the target mem-

Figure 8.9 Scheme of the hypothetical synaptic vesi-cle cycle in pre-synaptic terminals. (Top) The diagram represents the same synaptic vesicle at different stages. Sites of docking, fusion and retrieval have been sepa-rated for clarity. The integral membrane proteins (■, □) involved in docking have been omitted in the subsequent steps. (Bottom) The 20S fusion parti-cle involved in docking and fusion steps. nT, neuro-transmitter. See text for explanations. (Adapted from Südhof TC and Jahn R, 1991. Proteins of synaptic vesicles involved in exocytosis and membrane recy-cling, *Neuron* **6**, 665–677, with permission, and from Stanley EF, 1993. Single calcium channels and acetyl-choline release at a presynaptic nerve terminal, *Neuron* **11**, 1007–1011, with permission.)

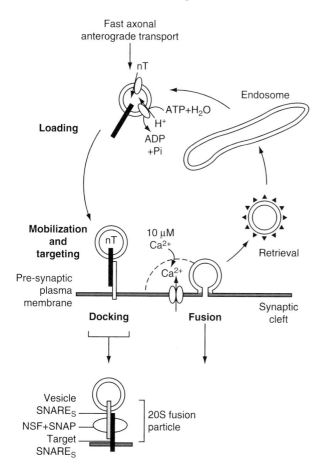

(Soluble NSF-Attachment Protein or SNAP) to attach to Golgi membranes. It is therefore found in the cytosol and in a membrane-bound form which is released from the membrane by ATP hydrolysis. This property was used to purify the proteins that attach the NSF protein to membranes. Thus, in the presence of Mg-ATP-γS (a non-hydrolyzable analog of ATP), the stable complex [NSF–SNAP–membrane proteins] is isolated. The membrane proteins are named SNAREs (**S**oluble **N**SF-**A**ttachment protein **RE**ceptors) (Figure 8.9 inset).

This complex migrates in velocity centrifugation with a sedimentation coefficient of 20S and is thus called the 20S fusion particle (Figure 8.9, inset). The soluble proteins are released from the complex by ATP hydrolysis. The SNAREs can thus be purified. Performing these experiments in the synapse led to the identification of membrane proteins involved in synaptic vesicle docking. In the vesicle membrane the synaptobrevin or VAMP are vSNAREs (v = vesicle) and in the pre-synaptic membrane the syntaxin is a tSNARE (t = target) (Figure 8.10). Both proteins are integral membrane proteins with a short extracellular domain. These proteins are also the selective target proteins of toxins such as botulinum and tetanus tox-ins known to block synaptic transmission (see Section 8.4.2). These toxins are Zn^{2+}-dependent endopepti-dases (metalloproteases). They cleave VAMP or syn-taxin at a specific site leading to their inactivation and block of neurotransmitter release. VAMP and syntaxin are two examples of SNAREs in the synapse. Other proteins might share this role.

In summary, NSF proteins and soluble NSF attach-ment proteins are very general cytoplasmic proteins. In contrast the integral membrane proteins to which they bind, the SNAREs, differ from one secretion system to the other. VAMP and syntaxin are synaptic SNARE proteins specific for the exocytosis of small synaptic vesicles. One of the many questions that remains to be answered is why ATP hydrolysis by NSF is required for targeting/docking to occur?

How and when do the synaptic vesicles fuse with the target pre-synaptic plasma membrane?

In constitutive exocytosis models, once the vesicles are docked to the target membrane they fuse with it and release their contents. Thus, NSF proteins, soluble

brane. This enabled the purification and identification of an NEM-sensitive fusion (NSF) protein on the basis of its ability to restore intercisternal Golgi transport in a cell-free system. NSF protein is a water soluble ATPase. It requires additional cytoplasmic proteins

Figure 8.10 Structural models of synaptic vesicle-associated proteins. See text for explanation. The neurotransmitter transporters are integral membrane proteins responsible for vesicle loading with neurotransmitter. The proton pump is omitted. (Adapted from Jahn R Südhof TC, 1993. Synaptic vesicle traffic: rush hour in the nerve terminal, *J. Neurochem.* **61**, 12–21, with permission.)

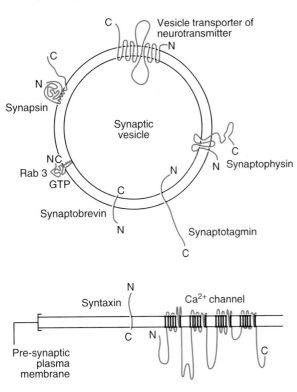

NSF attachment proteins and SNARE proteins would be involved in *docking and fusion* of vesicles. In synapses, the docked vesicles do not fuse with a high probability to the pre-synaptic membrane in the absence of an adequate local Ca^{2+} concentration. It therefore appears that constituents which operate a negative regulation of fusion, a 'fusion clamp', would be present in synaptic terminals to restrain constitutive exocytosis. This fusion clamp would be a Ca^{2+} sensor with a low affinity since we learned above that the local Ca^{2+} concentration in the active zone is around 10^{-4} M. One of the candidate proteins for the role of fusion clamp is synaptotagmin, another integral synaptic vesicle protein (Figure 8.10): synaptotagmin binds to the complex [VAMP–syntaxin]. Other proteins present in the vesicle membrane or

associated with it, such as synaptophysin, have also been shown to play a role in neurotransmitter release but this role is not yet clearly identified. The molecular events occurring before and just after Ca^{2+} entry, i.e the regulation of the fusion step, remain to be precisely understood.

8.2.3 Neurotransmitter Release: a Ca^{2+}-Regulated Multiprotein Process

As seen above, several proteins of the pre-synaptic element participate in different aspects of the release cycle. They fall into different groups: proteins such as synapsin that are thought to control the mobilization of vesicles and proteins that are thought to control the docking of synaptic vesicles and the formation of the fusion pore (Figure 8.10).

Synapsin I

Synapsins, discovered by Greengard's laboratory, are a family of phosphoproteins that are specifically associated with the cytoplasmic surface of the synaptic vesicle membrane. They comprise homologous proteins, synapsins I and II. The mechanism of membrane anchoring occurs via hydrophobic interactions involving amphiphilic helices (Figure 8.10). They are physiological substrates for both cAMP-dependent protein kinase (PKA) and for Ca^{2+}-calmodulin-dependent protein kinase I (CAM kinase I) which phosphorylate them. In addition, synapsin I but not synapsin II is a physiological substrate for Ca^{2+}-calmodulin-dependent protein kinase II.

Synapsin I (labeled with a specific antibody) is found in high concentration in the pre-synaptic terminals, close to the synaptic vesicles. The structure of synapsin I, as observed by electron microscopy, is similar in shape and size to the numerous small filaments present around the synaptic vesicles: a globular head and a total length of about 35 nm. The numerous filaments could thus be synapsin I.

Synapsin I exists in two forms: a dephosphorylated form (dephosphosynapsin I) and a phosphorylated form (phosphosynapsin I). Exogenous dephosphosynapsin I binds with high affinity synaptic vesicles and elements of the cytoskeleton whereas exogenous phosphosynapsin I has an affinity for these structures that is five times lower. Thus, the binding of synapsin I to both vesicles and actin filaments is weakened upon phosphorylation by Ca^{2+}/calmodulin-dependent protein kinase II. *In vivo*, neuronal depolarization potentiates the phosphorylation of synapsin I by increasing $[Ca^{2+}]_i$.

In the squid giant synapse, injection of the dephosphorylated form of synapsin I (or vesicle binding form) into the pre-synaptic element causes a gradual reduction of the amplitude of the post-synaptic depolarization whereas the pre-synaptic Ca^{2+} current is unchanged (Figure 8.11a). Injection of the Ca^{2+}-calmodulin-dependent protein kinase II into the pre-synaptic element causes an increase of the amplitude and rising time of the post-synaptic depolarization (the pre-synaptic Ca^{2+} current is also unchanged) (Figure 8.11b).

The results of these experiments suggest that:

- When the pre-synaptic element is at the resting state, the majority of synapsin I would be in the dephosphorylated form, thus being bound to the synaptic vesicles and cytoskeleton. This would decrease the possibility that the synaptic vesicles move in the cytoplasm: the synaptic vesicles are 'sequestered'. In other words, the dephosphorylated form provides an inhibitory constraint for synaptic vesicle exocytosis.
- When the pre-synaptic element is excited, the Ca^{2+}-calmodulin-dependent protein kinase II, activated by the entry of Ca^{2+}, would phosphorylate synapsin I. The synaptic vesicles are no longer bound to the cytoskeleton, and they can move to and from the active zone: the synaptic vesicles are 'unsequestered'.

This model predicts that synapsins would regulate neurotransmitter release by determining the availability of synaptic vesicles for exocytosis.

However, these electrophysiological experiments do not provide complete proof of the hypothesis. Does the injected Ca^{2+}-calmodulin-dependent protein kinase II only phosphorylate synapsin I, and is the increase of neurotransmitter release a direct consequence of synapsin I phosphorylation? This could be shown using anti-synapsin I antibodies. Their injection, along with that of the protein kinase, should void the effect of the kinase.

Figure 8.11 Modulation of synaptic transmission by synapsin I. (a) Recordings of I_{Ca} (five superimposed traces) and post-synaptic excitatory potentials (lower traces) in the squid giant synapse, generated by 40 mV depolarizing voltage steps (V_{pre}) delivered immediately before intracellular injection of dephosphosynapsin I into the pre-synaptic terminal and after this injection at the indicated times. Injection of dephosphosynapsin I decreases the post-synaptic response without affecting I_{Ca}. (b) Recordings of I_{Ca} (four superimposed traces) and post-synaptic excitatory potentials (middle traces) generated by 28 mV depolarizing voltage steps (V_{pre}) delivered at the indicated times following injection of Ca/calmodulin dependent-protein kinase II into the pre-synaptic terminal. The kinase increases the post-synaptic response. (From Llinás R, McGuinness TL, Leonard CS, Sugimori M and Greengard P, 1985. Intraterminal injection of synapsin I or calcium/calmodulin-dependent protein kinase II alters neurotransmitter release at the squid giant synapse, *Proc. Natl Acad. Sci. USA* **82**, 3035–3039, with permission.)

(a) Dephosphorylated synapsin I (dephosphosynapsin I)

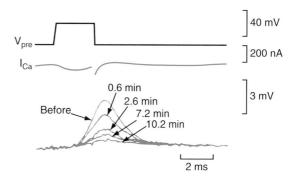

(b) Ca/Calmodulin – dependent protein kinase II

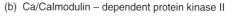

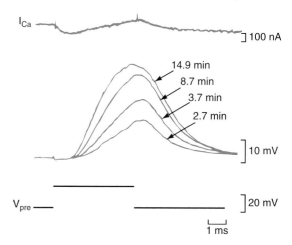

VAMPs, synaptobrevins, syntaxin and synaptotagmin

VAMPs (vesicle associated membrane proteins) and synaptobrevins are small 18 kDa proteins anchored to the vesicle membrane via a single transmembrane region located at its carboxyl terminus. It exists as two isoforms referred to as VAMP1 and VAMP2.

Synaptotagmin is the first intrinsic membrane protein of small synaptic vesicles to be identified and characterized. It has a single transmembrane region with an intraluminal amino-terminus. It is specifically localized in the membrane of synaptic vesicles. It is a phospholipid-dependent Ca^{2+} binding protein. There are at least eight isoforms of synaptotagmin cloned with variable Ca^{2+} affinities and distributions, including several that are not neuronal.

Syntaxin, named from the Greek word meaning 'putting together in order', is an integral membrane protein localized in the pre-synaptic membrane that appears to be associated with pre-synaptic N and P/Q but not L-type Ca^{2+} channels and synaptotagmin. It is supposed to play a role in vesicle docking: it would participate in putting into close proximity the two membranes, the vesicle membrane and the pre-synaptic plasma membrane, to ensure that exocytosis occurs both at restricted sites and with an extremely rapid time course. Syntaxin is not exclusively found at active zones.

Synaptophysins

Synaptophysins are a major integral membrane glycoprotein of the synaptic vesicle membrane, characteristically found in neuronal or endocrine vesicles and having a small diameter (30–80 nm). The primary sequence inferred from its cDNA (see Appendix 5.2) has allowed a model of its organization across the membrane to be established (Figure 8.10). It contains four putative transmembrane domains, each made of 24 amino acids and a cytoplasmic carboxyl terminus consisting of 10 copies of a tyrosine rich repeat. This model bears a high resemblance with that of a hemigap junction (see Figure 5.8). It is a substrate for Ca^{2+}/calmodulin-dependent protein kinase II and for tyrosine kinases.

Antibodies against synaptophysin, when injected into *Xenopus* spinal neurons, inhibit both spontaneous and evoked transmitter release. In mast cells and probably also in neurons, exocytosis involves, when the vesicle membrane merges with the pre-synaptic membrane, the formation of a transient fusion pore, involving two proteins, one in the vesicular membrane, the other in the pre-synaptic membrane. Since synaptophysin oligomers form channels when incorporated in planar lipid bilayers, it is postulated that synaptophysin is involved in forming the fusion pore when interacting with a still unidentified pre-synaptic plasma membrane protein.

8.2.4 Summary

Comparison of neurotransmitter release with other secretory systems shows that targeting, docking and fusion of vesicles involve common mechanisms: synaptic transmission makes use of a mechanism that is common to biology. The specificity of the targeting of a type of vesicle (a Golgi vesicle or a synaptic vesicle) to its target membrane (a Golgi stack membrane or the pre-synaptic plasma membrane) results from the pairing of proteins specific for each type of vesicle and target membranes. For example, in synaptic transmission, the VAMP and the pre-synaptic plasma membrane protein syntaxin are proteins capable of pairing. In regulated exocytosis (Ca^{2+}-triggered exocytosis), the fusion of docked vesicles is prevented in the absence of an adequate increase of $[Ca^{2+}]_i$. It is suggested that specific proteins would restrain the constitutive pathway until the Ca^{2+} signal is perceived. The identification of the proteins and processes involved in the fusion step is under study.

8.3 The Probabilistic Nature of Neurotransmitter Release

Neurotransmitter release is probabilistic. In response to an action potential, each synaptic vesicle has a probability p of merging with the plasma membrane and undergoing exocytosis. This probability p varies from 0 to 1 ($0<p<1$).

8.3.1 The Neuromuscular Junction as a Model

The first studies concerning the quantal release of neurotransmitters were performed on the neuromuscular

Figure 8.12 Demonstration of the probabilistic nature of acetylcholine release at the neuromuscular junction. (a) Recordings of spontaneous potentials (miniature potentials) and of post-synaptic potentials (motor end plate potentials) evoked by a pre-synaptic depolarization. The nerve–muscle preparation is bathed in a low Ca^{2+} concentration medium. In such conditions, the spontaneous potentials always have the same amplitude, whereas end plate potentials have an amplitude that is a multiple of the miniature potential amplitude. (b) The average recorded amplitude of spontaneous potentials or average quantal amplitude is $q = 0.4$ mV. (c) Histogram of end plate potentials generated by a pre-synaptic depolarization. The cases where the pre-synaptic depolarization is insufficient to trigger a response are represented at the 0 mV peak (18 cases here). The adjustment of the bar chart calculated from the Poisson distribution is represented by the blue line. (a: From Liley AW, 1956. The quantal component of the mammalian end plate potential, *J. Physiol. (Lond.)* **133**, 571–587, with permission. b, c: From Boyd IA and Martin AR, 1956. The end plate potential in mammalian muscle, *J. Physiol. (Lond.)* **132**, 74–91, with permission.)

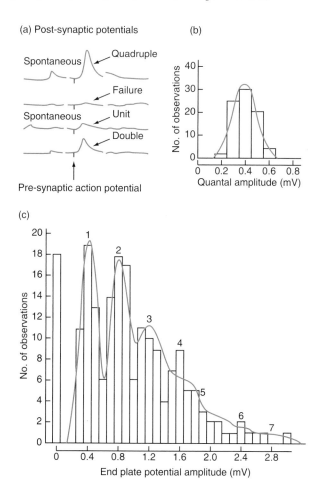

(a) Post-synaptic potentials

(b)

(c)

junction or motor end plate, this preparation offering the possibility of simultaneously recording both pre- and post-synaptic elements and of manipulating the parameters related to neurotransmitter release, in this case, the release of acetylcholine. At the motor end plate level, the number of active zones is estimated at about 500–1000. For this reason, the recorded post-synaptic response is global, representing the summation of evoked responses at each active zone.

In the absence of any nerve stimulation, miniature end plate post-synaptic potentials of 0.5 mV average amplitude are recorded (Figure 8.12a, b). They occur randomly at a frequency of about 1 per second (see Appendix 8.1 and Section 9.4). These miniature end plate potentials, being the smallest recorded event and having a relatively constant amplitude, were named quanta (with reference to quantal physics) by Del Castillo and Katz (1954). They proposed that each quantum corresponds to the content of one synaptic vesicle. The size of a quantum is q.

In the neuromuscular junction preparation, the probability of synaptic vesicle exocytosis in response to nerve stimulation is very high. When the preparation is immersed in an extracellular medium containing a low Ca^{2+} concentration, the amplitude of the EPSP decreases. Following nerve stimulation in these conditions, one can record post-synaptic depolarizations (motor end plate potentials) having a low and variable amplitude and also numerous failures (absence of post-synaptic response). In response to the same pre-synaptic depolarization, the post-synaptic potentials present variations in their amplitude (Figure 8.12a). These amplitude variations are in graduated steps, each step corresponding to a quantum of amplitude q (Figure 8.12b). The post-synaptic response is constantly a multiple of 0, 1, 2, 3 ... or x quanta, x always being a whole number. If one admits that a quantum corresponds to the release of a synaptic vesicle, it appears that 0, 1, 2, 3 ... or x synaptic vesicles are released (x being a natural number as each synaptic vesicle is an entity). This produces fluctuations in the amplitude of the post-synaptic response. The distribution of these fluctuations on a graph shows the presence of regularly spaced peaks, the first three peaks clearly corresponding to amplitudes $1q$ (0.4 mV), $2q$ (0.8 mV) and $3q$ (1.2 mV) but the presence of other peaks ($4q$, $5q$, ... xq) is less evident. The first two amplitudes ($1q$ and $2q$) are more frequent than others. In other words, the probability of recording post-synaptic potentials of amplitude $1q$ or $2q$ is greater than the probability of observing potentials of amplitude $3q$, $4q$, ... in the presence of a low external Ca^{2+} concentration.

The demonstration that post-synaptic potentials are composed of discrete units has necessitated the application of statistical tests, here the Poisson distribution, to the experimental data. As stated earlier, the results shown in Figure 8.12 were obtained under conditions where p is reduced (reduced extracellular Ca^{2+} concentration). This is a necessary condition for the use of the Poisson distribution, in particular for the binomial distribution (Section 8-3-2). In the Poisson distribution, the probability of observing a post-synaptic potential composed of x miniature potentials (due to the release of x synaptic vesicles), $p(x)$ is:

$$p(x) = e^{-m} \cdot m^x / x! = n(x) / N$$

where m is the average number of vesicles released at the neuromuscular junction by a pre-synaptic spike; N the total number of experiments, i.e. the number of recordings of the post-synaptic potential in response to a pre-synaptic spike and $n(x)$ the number of times where the recorded post-synaptic potential is composed of x miniature potentials (amplitude of the post-synaptic response $= xq$). The probability that a post-synaptic potential is composed of x miniature potentials, $p(x)$, is equal to the number of times this event is observed, $n(x)$, over the total number of experiments, N.

The difficulty here is to determine the value of m, the average quantal content. To determine m, two methods can be used:

- Knowing that the amplitude of miniature potentials is a unit, one can calculate (this method is used in Chapter 9):

$$m = \frac{\text{average amplitude of evoked responses}}{\text{average amplitude of miniature potentials}}$$

- Failure method: in conditions where p is artificially reduced (low external Ca^{2+} concentration), the number of times where the synaptic transmission fails is high: numerous influxes are not followed by vesicle release. In these cases (failure), $x = 0$ (the post-synaptic responses of null amplitude are composed of 0 miniature potentials) $n(x) = n(0)$ and

$p(0)$, the number of failures over the total number of influxes, is large and equal to:

$$p(0) = \frac{\text{number of failures}}{\text{total number of influx}} = \frac{n(0)}{N} = e^{-m}$$

consequently, $m = -\log p(0) = \log \dfrac{N}{n(0)}$

The $n(0)/N$ ratio, determined with experimental results (Figure 8.12c), leads to an easy deduction of m.

With m known, p can be calculated for each value of x, and a theoretical curve is drawn, showing the distribution of post-synaptic potentials. Figure 8.12c shows a good correlation between experimental data and Poisson distribution. Quantal acetylcholine release at the neuromuscular junction is a valid model.

Acetylcholine release is a discontinuous quantal phenomenon, each quantum corresponding to the total content of one synaptic vesicle. The probability p that the post-synaptic response will be composed of 1, 2, 3, or ... x quanta depends on the experimental conditions (composition of the extracellular medium), the intensity and frequency of pre-synaptic activity. Once again, the results in Figure 8.12 have been obtained in a medium where p is reduced, a condition necessary for the use of the Poisson distribution. We will see in Section 8.3.2 that the binomial distribution permits a more general description of p.

8.3.2 Inhibitory Synapses Between Interneurons and the Mauthner Cell in the Teleost Fish Bulb, as a Model

To determine if the theory on the quantal release of neurotransmitters is applicable to central synapses, and to describe the release probability, the inhibitory synapses between inhibitory afferent neurons and the Mauthner cell (M cell) was the chosen model (Figure 8.13a). Glycine is the neurotransmitter and it opens receptor channels in the post-synaptic membrane that are selectively permeable to Cl^- ions.

In this preparation, one can identify electrophysiologically the pre-synaptic neurons making inhibitory synapses with the Mauthner cell, make simultaneous intracellular recordings of the pre-synaptic axon and

Figure 8.13 Demonstration of quantal release of neurotransmitter in a central synapse. (a) Experimental design. The Mauthner cell (M cell) in teleost fish bulb receives afferents from inhibitory glycinergic neurons (PHP cell). Antidromic activation (stim) allows the identification of cells whose activity is recorded in current clamp. The recording electrodes are filled with a solution of KCl. The Cl^- ions diffuse in the intracellular medium, thus changing the reversal potential of Cl^- ions and consequently the potential at which the glycine response reverses polarity (glycine opens receptor channels selectively permeable to Cl^- ions). For this reason, the recorded post-synaptic response is not a hyperpolarization but a depolarization, called inverted IPSP, since E_{Cl} had moved to a more positive value and Cl^- ions are now moving outward at the recorded membrane potential. At the end of the experiment, HRP is injected into the pre-synaptic neuron to study its synaptic contacts with the Mauthner cell at the electron microscopic level. (b) Following a pre-synaptic spike (lower trace), inverted IPSPs having variable amplitudes are recorded (arrows, top three traces). The measure of the amplitudes of post-synaptic responses necessitates the elimination of thermal noise by mathematical calculations. (c) Distribution of amplitudes of post-synaptic potentials generated by a pre-synaptic spike. This histogram is adjusted by binomial distribution of $n = 6$, $p = 0.47$ and $q = 300$ µV parameters (see text). In this preparation, the number n of synaptic contacts between the pre-synaptic neuron and the Mauthner cell is also 6. This suggests that each synaptic contact is characterized by a single vesicular exocytosis event (there is a single active zone for each of the synaptic contacts). Adapted from Korn H and Faber DH, 1987. Regulation and significance of probabilistic release mechanisms at central synapses. In Edelman GM, Gall WE and Cowan WM, eds. *Synaptic function*, pp. 57–107, Neuroscience research foundation, Wiley, with permission.

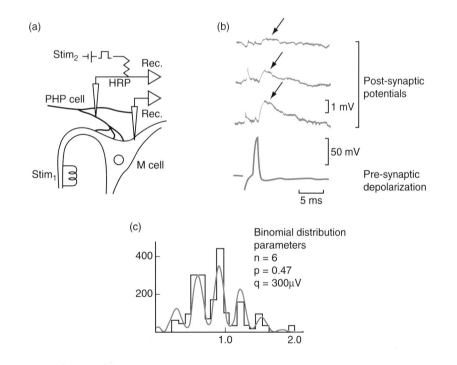

the post-synaptic Mauthner cell, and also inject HRP (a marker) in the pre-synaptic neurons in order to establish the number of synaptic contacts (Figure 8.13a). Morphological data have shown that the afferent inhibitory neurons make between 3 and 60 synaptic boutons, and that *one and only one* active zone is associated with each bouton.

As in the neuromuscular junction model, the distribution of amplitudes of evoked responses has been confronted by the predictions of a mathematical model to determine if the response fluctuations are in graduated steps and discrete and to also determine the fluctuations' parameters. For the analysis of the Mauthner cell synapse, the binomial distribution was used because the Poisson distribution cannot be used when the variable p has a high value, in other words when a large number of synaptic vesicles are released in each assay. The binomial distribution indicates that there are two possible results for each assay. In this case, the synaptic vesicle is released or it is not released.

In both the Poisson and binomial distributions, one considers that an event (vesicle exocytosis) may occur at n places with a probability p. The Poisson distribution is used when p is small (low extracellular Ca^{2+} concentration) and n not measurable. In cases where p is not too small, the binomial distribution permits the evaluation of both p and n. The variable m is therefore equal to the multiplication of n and p, $m = np$, where m is, as described above, the average number of released quanta, n is the number of quanta that can actually be released and p is the average probability for each quantum to be released. When the binomial distribution is used, n can be calculated.

The question now becomes: can we give a biological significance to n?

The binomial distribution can predict the distribution of events, i.e. the $p(x)$ probability of having a post-synaptic response of x amplitude:

$$p(x) = \left(\frac{n}{x}\right) p^x (1-p)^{n-x}$$

The experimental results have indeed shown that the distribution of amplitudes of post-synaptic responses is best described by the binomial distribution (Figure 8.13c). Moreover, these results, when compared with morphological data on active zones, show that the value of n which best describes the response bar graph corresponds to the number of active zones in the pre-synaptic terminal. This means that the exocytosis of only a single synaptic vesicle could occur at each active zone.

Figure 8.14 illustrates the conclusions drawn. The

Figure 8.14   Diagram showing the hypothesis on quantal release of neurotransmitter at central synapses. (a)The pre-synaptic neuron makes six synaptic contacts with the Mauthner cell. After each pre-synaptic spike (8 trials), a variable number x of boutons release neurotransmitter in the synaptic cleft (success, indicated by a cross, whose probability is p) whereas other contacts remain inactivated (failure, whose probability is $1-p$). Cases where exocytosis occurs (success) are represented with an opened vesicle and correspond to the first line of the table. Seven other cases are presented in this table. In the experiment, the average probability p is 0.5 (one failure in two trials), thus an average three active and three inactive contacts with various possible combinations. (b) Variations of the amplitude of the post-synaptic response. The amplitude depends on the number of released quanta after each pre-synaptic activation. Responses composed of three quanta are the most frequent (average quantal content = $m = np = 3$), whereas responses of amplitude $np = 2$, 4 or 5 are rare. Binomial distribution allows the calculation of the $p(x)$ probability that a response will be composed of x quanta. Adapted from Korn H, 1988. Libération des neurotransmetteurs dans le système nerveux central, *Médecine Sciences* 8, 476–483, with permission.

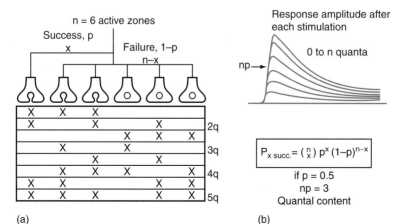

(a)   (b)

schematized neuron makes contacts with six synaptic boutons and with an equal number of active zones. Each action potential can provoke the release of synaptic vesicles at 1, 2, 3 or ... 6 boutons. Electrophysiological data analyzed along with morphological data revealed that n, the number of quanta that can actually be released, is equal to the total number of active zones established by a neuron on the Mauthner cell. In other words, only one synaptic vesicle can be released at one active zone.

Thus n is now a physical reality: the number of active zones established by a neuron on a target cell (also corresponding to the number of synaptic contacts). The parameter q, being the size of a quantum or average content of a synaptic vesicle, also has a physical reality: it corresponds to the amount of neurotransmitter released by a synaptic complex, and for an influx this amount is the same for each complex. Only the parameter p has yet to have a physical counterpart. n and q have constant values and thus p is the only variable of synaptic activity.

8.4 Pharmacology of Neurotransmitter Release

8.4.1 Agents Blocking K+ Currents Increase the Duration of Pre-synaptic Action Potentials and Potentiate Neurotransmitter Release

At the neuromuscular junction, the quantitative description of the chemical potentiation of release can be undertaken by comparing m, the quantal content of the post-synaptic response, before and after treatment. The quantal content, m, can be estimated in two ways:

- by calculating the ratio: $m_1 =$

$$\frac{\text{intensity of motor end plate current}}{\text{intensity of miniature current}}$$

- or by taking into account the intensity and duration of both currents and calculating the ratio: $m_2 =$

$$\frac{\text{intensity} \times \text{duration of end plate current}}{\text{intensity} \times \text{duration of miniature current}}$$

Potassium channels blockers such as TEA and 3,4-diaminopyridine, when used at the neuromuscular junction in conjunction with TTX (blocking the action potential Na+ channels), prolong the duration of the pre-synaptic calcium spike (evoked by electrical stimulation of the pre-synaptic terminal). Consequently, there is potentiation of acetylcholine release. Figure 8.15 shows voltage clamp recording of the end plate current or excitatory post-synaptic current in the presence of TTX and 3,4-diaminopyridine. However 3,4-diaminopyridine has a post-synaptic effect on nicotinic receptors as it decreases by 50% the amplitude of miniature end plate potentials. Because the calculation of m is based on a ratio, one can compare m, the control average quantal content with m', the quantal content in the presence of 3,4-diaminopyridine. In the cases shown in Figure 8.15a, b: $m_1 = 288$ and $m_2 = 390$; $m'_1 = 2870$ and $m'_2 = 46\ 200$.

In the presence of K+ blocking agents, the end plate current has an average time of decline much larger

Figure 8.15 Diaminopyridine (DAP) increases the duration and amplitude of motor end plate current. The activity of a frog sartorius muscle cell is recorded in normal Ringer solution ($V_m = -90$ mV). (a) The motor end plate current is evoked by stimulation of the motor nerve (2 µA intensity, 5 ms duration). The average current intensity in response to the stimulation is 0.5 µA. (b) The response to the same stimulation is now recorded in presence of diaminopyridine (DAP 1 mM). The current intensity of the motor end plate is always greater than 1 µA and can reach 3.3 µA. The inward currents are represented upwardly, which is unusual. Adapted from Katz B and Miledi R, 1979. Estimates of quantal content during chemical potentialization of transmitter release. *Proc. R. Soc. Lond.* B **205**; 369–378, with permission).

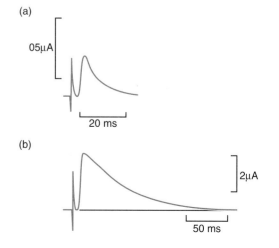

(a)

05µA

20 ms

(b)

2µA

50 ms

than that of the miniature current. This is due in part to the fact that, in this case, the release of vesicles is asynchronous and there is a temporal spread of quantal release during the entire pre-synaptic calcium spike. On the other hand, the massive release possibly saturates the enzyme acetylcholinesterase and as a result there is a repeated activation of post-synaptic nicotinic receptors. Therefore, if the first mode of calculation of m (m_1 and m'_1) underestimates it, the second mode (m_2 and m'_2) overestimates it.

In summary, K^+ channel blocking agents potentiate from 10 to 100 times acetylcholine release following a pre-synaptic spike. These agents are used to estimate the total quantal content of a terminal. The potentiating effect of TEA and 3,4-diaminopyridine has been shown at the neuromuscular junction and is also valid for all chemical synapses.

8.4.2 Toxins: Example of the Botulinum Toxin

The botulinum toxin derived from the microorganism *Clostridium botulinum* is a powerful neurotoxin made up of seven different toxins (A to G). These proteins have a heavy chain (100 kDa, responsible for selective binding of the toxin to neuronal cells and penetration of the light chain into neurons) joined by a single disulfide bond to a light chain (50 kDa) which bears the activity. Botulinum toxin blocks synaptic transmission at all peripheral cholinergic synapses. The transmission is blocked for several months. The patient usually dies from asphyxia (paralysis of respiratory muscles) and, in cases where the patient survives, muscle atrophy results from the non-functioning of muscle cells.

Botulinum toxin decreases the number of acetylcholine vesicles released in the synaptic cleft without affecting acetylcholine synthesis or conduction in the motor nerve. In cases where the decrease is not total, the effect of the toxin can be reversed by increasing the Ca^{2+} concentration in the extracellular medium or by adding TEA or 3,4-diaminopyridine, agents that potentiate Ca^{2+} ion influx. Aminopyridines are used to cure patients poisoned by the botulinum toxin contained, for example, in damaged preserves.

Knowing these facts, it appeared that botulinum toxin had an effect on Ca^{2+} entry, or at the level of the coupling between intracellular Ca^{2+} concentration increase and exocytosis of synaptic vesicles. To verify the first proposition, Ca^{2+} entry was recorded on terminals 'paralysed' by the botulinum toxin. The results showed that the Ca^{2+} current is not significantly changed. The botulinum toxin would therefore act at the pre-synaptic level to decrease acetylcholine release, after the entry of Ca^{2+} ions.

In order to identify the intracellular target of botulinum toxin, synaptic vesicles from rat cerebral cortex were purified. Of the many proteins detected in these purified synaptic vesicles, one protein band was altered by incubation of the vesicles with botulinum toxin. The electrophoretic mobility of this band corresponds to that of synaptobrevins (VAMPs), one of the vesicle proteins thought to play a role in vesicle docking (see Figure 8.10). Syntaxins are also a target for botulinum toxin. The light chain of botulinum toxin contains a consensus sequence of the catalytic site of metallopeptidase. It has a Zn^{2+}-dependent endopeptidase activity and is able to cleave synaptobrevins and syntaxin. Toxins D, F and G are specific for VAMPs, toxin C cleaves syntaxin and SNAP-25 and toxins A and E are specific for SNAP-25.

Appendix 8.1
Different Modes of Neurotransmitter Release

The first studies dealing with neurotransmitter release were performed on acetylcholine release at the neuromuscular junction. Acetylcholine is synthesized in the cytoplasm of axon terminals and then stored in synaptic vesicles. However a percentage of acetylcholine stays in the cytoplasm. Thus, released acetylcholine can come from two sources, one vesicular and one cytoplasmic. Arguments in favor of the vesicular release of acetylcholine (spontaneous and evoked release) will be briefly discussed and data proving the existence of non-vesicular release (evoked, spontaneous) will be described in detail.

A8.1.1 Equilibrium Between Cytoplasmic and Vesicular Acetylcholine Compartments

Acetylcholine (ACh) is synthesized in the cytoplasm of axon terminals from choline and acetylCoA. Choline comes from either the synaptic cleft, following degradation of ACh released before, or from the blood. It is taken up by axon terminals by a process using the energy of the Na$^+$ ion gradient. AcetylCoA is synthesized from acetate, which comes from the synaptic cleft (for neuromuscular junctions), or from degradation of glucose (citric acid cycle). ACh is then stored in synaptic vesicles by an active mechanism (see Appendix 2.1). In the absence of evoked release of ACh in the synaptic cleft, ACh concentration in the cytoplasmic compartment thus depends on: (i) the enzymatic reactions equilibrium (law of mass action), (ii) equilibrium between entrance of ACh precursors and ACh leak in the synaptic cleft, and (iii) the exchange equilibrium with the vesicular compartments. In the same way, ACh concentration in the vesicular compartment depends on the exchange equilibrium with the cytoplasmic compartment (Figure A8.1).

A8.1.2 Vesicular Spontaneous and Evoked Release

ACh release evoked by motor nerve stimulation and Ca^{2+} entry into the pre-synaptic terminal induces a post-synaptic response composed of quanta. This result has been shown for various synapses in vertebrates and invertebrates (see Section 8.3). At the neuromuscular junction, a quantum produces a 1 m V miniature potential and, normally, hundreds of quanta are released simultaneously in response to a pre-synaptic depolarization. The observation of synaptic vesicles in the pre-synaptic element along with the observation of exocytosis at active zones (Couteaux and Pécot-Dechavassine, 1974) has led to the hypothesis that one quantum equals one vesicle. Therefore, the evoked release of ACh at the neuromuscular junction depends on the extracellular Ca^{2+} concentration and generates post-synaptic potentials called motor end plate potentials. The vesicular release of ACh may also be spontaneous (in the absence of a pre-synaptic spike). This spontaneous release is primarily unsensitive to the extracellular Ca^{2+} concentration and generates miniature post-synaptic potentials, thus called because of their small amplitude.

In order to demonstrate the fusion of synaptic vesicles with the pre-synaptic membrane (exocytosis), new

Figure A8.1   Cytoplasmic and vesicular compartments of acetylcholine. (From Israël M and Morel N, 1987. La transmission synaptique chimique cholinergique; mécanismes de contrôle, *Rev. Neurol. (Paris)* **143**; 89–97, with permission.)

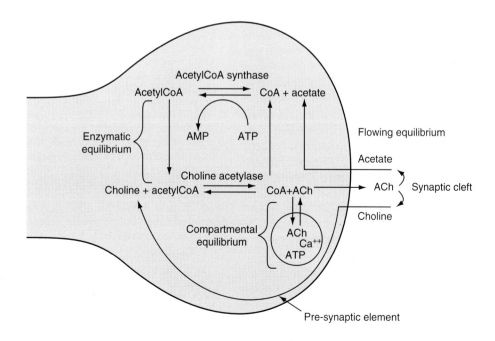

methods to rapidly freeze nerve terminals have been developed (Heuser *et al.*, 1979). The tissue is freeze-fractured during synaptic activity, and a metal replica of the pre-synaptic membrane after fracture is observed under the electron microscope. Images showing exocytosis were observed while important ACh release occurred in the presence of 4-aminopyridine (a blocker of K^+ channels that depolarizes the membrane). In the absence of drugs, rearrangement of pre-synaptic intra-membranous particles is the most common ultrastructural observation.

This low probability of exocytosis observation in the absence of 4-aminopyridine is not surprising, knowing the low probability of exocytosis at a synaptic complex at a given time (see Section 8.3).

A8.1.3 Spontaneous Leak of Neurotransmitter: Non-quantal Spontaneous Release

This is a diffuse and continuous release of neurotransmitter shown at the neuromuscular junction: neuromuscular junctions are treated with high doses of DFP, an irreversible inhibitor of ACh degradation, and TTX to prevent spontaneous neural (pre-synaptic) or muscular (post-synaptic) activity. In these conditions, the effect of curare on the post-synaptic membrane potential is recorded. The addition of curare provokes the disappearance of miniature potentials and a 0.04 mV post-synaptic membrane hyperpolarization at the motor end plate. This effect suggests the existence of a continuous ACh leak, from the cytoplasmic compartment of nerve terminals in the synaptic cleft, bringing ACh concentration in the cleft to 10^{-8} mol/l, responsible for the small post-synaptic depolarization abolished in curarized post-synaptic membrane. In normal conditions, this concentration is not 'seen' by the post-synaptic membrane owing to the efficacy of acetylcholinesterase, the enzyme that quickly degrades ACh.

A8.1.4 Non-vesicular Evoked Release (Israël *et al.*)

The experiments leading to the non-vesicular theory for evoked transmitter release were carried out on *Torpedo* electric organ (entire tissue, see Figure 9.1a) and on synaptosomes isolated from this tissue.

The model of Torpedo synaptosomes

The electrical organs of *Torpedo* are densely innervated (two billion nerve terminals per gram of electric organ, the two organs weighing up to 300 g). This dense innervation is homogeneous, all synapses being cholinergic. It is possible to obtain fractions of isolated nerve terminals or synaptosomes: during tissue homogenization nerve terminals can be extracted with their contents, notably the cytoplasm and synaptic vesicles. The synaptosomes are deprived of the post-synaptic membrane but retain all their normal functional properties.

Released ACh originates from the cytoplasmic compartment

To demonstrate the origin of ACh after stimulation, ACh levels are measured in both cytoplasmic and vesicular compartments before and after stimulation of synaptosomes by Ca^{2+} influx (in the presence of A23187, a calcium ionophore). ACh release is measured by chemoluminescence (Figure A8.2) in two experimental conditions (Figure A8.3):

- freeze-thaw: this breaks the membrane of nerve terminals, but the vesicles are intact. In this condition, the ACh level in the cytoplasmic compartment can be estimated;

Figure A8.2 Chemoluminescent measurement of ACh content. Released ACh at a nerve terminal is degraded into acetate and choline by the enzyme acetylcholinesterase. In the presence of choline oxidase, choline is oxidated to form betaine, and hydrogen peroxide which reacts with luminol to emit blue light in the presence of a catalyst, peroxidase. One can thus measure ACh release in response to Ca^{2+} ion influx. ACh release is then standardized by injection of a standard solution (150 pmol/l for example). (From Israël M and Morel N, 1987. La transmission synaptique chimique cholinergique; mécanismes de contrôle, *Rev. Neurol.* (Paris) **143**, 89–97, with permission.)

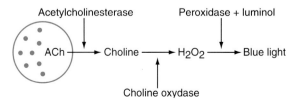

Figure A8.3   Cytoplasmic and vesicular measurements of ACh content. Synaptosomes are freeze-thawed in the presence of reagents described in Figure A8.2 to measure ACh content. ACh released gives a first light emission. A detergent is added (Triton X 100) and a second light emission is measured corresponding to the ACh release in vesicles spared by the freeze-thaw process. (From Israël M and Morel N, 1987. La transmission synaptique chimique cholinergique; mécanismes de contrôle, *Rev. Neurol. (Paris)* **143**, 89–97, with permission.)

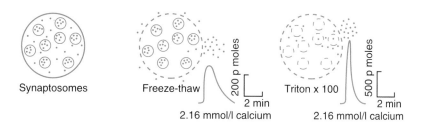

- addition of detergent after freeze-thaw: this breaks the vesicles. The vesicular content of ACh can thus be measured.

By comparing results obtained in both experimental conditions before (control) and after introduction of A23187, Israël *et al.* have shown that the ACh content of the cytoplasmic compartment decreases by a quantity equal to ACh released: evoked ACh release in this model is cytoplasmic (not vesicular). These results are in agreement with results obtained on the entire tissue. One must keep in mind that Ca^{2+} ion influx may have provoked ACh release from a subpopulation of vesicles destroyed or rendered fragile by freeze-thaw.

A pre-synaptic membrane protein, the mediatophore, assures ACh outflow

The increase of pre-synaptic membrane proteins during neurotransmitter release led many authors to propose that the Ca^{2+}-dependent ACh outflow would result from the passage of ACh through pre-synaptic membrane proteins. A 200 kDa pentamerous structure, called the mediatophore, has been isolated and purified from pre-synaptic membrane. Further investigations are needed to clarify the role of this protein.

Conclusion

Numerous arguments, notably the quantal composition of the post-synaptic response, are in favor of the vesicular theory of neurotransmitter release.

Moreover, it is difficult to speculate on the role of synaptic vesicles in the non-vesicular theory (in this case, the vesicles are considered as storage compartments, involved only in the regulation of cytoplasmic ACh content).

However, if the non-vesicular theory of evoked neurotransmitter release cannot be applied to all synapses, certain data must be taken into account: recent experiments have shown that during exocytosis, when the vesicle fuses with the membrane, a fusion pore is formed, linking the lumen of the vesicle to the extracellular medium (see Figure. 5.11, a_3). The formation of this fusion pore implies the interaction of a vesicular protein with a membrane protein. The latter protein could be associated to the mediatophore.

A8.1.5 Non-vesicular Release by Reverse Uptake

In certain conditions, both physiological and pathological, the transmitter uptake carriers (see Section 5.5.2) can run backward, carrying transmitters out of axon terminals and serving as a Ca^{2+}-independent, non-vesicular mechanism for transmitter release. We will present evidence supporting this idea for GABA.

The synaptic action of GABA released by axon terminals is taken up into neurons and glial cells. The GABA uptake carrier is a protein that transports GABA against its concentration gradient by using the energy of the Na^+ electrochemical gradient (Figure A8.4a). It co-transports two Na^+ ions and one Cl^- ion into the cell with each GABA molecule. This transport can theoretically reverse if the intracellular concentration of Na+ rises high enough. Indeed, in central synaptosome preparations incubated in the presence of ^{3}H, tritiated GABA release can be evoked by depolarization of the membrane by perfusing a high K+ concentration extracellular medium or glutamate (Figure A8.4b). The functional significance of this Ca^{2+}-independent release of neurotransmitter mediated by reversed uptake of neurotransmitter from the cytoplasm to the synaptic cleft depends on (i) the variations of Na+ concentration in the synaptic cleft in

physiological or pathological conditions, and (ii) the speed with which reversed uptake can raise the neurotransmitter concentration in the synaptic cleft to a level that will activate the receptors. In fact, the neurotransmitter will activate post-synaptic receptors if its concentration in the synaptic cleft is in the order of receptor K_D and if this concentration is achieved quickly so that post-synaptic receptors do not desensitize before. In anoxic conditions, it has been shown that glutamate is released by reversed uptake. Its concentration rises above 100 µM and depolarizes post-synaptic membrane. The consequent influx of Ca^{2+} ions is supposed to trigger delayed neuronal death after anoxia.

Figure A8.4   GABA uptake from the synaptic cleft (a) and GABA release in the synaptic cleft by reversed uptake (b). GABA is actively taken up into synaptic terminals and surrounding astrocytes by co-transport with 2 Na+ ions and 1 Cl$^-$ ion (a). The [Na+]i increase, induced for example by glutamate, reverses the operation of the GABA uptake carrier which therefore releases GABA into the synaptic cleft. (b) Adapted from Attwell D, Barbour B and Szatkowski M, 1993 Non-vesicular release of neurotransmitter, *Neuron* **11** 401–407, with permission.)

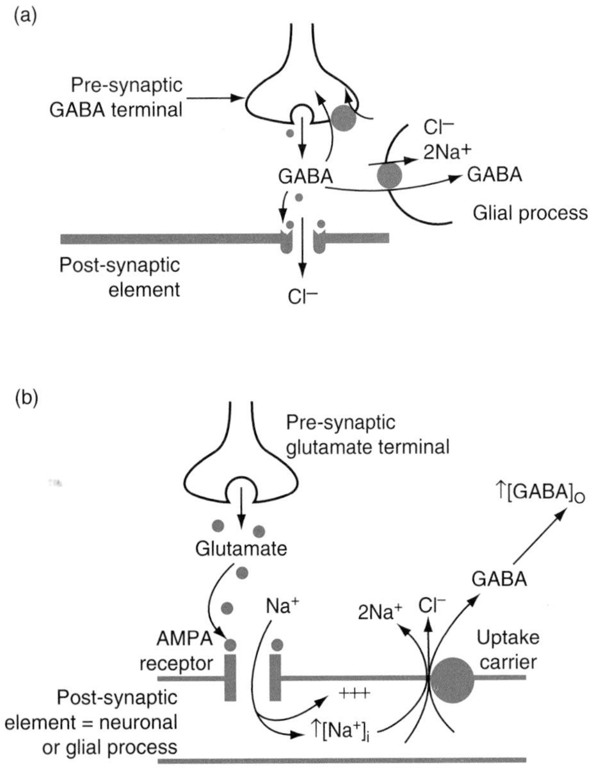

Further Reading

Augustine, G.J. (1990) Regulation of transmitter release at the squid giant synapse by presynaptic delayed rectifier potassium current. *J. Physiol. (Lond.)* **431**, 343–364.

Betz, W.J. and Bewick, G.S. (1992) Optical analysis of synaptic vesicle recycling at the frog neuromuscular junction. *Science* **255**, 200–203.

Betz, W.L. Bewick, G.S. and Ridge R.M.A.P. (1992) Intracellular movements of fluorescently labeled synaptic vesicles in frog motor nerve terminals during nerve stimulation. *Neuron* **9**, 805–813.

Cheek, T.R. and Burgoyne, R.D. (1992) Cytoskeleton in secretion and neurotransmitter release. In: Burgoyne, R.D. (Ed), *The Neuronal Cytoskeleton*, pp. 309–326, Wiley-Liss, New York.

Del Castillo, J. and Katz, B. (1954) Quantal components of the end plate potential. *J. Physiol. (Lond.)* **124**, 560–573.

Dunlap, K., Luebke, J.I. and Turner, T.J. (1995) Exocytotic Ca^{2+} channels in mammalian central neurons. *Trends Neurosci.* **18**, 89–98.

Jahn, R. and Südhof, T.C. (1994) Synaptic vesicles and exocytosis. *Ann. Rev. Neurosci.* **17**, 219–246.

Katz, B. and Miledi, R. (1979) Estimates of quantal content during chemical potentiation of transmitter release. *Proc. R. Soc. Lond. B* **205**, 369–378.

Littleton, J.T. and Bellen, H.J. (1995) Synaptotagmin controls and modulates synaptic vesicle fusion in a Ca^{2+}-dependent manner. *Trends Neurosci.* **18**, 177–183.

Liu, G. and Tsien, R.W. (1995) Properties of synaptic

(a)

(b)

transmission at single hippocampal synaptic boutons. *Nature* 375, 404–408.

Llinas, R., Sugimori, M. and Silver, R.B. (1995) The concept of calcium concentration microdomains in synaptic transmission. *Neuropharmacology* 34, 1443–1451.

Penner, R. and Neher, E. (1989) The patch clamp technique in the study of secretion. *Trends Neurosci.* 12, 59–63.

Popov, S.V. and Poo, M. (1993) Synaptotagmin: a calcium-sensitive inhibitor of exocytosis. *Cell* 73, 1247–1249.

Redman, S. (1990) Quantal analysis of synaptic potentials in neurons of the central nervous system. *Physiol. Rev.* 70, 165–198.

Regehr, W.G. and Mintz, I.M. (1994) Participation of multiple calcium channel types in transmission at single climbing fiber to Purkinje cell synapses. *Neuron* 12, 605–613.

Robitaille, R., Garcia, M.L., Kaczorowski, G.J., and Charlton, M.P. (1993) Functional colocalization of calcium and calcium-gated potassium channels in control of transmitter release. *Neuron* 11, 645–655.

Schweizer, F.E., Betz, H. and Augustine, G. (1995) From vesicle docking to endocytosis: intermediate reactions of exocytosis. *Neuron* 14, 689–696.

Seward, E.P., Chernevskaya, N.I. and Nowycky, M. (1995) Exocytosis in peptidergic nerve terminals exhibits two calcium sensitive phases during pulsatile calcium entry. *J. Neuroscience* 15: 3390–3399.

Sheng, Z.H., Rettig, J., Takahashi, M. and Catterall, W.A. (1994) Identification of a Ca^{2+} binding site on N-type Ca^{2+} channels. *Neuron* 13, 1303–1313.

Söllner T., Whiteheart W., Brunner M., Erdjument-Bromage H., Geomanos S., Tempst P. and Rothman E. (1993) SNAP receptors implicated in vesicle targeting and fusion *Nature* 362, 318–324.

Südhof, T.C. (1995) The synaptic vesicle cycle: a cascade of protein-protein interactions. *Nature* 375, 645–653.

Part III

Ionotropic Receptors in Synaptic Transmission and Sensory Transduction

The Nicotinic Acetylcholine Receptor

The nicotinic acetylcholine receptor (nAChR) is a glycoprotein present at nicotinic cholinergic synapses (Figure 9.1). In mammals, they have been mostly studied in the peripheral nervous system (neuromuscular junction and synapses between pre- and post-ganglionic neurons of the autonomic nervous

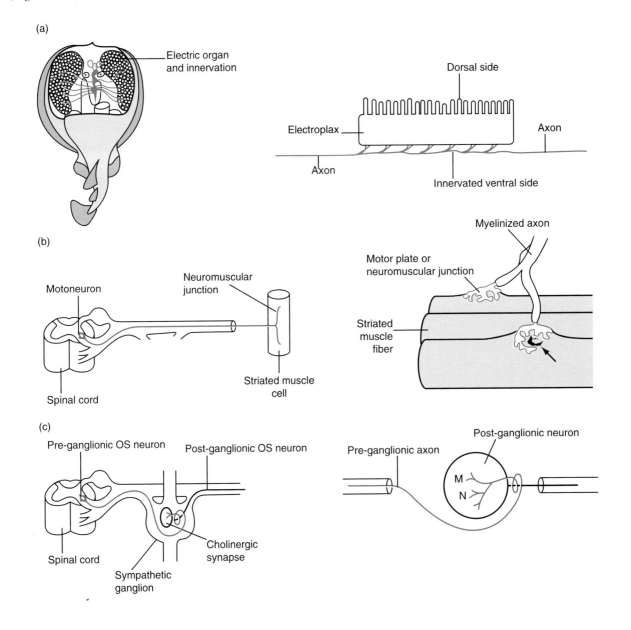

system) (Figure 9.1b, c), but they are also present in the central nervous system. The preparation that has been used most extensively to study the nicotinic receptor is the electric organ of the electric ray, *Torpedo* (Figure 9.1a), or of the electric eel. This preparation is extremely rich in nicotinic receptors, which are located in the membranes of the electroplax ventral face where there are numerous synapses between axon and electroplax. It is from this preparation that the receptor has been isolated and purified.

The nicotinic acetylcholine receptor of *Torpedo* is composed of four transmembrane subunits assembled as a pentamer, $\alpha_2\beta\gamma\delta$. This pentamer presents two acetylcholine receptor sites on its surface, contains the elements to form an ionic channel, and contains all the necessary structural elements for the required interactions between the different functional domains. The acetylcholine receptor sites and the ionic channel controlled by acetylcholine are, therefore, part of the same protein: the nicotinic receptor is a receptor channel or an ionotropic receptor.

The function of the nicotinic receptor is to ensure rapid synaptic transmission. This is achieved by converting the binding of two acetylcholine molecules to the receptor into a rapid and transient increase in cationic permeability. This permeability increase is made possible by conformational changes of the receptor channel: it transiently switches from the state in which the channel is closed into a state in which the channel is open. The nicotinic acetylcholine receptor

also presents allosteric binding sites, topographically distinct from the neurotransmitter binding site, to which a variety of pharmacological agents and physiological ligands can bind. In doing so they regulate the transitions between the different states of the nAChR.

The nicotinic receptors present in the different synapses shown in Figure 9.1a–c have comparable structures and functions. For this reason we will present them simultaneously throughout this chapter. Acetylcholine also activates another type of receptor, the muscarinic receptors, also termed metabotropic cholinergic receptors (mAChR) which belong to the family of receptors linked to G-proteins (see Table 5.1). They will not be studied in this chapter.

9.1 The Nicotinic Receptor is a Heterologous Pentamer $\alpha_2\beta\gamma\delta$

9.1.1 Nicotinic Receptors have a Rosette Shape with an Aqueous Pore in the Center

Under the electron microscope, the nicotinic receptor of the neuromuscular junction, located in the post-synaptic muscular membrane, has a rosette shape with an 8–9 nm diameter and a central depression 1.5–2.5 nm in diameter. This depression corresponds to the channel portion of the protein (Figure 9.2). Each rosette is made up of five regions of high electronic density arranged around an axis perpendicular to the

Figure 9.1   Nicotinic receptors have been most extensively studied in the following three preparations. (a) The electric organ of the electric ray. On a dissected *Torpedo* (left) we can see the electric organs and their innervation. These organs are constituted by electroplax membranes (right) which are modified muscle cells that do not contract. Nicotinic receptors are present at the command neuron's synapse level, on the ventral side of the post-synaptic membrane of the electroplax. The electroplax are simultaneously activated and the summation of their electric discharges can be of the order of 500 V. (b) The neuromuscular junction. Striated muscle cells are innervated by motoneurons whose cell bodies are located in the ventral horn of the spinal cord (horizontal section, left). In mammals, each muscle cell is innervated by one nerve fiber. As the axon makes contact with the muscle cell, it loses its myelin sheath and divides into several branches that are covered by unmyelinated Schwann cells. The thick arrow (right) points to one terminal that has been lifted to show the post-synaptic folds where nicotinic receptors are located (see also Section 2.3 and Figures 2.9 and 2.10). (c) The amphibian sympathetic ganglion. Diagram (left) representing a horizontal section of the spinal cord and a sympathetic ganglion. The orthosympathetic (OS) pre-ganglionic neuronal cell bodies are located in the medial horn of the spinal cord. The axons of these neurons, or pre-ganglionic fibers, exit the spinal cord through the ventral root and end in the sympathetic ganglion. At that level, they establish synaptic contacts with the post-ganglionic orthosympathetic (OS) neurons (see also Figure 4.5b). In amphibians (right) each post-ganglionic neuron receives one or two pre-ganglionic fibers which wrap around the initial segment of the axon and establish multiple cholinergic synaptic endings. Acetylcholine released at each pre-ganglionic terminal binds to the post-synaptic nicotinic and muscarinic (metabotropic) receptors, both of which are present on post-ganglionic neurons. Since nicotinic and muscarinic synaptic effects are very different and well separated in time, they can be studied independently.

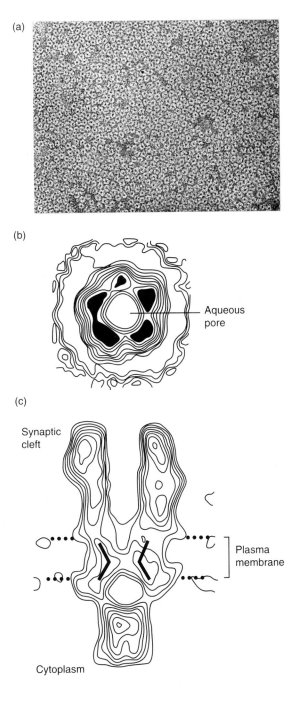

(a)

(b)

Aqueous
pore

(c)

Synaptic
cleft

Plasma
membrane

Cytoplasm

plane of the plasma membrane. In transverse section the rosette appears as a cylinder 11 nm long, extending beyond each side of the membrane (6 nm towards the synaptic cleft and 1.5 nm towards the cytoplasm).

Figure 9.2 The nicotinic receptor has a rosette shape. (a) Membrane surface of *Torpedo* electric cells (electroplax). Each rosette constitutes one nicotinic receptor. (b) The computer reconstructed image of a single nicotinic receptor provides a more detailed view (superior view). (c) Electron microscopy analysis of tubular crystals of *Torpedo* nAChR viewed from the side. (a: From Cartaud J, Benedetti EL, Sobel A, Chargeux JP, 1978. A morphological study of the cholinergic receptor protein from Torpedo narmorata in its membrane environment and in its detergent-extracted purified form, *J. Cell Sci.* **29**: 313–337. b: From Bon F *et al*, 1982. Orientation relative de deux oligomères constituant la forme lourde du récepteur de l'acétylcholine chez la torpille marbrée, *C. R. Acad. Sci.* **295**, 199, with permission. c: From Unwin N, 1993. The nicotinic acetylcholine receptor at 9 A resolution, *J. Mol. Biol.* **229**, 1101–1124, with permission.)

9.1.2 The Four Subunits of the Nicotinic Receptor are Assembled as a Pentamer $\alpha_2\beta\gamma\delta$

The nicotinic receptor is normally purified from the electric organ of *Torpedo* or the electric eel. A 290–300 kD glycoprotein is obtained when this purification is performed on an affinity column using an agarose bound cholinergic ligand (Figure 9.3). When this glycoprotein is incorporated into a planar lipid bilayer or into lipid vesicles (see Appendix 9.1), it presents the same functional characteristics as the native receptor: if acetylcholine is present in the extracellular side at a concentration of 10^{-5}–10^{-4} moles/l, it allows the passage of cations across the bilayer.

The nicotinic receptor is composed of four glycopolypeptide subunits $\alpha, \beta, \gamma, \delta$

In the presence of the detergent SDS (sodium dodecyl sulfate), the 290–300 kD protein dissociates into four different subunits, which migrate on a polyacrylamide gel as molecules with apparent molecular weights of 38 kD (α), 49 kD (β), 57 kD (γ) and 64 kD (δ) (Figure 9.4a). The same experiment carried out with nicotinic receptors obtained from the neuromuscular junction shows very similar results (Figure 9.4b).

Genes coding for each subunit of the nicotinic receptor of the electric ray and of the mammalian receptor have been cloned. When the corresponding mRNAs are injected into *Xenopus* oocytes (Appendix 9.2) functional nicotinic receptors are synthesized and incorporated into the oocyte membrane. It has, there-

Figure 9.3   Different stages of affinity column purification of the nicotinic receptor. (a) The electric organ of the electric ray is homogenized and membrane proteins solubilized. The resulting extract is run through an affinity column, onto whose sepharose (^^^=) a nicotinic cholinergic ligand α-bungarotoxin (α-BTX) has been covalently bound. Owing to their affinity to α-BTX, the nicotinic receptors bind to it. (b) In order to recover the nicotinic receptors, another nicotinic ligand, carbamylcholine (Carb), is run in excess through the column to displace the binding of α-BTX to the receptor. Carbamylcholine-bound nicotinic receptor is obtained at the outflow of the column. Carbamylcholine is eliminated by dialysis and the nicotinic receptor is thus obtained in an isolated form. The nicotinic receptor can then be reincorporated into a lipid bilayer (Appendix 9.1) to study its functional characteristics. It may also be treated with a detergent (SDS) to dissociate its different subunits (Figure 9.4).

Figure 9.4   Separation of the different nicotinic receptor subunits on a gel. The subunits of the purified nicotinic receptor have been dissociated with the detergent sodium dodecyl sulfate (SDS) and separated on a polyacrylamide gel: subunits of the nicotinic receptor of electric organ (a), and of the calf neuromuscular junction (b). The four subunits obtained, α, β, γ, δ and α', β', γ', δ', have similar molecular weights. (From Anholt R, Lindstrom J and Montal M, 1984. The molecular basis of neurotransmission: structure and function of the nAChR. In Martinosi A, ed., *The Enzymes of Biological Membranes*, pp. 335–401, Plenum Press, New York, with permission.)

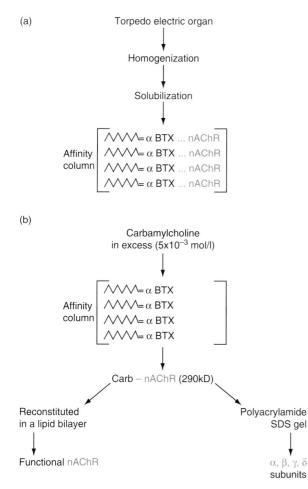

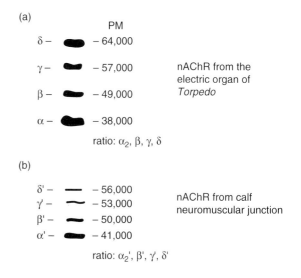

fore, been confirmed that the subunits α, β, γ and δ are sufficient to obtain a functional nicotinic receptor containing the acetylcholine receptor sites and the elements that form the ionic channel. The receptor also contains the necessary elements for the interactions between the different functional domains.

Organization of the different subunits: the nicotinic receptor model

Images observed under the electron microscope, and results obtained with biochemical techniques, have shown that the nicotinic receptor is made up of five units. However, they did not show in which proportion and in which order the subunits α, β, γ and δ are assembled.

The molecular weight of the isolated and purified nicotinic receptor is consistent with the existence of two α chains for each β, γ or δ subunit. This stoichiometry has been confirmed by quantitative analyses of the different chains extracted from an electrophoresis gel (see Figure 9.4). Likewise, when the purified nicotinic receptor is centrifuged in a sucrose gradient in the presence of monoclonal antibodies directed against the α subunit, it appears that two α chains exist per receptor channel.

Using various procedures to label both α subunits (notably α-bungarotoxin) it has been possible to show that both subunits subtend an angle of 150°. This means that the two α chains are not adjacent (Figure 9.5a).

Figure 9.5   Nicotinic receptor (nAChR) model. (a) Viewed from above, the nAChR has a rosette shape. Both α-subunits carry one acetylcholine (ACh) receptor site each. The subunits are attached to each other by non-covalent interactions. αβαγδ or αγαβδ are the two possible orders of the subunits around the symmetrical axis. (b) Profile view of the nAChR *in situ* (cut along the plane aa'). Binding of two acetylcholine molecules to the α-subunits promotes a conformational change of the pentamer, leading to a state in which the channel is open (not shown). (From Changeux JP and Revah F, 1987. The acetylcholine receptor molecule: allosteric sites and the ion channel, *TINS* **10**, 245–250, with permission.)

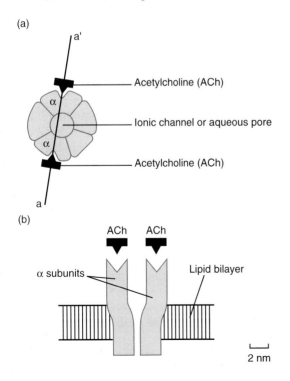

9.1.3 Each Subunit Presents Two Main Hydrophilic Domains and Four Hydrophobic Domains

The amino acid sequence of each subunit α, β, γ and δ has been deduced from the corresponding DNA nucleotide sequence. This has shown that the subunits exhibit among themselves a high percentage of sequence homology and a very similar organization (Figure 9.6a, b). For each subunit one finds:

- an NH_2 terminal region which forms a large hydrophilic domain of 210–224 amino acids and carries the glycosylation sites;
- it is followed towards the COOH end by three hydrophobic sequences (M1, M2 and M3) of 20–30 residues each with short connecting hydrophilic loops;
- a second large hydrophilic domain of about 150 residues containing functional phosphorylation sites;
- finally a fourth hydrophobic sequence and a short carboxy terminal tail.

A model of the transmembrane organization common to all subunits has been proposed (Figure 9.6c): the hydrophilic NH_2 terminal domain is located on the extracellular side of the membrane (in the synaptic cleft), the second hydrophilic domain is located on the cytoplasmic side and the four hydrophobic sequences are membrane-spanning segments. Each subunit therefore crosses the membrane four times and the carboxy terminal tail is oriented towards the synaptic cleft.

9.1.4 Each α Subunit Contains One Acetylcholine Receptor Site Located in the Hydrophilic NH_2 Terminal Domain

Before the structure of the nicotinic receptor was known, it had been demonstrated that two acetylcholine molecules had to be bound to the receptor in order to initiate an ionic flux (see Section 9.2). It seemed logical that these two sites had to be located on identical subunits, i.e. one on each α subunit. Additionally, based on the organization of the hydrophilic sequences (Figure 9.6), it was proposed that this site would be located in the large hydrophilic

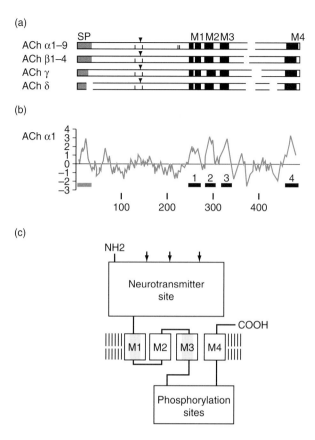

Figure 9.6 Diagrammatic representation of the primary structure of nicotinic acetylcholine receptor subunits from electric organ, muscle cells and neurons. (a) The sequences are aligned to bring homologous regions into phase; gaps in sequences are indicated by blank spaces (polypeptide lengths are normalized), and cysteinyl residues by vertical bars. SP, signal peptide; α, β, γ and δ chains. One can distinguish two hydrophilic domains, the largest of which is located in the NH_2 terminal, and four hydrophobic segments M1, M2, M3 and M4. This observation has led to the assumption that all four subunits have identical transmembrane organizations. (b) Hydropathy plot of the $\alpha1$ subunit from *Torpedo* electric organ receptor showing the four hydrophobic segments assumed to span the lipid bilayer, the large hydrophilic amino terminal domain and the hydrophilic domain separating M3 from M4. (c) Model of subunit transmembrane organization. The large hydrophilic amino-terminal domain of receptor subunits is exposed to the synaptic cleft and carries the neurotransmitter site and glycosylation sites (arrows). Each subunit spans the membrane four times (M1, M2, M3 and M4). The hydrophilic domain separating M3 from M4 faces the cytoplasm. It contains functional phosphorylation sites. (Adapted from Changeux JP, 1994. Functional architecture and dynamics of the nicotinic acetylcholine receptor: an allosteric ligand-gated ion channel, Fidia Research Foundation Neuroscience Award Lecture, pp. 21–168, Raven Press, New York, with permission.)

NH_2 terminal domain which is exposed to the synaptic cleft.

This proposal has been confirmed by covalent binding studies of cholinergic agonists on α subunits, isolated either from nicotinic receptor rich membranes, or expressed in frog oocytes from the corresponding mRNA (Appendix 9.2). Of the four subunit types α, β, γ and δ, the α subunits have been shown to be the main contributors to cholinergic agonist binding.

The next step was to determine which amino acids are part of the acetylcholine receptor site. To this end, labeled cholinergic ligands were used. These ligands are able to bind covalently to the acetylcholine receptor sites. One of the most used is MBTA (4-(N-maleimido) benzyl trimethylammonium iodide) which binds covalently to α subunit receptor sites after reduction of disulfide bridges. Once labeled, the α chain is sequenced and the labeled regions identified. In this way a region containing cysteines 192 and 193 was identified and proposed as one of the potential sites of interaction with cholinergic ligands (Figure 9.7).

Other data have provided additional evidence of the participation of cysteine residues 192 and 193 in the acetylcholine receptor site. In the first place, these cysteine residues are present only in the α subunits. Furthermore, when frog oocytes are injected with mRNA coding for α subunits that have been mutated at the level of cysteines 192 and 193 (serines replaced for cysteines), α subunits are obtained that are unable to bind cholinergic ligands.

However, all these results have the shortcoming of having been obtained from preparations previously treated with disulfide bond reducing agents (such as dithiothreitol). This treatment is necessary in order to allow the covalent binding of the cholinergic ligand MBTA to the receptor site. However, this treatment alters the receptor site selectivity for cholinergic ligands.

In order to obtain a more detailed map of the native protein's acetylcholine receptor site, a labeled photo-activated cholinergic ligand has been used: ^{3}H-DDF (para N,N dimethylamino benzene diazonium fluoro-

Figure 9.7   Model of the acetylcholine binding site. (a) The amino acids labeled with the nicotinic antagonist
³H-DDF are localized on different regions of the α chain. In the three-dimensional structure of the protein,
these regions fold into positions that are close to each other. (b) More precise view of the labeling of the receptor site. The acetylcholine binding site is located at the interface between α- and γ- or δ-subunits. The amino
acids covalently labeled with ³H-DDF are in the α-subunit: W86 and Y93 in loop A, W149 and Y151 in loop
B, Y190, C192, C193 and Y198 in loop C. d-Tubocurarine, an antagonist of nAChR, labels one amino acid
in loop D of the γ- or δ-subunit. C, cysteine; W, trytophan, Y, tyrosine. (a: Adapted from Dennis M, Giraudat
J, Kotzyba-Hibert F, *et al.*, 1988. Amino acids in the *Torpedo marmorata* acetylcholine receptor α subunit
labelled by a photoaffinity ligand for the acetylcholine binding site, *Biochemistry* **27**, 2346–2357, with permission. b: Adapted from Galzi JL and Changeux JP, 1994. Neurotransmitter-gated ion channels as unconventional allosteric proteins, *Curr. Opin. Struct. Biol.* **4**, 554–565, with permission.)

(a)

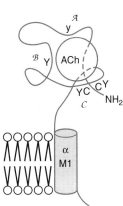

(b)

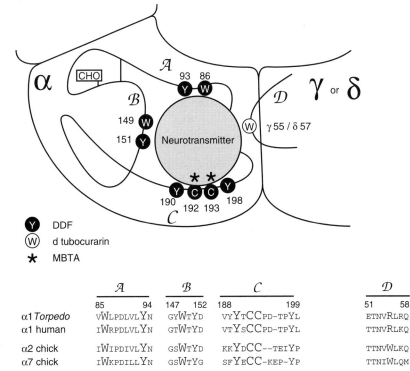

	A		*B*		*C*		*D*	
	85	94	147	152	188	199	51	58
α1 *Torpedo*	vWLPDLVL	Yn	GYWTY	D	vYYtCCPD-TPYL		ETNVRLRQ	
α1 human	iWRPDLVL	Yn	GTWTY	D	vTYsCCPD-TPYL		TTNVRLKQ	
α2 chick	iWIPDIVL	Yn	GSWTY	D	kkYDCC--TEIYP		TTNVWLKQ	
α7 chick	iWKPDILL	Yn	GSWTY	G	sFYeCC-KEP-YP		TTNIWLQM	

borate). ³H-DDF is a competitive antagonist of acetylcholine which, once photoactivated, binds covalently (irreversibly) to the acetylcholine receptor sites (Appendix 9.3). This reaction is carried out on the whole nicotinic receptor channel and the α subunits are then isolated, the segments labeled by ³H-DDF are purified and their sequence analyzed (Figure 9.7). This led to the demonstration that the residues tyr 93, trp 149, tyr 190, cys 192 and cys 193, all labeled by ³H-DDF, are part of the acetylcholine receptor site. This labeling is in fact inhibited by other nicotinic agonists and competitive antagonists. This result is valid for the nicotinic receptor of the electric organ as well as for that of the neuromuscular junction.

9.1.5 The Pore of the Ion Channel is Lined by the M2 Transmembrane Segments of Each of the Five Subunits

The ion channel can be considered as functionally equivalent to the active site of allosteric enzymes: its states (open, closed, blocked, see Sections 9.2 and 9.5.3) are determined by the effectors of the receptor (binding of agonists, competitive antagonists and noncompetitive antagonists, see Appendix 2.1). Concerning the channel structure, the question was which of the four hydrophobic membrane-spanning segments M1 to M4 (Figure 9.6b) are part of the walls of the ionic channel? On the basis of the hypothesis that noncompetitive inhibitors bind to a high affinity site located inside the open ion channel (channel blockers, Section 9.5.3), photoactivable non-competitive inhibitors were used to label residues participating in the walls of the ion channel (this is a similar approach to that used for determination of the ACh binding site). Radioactive chlorpromazine activated with ultraviolet light labels serine, leucine and threonine residues from the M2 membrane-spanning segment from all subunits of the *Torpedo* acetylcholine receptor. These results point to a contribution of the M2 membrane-spanning segment to the walls of the ion channel.

In the M2 segments of nAChR subunits there are remarkable amino acids which, in the proposed model, form rings, assuming that the M2 segments of each of the subunits are symmetrically arranged around the central axis of the molecule (Figure 9.8): a cytoplasmic ring of negatively charged amino acids that repel negative ions, a hydrophobic ring of

leucines, a ring of serines, a ring of threonines and again a ring of negatively charged amino acids that repel negative ions.

Site-directed mutagenesis of some amino acids located in the M2 segment confirmed the contribution of M2 segments to the regulation of ion transport through the nicotinic channel. Chimeric cDNAs were constructed to add or substitute amino acids in the M2 segment. The results obtained will be explained in

Figure 9.8 Characteristic amino acid residues along the M2 segment of the subunits of the nAChR. The M2 membrane-spanning segments are symmetrically arranged around the central axis of the molecule (two of them are represented). The relative position of the α-carbons of the amino acids is shown as one letter code. E, glutamic acid, S, serine, T, threonine, L, leucine, Q, glutamine. (Adapted from Revah F, Galzi JL, Giraudat J, Haumont Y, Lederer F and Changeux JP, 1990. The noncompetitive blocker [³H]-chlorpromazine labels three amino acids of the acetylcholine receptor gamma subunit: implications for the alpha-helical organization of the M2 segments and the structure of the ion channel, *Proc. Natl. Acad. Sci. USA* 87, 4675–4679, with permission.)

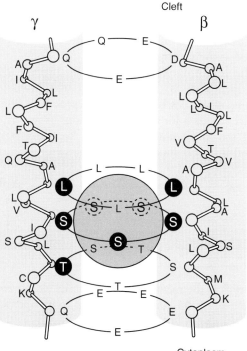

detail in the section describing the study of ionic selectivity (Section 9.2.2).

9.2 Binding of Two Acetylcholine Molecules Favors Conformational Change of the Protein Towards the Open State of the Cationic Channel

9.2.1 Demonstration of the Binding of Two Acetylcholine Molecules

It has been demonstrated that two acetylcholine molecules must bind to the receptor to trigger the opening of the channel and allow cations to flow through. The proof of this has been obtained from dose–response curves. The response to acetylcholine, i.e. the flux of cations measured at very short intervals after the application of acetylcholine (Appendix 9.4), or the opening probability of the channel (see below), is proportional to the square of the acetylcholine concentration:

$$\text{response} = f(ACh)^2$$

However, this demonstration is obscured by the consequences of receptor desensitization, which have to be eliminated from the recordings (see Section 9.3). For this reason this demonstration will not be presented in detail here.

The conformational change of the protein towards the open state is clearly favored when two acetylcholine molecules bind to the receptor. The following model accounts for these observations (however, as we shall see in Section 9.3 and in Appendix 9.5, this model is in fact much more complex):

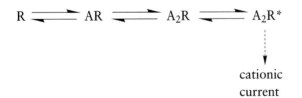

where R is the nicotinic receptor in its closed configuration; R* is the nicotinic receptor in its open configuration; and A is acetylcholine.

The rate of isomerization between R and R* lies in the microsecond to millisecond time scale. The passage of cations through the open channel is the result of the conformational change ($A_2R \rightleftharpoons A_2R^*$). Biochemical (quench flow, Appendix 9.4) or electrophysiological techniques (patch clamp recordings of the unitary cationic current flowing through a single channel, Appendix 7.3) can be used to study this flow of cations. Based on the results obtained with electrophysiological techniques, we shall describe the properties of the nicotinic channel and of the protein conformational changes.

9.2.2 The Nicotinic Channel has a Selective Permeability to Cations: Its Unitary Conductance is Constant

When the unitary current crossing a nicotinic channel in the presence of acetylcholine is recorded in patch clamp, all the preparations tested show an inward current at negative voltage (and under physiological ionic conditions) (Figure 9.9).

The nicotinic current reverses at 0 mV

If the imposed membrane potential (V_m) is varied between −100 mV and +80 mV while recording unitary currents with the patch clamp technique (i_{ACh}), one can trace an i_{ACh}/V curve (Figure 9.10). This curve is approximately linear between −80 and +80 mV. The

Figure 9.9 Patch-clamp recording of nicotinic receptor activity in rat sympathetic neurons. Channel activity is recorded in the attached-cell configuration. While the membrane is kept at a negative potential an inward current is recorded in the presence of acetylcholine under physiological conditions. C, closed channel; O, open channel. (Adapted from Colquhoun D, Ogden DC and Mathie A, 1987. Nicotinic acetylcholine receptors of nerve and muscle: functional aspects, *TIPS* 8, 465–472, with permission.)

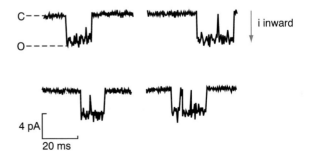

Figure 9.10 Nicotinic unitary current recorded in patch clamp (outside-out configuration) at different membrane potentials (from −80 mV to +80 mV). (a) Nicotinic unitary current recorded at different membrane potentials in response to the application of acetylcholine (ACh). A downward deflection indicates an inward current and an upward deflection indicates an outward current. (b) i_{ACh}/V curve obtained from the average values of i_{ACh} at each membrane potential V_m. The curve reverses at 0 mV and the slope corresponds to the unitary conductance γ.

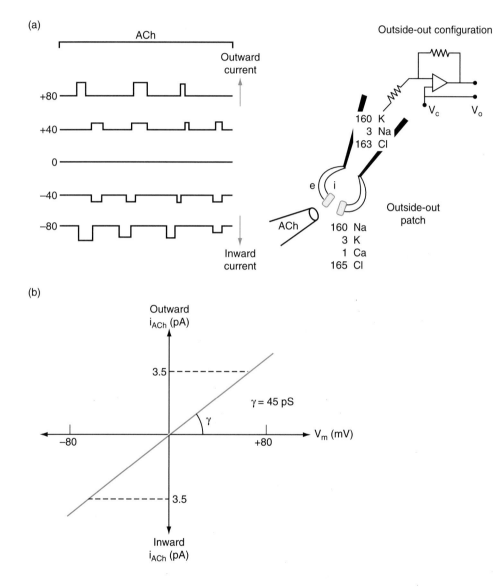

measured current is inward for negative voltages and outward for positive voltages.

The i_{ACh}/V curve crosses the voltage axis at a value where the current is zero. This value is called the reversal potential of the nicotinic response, or E_{ACh}.

The value of this reversal potential is close to 0 mV in the experimental conditions of Figure 9.10 but may vary slightly towards negative voltages depending on the preparation.

The unitary conductance is constant

The linear i_{ACh}/V relationship observed in Figure 9.10b (between −80 and +80 mV) is described by the equation $i_{ACh} = \gamma_{ACh} (V_m − E_{ACh})$, where V_m is the membrane potential, E_{ACh} is the reversal potential of the nicotinic response, and γ_{ACh} is the conductance of a single nicotinic channel, or its unitary conductance. The value of γ_{ACh} is given by the slope of the linear i_{ACh}/V curve. It has a constant value at any given membrane potential. This value varies between 35 and 55 pS depending on the preparation and is a fundamental property of a nicotinic channel.

The nicotinic channel is a cationic channel

The reversal potential of the nicotinic response ($E_{ACh} = 0$ mV) does not correspond to the equilibrium potentials of any of the ions in solution (Figure 9.10). It is not an Na^+ channel because, in the experimental conditions of Figure 9.10, $E_{Na} = 58 \log 160/3 = +100$ mV. It is not a K^+ channel either, since $E_K = 58 \log 3/160 = −100$ mV. And it is not a Cl^- channel because, if the chloride ions are replaced by large anions that cannot cross the channel, such as SO_4^{2-}, no reversal potential change of the nicotinic response is observed.

By performing extracellular ionic substitution experiments, it has been shown that the nicotinic channel is permeable to Na^+, K^+, Ca^{2+} and Mg^{2+} ions. However, Ca^{2+} and Mg^{2+} ions only contribute a small fraction to the nicotinic current, which is essentially due to the flux of Na^+ and K^+ ions through the open channel. If different cations cross the same channel and have similar permeabilities, we define:

$$E_{cations} = 58 \log [cations]_e/[cations]_i$$

where $[cations] = [Na^+] + [K^+]$. In our case we obtain $E_{cations} = 0$ mV. In other words, $E_{cations} = E_{ACh} = 0$ mV.

In what direction do Na⁺ and K⁺ ions cross the open nicotinic channel at different membrane potentials?

When the membrane is at a voltage of −80 mV, the Na^+ ion driving force is inward and equal to −180 mV,

while the K^+ ion driving force is outward and equal to +20 mV (Figure 9.11). If channels open, more Na^+ will enter the cell than K^+ ions will leave it. The net flux of positively charged ions is, thus, inward: an inward current is recorded (Figures 9.9 and 9.10a).

Figure 9.11 Determination and vectorial representation of the Na^+ ion driving force ($V_m − E_{Na}$) and K^+ ion driving force ($V_m − E_K$) for a membrane potential of −80 mV. One observes that 90% of the current is due to Na^+ ions. The net flux of positive charges is inward. This explains why ACh induces an inward current at $V_m = −80$ mV (see also Figure 9.10).

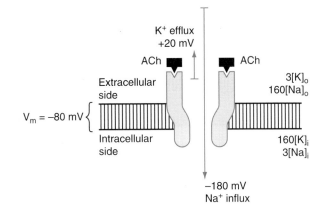

If the same reasoning is followed for different membrane potential values, the same result is obtained as with the i_{ACh}/V curve: the unitary current is inward for negative membrane potentials (net flux of positive charges is inward), and the unitary current is outward for positive membrane potentials (net flux of positive charges is outward) (Figure 9.12).

Effect of a decrease in [Na⁺]ₑ

When extracellular Na^+ ions are partially replaced with a non-permeant substance such as sucrose (without changing the osmotic pressure), the reversal potential of the nicotinic response shifts towards more negative potentials (Figure 9.13). This is explained by the fact that, at this point, extracellular Na^+ ions contribute less to the nicotinic current, and the nicotinic reversal potential E_{ACh} shifts towards the K^+ equilibrium potential (E_K).

Figure 9.12   Evolution of sodium and potassium currents (i_{Na} and i_K) through the nicotinic channel as a function of membrane potential V_m. The current induced by acetylcholine i_{Ach} corresponds to the sum of two currents: $i_{ACh} = i_{Na} + i_K$. When $i_{Na} = -i_K$ the current is zero. This occurs at the reversal potential of the nicotinic response ($V_m = E_{ACh}$). A deflection of the traces (left) or an arrow of the chart (right) in the downward direction represents an inward current, and in the upward direction an outward current.

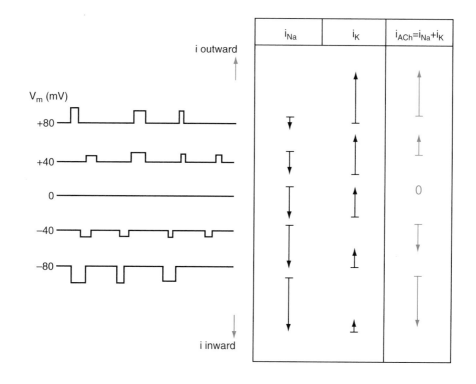

Substitution of K^+ ions for extracellular Na^+ ions

When almost all extracellular Na^+ ions are replaced with K^+ ions, the I/V curve obtained superposes on the control I/V curve (Figure 9.14). Thus, extracellular K^+ ions can replace extracellular Na^+ ions, i.e. the nicotinic channel does not distinguish between Na^+ and K^+ ions. In other words, it presents similar permeabilities for both ions. For this reason the reversal potential of the nicotinic response is independent of the relative concentrations of extracellular Na^+ and K^+ ions. It depends solely on the sum of these concentrations.

Mutations in the M2 membrane-spanning segment can convert ion selectivity from cationic to anionic

The question was: do substitutions and/or additions of amino acids within (or near) the M2 segment from a nicotinic α subunit (neuronal α_7 subunit) with homologous amino acids of the glycine receptor suffice to convert α-ion channel selectivity from cationic to anionic? (The glycine receptor is a receptor channel selectively permeable to anions, Cl^- ions, see Table 5.1.) A comparison of the M2 sequence of α subunits of a cationic channel (nAchR) and anionic channels (GlyR and $GABA_A R$) show similarities at the level of the threonine (244) and leucine (247) rings and differences at the level of rings of negative amino acids, Glu 237 and Glu 258 (Figure 9.15a). A chimeric cDNA encoding the α_7 subunit of neuronal nAChR was constructed in which in the M2 segment, a proline residue, was added at position 236 bis and amino acids at positions 237, 240, 251, 254, 255 and 258 were exchanged with those found in the M2 segment of the glycine receptor α subunit (Figure 9.15a). Interestingly, glutamates (E) 237 and 258 which

Figure 9.13 Effect of lowering the external Na⁺ concentration $[Na^+]_c$ on the I_{ACh}/V curve. The composition of the external environment is: 5 mmol/l K⁺, 0.1 mmol/l Ca²⁺ and 146 mmol/l Na⁺ (●), 21 mmol/l Na⁺ (□), 46 mmol/l Na⁺, (▼), 96 mmol/l Na⁺ (▽), and again 146 mmol/l Na⁺ (○). Each point represents the average of 25 measurements of I_{ACh}. When $[Na^+]_e$ decreases, the reversal potential of the nicotinic response shifts towards the K⁺ equilibrium potential.

Control: ○● $E_{ACh} = 58 \log (146 + 5)/[\text{cations}]_i$

$\triangle \, E_{ACh} = 58 \log (96 + 5)/[\text{cations}]_i$

$\blacktriangle \, E_{ACh} = 58 \log (46 + 5)/[\text{cations}]_i$

□ $E_{ACh} = 58 \log (21 + 5)/[\text{cations}]_i$

(Adapted from Linder TM and Quastel DMJ, 1978. A voltage clamp study of the permeability change induced by quanta of transmitter at the mouse end plate, *J. Physiol. (Lond.)* **281**, 535–556, with permission.)

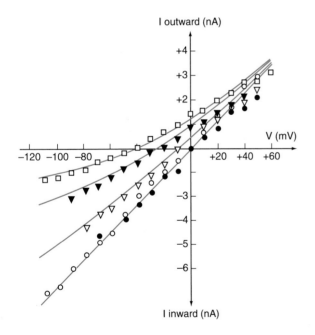

Figure 9.14 Replacing external K⁺ for Na⁺ ions has no effect. Control I/V curve (●) 146 mmol/l Na⁺ and 5 mmol/l K⁺, and (I) 2 mmol/l Na⁺ and 149 mmol/l K⁺. We observe that K⁺ ions can replace Na⁺ ions without affecting the I/V curve. The nicotinic channel does not distinguish between these two cations. (Adapted from Linder TM and Quastel DMJ, 1978. A voltage clamp study of the permeability change induced by quanta of transmitter at the mouse end plate, *J. Physiol. (Lond.)* **281**, 535–556, with permission.)

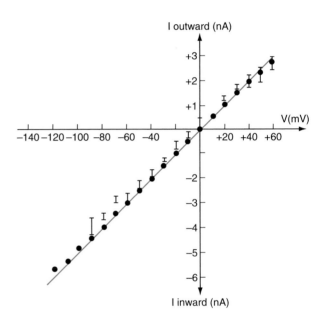

form negative rings in the nAChR (repeling negative ions) are exchanged with alanine (A) and asparagine (N) residues, respectively. The chimeric cDNA was injected into oocytes that expressed homomeric mutated nAChR (formed by five identical mutated α_7 subunits). The current recorded with double electrode voltage clamp (Appendix 7.2) was compared with

that recorded in oocytes expressing wild-type (non-mutated) homomeric AChR.

Ionic currents recorded in response to ACh application (100 μM, 2 s duration) from oocytes expressing wild-type homomeric αnAChR (in the presence of a Ca²⁺ chelator inside the oocyte, see Figure 9.15b caption) reversed around +3 mV. Substitution of 90% of the external chloride ions did not change the value of the reversal potential. These data thus support the conclusion that wild-type homomeric αnAChR, like native nAChR, is selective for cations.

Ionic currents recorded in response to ACh application (100 μM, 2 s duration) from oocytes expressing mutated homomeric α*nAChR reversed around −20 mV. Substitution of 90% external chloride ions by isethionate (an impermeant anion) shifted the reversal potential towards positive voltage (around +30 mV)

Figure 9.15   Mutations in the M2 segment of an α-subunit of the nAChR convert ion selectivity of the homomeric nAChR from cationic to anionic. (a) Comparison of M2 sequences from subunits of the cation selective nicotinic α7 receptor subunit with those of the anion-selective glycine α1, GABA$_A$ α1 and β1 and mutated nicotinic α7* receptor subunits. (b left) I–V relationship of the α7* mutant receptor is first determined in control conditions (control) with 2 s ACh (100 μM) applications (outside-out patch clamp recordings of a patch of membrane containing a large number of nicotinic receptors called macropatch). Then, 90% of chloride ions of the extracellular medium were replaced by the non-permeant anion isethionate and the I–V curve determined (isethionate). This last experiment is also performed in the presence of a chelator of Ca^{2+} ions (BAPTA) injected inside the cell (iset-BAPTA) in order to reduce secondary currents that could be triggered by the entry of Ca^{2+} ions through the nicotinic receptors. (b right) Reversal potential values as a function of the logarithm of external chloride concentration (92, 50.5, 19.75 and 9.5 mM external chloride after substitution of NaCl by mannitol or isethionate). The solid line corresponds to the theoretical Nernst relation. (From Galzi JL, Devillers-Thiéry A and Hussy N, 1992. Mutations in the channel domain of a neuronal nicotinic receptor convert ion selectivity from cationic to anionic, *Nature* 359, 500–505, with permission.)

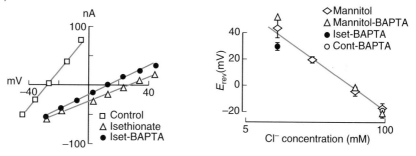

(Figure 9.15b left). This shift is well described by the Goldman–Hodgkin relationship for chloride specific channels (Figure 9.15b right). This indicates that ACh-activated currents are almost entirely carried by chloride ions in oocytes expressing mutated homomeric α*nAChR. Then, introducing appropriate amino acid residues from the putative channel domain of a chloride-selective GlyR α subunit into that of a cation selective nAChR α subunit allows the design of an ACh-gated channel now selective for chloride. This confirms that the M2 segment forms the walls of the channel and strongly suggests that the exchanged residues face the lumen of the channel.

9.2.3 The Time During Which the Channel Stays Open Varies Around an Average Value τ$_o$, the Mean Open Time, and is a Characteristic of Each Nicotinic Receptor

When recording in patch clamp from myotubes (embryonic muscle cells) or from denervated muscle cells, in the presence of very small doses of acetylcholine, openings of the nicotinic channels separated by periods of silence are observed (Figure 9.16a). The nicotinic receptor switches between states in which the channel is closed and the unitary current is zero (R, AR, A_2R), and a state in which the channel is open and shows a measurable unitary current (A_2R^*) (Figure 9.17). These conformational changes can be modeled as:

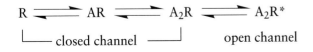

Figure 9.16 Patch clamp recording (attached-cell configuration) of myotube nicotinic receptor channel activity ($V_m = -170$ mV). (a) Myotubes (embryonic muscle cells) are recorded in the presence of a low concentration of acetylcholine (200 nmol/l). At this concentration, the channels open during periods t_o. This recording does not correspond to a single nAChR because one finds approximately 100 000 nAChR per patch. The repeated openings (downward deflections) correspond, therefore, to the opening of different nAChR. However, all the nAChR being identical, it seems as though the activity of the same nAChR was recorded from. The mean open time τ_o can thus be calculated (b). C, closed channel; unitary current is zero. O, open channel; inward unitary current (downward deflections).

Figure 9.17 Correlation between the nicotinic current and the different states of the channel. The channel only opens (inward current, lower trace) when the protein is in the A_2R^* state. The rapid fluctuations between states A_2R^* and A_2R correspond to short-lived closures. When the receptor channel loses one or two of its acetylcholine molecules, the closures last longer. (Adapted from Colquhoun D, Ogden DC and Mathie A, 1987. Nicotinic acetylcholine receptors of nerve and muscle: functional aspects, *TIPS* 8, 465–472, with permission.)

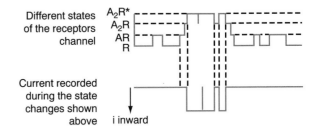

where A is acetylcholine or any nicotinic agonist; R is the receptor in the closed conformation; and R* is the receptor in the open conformation.

In Figure 9.16a one observes that the periods during which the channel is open, t_o, are variable. To obtain the mean open time of the channel, τ_o, one can build a frequency histogram of the different t_o. The exponential curve obtained provides the value of τ_o (Figure 9.16b and Appendix 7.3). The functional significance of this value is as follows: during a time equal to τ_o the channel has a high probability of being open.

τ_o is a characteristic of the nicotinic receptor channel type

Nicotinic receptors from the electric organ of *Torpedo* and from the calf neuromuscular junction can be studied in patch clamp after the expression of the corresponding mRNA injected into *Xenopus* oocytes (outside-out configuration) (Appendix 9.2). Recording of such channels have shown that electric organ and neuromuscular junction channels present very similar conductances (40 pS and 42 pS) but very different mean open times ($\tau_o = 0.6$ ms and 7.6 ms, respectively).

Another example is given by the study of nicotinic receptors from fetal or adult bovine muscle. A study of the subunit structure of the bovine muscle nAChR showed the presence of the α, β, γ and δ subunits as in

(a)

C

O i inward

t_o t_o t_o t_o t_o

6 pA

40 ms

(b)   100

No. of events

$\tau_o = 8.9$ ms

0

150

Open state time (t_o) (ms)

the case for *Torpedo* electroplax nAChR. In addition, a novel subunit termed ε-subunit, has been discovered by cloning and sequencing the DNA complementary to the muscle mRNA encoding it. The ε-subunit shows higher sequence homology with the γ-subunit than with any other subunit. In order to study the properties of the γ- and ε-subunits, various combinations of the subunit-specific mRNAs are injected in *Xenopus* oocytes (Appendix 9.2) and their functional properties are studied in the presence of acetylcholine.

Figure 9.18a shows recordings of ACh-activated single channels from outside-out patches isolated from oocytes injected with the α, β, γ and δ subunit-specific mRNAs (left) or with the α, β, ε and δ subunit-specific mRNAs (right). The conductance and mean open time τ_o (Figure 9.18c, d) of the channels formed in a given oocyte differ in relation to the mRNA combination with which it was injected. This suggests that a single subunit can change the conductance and gating properties of the nAChR channel.

To compare the two classes of nAChR channels produced in *Xenopus* oocytes with native bovine nAChR channels, the ACh-activated channels of fetal and adult bovine muscle are recorded. Figure 9.18b shows ACh-activated single currents from outside-out patches of fetal (left) and adult (right) bovine muscle. The results show that the nAChR channel in fetal muscle is similar to the nAChRγ whereas the nAChR channel in adult muscle is similar to the nAChRε (compare Figures 9.18a, 9.18b). This suggests that the nAChR channel in fetal muscle is assembled from α, β, γ and δ subunits whereas the end plate channel in adult muscle is assembled from the α, β, ε and δ subunits. To study this developmental change in the contents of the five nAChR subunit mRNAs in bovine muscle, total RNA is extracted from the diaphragm muscle at various stages of fetal and postnatal development. It is then subjected to blot hybridization analysis using the respective cDNA probes. The results show that the contents of the γ- and ε-subunit mRNAs varies markedly during muscle development showing reciprocal changes: the γ-subunit mRNA is abundant at earlier fetal stages (3–5 months gestation), but is hardly or not detectable after birth; conversely, considerable amounts of ε-subunit mRNA appear only at postnatal stages and is not detectable at earlier fetal stages (3–4 months gestation). Therefore, the replacement of the γ-subunit by the ε-subunit in the nAChR complex is responsible for the changes in the properties of the nAChR channel that occur during muscle development. This phenomenon of subunit replacement during development cannot be generalized to all the other mammalian nAChR.

9.3 The Nicotinic Receptor Desensitizes

During the recording of a nicotinic receptor channel with the patch clamp technique (whole-cell configuration) in the presence of a high and constant concentration of acetylcholine, there is a progressive diminution of the total current I_{ACh} (Figure 9.19a). This decrease in current corresponds to the progressive desensitization of the nicotinic receptor present in the membrane.

When recording unitary nicotinic currents (outside-out or cell-attached configuration) in the presence of a strong concentration of acetylcholine, there are repeated openings separated by long periods of silence (Figure 9.19b). These sequences of openings are known as unitary current bursts. Within a burst, the protein rapidly fluctuates between the closed and open states, symbolized as follows:

$$R \rightleftharpoons AR \rightleftharpoons A_2R \rightleftharpoons A_2R^*$$

$$\underbrace{\qquad\qquad}_{\text{closed channel}} \qquad \underbrace{\qquad}_{\text{open channel}}$$

The long silent periods correspond to desensitization of the receptor in the presence of acetylcholine. In the desensitized state, the nicotinic receptor is refractory to activation. Consequently, the channel does not open despite the fact that two molecules of ACh are bound to the receptor. In summary, desensitization is a phenomenon that renders the nicotinic receptor incapable of being activated by its agonists. The desensitized nicotinic receptor presents two main characteristics: (i) a high affinity for acetylcholine; and (ii) a closed ionic channel: the unitary current is zero (long silent periods).

At least two desensitized states exist: D_1 and D_2, or according to other authors, I and D, so that:

$$A_2R \underset{}{\overset{}{\rightleftharpoons}} A_2R^* \underset{k_{-3}}{\overset{k_3}{\rightleftharpoons}} A_2D_1$$

$$A_2R^* \underset{k_{-4}}{\overset{k_4}{\rightleftharpoons}} A_2D_2$$

Figure 9.18 The subunit structure participates in determining the nicotinic channel conductance and mean open time. See text for explanations. C, closed channel; O, open channel. (Adapted from Mishina M, Takai T, Imoto K, Noda M, Takahashi T, Numa S, Methfessel C and Sackman B, 1986. Molecular distinction between fetal and adult forms of muscle acetylcholine receptor, *Nature* **321**, 406–411, with permission.)

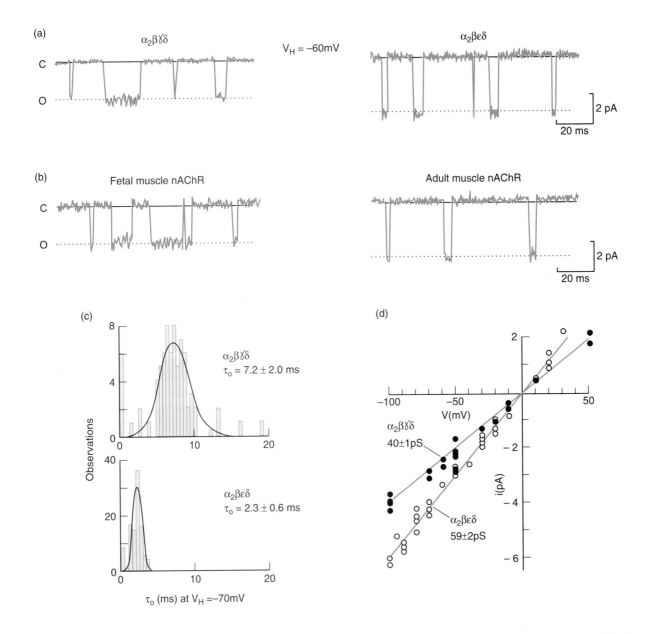

These two states D_1 and D_2 are distinguished from each other and also from the R state by their affinity constants for acetylcholine (Table 9.1) and by the rate constants $k_3 = 0.01$ s^{-1} and $k_4 = 1$ s^{-1}.

The concept of nicotinic receptor desensitization had been proposed by different authors, notably by Katz and Thesleff, from measurements of the time course of the global synaptic response during an iontophoretic application of acetylcholine.

The process of desensitization appears slowly and is

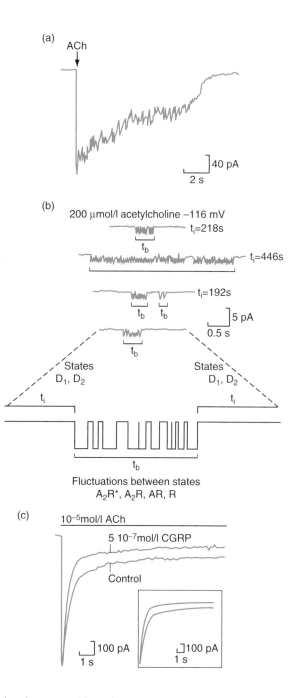

Figure 9.19 Nicotinic receptor desensitization. (a) Patch clamp recording (whole-cell configuration) of the nicotinic current from adrenal chromaffin cells (V_m = −70 mV). In the presence of a high concentration of acetylcholine (20 µmol/l) the inward current reaches a peak of 235 pA, and then decreases despite a constant acetylcholine concentration. This current corresponds to the sum of several unitary currents crossing all the activated nicotinic channels. The decrease in current is due to the desensitization of a large fraction of cellular nicotinic receptors. (b) Single channel recordings (cell-attached or outside-out configurations) illustrating another consequence of desensitization. The membrane patch is exposed to a high concentration of acetylcholine (200 µmol/l) for an extended period. Under these conditions, nicotinic receptors present in the patch desensitize. After a certain time, one of the channels reopens and fluctuates between the states A_2R^*, A_2R, AR and R during a time t_b (duration of the burst of openings) before desensitizing again for a duration t_i (interburst duration). The traces shown correspond to segments of a continuous recording. The duration of the desensitized periods t_i between two successive traces is indicated at the end of each trace (218 s, 446 s and 192 s). (c) Cultured muscle cell recording (whole-cell configuration). Nicotinic current evoked by the application of 10 µmol/l acetylcholine recorded in the presence of 500 nmol/l CGRP (calcitonin gene related peptide) and in the absence of the peptide (control) (V_m = −60mV). The nicotinic current reaches a peak with a 200 ms delay and then begins to decrease. The sum of two exponentials can describe this decrease in current. CGRP increases the speed of the fast component. (a: From Clapham DE and Neher E, 1984, Trifluoperazine reduces inward ionic currents and secretion by separate mechanisms in bovine chromaffin cells, *J. Physiol.* (*Lond.*) **353**, 541–564, with permission. b: From Colquhoun D, Ogden DC and Mathie A, 1987. Nicotinic acetylcholine receptors of nerve and muscle: functional aspects, *TIPS* **8**, 465–472, with permission. c: From Mulle C, Benoit P, Pinset C, Roa M and Changeux JP, 1988, Calcitonin generelated peptide enhances the rate of desensitization of the nicotinic acetylcholine receptor in cultured mouse muscle cells, *Proc. Natl Acad. Sci. USA* **85**: 5728–5732, with permission.)

slowly reversible. This is an intrinsic property of the protein. In order to study in patch clamp the states R and R* of the nicotinic receptor channel, it is necessary to choose conditions under which desensitization is negligible. To this end, researchers work with very low doses of acetylcholine (of the order of the nanomoles/liter) (see Figure 9.16) because high doses

favor the conformational change of the protein into desensitized states. An alternative solution is the use of high doses of acetylcholine (in the order of micromoles/liter, see Figure 9.19b). In this case, the receptors desensitize (silent periods known as interburst periods) and eventually one or several of the channels open and close repetitively (opening bursts) before

Table 9.1   Affinity constants for acetylcholine

State	Affinity constant for ACh K_D
R	10 µmol/l to 1 mmol/l
D_1	1 µmol/l
D_2	3–10 nmol/l

re-desensitizing. Desensitization can be minimized by excluding the first and the last opening during the bursting periods, and thus the values calculated for τ_o are then only related to the R* state.

The rate of desensitization of the nicotinic receptor seems to be related to its state of phosphorylation. In fact, studies of the ionic flux through nicotinic receptors incorporated into liposomes (Appendix 9.4) have shown that an increase in the level of phosphorylation of the receptors by cyclic AMP augments the desensitization rate of these receptors. In the neuromuscular junctions a peptide present in the motoneurons is released at the same time as acetylcholine. This peptide, CGRP (calcitonin gene related peptide), is capable of increasing the level of cyclic AMP in cultured embryonic muscle cells, consequently increasing the number of phosphorylated nicotinic receptors. In patch clamp recordings (whole-cell configuration) of embryonic muscle cells, the simultaneous application of this peptide and acetylcholine accelerates the rapid phase of desensitization of the nicotinic receptors (Figure 9.19c). In unitary recordings (cell-attached configuration) CGRP decreases the opening frequency

of the nicotinic channels (while at the same time leaving unaffected their mean open time and unitary conductance). These effects are mimicked by the application of substances that augment the intracellular cyclic AMP level (such as forskolin). The following hypothesis has been proposed: CGRP activates a specific membrane receptor. This leads to an increase in the intracellular cyclic AMP concentration and an activation of protein kinase A. Protein kinase A, directly or indirectly, phosphorylates certain subunits of the nicotinic receptor leading to a rapid desensitization of the receptors.

9.4 Nicotinic Cholinergic Synapses

A nicotinic synaptic current is evoked by a brief augmentation of the concentration of acetylcholine in the synaptic cleft. This increase, caused by the asynchronous release of synaptic vesicles, is brief because (Figure 9.20a): (i) the release is brief; and (ii) acetylcholine rapidly disappears from the synaptic cleft. In fact, when acetylcholine is released into the synaptic cleft, it may either bind to nicotinic receptor channels, diffuse out of the synaptic cleft, or be degraded by acetylcholinesterase.

During the analysis of synaptic currents induced by the release of endogenous acetylcholine, the desensitized states of the receptor can be neglected because of the rapid elimination of acetylcholine from the synaptic cleft (in the order of microseconds). The model for this is:

Figure 9.20   Miniature current (a) Functional scheme of the pre-synaptic component of the neuromuscular nicotinic cholinergic synapse. The enzymes choline acetyl transferase (CAT) and acetylcholinesterase (AChE) (see Figure 2.10b) are synthesized in the cell body of the motoneuron and carried to axon terminals via anterograde axonal transport. Acetylcholine (ACh) is synthesized in axon terminals from choline and acetyl coenzyme A (acetylCOA). About 50% of the released choline is recaptured by the pre-synaptic terminals. Acetylcholine is actively transported from the cytoplasm into synaptic vesicles via a vesicular ACh carrier using the H+ gradient as an energy source (antiport). (b) Miniature current recorded in two-electrode voltage clamp from a normally innervated muscle fiber in the absence of stimulation. (c) The neuromuscular junction miniature current I_{ACh} is the current crossing N nicotinic channels activated by spontaneously released endogenous acetylcholine. The current rising phase is fast due to the quasi synchronous activation of the N nicotinic channels. The exponential falling phase of the current is slower ($V_m = -90$ mV). (d) Since the opening of the channels is synchronous, their closure appears after a variable time t_o whose distribution is exponential. The mean open time of the N channels is $\tau_o = 3.2$ ms. (e) The same value of τ_o is obtained for the time constant of the falling phase (τ) of the total current I_{ACh}. In the example given in (d), N = 5, but N is in fact always larger (see text). c, d: Adapted from Colquhoun D, 1981. How fast do drugs work? TIPS 2: 212–217. with permission.)

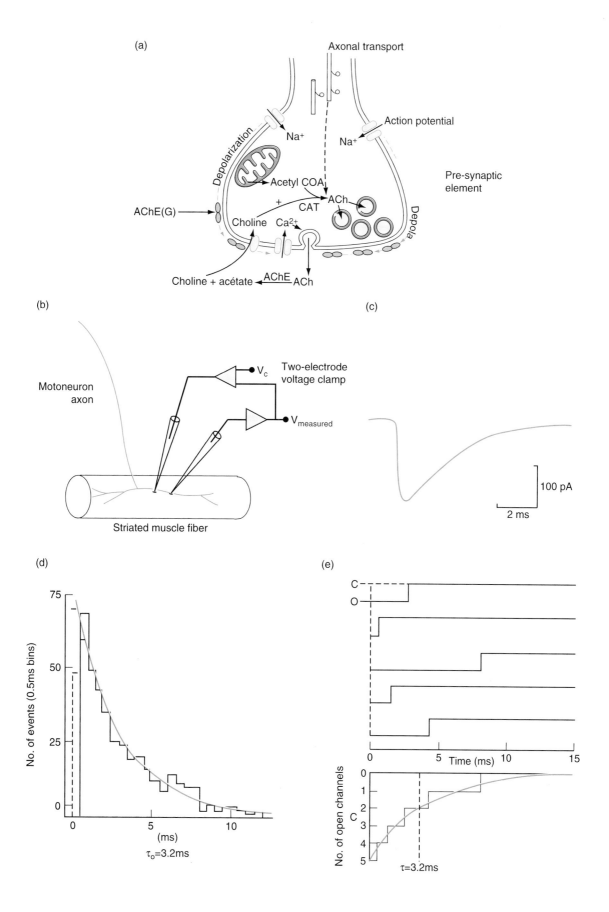

(a)

Axonal transport

Action potential

Na⁺

Depolarization

Na⁺

Acetyl COA

Pre-synaptic
element

AChE(G)

ACh

CAT

Choline

Ca²⁺

Depola

Choline + acétate ←AChE← ACh

(b)

Motoneuron
axon

Two-electrode
voltage clamp

V_c

V_measured

Striated muscle fiber

(c)

100 pA

2 ms

(d)

No. of events (0.5ms bins)

(ms)

τ_o=3.2ms

(e)

C

O

Time (ms)

No. of open channels

C

τ=3.2ms

diffusion

acetylcholine
release   ----→ A +R ⇌ AR ⇌ A₂R ⇌ A₂R*

degradation

This is very different from what occurs during the recording of the activity of a nicotinic receptor in a patch of membrane in the inside-out configuration, in response to the continuous presence of acetylcholine in the patch pipette. Likewise, during the recording of the activity of a nicotinic receptor channel in a patch of membrane in the outside-out configuration in response to acetylcholine pressure applied from another pipette. Even the shortest applications in this case are of the order of tens of milliseconds.

9.4.1 The Synaptic Current is the Sum of Unitary Currents Appearing with Variable Delays and Durations

There is a variable delay in the appearance of current flow through each one of the post-synaptic receptor channels. The reason for this is that the synaptic vesicles are released in an asynchronous manner. Furthermore, acetylcholine molecules must diffuse for a certain time before they reach a free receptor channel. We have seen that the concentration of acetylcholine in the synaptic cleft decreases so rapidly that a receptor channel has very few chances of being reopened a second time by binding again two acetylcholine molecules.

Determination of the value of the total synaptic current, I_{ACh} at steady state is

$$I_{ACh} = N \times p_o \times i_{ACh}$$

where N is the number of nicotinic channels in the membrane; i_{ACh} is the unitary current; and p_o is the open state probability of the channel and depends on the acetylcholine concentration and on the receptor channel opening (β) and closing (α) rate constants.

In model (1), we have the following rate constants:

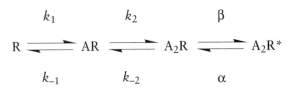

where α is the closing and β is the opening rate constants of the channel. The channel's probability of being in the open state at steady state (see Appendix 7.3) is then:

$$p_o = \beta' / (\beta' + \alpha)$$

where β' is the apparent opening rate constant of the channel, which depends on β but also on the rate constants of the preceding stages k_1 and k_2 ($\beta' = f[ACh]$). Thus, if α is short (i.e. the mean open time τ_o is long, because $\tau_o = 1/\alpha$), then p_o is high (it approaches its maximum value), and I_{ACh} is large.

The falling phase of the total current is exponential, with a time constant equal to τ_o

Let us assume that at a time t a certain number of ionic channels are opened more or less synchronously (this is the case of miniature currents, see Section 9.4.2). Because acetylcholine disappears very rapidly from the synaptic cleft, a channel has very few chances of reopening. Each one of the open channels has an opening duration t_o. We have seen that the duration t_o during which each channel remains open can be described by an exponential distribution (Figure 9.16). Figure 9.20e shows that the total current crossing N channels decreases exponentially with a time constant equal to τ_o.

In conclusion, the falling phase of the total current is not due to the progressive disappearance of acetylcholine from the synaptic cleft (because it disappears with a time constant of the order of microseconds) but depends only on τ_o, an intrinsic property of the channel.

9.4.2 Synaptic Currents Recorded from the Neuromuscular Junction

Miniature currents

Miniature currents are the currents recorded at the neuromuscular junction in the total absence of stimulation of the motor nerve (Figure 9.20b). These currents are evoked by the spontaneous liberation of acetylcholine from the pre-synaptic terminal. Thus, if an innervated muscle fiber in the absence of nerve

stimulation is recorded from under voltage clamp (Figure 9.20b), from time to time a miniature current will be recorded (Figure 9.20c). The recorded current is due to the spontaneous release of a synaptic vesicle or quantum of acetylcholine (1 vesicle = 1 quantum, see Chapter 8). This current is inward at −80 mV and has a maximum amplitude of about 4 nA.

Determination of the number of receptor channels opened by acetylcholine at the peak of a miniature current. Knowing the amplitude of the unitary current

Figure 9.21   Motor end plate current. (a) Current recorded in response to a stimulation of the nerve fiber under two-electrode voltage clamp. (b) This current is inward for negative membrane potentials and outward for positive voltages. As in the case of the unitary current, the motor end plate current reverses around 0 mV (frog's neuromuscular junction). Muscular action potentials are blocked by voltage clamping the corresponding muscle region. The muscle contraction induced by the inward current can be blocked by the destruction of T tubules (with a hyperosmotic shock). (Adapted from Magleby KL and Stevens CF, 1972. A quantitative description of end plate currents, *J. Physiol. (Lond.)* **223**: 173–197, with permission.)

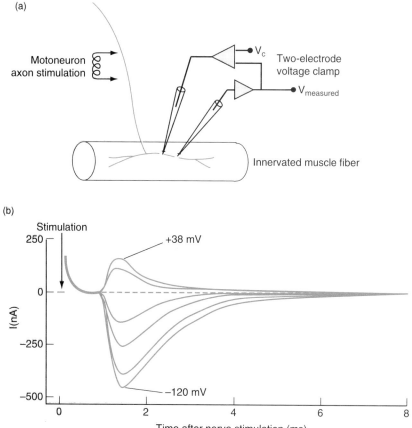

and the amplitude of a miniature current at the same membrane potential, we can calculate the number of nicotinic receptor channels opened by acetylcholine at the peak of the miniature response. At $V_m = -80$ mV, we have:

$i = 2.5$ pA, and $I = 4$ nA $= 4 \times 10^3$ pA

i.e. $4 \times 10^3/2.5 = 1600$ nicotinic receptor channels opened by acetylcholine.

Since two molecules of acetylcholine are needed to open one channel, the average number of acetylcholine molecules released is $1600 \times 2 = 3200$ molecules of ACh per vesicle. In other words, 1 quantum = about 3000 molecules of ACh.

Time course of a miniature current. The time it takes to reach the maximal amplitude of the miniature current is approximately 100 μs while it takes longer to disappear. The decrease of the current has an exponential time course with a time constant of the order of milliseconds (Figure 9.20e). This current decrease depends solely on τ_o (Figure 9.20d, e).

Motor end plate current

The end plate current is recorded (in voltage clamp) at the neuromuscular junction while the motor nerve is being stimulated (Figure 9.21). At $V_m = -80$ mV the current is inward and has an amplitude of approximately 400 nA.

Determination of the number of open channels at the peak of the motor end plate current. The motor end plate current is composed of 400 nA/4 nA = 100 miniature currents produced by $1600 \times 100 = 16 \times 10^4$ nicotinic receptors opened by released acetylcholine.

Time course of the motor end plate current. Approximately 100 vesicles are released in an asynchronous manner by the stimulated pre-synaptic terminal. This is the reason why the time it takes to reach the maximal or peak amplitude of this current is relatively longer than the time it takes to reach the peak of a miniature current (300 μs instead of 100 μs).

9.5 Nicotinic Transmission Pharmacology

9.5.1 Nicotinic Agonists

Nicotinic receptor agonists (see Appendix 2.1) bind to the same receptor site as acetylcholine and favor the conformational changes of the protein towards the open state. These agonists are, for example, suberyldicholine, carbachol and PTMA (phenyl trimethyl ammonium) (Figure 9.22a). The application of one of these on a patch of muscle membrane (outside-out configuration) leads to the onset of a current whose amplitude at each membrane potential tested is equal to the current evoked by acetylcholine. However, the duration of the openings of the channel depends on the agonist used (see Figure 9.22b, c).

9.5.2 Competitive Nicotinic Antagonists

Competitive antagonists (see Appendix 2.1) bind to the same receptor site as acetylcholine but *do not favor* its conformational change towards the open state. By binding to the acetylcholine receptor sites, competitive antagonists prevent acetylcholine from binding to its receptor sites and activating the nAChR. They decrease the number of sites available to acetylcholine and, therefore, decrease or completely block (depending on the dose used) the nicotinic cholinergic response. A distinction is made between competitive antagonists whose effect is reversible ((+)tubocurarine) from those whose effect is irreversible (DDF).

The application of (+)tubocurarine on a patch of muscle membrane in the outside-out recording configuration and in the presence of a low dose of acetylcholine causes a drop in the opening frequency of the channels. This occurs because (+)tubocurarine reduces the number of receptor sites available for acetylcholine. It should be noted, however, that the amplitude of the unitary current i_{Ach} evoked in the presence or absence of (+)tubocurarine is identical. The application of (+)tubocurarine on an isolated nerve–muscle preparation induces a reduction in the amplitude of the spontaneous miniature currents (currents evoked by the endogenous and spontaneous liberation of acetylcholine). The effect of (+)tubocurarine can be reversed by elevating the concentration of acetylcholine applied or released. Since the binding of (+)tubocurarine to the nicotinic receptor is reversible, increasing the acetyl-

Figure 9.22 Unitary currents evoked by nicotinic agonists (a) Structure of the different nicotinic agonists tested. (b) Inward unitary currents evoked by different nicotinic agonists ($V_m = -80$ mV) recorded in patch clamp (outside-out configuration) from isolated rat myotubes. Solutions (in mmol/l): intracellular 150 KCl, 5 Na$_2$EGTA, 0.5 CaCl$_2$, and extracellular 135 NaCl, 5.4 KCl. (c) i/V curves built from results similar to those shown in (b), but at different membrane potentials, are completely superimposable. The slope of each curve gives a unitary conductance γ of approximately 34 pS. (Adapted from Gardner P, Ogden DC and Colquhoun D, 1984. Conductances of single ion channels opened by nicotinic agonists are indistinguishable, *Nature* **289**, 160–163, with permission.)

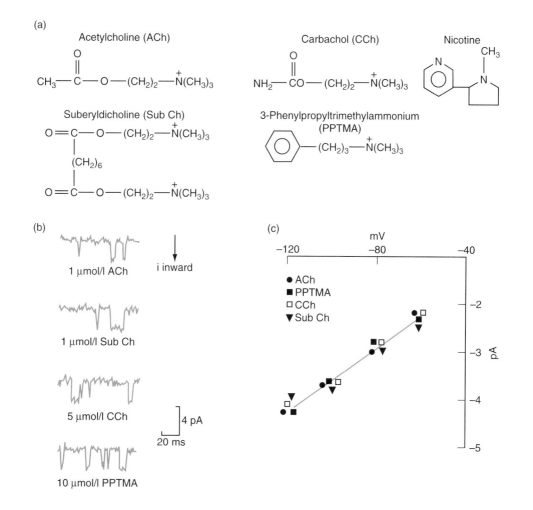

choline concentration will increase the probability that the receptor sites are occupied by acetylcholine.

The binding of α-bungarotoxin (venom from the snake *Bungarus multicinctus*) to the nicotinic receptor of the neuromuscular junction is very stable. For this reason, this toxin is used as a marker of acetylcholine receptor sites in this preparation. This labeling permits localizing and counting of these receptors. Labelled α-bungarotoxin also allows the identification of the receptor during its purification process (Figure 9.3).

9.5.3 Channel Blockers

Channel blockers are substances that bind to the aqueous pore of the open receptor, preventing the passage of cations through it. Among these substances are procaine and its derivatives (QX 222, lidocaine, benzocaine), and also histrionicotoxin and chlorpromazine.

The application of acetylcholine in the presence of benzocaine to a muscle membrane patch in the outside-out recording configuration evokes the onset of opening bursts. These bursts of unitary currents are due to the numerous fluctuations of the receptor between its open and its closed state (Figure 9.23a). The following model describes this process:

$$R \rightleftharpoons R^* \rightleftharpoons R^*B$$

where R represents the nicotinic receptor in its closed state, R^* the nicotinic receptor in its open state, and R^*B the nicotinic receptor in the open but blocked

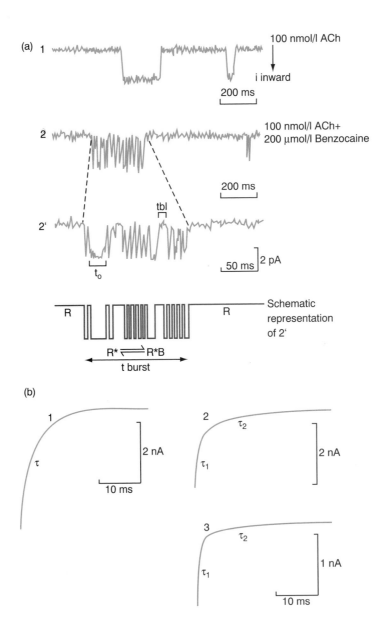

state. In the R* state, the cations cross the aqueous pore, while in the states R and R*B the ions cannot cross it.

In the presence of benzocaine, a change in the kinetics of the falling phase of the current (Figure 9.23b) is observed during the recording of spontaneous miniature currents of an isolated nerve–muscle preparation (V_m = –100 mV). In the absence of benzocaine, the falling phase is described by a single exponential with a time constant of τ = 3.8 ms. In the presence of benzocaine, the falling phase is described by two exponentials with time constants τ_1 = 1.0 ms and τ_2 = 7.6 ms. The explanation of this effect is that the channels opened by acetylcholine are very rapidly blocked by benzocaine, which quickly blocks the unitary current. Thus, one observes a fast initial decrement of the miniature current (with a shorter time constant than in the absence of benzocaine). The channels then reopen and reblock repeatedly. This increases the duration of the miniature current and one observes a second slower decrementing phase (with time constant τ_2).

9.5.4 Acetylcholinesterase Inhibitors

These inhibitors have a reversible effect, as in the case of prostigmine, or an irreversible effect, as in the case of DFP (difluorophosphate). The application of prostigmine to an isolated nerve–muscle preparation significantly increases the miniature current duration (Figure 9.24). In the presence of prostigmine, acetylcholine molecules degrade much more slowly, and thus are able to bind repeatedly and trigger the reopening of nicotinic receptors. This repeated binding considerably increases the duration of the miniature current falling phase. As we have already seen (Section 9.4) the miniature current time constant in the absence of acetylcholinesterase inhibitors reflects the nicotinic receptor average open time. However, the average open time of the nicotinic receptor is clearly not the same in the presence of prostigmine.

Figure 9.24 Effect of the acetylcholinesterase inhibitor prostigmine (10^{-6} g/ml) on the duration of miniature currents. Recordings in the absence (a) and presence (b) of prostigmine, showing that prostigmine augments the duration of the miniature current. (Adapted from Katz B and Miledi R, 1973. The binding of acetylcholine to receptors and its removal from the synaptic cleft, *J. Physiol. (Lond.)* **231**, 549–574, with permission.)

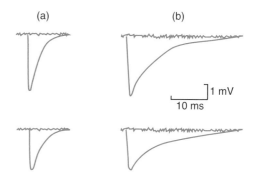

Figure 9.23 Benzocaine effect on the time course of ACh evoked unitary and miniature nicotinic currents. (a) Patch clamp recording (cell-attached configuration) of nicotinic unitary currents evoked by the application of ACh (i_{ACh}). (1) In the presence of 100 nM ACh, the channels open for a mean duration of τ_o = 19 ms (V_m = –110 mV). (2) In the presence of 100 nM ACh + 200 µM benzocaine bursts of openings (V_m = –130 mV) are recorded. (2') The same recording as (2) but with a different time scale and with an added diagram of the openings and closings of the channel. t_o, time during which the channel stays open; t_{bl}, time during which the channel is blocked by benzocaine; t_{burst}, duration of a burst of openings. The histograms of t_o and of t_{bl} are described by a single exponential with the following average values: τ_o = 2.8 ms, and τ_{bl} = 3.5 ms (extrajunctional muscle membrane of 4- to 6-week-old muscle cells). (b) Two-electrode voltage clamp recording of miniature nicotinic currents. Each curve corresponds to the average of 8 to 14 miniature currents (V_m = –100 mV). (1) In the absence of benzocaine, the miniature currents reach their maximum in approximately 1 ms. Their decrement is described by a single exponential with a time constant τ = 3.8 ms. (2) In the presence of extracellular benzocaine (300 µM, 15 min), the peak amplitude of miniature currents decreases, and the falling phase is described by two exponentials with time constants τ_1 = 1.0 ms and τ_2 = 7.6 ms. (3) In the presence of a higher concentration of benzocaine (500 µM, 17 min), the amplitude of the miniature current peak is further diminished and the time constants of the falling phase become τ_1 = 0.7 ms and τ_2 = 11.6 ms (frog cutaneous pectoris muscle). (a, b: Adapted from Ogden DC, Siegelbaum SA and Colquhoun D, 1981. Block of acetylcholine-activated ion channels by an uncharged local anesthetic, *Nature* **289**, 596–598, with permission.)

Appendix 9.1
Incorporation of Purified Nicotinic
Receptors into Liposomes

Nicotinic receptor channels (nAChR) found in elec-troplax membranes of the electric ray *Torpedo* are solubilized in the presence of a low concentration of detergent (2% cholate) (Figure A9.1). The detergent has a polar structure and surrounds membrane lipids still associated with the nicotinic receptors or which

have formed micelles. In order to enrich the prepara-tion with this protein, the receptor is purified.

Exogenous lipids are then added in excess, and the detergent is dialyzed. Under these conditions nicotinic receptors are incorporated into the liposomes. It is estimated that a 200 nm diameter vesicle encloses approximately 100 receptors. The liposome external and internal faces can be distinguished, and thus one can measure radioactive ion fluxes (see Appendix 9.4).

Figure A9.1   Nicotinic receptors are purified and incorporated into lipid vesicles or liposomes. (From Anholt R, Lindstrom J, and Montal M, 1981. Stabilization of acetylcholine receptor channels by lipids in cholate solu-tion and during reconstitution of vesicles, *J. Biol. Chem.* **256**, 4377–4387, with permission.)

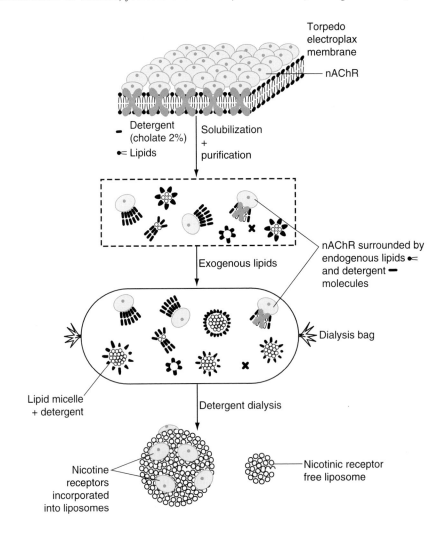

Appendix 9.2
The Contribution of Genetic Engineering to the Study of Ionic Channels – Example: The Nicotinic Acetylcholine Receptor

Genetic engineering techniques have proved to be remarkably useful in studying the structure–function relationship of ionic channels, the mechanisms of their assembly, and the regulation of their expression. For example, in the case of the nicotinic receptor (nAChR), which is an oligomer made up of different subunits, the following questions arise:

(a) What are the transmembrane, extracellular and cytoplasmic regions of each subunit?
(b) What is the degree of homology between peripheral and central nicotinic receptors, as indicated by the percentage of similarity of their sequence?
(c) Are all the α, β, γ and δ subunits necessary for the function of the nicotinic receptor?
(d) Are the α, β, γ and δ subunits sufficient to assemble correctly a functional pentamer $\alpha_2\beta\gamma\delta$, or are other proteins necessary?
(e) Does each subunit have a precise function?
(f) Which amino acids form the acetylcholine receptor site and which form the ionic channel?

To answer some of these questions we need to know the primary structure of each subunit. To answer others it is necessary to be able to compare the function of the native receptor with that of hybrid or modified (mutated) ones. Thanks to genetic engineering techniques we can produce hybrid receptors, i.e. receptors built from combinations of subunits of different animal species or from combinations of embryonic and adult receptor subunits, etc. We can also produce mutated receptors, made up of various combinations of native and mutated subunits.

The analysis of the function of native, hybrid or mutated receptors is mainly carried out using electrophysiological techniques, notably the patch clamp technique.

Figure A9.2   Methods of analysis of mutated (nAChR*) and non-mutated (nAChR) nicotinic receptor function when inserted in the plasma membrane of a host cell (electrophysiological, kinetic or biochemical studies).

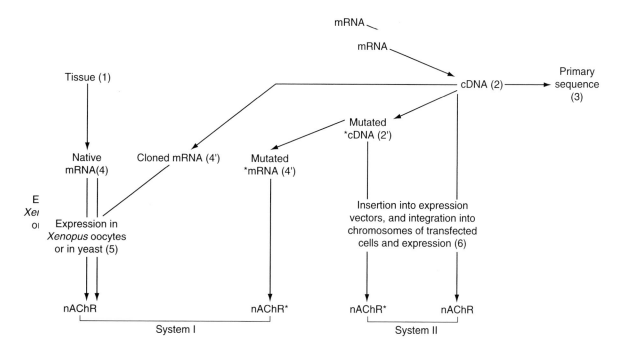

A9.2.1 Analysis of the Primary Structure of each Subunit

As a first step, genomic (Figure A9.2, (1)) or complementary (2) DNA coding for each subunit is cloned and its sequence determined. From this sequence, we can deduce the primary amino acid sequence of each subunit (3). It is in fact much easier to sequence a molecule of DNA than a protein. We can thus determine the hydrophobicity profile of each subunit (see Appendix 5.2) and propose a model of its transmembrane organization (Question a). We can also compare the primary structure of different subunits and look for sequence homologies (Question b).

If we want to modify the sequence of one of the subunits to analyze the relationships between its structure and function, mutations of the complementary DNA (cDNA) in precise places of its sequence can be obtained by using site-directed mutagenesis (2'). We can also interchange homologous regions from different subunits (α, β, γ, δ), from receptors of different origin (peripheral and central receptors), or from different species, in order to identify different functional roles of different structural domains (see Section 9.2.3).

A9.2.2 Analysis of the Function of Native, Hybrid or Mutated Nicotinic Receptors

Using an expression system we can produce different native or mutated subunits. Currently, two such expression systems are used, named I and II on Figure A9.2. Each system presents different advantages and disadvantages.

System I: Translation of Messenger RNA (mRNA) of Different Subunits in the Oocyte of Xenopus

Rationale

Mutated or native mRNA molecules are isolated and injected into a *Xenopus* oocyte. The enzymatic machinery of the oocyte is capable of translating these mRNA molecules, which are then assembled and inserted into the plasma membrane. This expression is fast (of the order of a few hours) but the synthesized molecules can be allowed to accumulate for several days.

- Normal mRNA (4) is either isolated from cells (1–4) or a cRNA is synthesized *in vitro* from cDNA (2–4').
- Alternatively, mutated mRNA (4') is obtained by *in vivo* or *in vitro* transcription of mutated cDNA (2'–4"). Mutations are produced on precise regions of the cDNA molecule by site-directed mutagenesis (2–2').
- Finally, native or mutated mRNA molecules from different subunits are injected into the oocyte of *Xenopus* (Figure A9.3) and are translated by these cells. The polypeptide subunits are assembled and inserted into the membrane of the host cells (5).

Conclusion

This expression system is fast but transient (it lasts for about 2 days). Because of its speed, it is particularly useful for the study of hybrid (Section 9.2.2) or mutated receptors, since it allows for a rapid screening of interesting mutations. It has allowed us to broach Question c (Section 9.1.2) and Question f (Sections 9.1.4 and 9.1.5).

System II: Expression of Genomic DNA or cDNA in Cell Lines (Transfected Cells)

This expression can be stable or transient.

Rationale of the stable transfection

Genomic DNA (1) or cDNA (2) is integrated into chromosomes of immortalized cells. This creates a new cell line originating from a single cell, which expresses the integrated DNA.

- Cloning of genomic (1) or complementary (2) DNA.
- Alternatively, cDNA (2) is first mutated in precise regions (2') and then cloned.
- Host cells are permeabilized in order to allow a vector-carried DNA (mutated or native) to enter the cytoplasm (transfection step). This DNA integrates into the genome of the host cell and is then contin-

Figure A9.3 Nicotinic receptor expression in *Xenopus* oocytes. The cDNAs of different subunits are cloned, and the corresponding mRNAs injected into *Xenopus* oocytes in the proportion 2 mRNA α, 1 mRNA β, 1 mRNA γ, 1 mRNA δ. It should be noted that the oocyte membrane normally does not express any nicotinic receptors. These mRNAs are translated by the enzymes and organelles present in the oocyte and the subunits thus produced assemble and are inserted in the plasma membrane. These nicotinic receptors can be studied after 2 to 4 days. One must remove the vitelline membrane that surrounds the oocytes if the recordings are to be carried out. In the outside-out patch clamp configuration the currents crossing a single channel (unitary currents can be recorded), whereas in the two-electrode voltage clamp configuration the macroscopic current crossing all the channels expressed can be recorded.

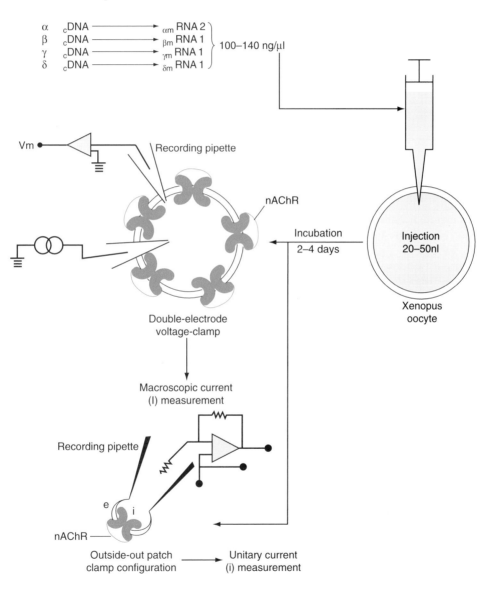

uously translated and transcribed (6). For this, a stable integration is necessary.

In order to isolate the cellular clones that may have incorporated a gene or genes into their genome (stable lineages) one uses a selection procedure: in this case the transfection procedure is carried out in the presence of a low concentration of an additional vector, which carries a selection gene. One assumes that a cell that has integrated the selection vector will, in general, also have integrated the vector that carries the gene of interest, because this gene is used at a much higher concentration (the limiting step is the DNA penetration). Two or three weeks are required to obtain these clones. Stable transfection is thus a lengthy procedure. However, it permits the systematic study of the proteins produced.

Conclusion

Despite the long time it takes to produce this system, it generates many identical cells and a continuous expression of the integrated DNA. Consequently, it is particularly useful for kinetic studies and studies of the mobility membrane receptors (receptor internalization and recycling).

Principle of transient transfection

In this case the plasmid vectors do not integrate into the cellular genome but can still multiply. This system allows for a very high level of expression over approximately 2 days. It offers the same advantages as the oocyte expression system.

Other Uses of Cloned DNA

Another use for cloned DNA is in the method of *in situ* hybridization (see Appendixes 2.2 and 2.3). This method uses labeled nucleic acid probes to highlight mRNA *in situ*. Therefore, it allows the identification of those cell bodies in which the synthesis of the proteins involved in nerve transmission takes place. The validity of this method is considerably extended because the hybridization of nucleic acid sequences across species is better conserved than the immunoreactivity of proteins across species.

Appendix 9.3
Principle of Acetylcholine Receptor Site Labeling Using Photoactivated Nicotinic Ligands

The nicotinic cholinergic receptor is incubated in the presence of a photosensitive nicotinic ligand, as for example ^{3}H-DDF (para N,N dimethylamino benzene diazonium fluorborate). As with all nicotinic ligands, ^{3}H-DDF binds non-covalently to the ACh receptor sites located on the two α-subunits. ^{3}H-DDF has to be photoactivated to allow its irreversible covalent binding to the ACh receptor sites. The amino acids involved in the receptor site are thus permanently labeled by radioactive hydrogen (^{3}H) and can then be identified.

[3]H-DDF is photoactivated by energy transfer from tryptophane residues located close to the receptor site

Nicotinic receptors are incubated in the presence of ^{3}H-DDF. The preparation is then irradiated with light of $\lambda = 290$ nm wavelength, the wavelength of excitation of tryptophane (Trp). The excited Trp residues emit at $\lambda = 320$ nm, and the energy of this 320 nm wavelength radiation activates the photosensitive nicotinic ligand ^{3}H-DDF. This means that there is an overlap between the emission spectrum of Trp and the absorption spectrum of ^{3}H-DDF. The Trp residues that are closer than 8 nm from the ACh receptor site, the site where ^{3}H-DDF is bound, are the only ones to participate in this energy transfer process. In order to activate only the ^{3}H-DDF molecules that are closer than 8 nm from the receptor site, photoactivation by energy transfer (explained above) is used instead of direct photoactivation.

What is the result of the photoactivation of the nicotinic ligand ^{3}H-DDF?

Photoactivation allows covalent binding between amino acids located at the receptor site and provides an easily identifiable marker, the radioactive hydrogen of ^{3}H-DDF.

When ^{3}H-DDF is photoactivated it forms an arylcation. This arylcation covalently binds to the nearest amino acids. Since the nicotinic part is labeled by radioactive hydrogen, the amino acids that participate in the binding site or are close to it are also labeled. The α-subunits are subsequently separated and purified, and the labeled amino acids are identified.

Control experiments

In order to eliminate all non-specific labeling by ^{3}H-DDF (labeling of sites located outside the ACh receptor site), these experiments are carried out in the presence of phencyclidine. Phencyclidine is a ligand of receptor sites for non-competitive cholinergic antagonists. Phencyclidine thus prevents ^{3}H-DDF from binding to these non-specific sites. Furthermore, some of the experiments are performed in the presence of high concentrations of carbamylcholine, a nicotinic ligand that binds to the ACh receptor site. The ^{3}H-DDF labelling obtained under these conditions corresponds only to non-specific binding and can be used to identify the sites of specific DDF incorporation. It can also be used to subtract non-specific from specific binding results.

Appendix 9.4
Rapid Measurement of Radioactive Ion Flow: Quench Flow

Example of Na+ ion flux through nicotinic channels (nAChR) (Figure A9.4)

Rationale of the method. A low concentration of a nicotinic agonist (carbamylcholine (1), for example) is applied onto nicotinic receptors that have been incorporated into radioactive sodium [Na*] loaded liposomes. This low concentration is sufficient to open the nicotinic channel receptors (nAChR). Na* ions exit towards the external environment (2). After a brief interval (10 ms) a strong concentration of carbamylcholine is added. Under these conditions, the nAChR desensitize: the cationic channel closes despite its high affinity for the agonist and Na* ions stop flowing out of the liposome (3). One can thus measure the passage of Na* ions or of any other cation during a short period of time (of the order of 10 ms).

Technique employed. Compartment (1) contains the liposomes into which nAChR have been incorporated. Compartment (2) contains carbamylcholine at a low concentration. Compartment (3) contains a high concentration of carbamylcholine. (1) and (2) are mixed at time t, and (3) is added at $t + 10$ ms. The time during which the nAChR are open is, therefore, approximately 10 ms.

An alternative use of this technique in the study of nicotinic receptor desensitization is to incubate the liposomes with carbamylcholine before stages (2) and (3).

Appendix 9.5
Additional States of the Nicotinic Receptor

Jackson *et al.* have shown the existence of spontaneous openings of nicotinic channels during patch clamp recordings of their activity in cultured muscle cells (cell-attached configuration). These openings occur even in the absence of acetylcholine from the patch pipette (Figure A9.5, A). In order to eliminate the possible activation of nicotinic receptors by acetylcholine or other nicotinic agonists that may be present at very low concentrations in the patch pipette, the preparation is previously treated with DTT (dithiothreitol) and N-ethylmaleimide, which denature the acetylcholine receptor sites. In spite of this treatment, one can still observe spontaneous openings of the nicotinic channels (Figure A9.5, B). To verify that the DTT treatment actually prevents possible openings triggered by residual acetylcholine, the authors compared the effect of acetylcholine application before (Figure A9.5, C) and after (Figure A9.5, D) the treatment. While acetylcholine triggers numerous openings in the non-treated cells (Figure A9.5, C) it evokes only a few openings in the treated cells (Figure A9.5, D). Furthermore, the frequency of openings of the treated cells is similar to the frequency of openings in DDT treated cells.

The following model has been proposed to account for the nicotinic channel opening when less than two ACh molecules are bound to its receptor sites:

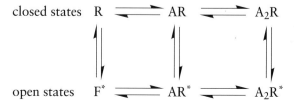

Figure A9.4   Example of Na⁺ flux through nicotinic cholinergic channels (nAChR).

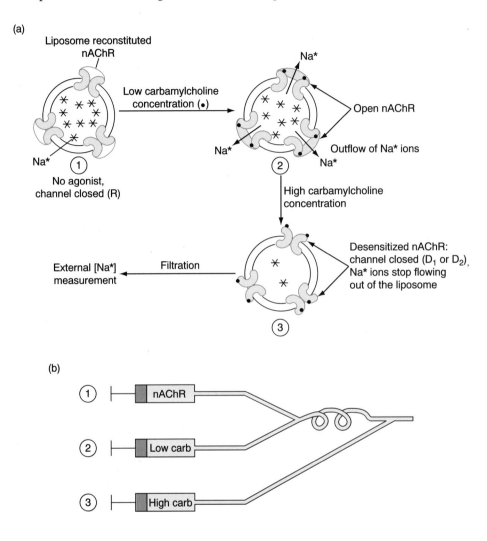

However, the opening durations of the receptor channel bound to only one or no ligand molecules are too short to contribute significantly to the end plate current.

This model has been expanded, and it has been suggested that the nicotinic receptor could desensitize in the absence of ACh (for instance in the presence of channel blockers). In the absence of ACh, a fraction (20%) of the nicotinic receptors from *Torpedo* electric organ is in the desensitized state. The model is the following:

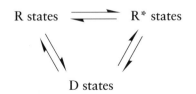

where closed states or R states are R, AR, A_2R; open states or R* states are R*, AR*, A_2R^*; and desensitized states or D states are D_1, AD_1, A_2D_1 and D_2, AD_2, A_2D_2.

Figure A9.5 Patch clamp recording (cell-attached configuration) of the activity of muscle cell nicotinic channels both in the presence and absence of acetylcholine (A, B, C, D). All the recordings are carried out in the presence of TTX to block the opening of voltage-sensitive Na⁺ channels, and in the absence of quaternary ammonium ions that might interact with the ACh receptor sites. (From Jackson MB, 1984. Spontaneous openings of the acetylcholine receptor channel, *Proc. Natl Acad. Sci. USA*; **81**, 3901–3904, with permission.)

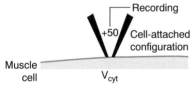

	Untreated muscle cells	Muscle cells treated with DTT
No ACh in the pipette	A	B
ACh in the pipette	C	D

50 pA

100 ms

Recording

+50 Cell-attached configuration

Muscle cell

V_{cyt}

Further Reading

Abakas, M.H., Kaufmann, C., Archdeacon, P. and Karlin, A. (1995) Identification of acetylcholine receptor channel-lining residues in the entire M2 segment of the α subunit. *Neuron* **13**, 919–927.

Bertrand, D., Devillers-Thiéry, A., Revah, F. *et al.* (1992) Unconventional pharmacology of a neuronal nicotinic receptor mutated in the channel domain. *Proc. Natl. Acad. Sci. USA* **89**, 1261–1265.

Couturier, S., Bertrand, D., Matter, J.M. *et al.* (1990) A neuronal nicotinic acetylcholine receptor subunit (α7) is developmentally regulated and forms a homo-oligomeric channel blocked by α-BTX. *Neuron* **5**, 847–856.

Czajikowski, C. and Karlin, A. (1995) Structure of the nicotinic acetylcholine-binding site: identification of acidic residues in the δ subunit with 0.9 nm of the α subunit-binding site disulfide. *J. Biol. Chem.* **270**, 3160–3164.

Edmonds, B., Gibb, A.J. and Colquhoun, D. (1995) Mechanisms of activation of muscle nicotinic acetylcholine receptors and the time course of end plate currents. *Ann. Rev. Physiol.* **57**, 469–493.

Galzi, J.L. and Changeux, J.P. (1995) Neuronal nicotinic acetylcholine receptors: molecular organization and regulation. *Neuropharmacol.* **34**, 563–582.

Karlin, A. and Akabas, M.H. (1995) Toward a structural basis for the function of the nicotinic acetylcholine receptors and their cousins. *Neuron* **15**, 1231–1244.

Katz, B. and Miledi, R. (1973) The binding of acetylcholine to receptors and its removal from the synaptic cleft. *J. Physiol. (Lond.)* **231**, 549–574.

Léna, C. and Changeux, J.P. (1993) Allosteric modulations of the nicotinic acetylcholine receptor. *Trends Neurosci.* **16**, 181–186.

Leonard, R.J., Labarca, C.G., Charnet, P. *et al.* (1988) Evidence that the M2 membrane-spanning region lines the ion channels pore of the nicotinic receptor. *Science* **242**, 1578–1581.

Murray, N., Zheng, Y.C., Mandel, G. *et al.* (1995) A single site on the ε subunit is responsible for the change in ACh receptor channel conductance during skeletal muscle development. *Neuron* **14**, 865–870.

The GABA$_A$ Receptor

The GABA$_A$ receptor channel (GABA$_A$R) is a ligand-gated channel activated by γ-aminobutyric acid (GABA), the neurotransmitter at numerous synapses in the mammalian central nervous system.

The GABA$_A$ receptor is a glycoprotein composed of several subunits, five of which have been described to date: α, β, γ, δ, and ρ. The GABA$_A$ receptor is comprised of the GABA receptor sites on its surface, the elements that make the ionic channel selectively permeable to chloride ions as well as all the elements necessary for interactions between different functional domains. Thus, the GABA receptor sites and the chloride channel are part of the same unique protein.

Aside from the GABA receptor sites, the GABA$_A$ receptor contains a variety of topographically distinct receptor sites capable of recognizing clinically active substances, such as the benzodiazepines (anxiolytics and anticonvulsants) and the barbiturates (sedatives and anticonvulsants) (Table 10.1). These substances interact allosterically with the GABA receptor sites and modulate the GABA$_A$ response. Recent data suggest the existence of several GABA$_A$ receptor types differing in their subunit composition. This leads not only to structural heterogeneity but also to pharmacological heterogeneity, especially regarding the sensitivity to benzodiazepines. The consequences of this heterogeneity remain poorly understood and will not be discussed in this chapter.

The function of the GABA$_A$ receptor in the adult vertebrate central nervous system is to mediate fast inhibitory synaptic transmission by converting the binding of two GABA molecules to a rapid and transient increase in permeability to chloride ions. In this chapter, we will present results obtained from isolated neurons and from synapses of the central nervous system: synapses between GABAergic interneurons and neurons of the spinal cord and synapses between GABAergic interneurons and pyramidal neurons in the hippocampus. The first demonstration of GABA as a neurotransmitter in the central nervous system was performed by K Krnjević in 1961.

It should be noted that GABA also acts via receptors coupled to G-proteins called GABA$_B$ receptors (GABAergic metabotropic receptors, see Table 5.1) and via GABA$_C$ receptors which are bicuculline-insensitive receptor channels (ionotropic receptors) permeable to Cl$^-$ions.

10.1 The GABA$_A$ Receptor is Hetero-oligomeric and has a Structural Heterogeneity

The GABA$_A$ receptor purified on affinity columns (see Figure 9.3) from calf, pig, rat or chick brain dissociates in the presence of a detergent into two major subunits which migrate on polyacrylamide gels and have apparent molecular masses of 53 kD (α subunit) and 56 kD (β subunit). However, electrophoretic

Table 10.1 Pharmacology of GABA receptors

	GABA$_A$ receptors	GABA$_B$ receptors
Agonists	GABA Muscimol Isoguvacine THIP	GABA Baclofen
Competitive antagonists	Bicuculline	Phaclofen
Channel blockers	Picrotoxin	—
Allosteric agonists	Benzodiazepines Barbiturates	—
Inverse agonist at the benzodiazepine site	β carboline (DMCM)	—
Antagonist at the benzodiazepine site	Ro 15 1788	—

THIP, 4,5,6,7-tetrahydroisoxazolopyridin-3-ol.

studies based on receptors purified from different regions of the central nervous system show the presence of multiple bands corresponding to apparent molecular masses of 48–53 kD and of 55–57 kD. This suggested the occurrence of several isoforms of α and β subunits.

The first demonstration of the structural heterogeneity of the GABA$_A$ receptor came from cloning of cDNAs for the different α subunits (named α$_1$, α$_2$ . . .) and β subunits (named β$_1$, β$_2$ . . .). The diversity of GABA$_A$ receptor subunits (α, β, γ, δ, ρ) was then revealed and for each subunit the existence of different isoforms (the ρ subunit is found in retina). All subunits are similar in size, containing about 450–550 amino acids and are strongly conserved among species. A high percentage of sequence identity (70–80%) is found between subunit isoforms (between α and between β isoforms, for example). Sequence identity is also found, but to a lesser extent (30–40%), between different subunit families (between α, β, γ, δ, and ρ).

The common elements of the subunit structure include (Figure 10.1a):

- a large NH$_2$-terminal hydrophilic domain exposed to the synaptic cleft;
- then four hydrophobic segments named M1 to M4, each composed of approximately 20 amino acids which form four membrane-spanning segments; the M2 segment of each of the subunits comprising the GABA$_A$ receptor is thought to line the channel (as for the nAChR) and to contribute to ion selectivity and transport. Apparently, a small number of amino acids within the M2 sequence is responsible for anionic versus cationic permeability (see Section 9.2.2);
- the M3 and M4 segments are separated by a large, poorly conserved hydrophilic domain located in the cytoplasm and which contains putative phosphorylation sites. Most of the divergence between the different subunits is found at the level of this domain.

To form a GABA$_A$ receptor, with the large number of known subunits taken four or five at a time, thousands of combinations are possible. Two approaches are currently used to elucidate which subunit combinations exist *in vivo*:

- a comparative study of the functional properties of receptors expressed in oocytes or in transfected

mammalian cells from known combinations of cloned subunits (with the restriction that *Xenopus* oocyte does not automatically assemble a channel composed of all injected subunits);
- a comparative study of the distribution of the various subunit mRNAs in the brain using the *in situ* hybridization technique (see Appendix 2.3).

Surprisingly, the transient expression in transfected cells of identical α or β subunits (see Appendix 9.2) gives functional homomeric GABA$_A$ receptors, i.e. receptors that induce chloride- (Cl$^-$) mediated currents in the presence of GABA or its agonists. This current is blocked by GABA$_A$ antagonists and potentiated by barbiturates but is unaffected by benzodiazepines. These properties can be attributed to the conserved structural features of all the subunits. However, the channels resulting from expression of single subunits are asssembled inefficiently (are rare and slightly detectable) and it is unlikely that native receptors are formed from identical subunits. Expression of a γ subunit together with an α and a β subunit in transfected cells gives rise to the expression of a GABA$_A$ receptor with all the features of the previous receptor in addition to its sensitivity to benzodiazepines (see Figure 10.8). This does not necessarily imply that the receptor site for benzodiazepines is situated on the γ subunit, but that expression of the latter is required for the action of benzodiazepines. The conclusion of these studies is that the combination αβγ (α1β1γ2 or α5β2γ2, for example) is the minimal requirement for reproducing consensus properties known for the vertebrate GABA$_A$ receptor channel *in situ*. Unfortunately, the exact subunit combination of not even one native GABA$_A$ receptor subtype is known at this time.

The amino acids identified by site-directed mutagenesis to affect channel activation by GABA are in the β2 subunit: tyrosine (Y) 157, threonine (T) 160, threonine (T) 202 and tyrosine (Y) 206 (Figure 10.1b, c). Mutations of the corresponding tyrosines in the α and γ subunits do not play a role in GABA-mediated activation. In the α1 subunit, the mutation of phenylalanine (F) 64 to leucine (L) also impairs activation of the GABA channel indicating a role for this α subunit residue in GABA binding (Figure 10.1c). Therefore, two identified domains (or loops B and C) of the β subunit and at least one domain (loop D) from a neighboring α subunit contribute to the GABA-binding site.

Figure 10.1   Transmembrane model of the GABA$_A$ receptor subunits. (a) Hydropathy plots of an α and a β subunit (see Appendix 5.2). The bars indicate the position of the hydrophobic segments (M1 to M4) assumed to span the lipid bilayer. The other regions are more hydrophilic. Note that the two subunits have similar hydropathic profiles. (b) Linear representation of the β$_2$ subunit (left). The amino acids (black dots) crucial for GABA-dependent gating are located in the N-terminal hydrophilic domain between the disulfide bridge and the first membrane-spanning segment M1. (Right) Model of transmembrane organization of GABA$_A$ receptor subunits. The large hydrophilic amino-terminal domain is exposed to the synaptic cleft and carries the neurotransmitter site and glycosylation sites (ψ). The four M segments span the membrane. The hydrophilic domain separating M3 and M4 faces the cytoplasm and contains phosphorylation sites. The COOH-terminus is extracellular. (c) Model of the GABA binding site. The amino acids labeled belong to different regions of the amino-terminal extracellular domain of β subunits and to one domain of subunits (see text for explanation). (a: Adapted from Barnard EA, Darlison MG and Seeburg P, 1987. Molecular biology of the GABA$_A$ receptor: the receptor channel superfamily, *TINS* **10**, 502–509, with permission. b, left: Adapted from Amin J and Weiss DS, 1993. GABA$_A$ receptor needs two homologous domains of the β subunit for activation by GABA but not by pentobarbital, *Nature* **366**, 565–570, with permission. b, right and c: Adapted from Galzi JL and Changeux JP, 1994, Neurotransmitter-gated ion channels as unconventional allosteric proteins, *Curr. Opin. Neurobiol.* **4**, 554–565, with permission.)

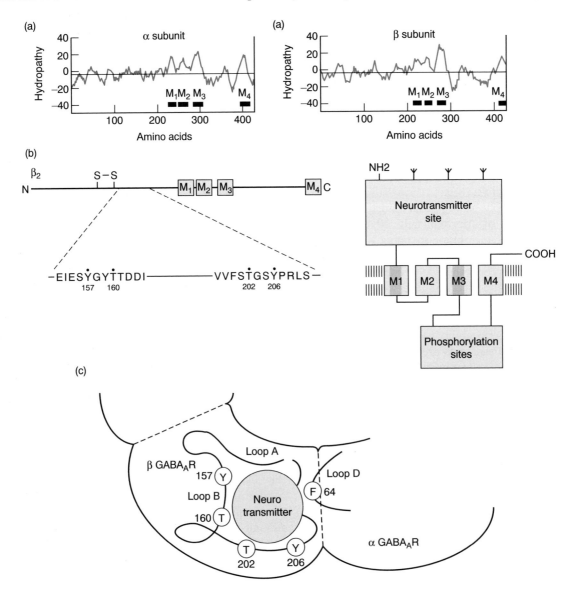

10.2 Binding of Two GABA Molecules Leads to a Conformational Change of the GABA$_A$ Receptor into an Open State

10.2.1 Evidence for the Binding of Two GABA Molecules

Analysis of dose–response curves suggests the binding of two GABA molecules prior to opening of the channel. The response studied, the peak amplitude of the total current I_{GABA} evoked by GABA in whole cell patch-clamp recording, was proportional to the square of the dose of GABA (but only at low doses of GABA):

$$I_{GABA} = f(GABA)^2$$

At low doses of GABA, when receptor desensitization is negligible, it seems that upon binding of two GABA molecules to the receptor, the conformational change of the receptor channel to an open state is favored. These observations can be accounted for by the following model:

$$2\,G + R \rightleftharpoons G + GR \rightleftharpoons G_2R \rightleftharpoons G_2R^*$$

where G is GABA; R is the GABA$_A$ receptor in closed configuration; GR or G$_2$R is the mono or doubly liganded GABA$_A$ receptor in the closed configuration; and G$_2$R* is the doubly liganded GABA$_A$ receptor in the open configuration.

10.2.2 The GABA$_A$ Channel is Selectively Permeable to Cl$^-$ Ions

The reversal potential of the GABA current varies with the Cl$^-$ equilibrium potential, E_{Cl}

The ionic selectivity of the channel has been shown in outside-out patch-clamp recording from cultured spinal neurons. This patch-clamp configuration allows control of the membrane potential as well as the composition of the intracellular fluid.

When the intracellular and extracellular fluids contain the same Cl$^-$concentration (145 mmM), the current evoked by GABA reverses at 0 mV (Figure 10.2a, c and 10.4a). In this case:

$$E_{inv} = E_{Cl} = -58 \log 145/145 = 0\ mV$$

If part of the intracellular Cl$^-$ is replaced with non-permeant anions such as isethionate (HO-CH$_2$-CH$_2$-SO$_3^-$), for a 10-fold change in intracellular Cl$^-$ concentration a shift in the reversal potential of approximately 56 mV is observed (Figure 10.2d). This value approaches very closely that of 58 mV predicted by the Nernst equation for E_{Cl} at 20°C.

$$E_{Cl} = -58 \log 145/14.5 = -58\ mV$$

Finally, changes in extracellular Na$^+$ or K$^+$ concentration have very little effect on the reversal potential of the GABA$_A$ response. Taken together, these results demonstrate that the GABA$_A$ channel is selectively permeable to Cl$^-$.

In physiological extracellular and intracellular solutions, the GABA$_A$ current recorded in isolated spinal neurons reverses at –60 mV

Using the technique of patch-clamp recording one can record the unitary currents (i_{GABA}) across the GABA$_A$ channel (spinal neurons in culture, cell-attached configuration). The GABA present in the solution inside the recording pipette (5 µM) evokes outward single channel currents at –30, 0 and +20 mV (Figure 10.3a). The magnitude of the single channel current increases with depolarization, suggesting that the reversal potential for the GABA$_A$ response is negative to –30 mV. The i/V curve, obtained by plotting the unitary current i_{GABA} against the membrane potential, shows in this experiment a reversal potential of the GABA-induced current of around –60 mV (Figure 10.2a, b). Thus, at a potential close to the resting membrane potential (–60 mV) the current evoked by GABA is not detectable. At potentials more positive than rest, an outward current is recorded whose magnitude increases with depolarization of the post-synaptic membrane.

As E_{Cl} is close to the resting membrane potential (–60 mV) in physiological intracellular and extracellular solutions, the electrochemical gradient for the Cl$^-$ ions ($V_m – E_{Cl}$) for $V_m = V_{rest}$ is close to 0 mV. The net flux of Cl$^-$ ions at a potential close to rest is therefore null or very small: no current is recorded even though the GABA$_A$ channels are open. On the other hand, as the membrane potential depolarizes, the net flux of Cl⁻ ions becomes inward. An inward net flux of negative charges corresponds to an outward current. At potentials more positive than V_{rest}, an outward current is recorded (compare Figures 10.3 and 10.4b).

10.2.3 The Single Channel Conductance of GABA$_A$ Channels is Constant in Symmetrical Cl⁻ Solutions but Varies as a Function of Potential in Asymmetrical Solutions

Experiments are performed on mouse spinal neurons in culture. Recordings are performed under conditions of equal intra- and extracellular Cl⁻ concentration (145 mM) to minimize rectification (variation of conductance γ as a function of membrane potential) resulting from the difference in Cl⁻ concentration on either side of the membrane. Histograms of single channel currents evoked by GABA and recorded at $V_m = +50$ mV (outward i_{GABA}) and $V_m = -90$ mV (inward i_{GABA}) show at each potential a single peak of current equal to +1.48 and −2.7 pA, respectively (Figure 10.2b). From these values of i_{GABA}, the mean single channel conductance γ can be calculated, as $i_{GABA} = \gamma_{GABA} (V_m - E_{rev})$ and $E_{rev} = 0$ mV in these conditions. A value of 30 pS is obtained for both experi-

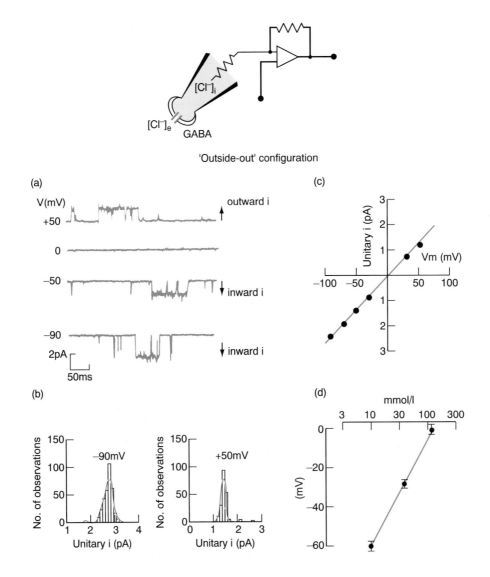

mental conditions. This value of γ_{GABA} is also the slope of the i_{GABA}/V curve obtained by averaging the most frequent single channel current i_{GABA} recorded at each membrane potential studied. This curve, based on the equation $i = \gamma (V_m - E_{rev})$ is linear between −90 mV and +50 mV and has a slope of 30 pS (Figure 10.2c).

However, in physiological conditions, when Cl⁻ concentration is approximately ten-fold lower in the intracellular than in the extracellular fluid, the unitary conductance varies with the membrane potential. The conductance in fact decreases progressively as the outward Cl⁻ current decreases (Figure 10.3b). This phenomenon is called rectification.

10.2.4 Mean Open Time of the GABA$_A$ Channel

With patch-clamp recording of GABA$_A$ channels (in chromaffin cells of the adrenal medulla or cultured hippocampal neurons, in outside-out configuration), two types of open times of the channel can be observed in the presence of low concentrations of GABA (Figure 10.5a): (i) brief openings; and (ii) longer duration openings interrupted by brief periods of closure: such a group of repeated openings and closures is called a burst of openings.

Brief openings

Brief openings have a mean duration, τ_o, of 2.5 ms and contribute little to the total current.

Bursts of openings

A burst is defined as a sequence of openings of duration t_o, separated by brief closures of duration t_c. Brief durations are defined as less than 5 ms in the example illustrated in Figure 10.5. The duration of each burst t_b is: $t_b = \Sigma t_o + \Sigma t_c$ and its mean duration is τ_b equal to 20–50 ms depending on the preparation used (Figure 10.5b). The openings and the brief closures observed within each burst in the presence of GABA are thought to correspond to fluctuations of the receptor between the double liganded open state and the double liganded closed state (before the two molecules of GABA leave the receptor site). Thus, upon a single activation by two molecules of GABA, the double liganded receptor would open and close several times:

Figure 10.2 Variations of the reversal potential of the GABA$_A$ response as a function of the Cl⁻ equilibrium potential. The single channel current i flowing across the GABA$_A$ channel is recorded in cultured mouse spinal neurons (outside-out patch-clamp recording; equal concentrations of Cl⁻ on both sides of the patch: [Cl⁻]$_i$ = 145 mM). (a) In the presence of GABA (10 μM), the single channel current i is outward at V_m = +50 mV (upward deflection), null at V_m = 0 mV and inward at V_m = −50 mV or −90 mV (downward deflections). (b) The distribution of single channel currents i in different patches of membrane held at V_m = −90 mV (left) and V_m = +50 mV (right) shows the existence of a single peak of current of −2.70 ± 0.17 pA and 1.48 ± 0.10 pA, respectively. These two values give a single channel conductance γ equal to 30 pS; $\gamma = i/V_m$ as E_{rev} = 0 mV. (c) i/V curve obtained by averaging the most frequently observed single channel currents. It is a straight line according to the equation $i = \gamma (V_m - E_{rev})$. The relationship is linear between V_m = −90 mV and V_m = +50 mV and the slope is γ = 30 pS. (d) Reversal potential of the GABA$_A$ response (in mV) as a function of the intracellular Cl⁻ concentration [Cl⁻]$_i$ (in mM). Each point represents the mean value of E_{rev} from four different cells. Note that, at the 3 [Cl⁻]$_i$ tested, E_{rev} (experimental value) is very close to E_{Cl} (calculated by the Nernst equation):

[Cl⁻]$_i$ (mM)	E$_{Cl}$ (mV)	E$_{rev}$ (mV)
14.5	−58	−56
45	−29	−28
145	0	0

(a, b and c: From Borman J, Hamill OP and Sakmann B, 1987. Mechanism of anion permeation through channels gated by glycine and γ-aminobutyric acid in mouse cultured spinal neurones, *J. Physiol. (Lond.)* 385, 246–286, with permission. d: From Sakmann B, Borman J and Hamill OP, 1983. Ion transport by single receptor channels, *Cold Spring Harbor Symp. Quant. Biol.* XLVIII, 247–257, with permission.)

Figure 10.3   Single GABA$_A$ receptor channel activity recording in physiological solutions. GABA$_A$-activated currents are observed with patch-clamp recording (cell-attached configuration) in rat spinal neurons. The activity of single GABA$_A$ channels is recorded. (a) At V_m = −30, 0 and +20 mV respectively, the GABA present in the patch pipette at a concentration of 10 μM elicits an outward current (upward deflection). This current increases with depolarization. At V_m = −60 mV, no current is recorded. (b) i/V curve obtained by plotting the amplitude of the recorded current i (pA) against the membrane potential V_m (mV). The current elicited by GABA reverses around V_m = −60 mV. The intracellular medium is the physiological cytosol and the extracellular or intrapipette solution has the following composition (in mM): 140 KCl, 1.8 CaCl$_2$, 1 MgCl$_2$ and 5 HEPES (K$^+$). The intracellular Cl$^-$ concentration is estimated at 13 mM, which gives a value of −60 mV for the Cl$^-$ reversal potential: E_{Cl} = −58 log 144.6/13 = −60 mV. As all the Na$^+$ ions are replaced by K$^+$ ions in the extracellular solution, the K$^+$ concentration is similar in both solutions, which gives a reversal potential for the K$^+$ current near 0 mV. The membrane potential values indicated in (a) and (b) are evaluated on the basis of a 0 mV value defined as the potential at which the K$^+$ currents across the K$^+$ channels are zero. (From Sakmann B, Bormann J and Hamill OP, 1983. Ion transport by single receptor channels, *Cold Spring Harbor Symp. Quant. Biol.* **XLVIII**, 247–257, with permission.)

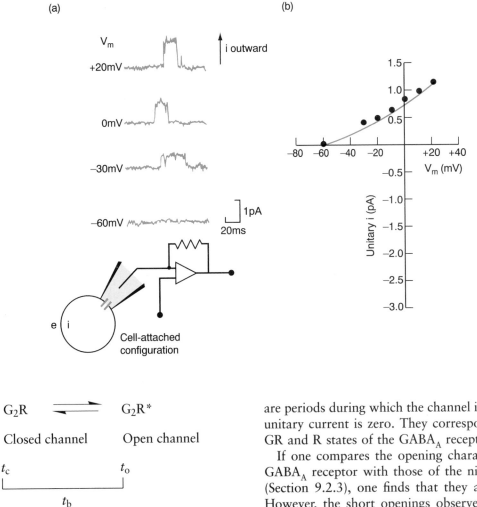

Silent periods separate single openings or bursts; they are periods during which the channel is closed and the unitary current is zero. They correspond to the G$_2$R, GR and R states of the GABA$_A$ receptor.

If one compares the opening characteristics of the GABA$_A$ receptor with those of the nicotinic receptor (Section 9.2.3), one finds that they are very similar. However, the short openings observed within bursts are approximately twice as abundant in the case of the GABA$_A$ receptor. This implies that opening (β) and

Figure 10.4 Variation of the electrochemical gradient of Cl$^-$ ions as a function of the membrane potential and intracellular and extracellular Cl$^-$ ion concentrations. The Cl$^-$ fluxes are: [ ], flux due to the Cl$^-$ concentration gradient; ↝, flux due to the electrical field across the membrane. (a) Symmetrical media: $[Cl^-]_e$ = $[Cl^-]_i$ = 145 mM; E_{Cl} = 0 mV; (b) physiological media: $[Cl^-]_e$ = 145 mM; $[Cl^-]_i$ = 14.5 mM; E_{Cl} = −58 mV.

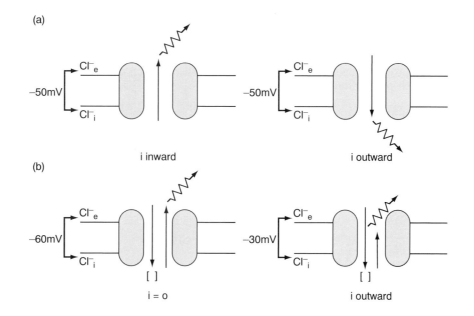

closing (α) rate constants have much closer values in the case of the GABA$_A$ receptor (Appendix 10.1) than in the case of the nicotinic receptor (Appendix 7.3).

10.3 The GABA$_A$ Receptor Desensitizes

When recording the total current I_{GABA} evoked by a prolonged application of GABA, one finds that the amplitude of the current decreases with time (Figure 10.6). This rundown of the GABA$_A$ response increases with increasing concentration of GABA. This phenomenon is attributed largely to desensitization of the GABA$_A$ receptors.

Recordings in outside-out configuration show a rundown of the frequency of opening of the GABA$_A$ channels upon prolonged application of GABA (0.5 µM), whereas neither the intensity of the unitary current nor the mean open time of the channels τ_o appears to be affected. Considering that $I = N \times p_o \times i$, if p_o (open probability of the channel) decreases as a result of a decrease in the frequency of opening events, the current I_{GABA} decreases even

though i_{GABA} remains constant. Similarly, G_{GABA}, the total conductance, decreases since $G = N \times p_o \times \gamma$. As the GABA$_A$ receptors gradually desensitize, p_o becomes progressively smaller with time, and I_{GABA} as well as G_{GABA} gradually decrease to practically zero.

10.4 Benzodiazepines and Barbiturates are Allosteric Agonists at the GABA$_A$ Receptor

Barbiturates and benzodiazepines (Figure 10.7) are two classes of clinically active agents. Barbiturates are hypnotic and antiepileptic agents and the benzodiazepines are anxiolytic agents, muscle relaxants and anticonvulsants.

10.4.1 Benzodiazepines and Barbiturates Bind to the GABA$_A$ Receptor

Benzodiazepines and barbiturates have the property of binding to the GABA$_A$ receptor at specific receptor sites. Photoaffinity labeling of the benzodiazepine

Figure 10.5   Mean open time of GABA$_A$ channels. (a, b) Patch-clamp recording of the activity of the GABA$_A$ receptor channels from chromaffin cells of the adrenal medulla (outside-out configuration). The intracellular and extracellular Cl$^-$ concentrations are similar and the membrane potential is maintained at –70 mV. (a) Inward unitary currents through GABA$_A$ channels evoked by GABA (10 μM). Brief openings (Δ) and bursts of openings (long duration openings interrupted by short closures defined in this experiment as less than 5 ms, O). (b) Histogram of open times measured in a homogeneous population of channels (mean value of i = –2.9 pA). The open times plotted on the graph represent the duration of short openings (t_o) and the duration of bursts of openings (t_b). The histogram is described by the sum of two exponentials with decay time constants of τ_o = 2.5 ms and τ_b = 20 ms. τ_o corresponds to the mean open time of short openings (Δ) and τ_b corresponds to the mean open time of bursts of openings (O). (From Borman J and Clapham DE, 1985. γ-aminobutyric acid receptor channels in adrenal chromaffin cells: a patch clamp study, *Proc. Natl. Acad. Sci. USA* **82**, 2168–2172, with permission.)

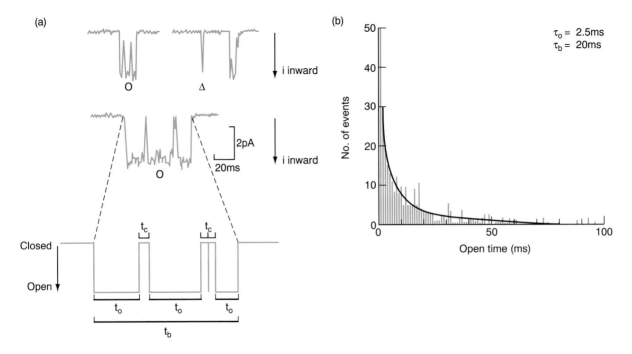

receptor site (Appendix 9.3) has shown binding of benzodiazepines on native GABA$_A$ receptors but also on receptors expressed in transfected cells with α, β and γ cDNA subunits. This demonstration of the presence of receptor sites for exogenous substances such as benzodiazepines or barbiturates on the GABA$_A$ receptor suggested the existence of endogenous ligands capable of binding to the barbiturate or benzodiazepine receptor sites. At first, research focused on the identification of endogenous ligands at the benzodiazepine receptor site. To this end, monoclonal antibodies were raised that recognize the epitopes of this site so that the secondary antibodies (anti-anti-epitope antibodies, see Appendix 2.3) would recognize other ligands.

10.4.2 Benzodiazepines and Barbiturates Potentiate the GABA$_A$ Response

Barbiturates and benzodiazepines have no effect when applied alone at low doses. On the other hand, when applied at low doses but together with GABA, they potentiate the effect of the latter. If one compares voltage clamp recordings of the current I_{GABA} in the presence or absence of benzodiazepines, one can see that the benzodiazepines (flunitrazepam or diazepam) increase the amplitude of the total current (Figure 10.8). The presence of benzodiazepines is also found to increase the rate of desensitization of the GABA$_A$ response. Similar results are obtained with barbiturates (pentobarbital) (Figure 10.8).

Figure 10.6 Desensitization of the GABA$_A$ receptor. (a) Patch clamp recording (whole-cell configuration, symmetrical Cl-concentration, V_m = –40 mV) from a chick cerebral neuron. The total current I_{GABA} recorded upon a prolonged application of GABA at high concentration (100 μM) decreases in amplitude with time to almost zero. The total current I_{GABA} corresponds to the sum of the unitary currents i, passing through the open GABA$_A$ channels, while the other currents have been blocked with TTX and TEA as well as with Cs$^+$ and Cd^{2+} ions. (b) Same experiment as in (a) but in the presence of 500 μM of GABA and with hyperpolarizing voltage steps applied at a constant rate. The decrease in amplitude of the step current during the GABA$_A$ response shows the rundown of I_{GABA} is associated with a decrease in G (as $i_{step} = G \times V_{step}$, V_{step} being constant, a decrease of i_{step} implies a decrease of G). (From Weiss DS, Barnes EM and Hablitz JJ, 1988. Whole-cell and single-channel recordings of GABA-gated currents in cultured chick cerebral neurons, *J. Neurophysiol.* 59, 495–513, with permission.)

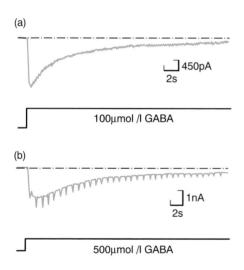

(a)

450pA
2s

100μmol /l GABA

(b)

1nA
2s

500μmol /l GABA

The *I/V* curves show that the total currents I_{GABA} evoked in the presence or absence of benzodiazepines or barbiturates reverse at the same potential. This indicates that the potentiation of the GABA$_A$ response by these drugs is not the result of a change in the ion selectivity of the channel.

In conclusion, benzodiazepines and barbiturates can be considered as allosteric agonists of GABA (Table 10.1) as they modulate the efficacy of activation of the receptor by GABA. However, the mechanism by which benzodiazepines and barbiturates produce this effect remains to be elucidated.

Figure 10.7 Common structure of benzodiazepines (a) and barbituric acid derivatives (b). For diazepam, the radicals are: R_1 = CH$_3$, R_2 = O, R_3 = H$_2$, R_4 is absent and R_7 = Cl. For phenobarbital, the radicals are: R_{5a} = ethyl, R_{5b} = H and R_3 = phenyl.

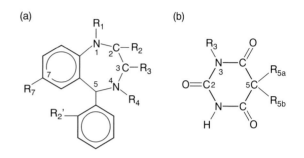

(a) (b)

10.5 GABAergic Synapses

10.5.1 Factors Affecting the Duration of the Post-synaptic GABA$_A$ Current at GABAergic Synapses

When GABA is released in the synaptic cleft, it can (Figure 10.9c):

- bind to the GABA$_A$ receptor;
- be taken up by pre-synaptic structures or by glial cells;
- diffuse away from the synaptic cleft.

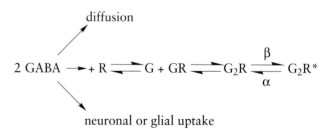

The duration of the synaptic current is determined by the period during which each activated GABA$_A$ receptor remains in the G$_2$R* state.

Two types of factors may determine the duration of the G$_2$R* state and therefore the time course of the post-synaptic GABA$_A$ response:

- the mean open time of the GABA$_A$ channel, τ_o, which is an intrinsic property of the protein;
- the removal of GABA from the synaptic cleft, due to neuronal or glial uptake or to diffusion.

Figure 10.8 Potentiation of the total current I_{GABA} by benzodiazepines and barbiturates. $GABA_A$ receptors are expressed in transfected cells with the α, β and γ cDNA subunits. This model is interesting because these cells do not normally express GABA receptors (neither $GABA_A$ nor $GABA_B$); the GABA applied in the bath activates therefore only the number (N) of $GABA_A$ receptors expressed. On the other hand, it is a model where the pre-synaptic release of GABA is excluded because of the absence of synapses. The total current I_{GABA} is recorded using the patch-clamp technique (whole-cell configuration). The intracellular or intrapipette solution contains (in mM): 130 CsCl, 1 $MgCl_2$, 0.5 $CaCl_2$, and the extracellular solution (in mM): 116 NaCl, 5.4 KCl, 0.8 $MgCl_2$, 1.8 $CaCl_2$, E_{Cl} is estimated to be near 0 mV. The total current I_{GABA} recorded at $V_m = -60mV$ (GABA, 10 µM) is inward and is significantly potentiated by the simultaneous application of diazepam (DZP, 1 µM), fluni-trazepam (FNZM, 1 µM) and pentobarbital (PB, 50 µM). (From Pritchett DB, Southeimer H, Shivers BD *et al.*, 1989. Importance of a novel $GABA_A$ receptor subunit for benzodiazepines pharmacology, *Nature* **338**, 582–585, with permission.)

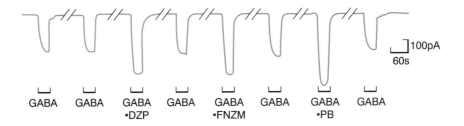

If the decay of the synaptic current is due to closure of the $GABA_A$ channel (first case), this implies that the concentration of GABA decreases very rapidly in the synaptic cleft after its release (as a consequence, for example, of rapid diffusion or very efficient uptake mechanisms). In this case, the channels have very little chance of being reactivated by the repeated binding of two molecules of GABA and the time constant of the decay of the post-synaptic current is then τ_o, i.e. mean open time of the channels which depends only on α, the closing time constant of the channels (in the absence of desensitization).

If the decay of the synaptic current is due to the slow disappearance of GABA from the vicinity of the receptors (removal due to GABA uptake and/or diffu-sion) (second case), this implies, on the contrary, a prolonged presence of GABA in the synaptic cleft. The prolonged presence of GABA may be due to increased GABA release in the synaptic cleft (due to repeated activation of pre-synaptic elements), to a slow mecha-nism of uptake or to a restricted diffusion of GABA away from the synaptic cleft. Hence, GABA may reactivate $GABA_A$ channels which have previously opened and the decay time constant will exceed the value of τ_o.

In the case of the nicotinic channel, the removal of acetylcholine is very rapid and it is the kinetic proper-ties of the channel that determine the time course of

the end plate current (see Section 9.4.1). In the case of the $GABA_A$ receptor, the situation appears to be more complex. For low amplitude post-synaptic currents, it appears that the mean open time of the $GABA_A$ channel determines their time course, the released GABA being rapidly removed by diffusion from the cleft (first case). However, for larger post-synaptic currents, evoked by a greater pre-synaptic release of GABA, the slower removal of GABA from the synap-tic cleft appears to determine the time course of the synaptic current (second case).

10.5.2 When E_{Cl} is more Negative than V_m, Activation of $GABA_A$ Receptors Leads to a Hyperpolarizing Post-synaptic Current and Inhibition of the Post-synaptic Activity (Figures 10.9 and 10.10)

In voltage clamp recordings with potassium acetate-filled electrodes, instead of potassium chloride, so as not to change the intracellular concentration of Cl^-, V_m is more positive than E_{Cl} and an outward synaptic current is recorded in response to stimulation of GABAergic afferent fibres. This current is inhibited by applications of bicuculline or picrotoxin (see Section 10.5.5) and potentiated by applications of benzodi-azepines and barbiturates (Table 10.1).

Figure 10.9   Characteristics of a monosynaptic IPSP due to activation of GABA$_A$ receptors and recorded in the hippocampus. *In vitro* recording from a pair of hippocampal neurons (guinea-pig hippocampal slices, intracellular recording in current clamp). (a) IPSP evoked in neuron 2 (post-synaptic pyramidal neuron) for each action potential of neuron 1 (pre-synaptic GABAergic interneuron). These IPSPs are blocked (not shown) by the application of picrotoxin (10^{-4} M), a GABA$_A$ channel blocker, which shows that they result from the activation of GABA$_A$ receptors. Their mean latency is 0.7 ± 0.2 ms. Note their variable amplitude (mean amplitude = -2.1 ± 0.7 mV). (b) Average of 20 IPSPs obtained by triggering each trace from the peak of the pre-synaptic action potential. (c) Functional scheme of a GABAergic synapse where the ionotropic (receptor channel) GABA$_A$ receptors and the metabotropic (G-protein linked) GABA$_B$ receptors are co-localized. Pre-synaptic receptors are omitted. In order to study in isolation the GABA$_A$ response, GABA$_B$ receptors can be selectively blocked (see Table 10.1). The enzymes glutamic acid decarboxylase (GAD) and GABA transaminase (GABAT) are synthesized in the soma and carried to axon terminals via fast anterograde axonal transport. (1) GABA is synthesized in the cytoplasm and transported actively into synaptic vesicles by a vesicular carrier. (2) A percentage of the GABA released in the synaptic cleft is taken up into pre-synaptic terminals and glial cells by GABA transporters which co-transport Na$^+$ and Cl$^-$. They are antagonized by nipecotic acid. (3) GABA degradation. (a, b: From Miles R and Wong RKS, 1984. Unitary inhibitory synaptic potentials in the guinea-pig hippocampus *in vitro*, *J. Physiol.* **356**, 97–113, with permission.)

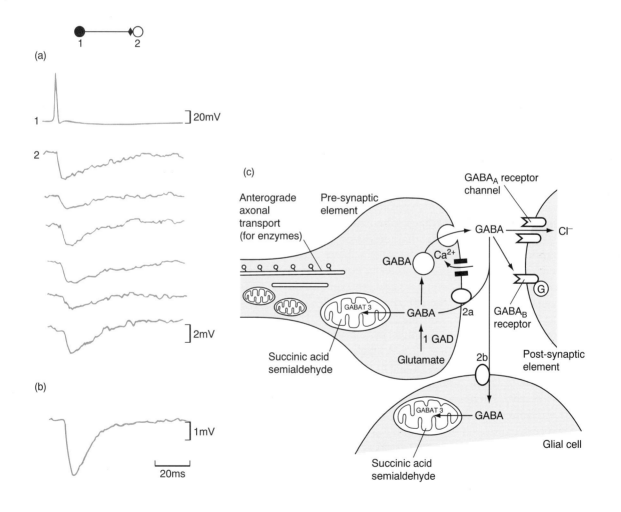

Figure 10.10   Schematic representation of current clamp recordings of the IPSP as a function of membrane potential where E_{Cl} is more negative (−70 mV), equal (−60 mV) or more positive (−50 mV) than the resting membrane potential of the neuron. A resting membrane potential for the neuron of −60 mV and a threshold for action potential generation at −40 mV are assumed. Action potentials are truncated owing to their large amplitude. In the three cases represented, inhibition of activity is produced during the IPSP (upper trace).

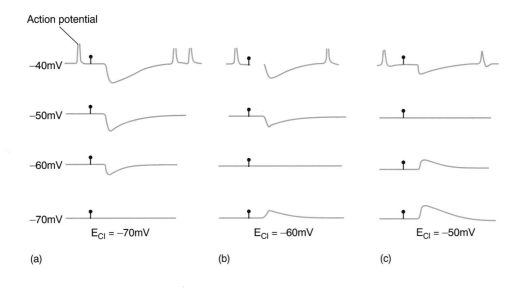

In hippocampal slices *in vitro*, simultaneous recordings can be made from pairs of neurones making GABA_A-type inhibitory monosynaptic contacts (Figure 10.9). In such simultaneous recordings, one can correlate pre-synaptic activity with the characteristics of the post-synaptic response. Different criteria have been used to demonstrate that the response is monosynaptic: short latency of the response; and, in contrast to polysynaptic responses, the ability to follow a high frequency of stimulation (100 Hz). The results obtained from intracellular recordings in current clamp mode are presented in Figure 10.9. A single pre-synaptic action potential (trace 1) is sufficient to evoke an inhibitory post-synaptic potential (IPSP, trace 2, $V_m = -62$ to -66 mV). However, the amplitude of this IPSP is very variable, from 0.6 to 4.2 mV, which suggests that a pre-synaptic action potential causes the release of a variable number of quanta from the population of activated axon terminals (see Section 8.3).

The conductance G_{IPSP} can be calculated knowing I, V and E_{Cl}. In this experiment, this conductance is 6.7 nS ± 2.3 nS. If G_{IPSP} is constant, knowing that the unitary conductance of the GABA_A channel is estimated in these neurons to be 20 pS, it can be deduced

that approximately 300 GABA_A channels are open at the peak of the IPSP (Figure. 10.9b) (recalling that $G_{IPSP} = N \times p_o \times \gamma$).

10.5.3 When E_{Cl} is near V_m, GABA_A Receptor Activation Leads to a 'Silent Inhibition' of Post-synaptic Activity (Figure. 10.10b)

If the post-synaptic membrane potential is close to the reversal potential of the GABA_A response, E_{Cl}, the electrochemical gradient for Cl⁻ being very weak or zero, no inhibitory post-synaptic current is observed and therefore no IPSP either, even though GABA_A channels are open. However, GABA still has an inhibitory effect on post-synaptic activity, as any EPSP occurring during the effect of GABA is strongly inhibited (see Section 16.2.3).

This inhibitory effect of GABA is called a shunting effect. It is due to an increase in the membrane conductance G_{IPSP}. If this effect is large (due to opening of GABA_A channels), the membrane resistance decreases and any other synaptic current evoked at this time will produce only a small change in membrane potential.

The silent GABA$_A$ inhibition reduces the amplitude of post-synaptic depolarizations and consequently prevents the generation of post-synaptic action potentials.

10.5.4 When E_{Cl} is more Positive than V_m but Below the Threshold for Action Potential Generation, GABA$_A$ Receptor Activation Leads to a Depolarizing Current and an Inhibition of Post-synaptic Activity (Figure 10.10c)

If E_{Cl} is more positive than V_m, the activation of GABA$_A$ receptors causes an inward current (outward flow of Cl$^-$ ions) and a depolarization of the membrane. As long as E_{Cl} remains below the threshold for activation of voltage-dependent Na$^+$ channels, post-synaptic activity is inhibited.

If E_{Cl} were more positive than the threshold for activation of voltage-dependent Na$^+$ channels, GABA$_A$ receptor activation would cause a post-synaptic depolarization or EPSP (by analogy with synaptic currents with reversal potentials more depolarized than threshold: nicotinic currents or currents evoked by excitatory amino acids). Note that this excitatory effect of GABA has not been shown for **adult** GABA$_A$ synapses.

10.5.5 Pharmacology of GABA$_A$ Synapses

Table 10.1 summarizes substances acting on GABA$_A$ receptors and their site of action.

Reversible competitive antagonists

The best-known is bicuculline. It is selective for the GABA$_A$ receptor and therefore serves as a good tool to identify GABA$_A$ responses: its presence in the extracellular space inhibits post-synaptic GABA$_A$ currents. Hence it is a potent convulsant when administered intravenously or intraventricularly.

Reversible non-competitive antagonists

The best-known is picrotoxin, which is a convulsant. It binds to the ionic channel (it is a channel blocker). Its binding site involves the M2 segment, the region

Figure 10.11   Benzodiazepines prolong the duration of post-synaptic GABA$_A$ currents but only slightly increase their intensity. Patch clamp recording of cultured neurons from rat cerebral cortex (whole-cell configuration). (a) Stimulation of a GABAergic pre-synaptic neuron by application of 15 µM of glutamate evokes an outward current in the post-synaptic neuron at $V_m = -40$ mV. (b) This current results from activation of GABA$_A$ receptors as it is blocked by application of bicuculline methiodide (25 µM). (c) Application of 4 µM of flunitrazepam prolongs the time course of this post-synaptic GABA$_A$ current but affects only slightly its intensity (d). [Cl$^-$]$_e$ = 154 mM and [Cl$^-$]$_i$ = 4 mM. Note the difference in time scale between (a) and (c) on one hand, and (b) and (d) on the other hand. (From Vicini S, Alho H, Costa E, Mienville JM, Santi MR and Vaccarino FM, 1986. Modulation of γ-aminobutyric acid-mediated inhibitory synaptic currents in dissociated cortical cell cultures, *Proc. Natl Acad. Sci. USA* **83**, 9269–9273, with permission.)

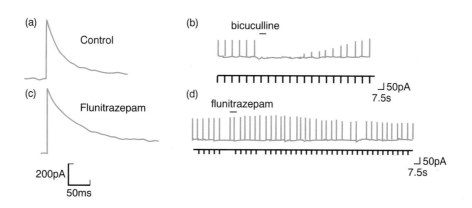

thought to line the chloride ion channel. In insects, resistance to picrotoxin (used as an insecticide) can be conferred to a single amino acid substitution in the M2 segment sequence: alanine 302 replaced by serine.

Allosteric agonists: barbiturates and benzodiazepines (see Section 10.4)

Allosteric agonists increase the amplitude and duration of GABA$_A$ inhibitory post-synaptic currents. In the example illustrated in Figure 10.11, GABA$_A$ synapses were studied in cultured neurons of the rat cerebral cortex. The activity of the post-synaptic neurons is recorded using the patch-clamp technique (whole-cell configuration) and pre-synaptic neurons are stimulated by the application of glutamate or by a depolarizing current pulse. To identify the synaptic responses of the GABA$_A$ type: (i) the effect of bicuculline is tested (Figure 10.11b) and (ii) the pre-synaptic neurons stimulated are localized in culture and tested by immunocytochemistry for their content in the GABA synthetic enzyme, glutamate decarboxylase (GAD). It has thus been demonstrated that an application of a benzodiazepine, flunitrazepam, significantly prolongs the duration of the GABA$_A$ inhibitory post-synaptic currents (by a factor of 3 to 5) but potentiates only slightly their intensity (Figure 10.11c, d). Because of the selective action of benzodiazepines on the GABA$_A$ channel, these substances can be used experimentally together with bicuculline to identify a GABA$_A$ response, but they are also widely used clinically.

Uptake inhibitors

Uptake inhibitors have very little effect on GABA$_A$ synaptic responses. The uptake of GABA is achieved by transport molecules present in the membrane of pre-synaptic profiles or glial cells. When applied by micro-iontophoresis in hippocampal slices, nipecotic acid, a neuronal and glial uptake inhibitor, has only a weak effect on the duration of the post-synaptic potential (IPSP) evoked by stimulation of GABAergic afferent fibres: it prolongs the later phase of the IPSP (Figure 10.12). Thus, as mentioned earlier (see section 10.5.1), the uptake process may be too slow to have much influence on the time course of the IPSP.

Figure 10.12   Effect of a GABA$_A$ uptake inhibitor, nipecotic acid, on GABA$_A$ synaptic responses. Current clamp recording from hippocampal neuron in rat brain slices. An orthodromic IPSP is recorded in response to stimulation of GABAergic afferent neurons. As this IPSP is bicuculline sensitive, it is likely to be mediated by activation of GABA$_A$ receptors. (a) Orthodromic IPSP recorded before and after (arrows) application of nipecotic acid (1 mM for 40 min). Each trace represents the average of six responses. Nipecotic acid decreases the amplitude of the IPSP, which obscures the analysis of its effect on the time course of the IPSP. However, after normalizing the IPSPs to the same peak (b), the analysis of their time course reveals that nipecotic acid prolongs the later phase of the repolarization. (From Dingledine R and Korn SJ, 1985. γ-aminobutyric acid uptake and termination of inhibitory synaptic potentials in the rat hippocampal slices, *J. Physiol. (Lond.)* **366**, 387–409, with permission.)

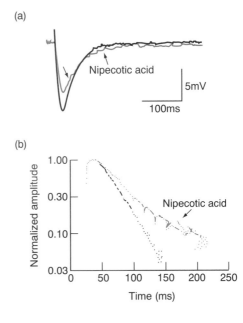

Appendix 10.1
Mean Open Time and Mean Burst
Duration of the GABA$_A$ Channel

The conformational changes of the GABA$_A$ channel are modelled as follows:

$$2\,G + R \underset{k_{-1}}{\overset{k_1}{\rightleftharpoons}} G + GR \underset{k_{-2}}{\overset{k_2}{\rightleftharpoons}} G_2R \underset{\alpha}{\overset{\beta}{\rightleftharpoons}} G_2R^*$$

Upon application of GABA, the conformational change of the GABA$_A$ receptor towards the G$_2$R* state is favoured (opening of the channel). However, it has been found that the GABA$_A$ receptor closes and opens rapidly several times upon opening: these are bursts of openings (Figure 10.5). The short duration closures represent the fluctuation of the receptor between the G$_2$R and G$_2$R* states. During these bursts, the receptor returns much less frequently to the GR state, and even less frequently to the R state, before reopening.

At steady state, the mean open time is $\tau_o = 1/\alpha$. When the receptor is in the G$_2$R* state, it can only transfer to the G$_2$R state with a rate constant of α (this is true when desensitization is negligible). The mean open time τ_o is calculated experimentally from the different open times t_o within each burst (Figure 10.5).

The mean closed time within bursts is $\tau_o = 1/(\beta + 2k_{-2})$. When the receptor is in the G$_2$R state, it can either reopen with the rate constant β or transfer to the GR state with a rate constant $2k_{-2}$. The average number of short closures per burst is $nf = \beta/2k_{-2}$ (see Colquhoun and Hawkes, 1977).

Once the values of τ_o, τ_i and nf are experimentally defined, the values of α and β can be deduced: $\alpha = 50$/s; $\beta = 330$/s.

Note that α and β differ by a factor of about 6 (whereas for the acetylcholine nicotinic receptor nAChR, they differ by a factor of 40). This illustrates numerically the fact that fluctuations between the double-liganded open and closed states are more frequent for the GABA$_A$ receptor, the probability that the channel opens in a given time being only six times greater than the probability that the channel closes.

Further Reading

Bormann, J. and Feigenspan, A. (1995) GABA$_C$ receptors. *Trends Neurosci.* **18**; 515–518.

Burt, D.R. and Kamatchi, G.L. (1991) GABA$_A$ receptor subtypes: from pharmacology to molecular biology. *FASEB J.* **5**, 2916–2923.

Jones, M.V. and Westbrook, G.L. (1995) Desensitized states prolong GABA$_A$ channel responses to brief agonist pulses. *Neuron* **15**, 181–191.

Kaila, K. (1994) Ionic basis of GABA$_A$ receptor channel function in the nervous system. *Prog. Neurobiol.* **42**, 489–537.

Macdonald, R.L. (1994) GABA$_A$ receptor channels. *Ann. Rev. Neurosci.* **17**, 569–602.

Perez-Velasquez, J.L. and Angelides, K.J. (1993) Assembly of GABA$_A$ receptor subunits determines sorting and localization in polarized cells. *Nature* **361**, 457–460.

Sieghart, W. (1992) GABA$_A$ receptors: ligand-gated Cl$^-$ ion channels modulated by multiple drug-binding sites. *Trends Pharmacol. Sci.* **13**, 446–450.

Silvilotti, L. and Nistri, A. (1991) GABA receptor mechanisms in the central nervous system. *Prog. Neurobiol.* **36**, 35–92.

Verdoorn, T.A., Draguhn, A., Ymer, S., Seeburg, P.H. and Sakmann, B. (1990) Functional properties of recombinant rat GABA$_A$ receptors depend upon subunit composition. *Neuron* **4**, 919–928.

Wafford, K.A., Bain, C.J., Quirk, K. *et al.* (1994). A novel allosteric modulatory site on the GABA$_A$ receptor β-subunit. *Neuron* **12**, 775–782.

Ionotropic Glutamate Receptors

Excitatory amino acids, such as glutamate and aspartate, are present in many synapses of the vertebrate central nervous system. From the original observations of Curtis *et al.* (1961) it was known that glutamate has a depolarizing effect on spinal cord neurons. This effect is rapid and can be mimicked by other amino acids (L-aspartate, L-homocysteate and L-cysteine sulfinate). The speed of this effect suggested that glutamate and its agonists evoke a depolarization by acting directly on receptor channels. Patch clamp recordings (outside-out configuration) have confirmed this hypothesis, since glutamate evokes its effect even in the absence of any intracellular messengers from the preparation.

We can distinguish two main groups of receptor channels activated by excitatory amino acids. This distinction is based on the affinity of the receptor for glutamate selective structural analogs (Figure 11.1), notably for N-methyl-D-aspartate (NMDA). Thus, the distinction is made between those glutamate receptor channels activated by NMDA (NMDA receptors) and those activated by AMPA or kainate (non-NMDA receptors). It should be noted that glutamate also acts via receptors coupled to G-proteins (glutamate metabotropic receptors, mGluR) (see Chapters 5 and 14).

Molecular cloning identified cDNAs in rat and mouse brain encoding AMPA receptor subunits (termed GluR-1 to GluR-4, also termed GluR-A to GluR-D), kainate receptor subunits (termed GluR-5 to GluR-7 and KA-1 and KA-2) and NMDA receptor subunits (termed NR1 and NR2). The hydropathy analysis of the deduced amino acid sequence of the proteins encoded by these cDNAs shows the presence of four putative transmembrane domains as for the other ligand-gated channels and the presence of a strikingly unusual large N-terminal extracellular domain such that glutamate receptor channels would have twice the molecular mass of those for GABA and acetylcholine receptors (see Figure A5.2).

NMDA and non-NMDA receptors are co-expressed in many neurons. Therefore, to study them separately, the patch clamp techniques and the use of selective agonists for each receptor type have proven to be particularly useful. Furthermore, the use of selective antagonists for NMDA or non-NMDA receptors (Figure 11.1) allows us to study each one of these receptors independently during synaptic responses mediated by endogenous excitatory amino acids.

11.1 Non-NMDA Channels are Classic Cationic Receptor Channels – Example: the AMPA Receptors

The class of non-NMDA receptors is further subdivided in two groups: the receptors activated by AMPA (and quisqualate) with a high affinity, and the receptors activated by kainate with a high affinity. We shall only describe here the properties of AMPA receptors.

11.1.1 The AMPA Channel is Permeable to Cations and has a Conductance of 8 pS

When quisqualate (1–10 µmol/l) is applied to the extracellular medium of cultured central neurons recorded in the outside-out patch clamp configuration, an inward unitary current, i_q, is observed at $V_m =$ –60 mV (Figure 11.2a). If the application of quisqualate is repeated on different membrane patches recorded at the same membrane potential, one observes that the recorded inward unitary currents are not a homogeneous population. However, one set of similar unitary currents appears with a higher frequency than the others (Figure 11.2b). Plotting the mean unitary current amplitude of this population as a function of the membrane potential, we obtain an i_q/V relation (Figure 11.2c) that follows the equation $i_q = \gamma_q (V_m - E_{rev})$. Between –80 mV and +80 mV this

Figure 11.1   Different molecules that act on excitatory amino acid receptor channels. (a) Table summarizing the agonists and antagonists of non-NMDA and NMDA receptor channels. (b) L-glutamate and its structural analogs, NMDA, quisqualate and kainate.

(a)

Receptor channels	Non-NMDA channels		NMDA channels
	AMPA receptors	KA receptors	
Most selective agonists	AMPA Quisqualate	Kainate	NMDA
Mixed agonists	Glutamate Aspartate	Glutamate Aspartate	Glutamate Aspartate
Competitive antagonists	CNQX NBQX	CNQX NBQX	D-APV (or DAP5) CPP
Channel blockers	—	—	MK801
Non-competitive antagonist at the glycine site			7-chlorokynurenate

AMPA:	α amino-3-hydroxy-5-methyl-4-isoxalone propionate.
D-AP5 or D-APV:	D 2-amino-5-phosphonopentanoate.
CNQX:	6-cyano-7-nitroquinoxaline-2,3-dione.
NMDA:	N-methyl-D-aspartate
MK801:	5-methyl-10,11-dihydro-5H-dibenzocyclohepten-5,10-imine maleate.
NBQX:	6-nitro-7-sulphamobenzoquinoxaline-2,3 dione.
CPP:	(2-carboxypiperazine-4-yl) propyl-1-phosphonic acid.

(b)

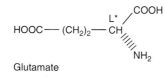

Glutamate

NMDA

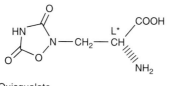

Quisqualate

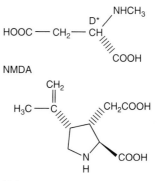

Kainate

Figure 11.2. Electrophysiological properties of the AMPA receptor channel. (a) Patch clamp recording (outside-out configuration) of a quisqualate activated channel. When the membrane is held at a voltage of −60 mV, the unitary current i_q is inward (downward deflection). At +60 mV or +80 mV, the current i_q is outward (upward deflection). (b) Unitary current (i_q) amplitude histogram (in pA). Currents recorded at the same voltage but from different membrane patches. The unitary conductance values corresponding to the four peaks are calculated from the equation $i_q = \gamma_q (V_m − E_{rev})$ given that $E_{rev} = 0$ mV. One observes that most channels have a conductance of 8 pS. (c) i_q/V curve obtained from the averages of unitary currents recorded from a homogeneous population of channels (8 pS population). The curve is described by the linear equation $i_q = \gamma_q (V_m − E_{rev})$ (between −80 mV and +80 mV). This curve shows that the unitary conductance is only slightly voltage dependent. Compositions of the solutions in (a) and (c): intrapipette or intracellular solution (in mmol/l): 140 CsCl, 5 K-EGTA and 0.5 CaCl$_2$; extracellular solution: 140 NaCl, 2.8 KCl and 1 CaCl$_2$. (a, c: From Ascher P and Nowak L, 1988. Quisqualate and kainate-activated channels in mouse central neurons in culture, *J. Physiol. (Lond.)* **399**, 227–245, with permission. b: From Cull-Candy SG and Usowicz MM, 1987. Patch clamp recording from single glutamate-receptor channels, *TIPS* **8**, 218–242, with permission.)

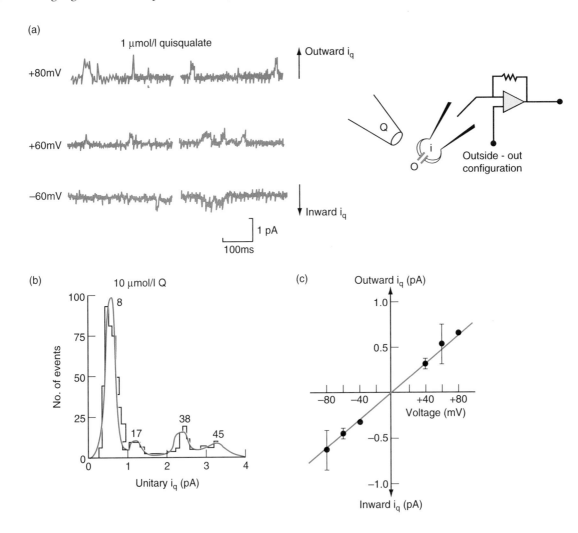

curve is linear, has a slope of 8 pS, and shows a quisqualate current reversal potential of approximately 0 mV.

These results show that most channels activated by quisqualate have a unitary conductance of 8 pS, and that this conductance is only slightly or not at all sensitive to membrane potential variations. Additionally, the unitary current i_q reverses at a value close to 0 mV if the extracellular and intracellular environments contain similar concentrations of monovalent cations (Figure 11.2c). This suggests that the quisqualate-activated channel is permeable to cations.

To test this hypothesis, the reversal potential of the current was recorded at different intracellular and extracellular concentrations of Na^+ and K^+ ions. When the extracellular Na^+ concentration is lowered from 140 to 50 mmol/l by replacing Na^+ ions with choline ions, the reversal potential becomes negative (it shifts from 0 mV to about –20 mV). When Cs^+ ions substitute for intracellular K^+ ions, the reversal potential is not affected. These results suggest that the quisqualate-activated channel is permeable to Na^+, K^+ and Cs^+ ions, and impermeable to choline ions.

This quisqualate-activated channel shows a low permeability to divalent cations, especially to Ca^{2+} ions. Thus, variations by a factor of 20 of the extracellular Ca^{2+} concentration have no effect on the reversal potential of the quisqualate current recorded from neurons in the whole-cell configuration. Likewise, only small changes of the photometrically recorded intracellular Ca^{2+} concentration (Appendix 11.1) can be measured during a quisqualate evoked response at a constant voltage of –60 mV (see Figure 11.5a). It should be noted that it is essential to carry out these recordings in cells maintained at membrane potentials lower than the activation threshold of the voltage sensitive Ca^{2+} channel in order to prevent Ca^{2+} inflow through these channels.

In conclusion, this quisqualate-activated channel, recorded in spinal neurons in culture, is permeable to monovalent cations: the application of quisqualate at a membrane potential of $V_m = -60$ mV evokes a unitary inward current that results from the inflow of Na^+ ions and an outflow of K^+ ions through the same channel (the Na^+ inflow is stronger than the K^+ outflow). This AMPA receptor is a classic cationic channel receptor: it has a negligible permeability to Ca^{2+} ions and its conductance is only weakly voltage dependent. However, studies performed in other preparations showed that some AMPA receptors are permeable to Ca^{2+} ions. These *princeps* electrophysiological experiments which characterized the properties of native AMPA receptor channels were carried out before molecular cloning of glutamate receptor subunits had been achieved, which suggest that the Ca^{2+} permeability of AMPA receptor channels varies with their subunit composition.

11.1.2 Molecular Biology of Non-NMDA Glutamate Receptors

Cloning studies demonstrated that AMPA selective ionotropic glutamate receptors are built from the four closely related subunits GluR-1 to GluR-4 (or GluR-A to GluR-D). The four predicted polypeptide sequences, each approximately 900 amino acids in length, revealed similarities of between 70% (GluR-1 and GluR-2) and 73% (GluR-2 and GluR-3). These subunits when expressed *in vitro* constitute a high affinity ^3H AMPA and low affinity kainate receptor type of glutamate-gated ion channels. These different subunits are abundantly and differentially expressed in the brain, as revealed by *in situ* hybridization studies (see Appendix 2.2). Although these different GluR subunits exhibit some ability to form homomeric channels when expressed by themselves in *Xenopus* oocytes or cultured mammalian cells, it is considered likely that channels are formed *in vivo* by different combinations of subunits. Thus with four receptor subunits there are already a very large number of potential combinations even if we do not yet know the precise stoichiometry of subunit association.

The diversity of GluR receptors results not only from subunit combinations but also from two genetic processes: *alternative splicing* and *editing* of the pre-messsenger RNA (or primary transcript). *Alternative splicing* concerns the 38 amino acid-long sequence preceding the most C-terminal putative transmembrane domain M4 of each of the four receptor subunits (Figure 11.3a). This small segment has been shown to exist in two versions (with different amino acid sequences) designated flip and flop and encoded by adjacent exons of the receptor genes. As a consequence, each of the four subunits exists in two molecular forms (GluR-1 flip and GluR-1 flop, GluR-2 flip and Glu R-2 flop . . .). When these splicing derivatives are expressed in oocytes, the proteins exhibit different

Figure 11.3   Molecular biology of AMPA receptor channels. (a) The predicted structure of AMPA receptors is shown in schematic form. Alternative splicing produces two forms (flip and flop) for each subunit which differ in a small domain preceding the M4 segment. The Q/R site is located in the M2 sequence. The gluR-2 subunit possesses an arginine (R) whereas in the GluR-1, -3 and -4 subunits, glutamine (Q) lies in the homologous position. (b) Whole cell recordings of the inward current evoked by rapid application of an L-glutamate agonist (300 µM) at a holding potential of –60 mV in cultured mammalian cells engineered for the transient simultaneous expression of the flip forms or the flop forms of GluR-1 and GluR-2. L-glutamate evokes a current of greater amplitude (measured at the steady state) when applied to the flip forms of the subunits. (c) Comparison of whole cell currents evoked by pulse application (25 s, bars) of a glutamate agonist to homomeric GluR-1(Q) (left) or heteromeric GluR-1(Q) + GluR-2(R) (right) channels expressed in oocytes and recorded in normal Ringer's (Na^+) and Ca^{2+}-Ringer's (Ca^{2+}) solutions. Oocytes were injected with a single GluR subunit cRNA (2 ng) or a combination of two types of GluR subunit cRNA (2 ng + 2 ng for 1:1 combination). Intrapipette or intracellular solution contains (in mM): 250 CsCl, 250 CsF, 100 EGTA. Normal Ringer's solution contains (in mM): 115 NaCl, 2.5 KCl, 1.8 $CaCl_2$, 10 Hepes; Ca^{2+}-Ringer's solution contains (in mM): 10 $CaCl_2$, Na^+, K^+-free, 10 Hepes. (b: From Sommer B, Keinänen K, Verdoorn TA, et al., 1990. Flip and flop: a cell-specific functional switch in glutamate-operated channels of the CNS, Science, 249, 1580–1585, with permission. c: From Hollmann M, Hartley M and Heinemann S, 1991. Ca^{2+} permeability of KA-AMPA-gated glutamate receptor channels depends on subunit composition, Science 252, 851–853, with permission.)

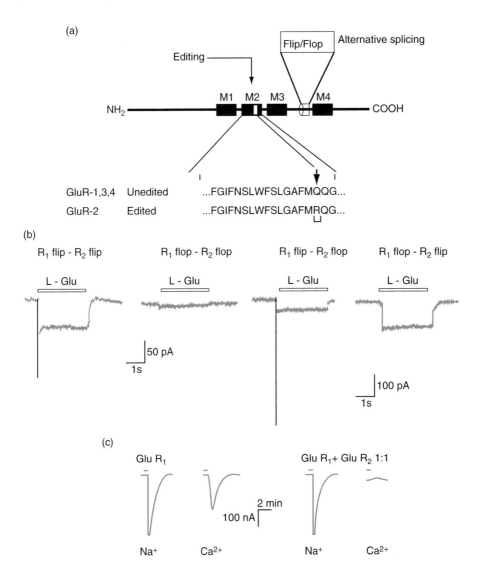

properties: GluR receptors incorporating the flip sequence would allow more current entry into the cell than receptors containing solely flop modules (Figure 11.3b). Native GluRs may be composed of heteromeric assemblies of different subunits which contain either flip or flop sequences.

Editing is a post-transcriptional change of one or more bases in the pre-mRNA such that the codon(s) encoded by the gene and that present in the mRNA differ. It has been established that the sequences necessary for editing lie in the introns. Thus only primary transcript can be edited. Therefore, editing is not a regulatory mechanism for mature mRNA. In AMPA receptors, editing only concerns the GluR-2 subunit. It has a consequence on the Ca^{2+} permeability of glutamate receptor channels. The GluR-2 subunit possesses in the M2 putative membrane-spanning segment an arginine (R) whereas in the GluR-1, 3 and 4 subunits glutamine (Q) lies in the homologous position (Figure 11.3a). This functional critical position is referred to as the Q/R site. The arginine codon (CGG) is not found in the GluR-2 gene and is introduced into the GluR-2 mRNA possibly by an adenosine to inosine conversion in the respective glutamine codon (CAG) of the GluR-2 transcript by an RNA editing process. Ninety-nine per cent of the native GluR-2 subunits are in the edited form.

The current response to glutamate application of homomeric GluR channels expressed in transfected cells is studied in extracellular solutions containing Na^+ or Ca^{2+} as the only cations. In cells expressing the GluR-2(R) subunit only, the glutamate-evoked current is present in high Na^+ solution and nearly absent in high Ca^{2+} solution thus indicating that this homomeric channel has a low divalent/monovalent permeability ratio. Moreover, heteromeric GluR-2(R) + GluR-3 subunit association forms Ca^{2+} impermeable oligomeric channels in oocytes (Figure 11.3c). The situation is different in the absence of the GluR 2(R) subunit since homomeric GluR-1, GluR-3 or heteromeric GluR-1 + GluR-3 channels allow the influx of Ca^{2+} (Figure 11.3c). Therefore, the presence of a positively charged side chain of one amino acid (R) would determine the divalent/monovalent permeability ratio and thus GluR-2(R) would dominate the properties of ion flow through the heteromeric GluR channel.

11.2 NMDA Receptors are Permeable to both Monovalent and Ca^{2+} Ions: They are Blocked by Mg^{2+} Ions at Voltages Close to the Resting Potential, which Confers a Strong Voltage Dependence

The NMDA receptor channels are activated by several agonists, of which NMDA is the most effective (Figure 11.1). They form cation selective channels with a high Ca^{2+} permeability, with unique voltage dependent sensitivity to Mg^{2+} and their activity is modulated by glycine.

11.2.1 Most of the Native NMDA Activated Channels have a Conductance of 40–50 pS

As we have already pointed out, the NMDA channel has the property of being blocked by extracellular Mg^{2+} ions at voltages close to the resting potential of the cell: Mg^{2+} ions block the channel in the open state thus preventing the passage of other ions. The concentrations of Mg^{2+} ions that produce a significant block are similar to the concentrations of Mg^{2+} ions normally present in the extracellular fluid. For clarity, we shall first study the conductance and permeability properties of the NMDA channel in the absence of extracellular Mg^{2+} ions (Sections 11.2.1 and 11.2.2). Subsequently we shall study the nature of the changes that occur in a medium containing Mg^{2+} ions (Section 11.2.3).

Let us look at patch clamp recordings (outside-out configuration) of cultured central neurons in the absence of Mg^{2+} ions. The application of NMDA (10 µmol/l) to the extracellular fluid at $V_m = -60$ mV induces an inward unitary current, i_N (Figure 11.4a). The i_N/V relation obtained under these conditions is linear (between –80 mV and +60 mV) and is described by the equation $i_N = \gamma_N (V_m - E_{rev})$ (Figure 11.4b). The slope of this curve corresponds to the unitary conductance of the NMDA channel, γ_N. The average value of γ_N is in the range of 40–50 pS.

11.2.2 The NMDA Channel is Permeable to Monovalent Cations and to Ca^{2+}

The i_N/V relation shows that i_N reverses at a membrane potential value close to 0 mV when the extra-

Figure 11.4 Electrophysiological properties of an NMDA receptor channel in the absence of extracellular Mg^{2+} ions. (a) Outside-out patch clamp recordings of an NMDA (10 µmol/l) activated channel. At −60 mV NMDA evokes an inward unitary current i_N (downward deflection), and at +40 mV the evoked current is outward (upward deflection). (b) i_N/V relation obtained from the averages of unitary currents i_N recorded from a homogeneous population of channels (a population that shows a 40–50 pS unitary conductance). This curve is described by the linear equation $i_N = \gamma_N (V_m − E_{rev})$ (between −80 mV and +60 mV) and shows that the unitary conductance of NMDA channels is only slightly voltage dependent in the absence of Mg^{2+} ions. Composition of the solutions: intrapipette or intracellular solution (in mmol/l): 140 CsCl, 5K-EGTA and 0.5 $CaCl_2$; extracellular solution: 140 NaCl, 2.8 KCl and 1 $CaCl_2$. (a: From Ascher P, Bregestovski P and Nowak L, 1988. N-methyl-D-aspartate-activated channels of mouse central neurons in magnesium free solutions, *J. Physiol.* (*Lond.*) **399**, 207–226, with permission. b: From Cull-Candy SG and Usowicz MM, 1987. Patch clamp recording from single glutamate receptor channels, *TIPS* **8**, 218–224, with permission.)

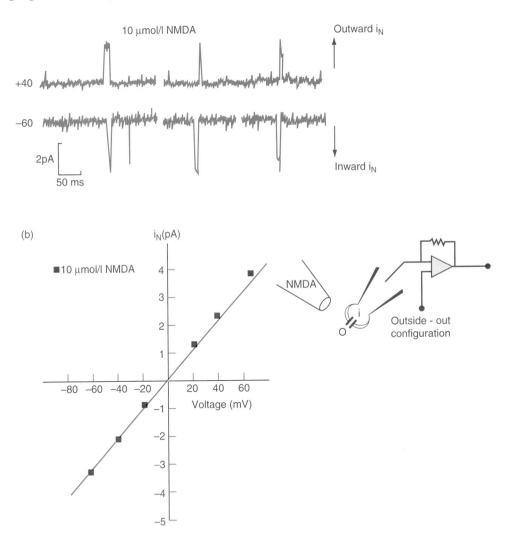

cellular and intracellular ion concentrations are similar. This value suggests that the NMDA channel is permeable to cations. If any of the monovalent cations (Na^+, K^+ or Cs^+) are replaced by another, only minor changes in the reversal potential are observed, i.e. the channel discriminates only slightly between the different monovalent cations.

During early experiments it seemed that the NMDA

channel was also permeable to Ca^{2+} ions. In order to establish whether the NMDA channel is permeable to Ca^{2+} ions or not, two types of experiments have been performed:

- The first type of experiment consisted of photometric measurements (Appendix 11.1) of the variations in intracellular Ca^{2+} ions. They showed an increase of the intracellular Ca^{2+} concentration during an NMDA evoked response. To carry out these experiments and to prevent the activation of voltage dependent Ca^{2+} channels, spinal neuron activity was recorded in patch clamp (whole-cell configuration) at a holding potential of -60 mV (Figure 11.5b). Under these conditions a strong increase of the intracellular concentration of Ca^{2+} is seen. This augmentation is selectively blocked by the antagonist APV and by the NMDA channel blocker MK 801 (see Figure 11.1). This increase clearly results from an influx of Ca^{2+} ions through the NMDA channels and is not due to a release of these ions from intracellular storage pools of Ca^{2+}, since it disappears in the absence of extracellular Ca^{2+} ions.

- A second type of experiment has shown that changes in the extracellular Ca^{2+} concentration is accompanied by changes in the reversal potential of the macroscopic NMDA current (Figure 11.5c). This indicates that Ca^{2+} ions actually carry part of the NMDA current. Furthermore, if an NMDA channel is recorded under conditions where Ca^{2+} ions are the only cations present in the extracellular environment, at -60 mV one can observe an inward current. Ca^{2+} ions are the only ions that can carry this current under these conditions.

11.2.3 NMDA Channels are Blocked by Physiological Concentrations of Extracellular Mg^{2+} Ions: This Block is Voltage Dependent

In order to show the block of the NMDA channel by Mg^{2+} ions, the unitary current evoked by NMDA (10 μmol/l) was recorded in the presence of increasing concentrations of extracellular Mg^{2+} ions (in μmol/l: 0, 10, 50 and 100) (Figure 11.6a). At $V_m = -60$ mV, NMDA evokes an inward unitary current whose amplitude remains constant at all the Mg^{2+} concentrations tested (see legend for 100 μmol/l). However, while in the absence of Mg^{2+} the NMDA channel opens for periods of several milliseconds, in the presence of Mg^{2+} the recordings show bursts of short openings during which the channel fluctuates between open (t_o) and blocked (t_{bl}) periods (Figure 11.6a). These repeated closures strongly diminish the average time during which the channel is open.

The most interesting aspect of this block is its voltage dependence. Mg^{2+} ions block the channel at negative potentials while at positive voltages (where the current i_N is outward) they have almost no effect at all (Figure 11.6a, $V_m = +40$ mV).

The same properties as those of the unitary current are observed in macroscopic recordings (whole-cell configuration). Let us remember that $I_N = N \times p_o \times i_N$. We know that i_N is approximately constant at a given membrane potential irrespective of the Mg^{2+} concentration, and that the mean open time of each channel (and therefore the open state probability p_o of the channel as well) decreases as a function of the Mg^{2+} concentration. From the recordings in Figure 11.6a we can predict that at negative potentials the macroscopic current I_N will be small.

In fact, the I_N/V curve in the presence of extracellular Mg^{2+} ions (500 μmol/l) is not linear. This nonlinearity appears at negative voltages, i.e. when the current is inward (Figure 11.6b). Furthermore, we observe that between $V_m = -35$ mV and $V_m = -80$ mV, the current amplitude diminishes instead of increasing, as would be expected from the increasing electrochemical gradients for Na^+ and Ca^{2+} and the decreasing electrochemical gradient for K^+. This peculiar property of the I_N/V curve in this region of voltage is due to the block of the channel by Mg^{2+}.

Since Mg^{2+} ions are normally found in the extracellular fluid at concentrations of approximately 1 mmol/l, at membrane potentials close to the resting potential most NMDA channels are blocked.

Mechanism of action of Mg^{2+} ion block: hypothesis

Mg^{2+} ions block *open* NMDA channels, thus preventing the passage of Na^+, Ca^{2+} and K^+ ions. The probability that an Mg^{2+} ion will enter the NMDA channel increases with the level of membrane hyperpolarization: the greater the electrical gradient, the stronger are the Mg^{2+} ions attracted into the channel. For this reason, the block of NMDA channels by Mg^{2+} is voltage sensitive. This block can be symbolized as follows:

Figure 11.5   Optic measurements of intracellular Ca^{2+} ion concentration changes during a quisqualate (a) or NMDA (b) evoked response. The Ca^{2+} sensitive dye arsenazo III was used. The absorption coefficient of this dye varies at certain wavelengths when it complexes Ca^{2+} ions (see Appendix 11.1). The activity of cultured spinal neurons is recorded in the whole-cell patch clamp configuration. (a) Pressure application of 100 µmol/l (15 ms) quisqualate evokes an inward current (top trace). The total recorded inward current I_q corresponds to the sum of the unitary currents i_q crossing non-NMDA channels opened by quisqualate. During this response only a slight increase in the intracellular Ca^{2+} concentration is observed (bottom trace, ΔCa^{2+}). (b) The pressure application of 1 mmol/l (20 ms) NMDA in the presence of 2.5 mmol/l Ca^{2+} in the extracellular solution evokes an inward current (top trace). The total recorded inward current I_N corresponds to the sum of the unitary currents i_N crossing all NMDA channels opened by NMDA. During this response one observes an increase in the intracellular Ca^{2+} concentration (bottom trace, ΔCa^{2+}). The holding potential is –60 mV and the extracellular solution does not contain Mg^{2+} ions. Solution compositions (a and b) in mmol/l, intrapipette or intracellular: 140 K-gluconate, 2 $MgCl_2$, 0.57–1.07 Na-arsenazo III; extracellular: 145 NaCl, 2.5 KCl, 2.5 $CaCl_2$, 0 $MgCl_2$. (c) Reversal potential of the NMDA current measurement as a function of extracellular Ca^{2+} ions. Whole-cell patch clamp recordings of total I_N current in cultured spinal neurons. Currents activated by the application of 1 mmol/l NMDA at different membrane potentials, in the presence of 1 mmol/l $[Ca^{2+}]_o$ (left) or 20 mmol/l $[Ca^{2+}]_o$ (right). One observes a shift in the reversal potential of the NMDA response at different extracellular Ca^{2+} concentrations. (a, b: From Mayer ML, MacDermott AB, Westbrook GL, Smith SJ and Barker JL, 1987. Agonist- and voltage-gated calcium entry in cultured mouse spinal cord neurons under voltage clamp using arsenazo III, *J. Neurosci.* 7, 3230–3244, with permission. C: MacDermott AB, Mayer ML, Westbrook GL, Smith SJ and Barker JL, 1986. NMDA-receptor activation increases cytoplasmic calcium concentration in cultured spinal neurons, *Nature* **321**, 519–522, with permission.)

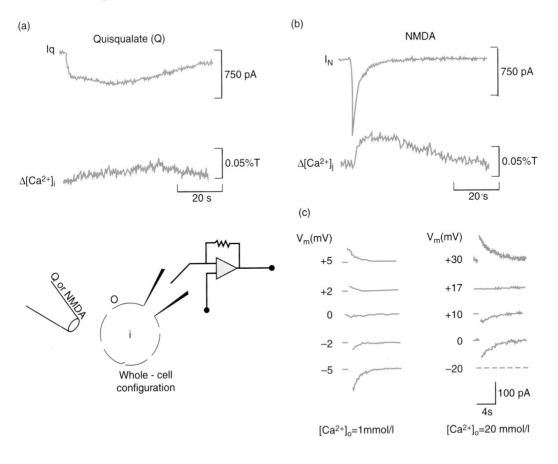

Figure 11.6 NMDA channel block by extracellular Mg^{2+} ions. (a): Outside-out patch clamp recording of the activity of cultured central neurons. The application of NMDA (10 µmol/l) evokes a unitary inward current with an amplitude $i_N = 2.7$ pA in the absence of Mg^{2+} ions (0). In the presence of extracellular Mg^{2+} ions (10, 50, 100 µmol/l) we observe that the unitary inward current has the same amplitude but that the channel opens in bursts (t_b), fluctuating between an open (t_o) and a blocked state (t_{bl}) with a variable frequency. For an Mg^{2+} concentration of 100 µmol/l the unitary current appears to have a lower amplitude. This is actually due to its higher closing frequency, which the recording system is unable to follow. The repeated closures of the channel (which actually correspond to fluctuations between the open and the blocked states) decrease the open time of the channel. Note that when the recorded unitary current is outward at +40 mV the presence of Mg^{2+} ions, even at a concentration of 100 µmol/l, has no effect on the channel open time. (b) Voltage sensitivity of the NMDA response in the presence of extracellular Mg^{2+} ions. The total current I_N is recorded in the whole-cell patch clamp configuration in the absence (O), and in the presence of 500 µmol/l (■) Mg^{2+} ions. The I_N/V relation obtained is described by the equation $I_N = G_N (V_m - E_{rev})$ is not linear at negative voltages in the presence of Mg^{2+} ions. Between -35 and -80 mV the curve shows a region of negative conductance. Let us recall that $I_N = N \times P_o \times i_N$, and that if τ_o decreases, p_o decreases, and consequently I_N also decreases. Solution compositions (in mmol/l): intrapipette or intracellular solution: 140 CsCl, 5 K-EGTA, 0.5 $CaCl_2$; extracellular solution: 140 NaCl, 2.8 KCl and variable concentrations of $MgCl_2$ (in µmol/l, see figure). (a: From Ascher P and Nowak L, 1988. The role of divalent cations in the N-methyl-D-aspartate responses of the mouse central neurons in culture, *J. Physiol. (Lond.)* **399**, 247–266, with permission. b: From Nowak L, Bregestovski P, Ascher P, Herbet A and Prochiantz A, 1984. Magnesium free glutamate-activated channels in mouse central neurones, *Nature* **307**, 463–465, with permission.)

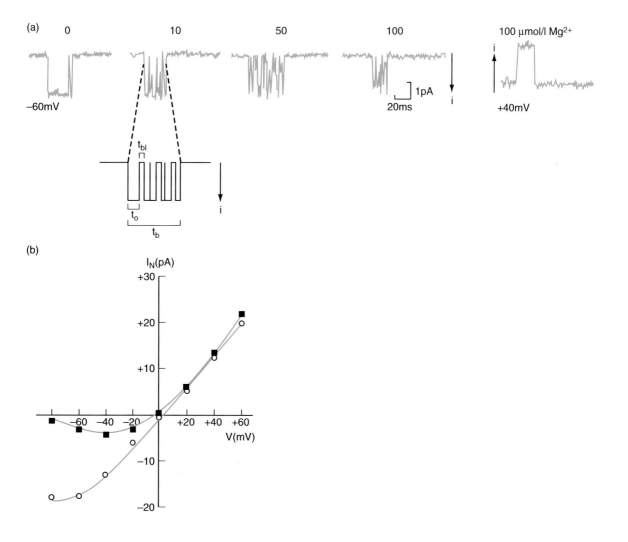

$$\text{R} + \text{NMDA} \rightleftharpoons \text{NMDA} - \text{R}^* \overset{\text{Mg}^{2+}}{\rightleftharpoons} \text{NMDA} - \text{R}^* - \text{Mg}$$

where R is the NMDA channel in the closed state, R^* is the NMDA channel in the open state, and R^*–Mg is the open NMDA channel blocked by Mg^{2+} ions, The reaction $R^* + Mg \rightleftharpoons R^*$–Mg is strongly favored to the right when $[Mg^{2+}]$ is increased and when $V_m < 0$ mV.

Why is the NMDA channel permeable to Ca^{2+} ions and blocked by Mg^{2+} ions?

One can separate the effects of cations into two groups:

- those, like Ca^{2+}, that pass through the NMDA channel, e.g. Ba^{2+}, Cd^{2+};
- those that mimic the Mg^{2+} effect, i.e. block the NMDA channel, e.g. Co^{2+}, Ni^{2+}, Mn^{2+}.

The difference between the ions that pass through the channel and those that block it coincides with the difference in the speed with which the water molecules surrounding these ions can exchange with other water molecules of the aqueous solution. In fact, this exchange is a thousand times faster for the group of permeable (Ca^{2+}-like) ions than for the group of blocking (Mg^{2+}-like) ions.

These differences have led to the suggestion that both ions can cross the channel but only in their dehydrated form. The following model of the channel has been proposed: the channel has a large extracellular entrance and presents a narrow constriction towards the intracellular side through which the ions can only cross in their dehydrated form. Because of the slow rate of dehydration of the cations from the Mg^{2+} group, these ions are trapped in the interior of the channel thus blocking it. Another hypothesis for the blockade by Mg^{2+} ions is the following: a high affinity binding site for Mg^{2+} ions could exist inside the channel so that Mg^{2+} ions would cross the channel slowly and thus block it for the time of passage.

11.2.4 Glycine Potentiates the NMDA Response

Glycine is an amino acid that acts as an inhibitory neurotransmitter at certain central nervous system synapses in vertebrates. However, this amino acid also plays a role in the NMDA response.

The effect of glycine on the NMDA receptor channel has been demonstrated in cultured central neurons recorded in the whole-cell patch clamp configuration. When NMDA was applied by slow perfusion the response was shown to be much larger than when NMDA was rapidly perfused into the bath. The following hypothesis was proposed: the cultured cells (neurons and glia) tonically release a substance that accumulates in the bath as a result of the slow perfusion and thus potentiates the NMDA response. In order to characterize the active substance present in the medium, a variety of treatments were applied. It was established that its activity was still present after heating the medium to 90°C, and that its molecular weight is less than 700 D. After testing the most common amino acids, glycine proved to be the most effective in reproducing the effects of the conditioning medium on the NMDA response (Figure 11.7).

Patch clamp outside-out recordings showed that glycine potentiates the NMDA response by augmenting the NMDA receptor channel opening frequency (thus increasing the open state probability of the channel, p_o). The molecular mechanisms of this potentiating effect remain to be determined. Nevertheless, the fact that glycine has an effect on excised outside-out patch clamp recorded NMDA receptor channels rules out the mediation of its effect by a diffusible second messenger.

It was then suggested that glycine would in fact be indispensable for activation of the NMDA receptor channel by its agonists. When the activity of NMDA receptor channels expressed in oocytes is recorded in the whole-cell patch clamp configuration, only a current is only observed in response to an application of NMDA when glycine is also present in the bath (Figure 11.7b).

How can these results be interpreted from a physiological perspective? This question still remains unanswered. Glycine is in fact present at relatively high concentrations in the cerebrospinal fluid (several micromoles per liter). This level is close to the concentration required to produce its maximum effect.

Figure 11.7   Potentiation of the NMDA response by glycine. (a) Whole-cell patch clamp recordings of cultured central neurons. The response to the application of 10 μmol/l NMDA or 10 μmol/l glutamate at −50 mV is potentiated by the application of 1 μmol/l glycine (Gly). The response evoked by quisqualate (Quis) or kainate (Kai) is not potentiated by Gly. It should be emphasized that glycine by itself does not trigger an inward current at any concentration through either NMDA or non-NMDA channels. (b) The application of 300 μmol/l NMDA at −60 mV to *Xenopus* oocytes which express NMDA channels (whole-cell patch clamp configuration) evokes a strong inward current (66 ± 13 nA) in the presence of 3 μmol/l glycine. On the same oocytes, the inward current evoked by NMDA in the absence of glycine is negligible (0.6 ± 0.3 nA). In (a) and (b) the extracellular solution is devoid of Mg^{2+} ions. (a: From Johnson JW and Ascher P, 1987. Glycine potentiates the NMDA response in cultured mouse brain neurons, *Nature* **325**, 529–531, with permission. b: From Kleckner N and Dingledine R, 1988. Requirements for glycine in activation of NMDA receptors expressed in *Xenopus* ovocytes, *Science* **241**; 835–837, with permission.)

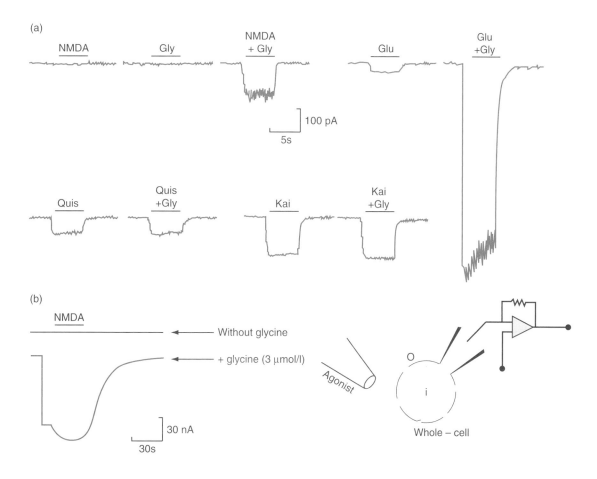

However, a high-affinity glycine pump may lower the extracellular glycine concentration to the level of glutamatergic synapses. The discovery of selective antagonists for the glycine receptor site should bring some insight into the role of glycine *in vivo*.

11.2.5 Molecular Biology of NMDA Receptors

The experiments described in the preceding section allowed the characterization of the electrophysiological properties of native NMDA channels. They were carried out before molecular cloning of NMDA receptor subunits had been achieved.

Molecular cloning has identified to date cDNAs encoding NR1 and NR2A, B, C, D subunits of the NMDA receptor, the deduced amino acid sequences of which are 20% (NR1 and NR2), 55% (NR2A and NR2C) or 70% (NR2A and NR2B) identical. The *Xenopus* oocyte system and transfected mammalian cells were used to study the functional properties of these subunits and large currents were measured only in oocytes co-expressing NR1 and NR2 subunits, a result that tends to predict that natural NMDA receptors would occur as hetero-oligomers like other ligand-gated channels. NR1 and NR2 subunits carry in their putative membrane-spanning M2 segment an asparagine residue in a position homologous to the Q/R site of AMPA receptors (Figure 11.8a). Expression of modified subunits in *Xenopus* oocytes showed that these asparagines are crucial for the particular properties of divalent ion permeation of NMDA channels.

What does molecular biology tell us about Mg^{2+} block?

The molecular substrate for the hypothesis of a high-affinity site in the NMDA channel for Mg^{2+} ion binding was analysed by exchanging (by site-directed

mutagenesis) either glutamine (Q) or arginine (R) for asparagine (N) in the M2 domain of NR1 or NR2A. Wild-type and mutant NR subunits were co-expressed by cells transfected with cDNAs. Whole cell currents were activated by application of L-glutamate to transfected cells expressing heteromeric wild-type or mutant NMDA receptors and differences in Ca^{2+} or Mg^{2+} permeability and channel block by extracellular Mg^{2+} were analysed. The presence of glutamine (Q) instead of asparagine (N) in the NR2A subunit generated 'wild-type NR1–mutant NR2A' channels with increased Mg^{2+} permeability and thus reduced sensitivity to block by extracellular Mg^{2+} (Figure 11.8b). The effect observed suggests that the M2 segment forms part of the channel of NMDA receptors. Replacing the asparagine (N) by arginine (R) in the NR1 subunit generated 'mutant NR1–wild type NR2A' channels that did not exhibit a measurable Ca^{2+} permeability (Figure 11.8c). Moreover, inward currents measured in divalent ion-free Ringer's solution were not measurably blocked when 0.5 mM Mg^{2+} was added to the extracellular solution. Thus, when the positively charged arginine (R) occupies the critical position in M2 of the NR1 subunit, divalent cations appear to be prevented from entering the channel, suggesting that the size and charge of

Figure 11.8   Molecular biology of NMDA receptor channels. (a): Linear representation of subunits of glutamate receptor channels is shown at the top. Predicted membrane spanning regions (M1 to M4) are boxed. The expanded M2 segment at the bottom lists sequences of subunits belonging to NMDA (NR1, NR2A, NR2C) and non-NMDA (GluR-1, GluR-2, GluR-6 and KA-2) receptor channels. NMDA receptor channels carry an asparagine residue (N) in a position homologous to the Q/R site of AMPA and KA receptor subunits. Amino acid residues in the shaded box of Figure 11.8a are likely to be in the path of ions permeating the glutamate-activated channel of the different receptors. (b) Difference in channel block by extracellular Mg^{2+} between wild-type and mutant NMDA receptor channels expressed in a cell line (293 cells). In the NR2A(N595Q) subunit, one asparagine (N) in the M2 segment was replaced by a glutamine (Q) by site-directed mutagenesis. The whole cell current evoked by glutamate is recorded in (a) divalent ion-free Ringer and (b) after addition of 0.1 mM Mg^{2+} as a function of membrane potential. The I/V relations show that the wild-type channel comprised of NR1 and NR2A subunits (left) is blocked by external Mg^{2+} ions while the mutant channel comprised of wild-type NR1 and mutant NR2A(N595Q) subunits is permeable to Mg^{2+} (right). (c) Reduction of Ca^{2+} permeability and channel block by extracellular Mg^{2+} in mutant channel where asparagine (N) in the M2 segment of the NR1 subunit is replaced by arginine (R). (Left) Whole cell current elicited by 100 μM glutamate (bar) at −60 mV in high Na$^+$ (Na$^+$, inward current) or high Ca^{2+} (Ca^{2+}, small outward current) extracellular solutions. Outward current at −60 mV in high Ca^{2+} solution indicates low Ca^{2+} permeability of the mutant channel. (Right) Whole cell I/V relations in (a) divalent ion-free external solution and (b) after adding 0.5 mM Mg^{2+} to the external solution. The two traces superimpose almost completely showing that the mutant channel is not blocked by external Mg^{2+} ions. Composition of the solutions (in mM). Intrapipette (intracellular) solution: 140 CsCl, 1 MgCl$_2$, 10 EGTA, 10 Hepes; extracellular solutions, high Na$^+$ solution: 140 NaCl, 5 HEPES; high Ca^{2+} solution: 110 CaCl$_2$, 5 HEPES; divalent ion-free Ringer's solution: 135 NaCl, 5.4 KCl, 5 HEPES. (a: From Wisden W and Seeburg PH, 1993. Mammalian ionotropic glutamate receptors, *Curr. Opin. Neurobiol.*, **3**, 291–298, with permission.) b: From Burnashev N, Schoepfer R, Monyer H *et al* (1992). Control of calcium permeability and magnesium blockade in the NMDA receptor, *Science* **257**, 1415–1419, with permission.)

the amino acid present at this critical position in the MII segment is important for cation permeability.

11.2.6 Conclusions

The NMDA receptor channel is unusual in that there are at least two conditions required for its activation:

the presence of a ligand (glutamate and perhaps also glycine) and depolarization of the membrane. It is a *doubly gated* channel.

It should be noted that the voltage sensitivity of the NMDA channels (a sensitivity resulting from an extrinsic ion, namely Mg^{2+} ions) differs radically from that of voltage-dependent Na^+ and Ca^{2+} channels. In the two latter cases, the voltage sensitivity is an

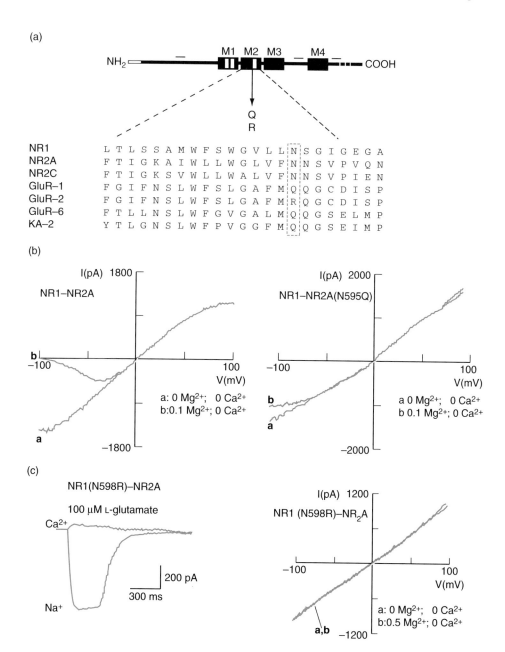

intrinsic property of the protein, which does not require extracellular or intracellular blocking ions.

The voltage sensitivity of the NMDA channel has important physiological implications. Since these channels are blocked by Mg^{2+} ions at voltages close to the resting potential of the cell, does the presence of the neurotransmitter in the synaptic cleft suffice to evoke a post-synaptic NMDA response? Knowing that the non-NMDA and NMDA receptors co-exist on the post-synaptic membrane, what is the fraction of the synaptic current that is due to the activation of NMDA receptors? These questions are analyzed in the following section.

11.3 Synaptic Depolarization Mediated by Excitatory Amino Acids: NMDA and Non-NMDA Components

There are many central nervous system synapses whose putative neurotransmitter is glutamate. We shall present results obtained from cultured neurons of the spinal cord and the hippocampus. These neurons form synapses in culture and their putative neurotransmitter is glutamate. This type of preparation is of interest compared with other *in vitro* preparations because one can perform patch clamp recordings (whole-cell configuration) of post-synaptic neurons connected to identified pre-synaptic neurons. One can thus study the effect of endogenous glutamate on NMDA or non-NMDA receptors.

The hypothesis is as follows: glutamate is released in the synaptic cleft where it will bind to post-synaptic NMDA as well as non-NMDA receptors (Figure 11.9d). When the membrane potential is near the resting potential of the cell, a large fraction of the NMDA receptors are blocked by Mg^{2+} ions present in the synaptic cleft. Therefore, the released glutamate mostly activates non-NMDA receptors. Is the depolarization thus evoked due only to the activation of non-NMDA receptors? If not, under which conditions are NMDA receptors activated by glutamate and how do they contribute to the post-synaptic depolarization?

In order to answer these questions, it is necessary to identify and separate the post-synaptic current components resulting from the activation of non-NMDA and of NMDA receptors.

11.3.1 The Inward Post-synaptic Current Resulting from the Activation of Excitatory Amino Acid Receptors has Two Components

To identify the NMDA and non-NMDA current components (or those of the post-synaptic depolarization) we can make use of the different properties of the non-NMDA and NMDA channels summarized in Figure 11.1. The non-NMDA component will not be affected by different concentrations of extracellular Mg^{2+} ions, nor by the presence of APV, but it will disappear in the

Figure 11.9 The post-synaptic inward current evoked by the stimulation of a glutamatergic pre-synaptic neuron shows two components. (a) While the post-synaptic membrane is held at a voltage of −46 mV, the inward current recorded in the absence of Mg^{2+} ions (whole-cell patch clamp configuration) shows two components. The decrement of the synaptic current can be described by two exponential functions, with time constants $\tau_1 = 4.2$ ms and $\tau_2 = 81.8$ ms. (b) In the presence of Mg^{2+} ions (100 µmol/1), the slow component is voltage sensitive whereas the rapid component is not. The peak of the early current (▼) has similar absolute values at symmetrical voltages around the reversal potential. However, the slow component (■) is much lower in amplitude at hyperpolarized potentials than at depolarized potentials. (c) In the presence of 33 µmol/1 APV and in the absence of extracellular Mg^{2+} ions the slow component (■) completely disappears at all voltages tested, whereas the early component (▼) is not affected. Solution compositions (in mmol/l): intrapipette or intracellular: 140 K^+ or cesium methyl sulfate; extracellular: 135 NaCl, 3 KCl, 1 or 2 $CaCl_2$, 0 or 0.1 $MgCl_2$. Picrotoxin (10–100 µmol/l) is added to the extracellular solution in order to block GABAergic inhibitory synaptic activity. (d) Functional scheme of a glutamatergic synapse where ionotropic and metabotropic glutamate receptors are co-localized. Pre-synaptic receptors are omitted. The enzymes (1 to 3) and mitochondria are synthesized in the soma and carried to axon terminals via anterograde axonal transport. Glutamate synthesized in mitochondria of the pre-synaptic element is transported actively into synaptic vesicles by a vesicular carrier. A percentage of the glutamate released in the synaptic cleft is taken up into pre-synaptic terminals and glial cells by an Na^+/K^+ dependent electrogenic transport. (a to c: From Forsythe ID and Westbrook GL, 1988. Slow excitatory postsynaptic currents mediated by N-methyl-D-aspartate receptors on cultured mouse central neurons, *J. Physiol. (Lond.)* **396**, 515–533, with permission.)

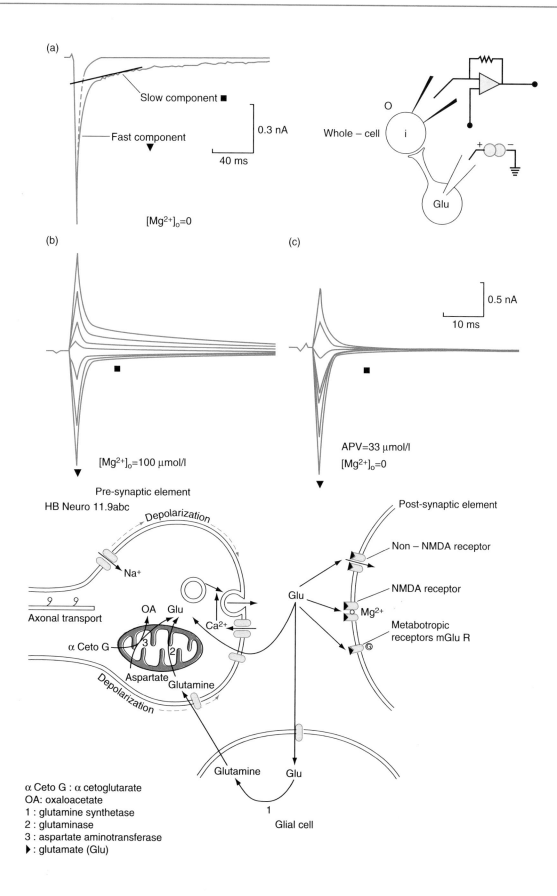

(a)

Slow component ■

Fast component ▼

0.3 nA

40 ms

$[Mg^{2+}]_o = 0$

Whole – cell

O

i

Glu

(b)

$[Mg^{2+}]_o = 100\ \mu mol/l$

(c)

0.5 nA

10 ms

APV = 33 $\mu mol/l$
$[Mg^{2+}]_o = 0$

Pre-synaptic element
HB Neuro 11.9abc

Depolarization

Na$^+$

Axonal transport

OA Glu

α Ceto G

3 2

Aspartate Glutamine

Depolarization

Ca^{2+}

Glu

Glutamine Glu

Glutamine Glu

1

Glial cell

Post-synaptic element

Non – NMDA receptor

NMDA receptor

Mg^{2+}

Metabotropic
receptors mGlu R

α Ceto G : α cetoglutarate
OA: oxaloacetate
1 : glutamine synthetase
2 : glutaminase
3 : aspartate aminotransferase
▶ : glutamate (Glu)

presence of CNQX, a selective antagonist of non-NMDA receptors. On the other hand, the NMDA component will be present in a medium devoid of Mg^{2+} ions but will disappear in the presence of APV, the competitive antagonist of NMDA receptors.

Figure 11.9a–c shows the patch clamp recordings (whole-cell configuration) of the post-synaptic inward current evoked by the stimulation of one of the pre-synaptic neurons. When the neuron is stimulated in the absence of extracellular Mg^{2+} ions and at –46 mV, an inward current showing two components is recorded:

- the early component: an initial peak of current of great amplitude and rapid inactivation; and
- the late component: a small current that inactivates slowly.

The initial inward current component or early component results from the activation of non-NMDA receptors

In the presence of Mg^{2+} ions (Figure 11.9b) or in the absence of Mg^{2+} ions and the presence of APV (Figure 11.9c) in the extracellular environment, the early component is not affected but clearly the late component is (see below). These experiments suggest that the early component is a consequence of the synaptic activation of non-NMDA receptors (Figure 11.9d).

The late component results from the activation of NMDA receptors

In order to identify the fraction of current resulting from the activation of NMDA receptors, the total synaptic inward current is recorded in the absence of Mg^{2+} ions. This current is compared with the current recorded in the presence of Mg^{2+} or, alternatively, in the absence of Mg^{2+} but in the presence of APV. In the presence of Mg^{2+} the late component is largely attenuated at negative potentials but is present at all positive voltages (Figure 11.9b). In the presence of APV, the late component disappears at all voltages tested (Figure 11.9c). These results strongly suggest that the late component of the inward synaptic current results from the activation of NMDA receptors (Figure 11.9d). When the recordings are made in the presence

of Mg^{2+} (when the current is outward), it should be noted that this late component is much clearer at positive voltages.

11.3.2 The Post-synaptic Depolarization (EPSP) Recorded in the Absence of Extracellular Mg^{2+} Ions Presents Two Components

Let us record in current clamp (i.e. leaving the voltage free to vary) the post-synaptic potential variations in response to stimulation of the pre-synaptic neurons (same preparation as before) in the absence of Mg^{2+} ions. Such stimulation evokes a post-synaptic depolarization (EPSP), which is a result of the evoked synaptic inward current crossing the non-NMDA and NMDA channels. As in the case of the synaptic current, the EPSP shows two identifiable components.

In the presence of APV the early component is only slightly affected or not at all (Figure 11.10a, c). This APV-insensitive early component is a result of the early synaptic inward current, i.e. the activation of non-NMDA receptors.

In the absence of Mg^{2+} ions and in the presence of APV, we observe that the duration of the EPSP is reduced (Figure 11.10a, c). The difference between the APV-insensitive component of the EPSP and the total EPSP corresponds to the APV-sensitive component, i.e. the component resulting from the activation of the NMDA receptors (Figure 11.10b, d).

In summary, the component resulting from the activation of the NMDA receptors has a slower rising phase and lasts longer than the component mediated by the non-NMDA receptors. Thus, when the NMDA receptors are activated, the peak of the EPSP is not always affected but the duration of the EPSP is much longer.

11.3.3 Synaptic Depolarization Recorded in Physiological Conditions: Factors Controling NMDA Receptor Activation

The extracellular physiological environment contains Mg^{2+} ions at concentrations of approximately 1 mmol/1. Since at this concentration of Mg^{2+} ions and at membrane potentials close to the resting potential of the cell most of the NMDA channels are closed, under

Figure 11.10   The excitatory post-synaptic potential (EPSP) evoked by endogenous glutamate in the absence of Mg^{2+} ions shows two components. (a) Current clamp recordings of cultured spinal neuron activity. The monosynaptic EPSP (a, control) has a fast rising phase and a very long duration, which can extend up to 500 ms. In the presence of APV (a, 33 µmol/l) a clear reduction in the EPSP duration is observed. The APV-insensitive component, which is most likely due to the activation of non-NMDA receptors, corresponds to the early phase or peak of the EPSP. The difference between the APV-insensitive component of the EPSP and the total EPSP corresponds to the APV-sensitive component, which probably results from the activation of NMDA receptors. This is a late component with a slow rising phase (b). (c, d) Very similar results are obtained from hippocampal neurons. Extracellular solution (in mmol/l): 135 NaCl, 3 KCl, 1 or 2 $CaCl_2$, 0 $MgCl_2$. Picrotoxin (10–100 µmol/1) is added to the extracellular solution in order to block GABAergic inhibitory synaptic activity. From Forsythe ID and Westbrook GL, 1988. Slow excitatory postsynaptic currents mediated by N-methyl-D-aspartate receptors on cultured mouse central neurons, *J. Physiol. (Lond.)* **396**, 515–533, with permission.)

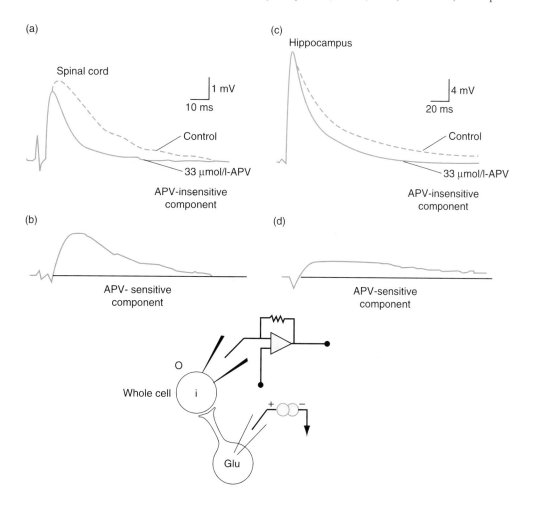

what conditions will NMDA receptors participate in synaptic transmission (see Figure 11.9d)?

It seems unlikely that the extracellular Mg^{2+} ion concentration *in vivo* will vary sufficiently to allow the 'unblocking' of NMDA receptors. However, depolarizations reduce the level of Mg^{2+} ion block of the NMDA channel. Thus, one can imagine that a depolarization of the membrane is precisely what allows the NMDA channels to become 'unblocked'. A depolarization can be the consequence of the activation of other receptors present in the post-synaptic membrane, such as non-NMDA receptors, for example. It can also result from the activation of a subpopulation of NMDA receptors that are not blocked at the resting potential. This hypothesis can be summarized as follows:

When the NMDA and non-NMDA receptors co-exist in the post-synaptic membrane

When the glutamate concentration is sufficiently high to activate non-NMDA receptor channels, a current is generated through these channels and an APV insensitive depolarization is recorded:

- If this non-NMDA mediated depolarization is not strong enough to allow the 'unblocking' of the NMDA receptors, only the early component of the depolarization (non-NMDA component) is recorded.
- If this non-NMDA mediated depolarization is sufficiently strong to unblock NMDA receptors, it triggers the activation of an inward current through these channels and an additional depolarization of the membrane. This depolarization allows the 'unblocking' of additional NMDA receptors which, activated by glutamate, evokes an enhanced depolarization. The more depolarized the membrane is, the higher is the number of NMDA receptors activated by glutamate. This regenerative phenomenon, due to the voltage sensitivity of the NMDA receptors (associated with the negative slope region of the I_N/V curve), reminds us of a similar phenomenon observed with the action potential generating Na^+ channels (see Chapter 7). In the present case,

an important post-synaptic depolarization made up of the non-NMDA early component and the NMDA late component is recorded (Figure 11.10). However, the NMDA component effect is not only to prolong the EPSP but also to allow a significant inflow of Ca^{2+} ions. These ions have numerous roles: one of them is the activation of channels sensitive to intracellular Ca^{2+} ions (see Chapter 5). Another role of intracellular Ca^{2+} is as a second messenger. Consequently it participates in the regulation of several intracellular Ca^{2+}-sensitive processes.

When the NMDA receptors are the only receptors present in the post-synaptic membrane

In certain preparations the post-synaptic depolarization recorded in response to the endogenous release of glutamate shows only one component, the NMDA component. This has led to the assumption that not all the NMDA receptors are blocked by Mg^{2+} ions at the resting potential. The activation mechanism of NMDA receptors in this case would be as follows: when the glutamate concentration in the synaptic cleft is high enough to activate the few NMDA receptors that are not blocked by Mg^{2+} at the resting potential, a small inward current is activated. This current produces a small depolarization of the membrane which allows the 'unblocking' of additional NMDA receptors and, as in the previous example, this triggers a regenerative phenomenon. The inflow of Ca^{2+} ions through the NMDA channels further triggers Ca^{2+} dependent processes.

Appendix
11.1 Flourescence Measurements of Intracellular Ca²⁺ Concentration

11.1.1 The Interaction of Light with Matter

Light is an electromagnetic radiation that oscillates both in space and time, and has electric and magnetic field components that are perpendicular to each other. If for the sake of simplicity one focuses only on the electromagnetic component, it can be seen that the molecule, which is much smaller than the wavelength of light, will be perturbed by light because its electronic charge distribution will be altered by the oscillating electric field component of the light. Without resorting to complicated quantum mechanical calculations we can say that light will interact with matter via a resonance phenomenon, i.e. the matter will only absorb light if the energy of the incoming photon is exactly equal to the difference between the potential energy of the lowest vibrational level of the ground state and that of one of the vibrational levels of the first excited state (Figure A11.1). The absorption of light therefore occurs in discrete amounts termed quanta. The energy in a quantum of light (a photon) is given by:

$$E = h\nu = h\ c/\lambda$$

Where h is Planck's constant, ν and λ are the frequency and wavelength of the incoming light and c is the speed of light in a vacuum. When a quantum of light is absorbed by a molecule a valence electron will be boosted into a higher energy orbit called the excited state. This phenomenon will take place in 10^{-15} s, resulting in conservation of the molecular coordinates. For the sake of simplicity the rotational energy levels are not taken into account and it is assumed that at room temperature the electrons will be at their lowest vibrational energy level. The difference of energy between the vibrational levels being typically in the order of 10 kcal mol⁻¹ there is not enough thermal energy to excite a transition to higher vibrational levels at room temperature. One might thus assume that most of the electrons will lie at the lowest vibrational level of the ground state. Because absorptive transitions occur to one of the vibrational levels of the excited state, had there been no interaction with the solvent molecules one could have mea-

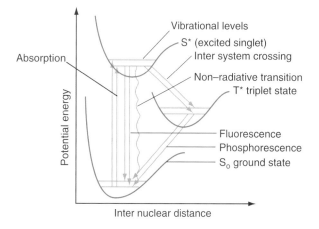

Figure A11.1 Pathways to excitation and de-excitation of an electron. The rotational levels between the vibrational levels and higher excited states are not shown for the sake of simplicity.

sured the energy difference between the ground state and each of the vibrational levels of the excited state. This type of spectra can only be obtained for chemical compounds in the gaseous state. The absorption spectra under those circumstances would resemble narrowly separated bands; however, the interaction of the orbital electrons with solvent molecules will broaden those peaks, producing the absorption spectra of the more familiar form.

The Return from the Excited State

The electrons that have been promoted to one of the vibrational levels of the excited state will lose their vibrational energy through interaction with solvent molecules by a process known as vibrational relaxation. This process has a time scale much shorter than the lifetime of the electrons in the excited state (10^{-9} to 10^{-7} for aromatic molecules). The electrons that have been promoted to the excited state will return to the ground state from the lowest lying excited vibrational state, by one of the following ways.

Fluorescence emission

Some of the electrons in the excited state will return to one of the vibrational levels of the ground state by a radiative transition, whose frequency will be a function of the energy difference separating these levels. If one simply assumes that the energy spacing of the vibrational levels of the excited and ground states are similar one expects the fluorescence emission spectrum to be a mirror image of the absorption spectrum (Figure A11.2).

Figure A11.2 The excitation (left) and emission (right) spectra of a hypothetical molecule. The excitation spectrum has the same peaks as the absorption spectrum; the separation between the individual peaks reflects the potential energy differences between the vibrational levels.

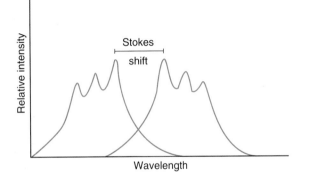

A further expectation will be that the $S_{v=0}$ to $S^*_{v=0}$ absorption will be at the same frequency as $S^*_{v=0}$ to $S_{v=0}$ emission; however, this is rarely the case, as the absorption process takes place in about 10^{-15} s. The orientation of the solvent molecules with respect to the electronic states will be conserved as well as the quantum coordinates of the molecule; however, as the excited level lifetimes are rather long, the solvent molecules will reorient favorably about the electronic levels, resulting in a difference in the zero–zero frequencies. This difference between $S_{v=0}$ to $S^*_{v=0}$ absorption and $S^*_{v=0}$ to $S_{v=0}$ emission is termed the Stoke's shift.

Non-radiative transition

In this process the excitation energy will be lost mainly by interactions with solvent molecules, resulting in some of the electrons of the excited state returning to the ground state with a non-radiative transition. This process is favored by an increase in temperature, and can explain why increasing the temperature causes a decrease in fluorescence intensities.

Quenching of the excited state

The excitation energy might be lost through interactions, in the form of collisions of quenchers with the electrons in the excited orbital. Typical quenchers such as O_2, I^- and Mn^{2+} ions will quench every time they collide with an excited singlet.

Intersystem crossing

Intersystem crossing is a mechanically forbidden quantum process that occurs by a spin exchange of the electron of the excited singlet state, resulting in an excited triplet state T^*. As this process involves a forbidden transition its probability of occurrence will be extremely low, nevertheless it will occur because the potential energy of the excited triplet is usually lower than that of the excited singlet state. The electron in the excited triplet state can then become de-excited by a non-radiative transition, quenching, or by a radiative transition termed phosphorescence (the light emitted will be of longer wavelength than fluorescence because of the lower potential energy of the excited triplet). One should note that the return to the ground state necessitates a novel forbidden transition $T^*_{v=0}$ to $S_{v=0}$. The probability of this transition will be extremely low, for the same reasons given above, resulting in a long lifetime of the excited triplet state (seconds to days). This long-lived triplet state will result in a very weak intensity of radiation, will be prone to quenching by collisions with quenchers, and the non-radiative processes will compete well with the phosphorescence. Phosphorescence in solution will rarely be observed. In order to observe phosphorescence at all, one must rigorously remove oxygen from the medium, and should use rigid glasses at very low temperatures, in order to minimize the competing non-radiative processes.

Delayed fluorescence

Some of the electrons that have undergone intersystem crossing, and therefore are in the T* state, may undergo a novel intersystem crossing to the S* level by the thermal energy provided by the solution, provided the energy difference between the T* and S* states is small; the return from the $S^*_{v=0}$ to $S_{v=0}$ level by fluorescence emission is called delayed fluorescence and has the effect of lengthening the fluorescence lifetime of the molecule beyond what is expected in normal fluorescence emissions.

Advantages of Fluorescence Measurements

When comparing the sensitivity of fluorescence to that of other techniques, it is notable that in the absence of a chromophore, provided there is no background fluorescence, the level of the signal will be zero, so even a very small change in concentration of the chromophore can be detected by a large amplification, limited by the noise level of the amplifier chain. In the case of an absorption measurement, however, the absence of the chromophore will translate itself by zero absorption, i.e. 100% transmission, therefore the maximum of the expected signal. The amplification factor will therefore be limited by the saturation of the amplifiers, and a small change in concentration of the chromophore will result in a small percentage change over the maximum signal level, which may not be detected. This difficulty can be overcome to some extent by the use of differential detection techniques, but even under these conditions the need for an extremely good match between the differential amplification chains will limit the sensitivity of the detection. As a rule of thumb, with absorption measurements, changes in the order of 1 ppm (parts per million) can be detected and with fluorescence techniques changes of 10^{-4}–10^{-5} ppm, a sensitivity that is comparable to radioactive tracers.

Observation of Fluorescence Emission

The fundamental principle underlying a fluorimeter is maximization of collection of the fluorescence emission and trying to minimize the collection of excitation light. This is usually accomplished by selecting a band of excitation wavelength that will not be present in the emission spectrum by the use of filters (interference or combination filters), or a monochromator on the excitation side and highpass or bandpass filters on the emission side. The emission side filters will pass wavelengths longer than the excitation wavelength (remember the Stoke's shift). For the measurement of fluorescence from individual cells the epi-illuminated fluorescence microscope is used, which is described below.

Epiluminescence Microscope

Most of the modern fluorescence microscopes will use the epiluminescence technique, which means that both the excitation and emission light has a common optical path through the objective. The key element of epi-illumination is the dichroic mirror; it is an interference mirror formed by successive depositions of dielectric layers on a transparent substrate. The dichroic mirror will reflect the wavelengths below its cutoff frequency and transmit those that are above the cutoff. This cutoff frequency should be chosen so that it will reflect all of the excitation wavelength, and transmit most of the emission wavelength. The Stoke's shift is an aid in this respect. One should note that the dichroic mirrors are far from being ideal: they may have bandpass characteristics at a different wavelength, and they are very sensitive to the angle of incidence of the light beam. It is now possible to find polychroic mirrors that allow the simultaneous detection of many chromophores (Figure A11.3).

Methods of Calcium Measurement by Fluorescence

The main requirement for an indicator to report the concentration of an ion is a change in its optical properties, and at the same time it should be highly specific for the ion in question, at the physiological pH values. Furthermore its binding and release from the ion must be faster than the kinetics of the intracellular ionic changes. One can therefore envisage the synthesis of probes that will change their absorption, bioluminescence (such as aequorin) or fluorescence properties. Fluorescence is the technique of choice because of its higher sensitivity. In fluorescence

Figure A11.3   Epi-illumination microscopy.

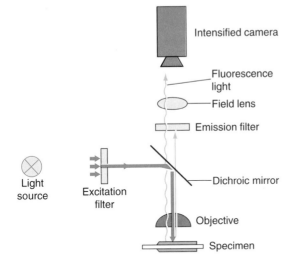

Figure A11.4   Chemical structure of FURA-2. Note the similarities between FURA-2 and the acetoxy-methylester variety FURA-2AM and EGTA. The AM variety is membrane permeant, and is de-esterified by intracellular esterases, liberating FURA-2, formaldehyde and acetate ions.

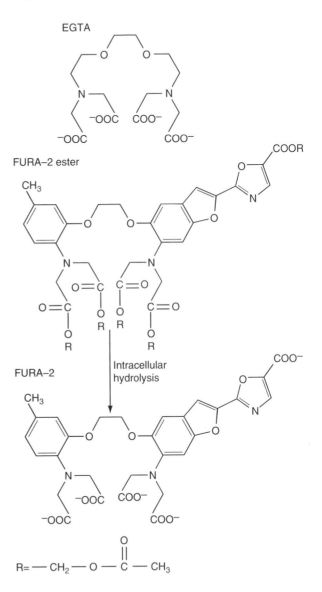

measurements the change in optical property sought to report an ionic concentration might be a change in quantum yield, excitation spectra or emission spectra.

This seemingly formidable task has been resolved by Tsien and colleagues, who have developed many probes sensitive to the free Ca^{2+} concentration. The common property of all of these probes is that they are all a fluorescent derivative of the calcium chelator BAPTA, which in turn is an aromatic analog of the commonly used calcium chelator (EGTA, ethylene-glycol bis (β-aminoether) -N,N,N',N' tetraaceticacid) (Figure A11.4). The probes form an octahedral complex, with the calcium ion at the center of the plane formed by the O^- groups of the carboxylic acid. The binding and unbinding of the ion will induce a strain or relaxation on the electron cloud of the aromatic groups, which will in turn result in changes of the spectral properties of the reporter chromophore. Three such reporter chromophores have found much use in the measurement of intracellular free calcium concentrations, namely INDO, FURA-2, and FLUO-3. Each of these probes have a certain number of advantages over the others, depending on the measurement technique sought. INDO and FURA-2 are ratiometric probes, i.e. the change in spectral properties will occur at two different wavelengths, and by measuring the fluorescence intensities at these two wavelengths and taking their ratio one can calculate the absolute value of the free calcium concentration

within the cytosol, given by the following formula (see Grynkiewicz et al., 1985):

$$[Ca] = \frac{R - R_{min}}{R_{max} - R} \times K_i$$

where R_{min} is the ratio at two wavelengths at 0 ion concentration, R_{max} is the ratio at 'infinite' ion concentration, R is the ratio of the measurement and K_i is an instrumental constant unifying instrumental parameters together with the K_D of the chromophore for calcium.

The major advantage of the ratiometric probes is the fact that they are insensitive to the intensity of the emitted light, which changes from the center to the periphery of most of the cells, because of differences in thicknesses at the center and towards the edges, thus more chromophores in the center than the edges.

INDO's emission properties at 405 nm and 480 nm change upon binding to Ca^{2+} (λ_{exc} = 350 nm). The two emission intensities can easily be measured by using a beam splitter, two interference filters and two photomultipliers; it is fairly difficult to envisage the use of two intensified cameras to form an image unless one uses a specifically split CCD array. Therefore INDO has found much application in processes that require either the rapid determination of the free calcium concentration, i.e. cell sorting, or where the kinetics of the free calcium change are fast.

FURA-2 (Figure A11.5) upon binding to calcium undergoes a change in its absorption spectrum and therefore in its excitation spectrum, namely the emission intensity (collected at λ_{em} = 520 nm and higher) increases at λ_{exc} = 340 nm and decreases at λ_{exc} = 380 nm. A typical property of all the indicators that undergo either an excitation or emission shift is the presence of an 'isosbestic point', namely the presence of a 'unique point' in the spectrum when the parameter sought is changed (calcium in the case of FURA-2). The isosbestic point will be present only when two species are in equilibrium (in our case calcium-bound and free forms of FURA-2 or of INDO). The absence of this point can be taken as an indication of contamination by another ion. This point appears at 360 nm for FURA-2 (Figure A11.5). As FURA-2 undergoes a change in its absorption properties, alternating the excitation filters at the two chosen wavelengths, mostly at 340 and 380 nm, and collecting the emission above 510 nm with an intensified camera, one can construct the free calcium image, or the time series of the changing free calcium in a living cell, by calculating the free calcium concentration at each pixel (picture element). One is not limited to these two wavelengths; it might even be advantageous to take the images at longer wavelengths than 340 nm as most

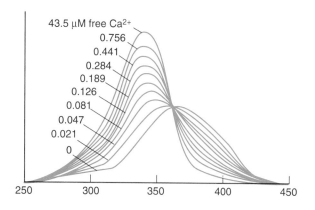

Figure A11.5   Excitation spectral changes of FURA-2 as a function of Ca^{2+} concentration.

of the old fluorescence microscopes are opaque to this wavelength. In cases where the kinetics of the intracellular calcium change are fast, one might use the property of the isosbestic point, and take an image at this point before stimulating the calcium increase and can image at the end of the experiment; taking the other images at 380 nm will allow the experimenter to follow calcium changes at video rates. These properties together with the high quantum efficiency and low bleaching made the FURA-2 the indicator of choice for imaging purposes.

With the advent of confocal microscopy, an indicator with absorption properties in the visible part of the spectrum were needed (the confocal microscopes use scanning lasers and lasers in the UV are rather sparse, or very expensive). FLUO-3 was developed to respond to those needs. The main disadvantage of FLUO-3 is that its quantum efficiency increases at one wavelength only (526 nm, when excited at 506 nm) upon binding to calcium. It is therefore not possible to measure absolute values of calcium directly; nevertheless, if the resting levels of the free calcium concentration in the cell are known, the values obtained before stimulation can be used to calculate an approximate value of free calcium concentration as calcium increase is stimulated.

Calcium-Imaging Hardware

Owing to the competing processes that cause a non-radiative transition, the fluorescence quantum yield is rather low, although for some molecules the fluorescence quantum yields are usually in the order of 50% or lower. The main loss of fluorescence emission will be from the collection optics. Because the fluorescence is emitted in all directions, the light collection efficiency of the best microscope objectives cannot be more than 10%. The detector photocathodes (usually poly metal alkali) will have quantum yields in the order of 20%. Even with this highly optimistic approach, it can be seen that for 100 molecules excited, one can expect at most one photon reaching the detector. In reality this figure is much lower. To cope with such low levels of light two resources can be used with a cooled CCD camera integrated for a long time, or an intensified CCD or SIT (silicon intensified target) camera. As the calcium changes in most cells will take few milliseconds, and the decay is in the seconds range, the use of cooled CCD cameras for such dynamics is impossible. The only resource remaining is therefore the use of an intensified CCD or SIT camera. Today the SIT or ISIT camera is rarely used, and the CCDs are gaining favor as microcircuit technology makes great progress.

The Intensifier

Most of the modern cameras use microchannel plates (MCP) as their intensifying entity (Figure A11.6). Basically a microchannel plate is made of millions of glass capillaries pulled together, whose interior surfaces are coated with a metal oxide of low work function. The work function can be thought of as the number of electrons released by electrons impinging on the surface. A large electric field applied to the front and back surfaces will make each of the channels work as an individual electron multiplier, and will accelerate them. With modern microchannel plates, typical gains of 10^4 are not uncommon. A gain beyond this value is not practical because of the noise created by random release of electrons. In summary the modern intensifier will have a photocathode which converts photons into photoelectrons; these electrons are multiplied by the microchannel plate and will fall on a fluorescent screen to form an image. This will be detected by either the camera (SIT) or the CCD coupled to the intensifier via fiberoptic links. Even with an intensified camera there may not be enough signal in most cases. There is the temptation to

increase the concentration of the reporter molecule within the cell, but in the case of calcium measurements, this will have the adverse effect of buffering the calcium and preventing its rise (all the molecules of interest were synthesized taking BAPTA as a model, which is a high affinity chelator for calcium). It is necessary to find a compromise between the signal level and the buffering of the molecule in general, the best approach being the minimal amount of indicator required for the job.

Figure A11.6   Image intensifier (a): the capillaries of the microchannel plate (b) are set at an angle of 14° so that the photoelectrons hit the walls of the capillaries.

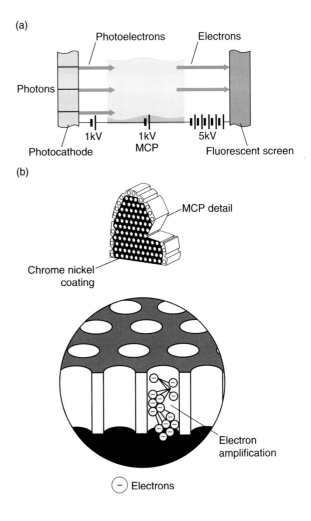

References

Grynkiewicz G, Poenie M, Tsien RY. A new generation of calcium indicators with greatly improved fluorescence properties. J. Biol. Chem. 1985; 260: 3440–3448.

Neher E, Augustine GJ. Calcium gradients and buffers in bovine chromaffin cells. J. Physiol. Lond. 1992; 450: 273–301.

Tsien RY. Fluorescent probes of cell signalling. Annu. Rev. Neurobiol. 1989; 12: 221–253.

Further Reading

Burnashev, N., Monyer, H., Seeburg, P.H. and Sakmann, B. (1992) Divalent ion permeability of AMPA-receptor channels is dominated by the edited form of a single subunit. *Neuron* **8**, 189–198.

Edmonds, B., Gibb, A.J. and Colquhoun, D. (1995) Mechanisms of activation of glutamate receptors and the time course of excitatory synaptic currents. *Ann. Rev. Physiol.* **57**, 495–519.

Huganir, R.L. and Greengard, P. (1990) Regulation of neurotransmitter receptor desensitization by protein phosphorylation. *Neuron* **5**, 555–567.

Jonas, P. and Burnashev, N. (1995) Molecular mechanisms controlling calcium entry through AMPA-type glutamate receptor channels. *Neuron* **15**, 987–990.

Keinänen, K., Wisden, W., Sommer, B. *et al.* (1990) A family of AMPA-selective glutamate receptors. *Science* **249**, 556–560.

McBain, C.J. and Mayer, M.L. (1994) NMDA receptor structure and function. *Physiol. Rev.* **74**, 723–759.

Nakanishi, S. (1993) Molecular diversity of glutamate receptor and implications for brain function. *Science* **258**, 597–603.

Raymond, L.A., Tingley, W.G., Blackstone, C.D., Roche, K.W. and Huganir, R.L. (1994) Glutamate receptor modulation by protein phophorylation. *J. Physiol.* **88**, 181–192.

Schneggenburger, R., Zhou, Z., Konnerth, A. and Neher, E. (1993) Fractional contribution of calcium to the cation current through glutamate receptor channels. *Neuron* **11**, 133–143.

Seeburg, P.H. (1993) The molecular biology of glutamate receptor channels. *Trends Neurosci.* **16**, 359–365.

12

Ionotropic Mechanoreceptors: The Mechanosensitive Channels

The detection of changes in local physical force by mechanosensitive cells plays many important roles in sensory physiology. Our ability to feel the external world via the sense of *touch* represents the most obvious case. Other familiar examples include: the sense of *hearing*, which is generated upon perception of vibrations in the tympanic membrane; the sense of *position*, which depends on proprioceptors in the body's muscles and joints; and the sense of *balance*, which arises from detection of head movements by vestibular hair cells.

In addition to having multiple roles in sensory perception, the detection of mechanical stimuli is also important for several involuntary physiological events. Thus, direct physical stress can modulate local processes such as structural plasticity in bone and the secretion of renin by renal glomerular mesangeal cells. Peripheral mechanosensors can also modulate homeostatic responses via connections with the central nervous system. For example, information concerning changes in vascular distension, detected at *baroreceptors* and *volume receptors*, is relayed to the brain from where it can modulate sympathetic outflow and the secretion of various hormones involved in the regulation of blood pressure and body fluid balance.

In all of these examples the perception of a sensation or the production of a homeostatic response only becomes possible once a physical stimulus has been detected and transduced into a signal that can be recognized by the mechanosensory cell itself, or by its extrinsic cellular targets. In this chapter we focus on the possible involvement of mechanosensitive ion channels as 'ionotropic mechanoreceptors' responsible for the transduction of mechanical stimuli into electrical signals.

12.1 Mechanoreception in Sensory Neurons is Associated with the Production of a Receptor Potential

Some of the cells specialized for the production of mechanically regulated effector responses are intrinsically sensitive to mechanical perturbation. Elongation of some muscle cells, for example, can provoke self-contraction. In such cases, local electrical or biochemical events resulting from the mechanical stimulus are sufficient to trigger an appropriate cellular response. In other instances, however, information concerning the stimulus must be relayed to distinct effector cells. This is particularly important in the nervous system, where the information must be processed by higher-order neurons in order to be perceived, or to produce a coordinated homeostatic response. In these cases mechanical stimuli first modify the frequency or pattern of action potential discharge in a mechanosensory neuron, which subsequently relays these signals to the brain.

Patterns of neuronal spike discharge are strongly influenced by the density and subtypes of ion channels present in the region of the cell responsible for the initiation of action potentials. In mechanosensory neurons, however, the principal factors governing stimulus-evoked changes in firing are the magnitude and time course of the receptor potential (see Figure 12.7), the primary change in membrane voltage provoked by the physical stimulus itself. The process by which a physical stimulus is converted into an ionic current and receptor potential is termed *mechanotransduction*. While the molecular basis for this process remains largely undefined, the introduction of the patch-clamp technique has led to the discovery of a category of ion channels that are uniquely suited to perform such a task: the mechanosensitive channels.

12.2 The Discovery of Mechanosensitive Ion Channels Provided a Potential Molecular Mechanism for Mechanotransduction

In 1984 Guharay and Sachs reported that during patch-clamp experiments on embryonic muscle cells they frequently encountered a cation-permeable channel whose probability of opening could be increased by applying suction to the inside of the recording pipette. The discovery of channels whose activity could be directly controlled by physical stimulation was exciting because it provided a potential molecular mechanism for mechanotransduction. Unfortunately, while mechanosensitive ion channels remain the most likely candidates, direct evidence of their involvement in mechanically regulated physiological processes has been difficult to obtain using single channel recording. This problem stems primarily from the fact that membranes responsible for mechanotransduction are usually embedded within complex cellular structures specialized for the capture and transfer of physical energy. Structural elements required for the channels to operate as mechanotransducers, therefore, are often destroyed by procedures related to cell isolation or patch-clamp recording.

12.3 Structural Basis for the Mechanical Gating of Ion Channels

The regulation of mechanosensitive channels does not result from physically evoked changes in the size of the ionic pore. Indeed, during single channel recordings, changes in activity are observed as variations in the rate of transitions between discrete closed and open states. Thus, as for other types of channels, ion flux through mechanosensitive channels appears to be regulated as if controlled by an all-or-none gate. In ligand- and voltage-sensitive channels the energy

Figure 12.1 Channels with orthogonally anchored gating springs. The channel on the left features a gating mechanism regulated via a coupling molecule attached to an extracellular anchoring site, in this case a membrane-bound protein in an adjacent cell. An arrangement of this type is believed to regulate the mechano-receptor channels of vertebrate hair cells (see Gillespie PG, 1995. Molecular machinery of auditory and vestibular transduction, *Curr. Opin. Neurobiol.* 5, 449–455). The gating apparatus of the channel shown on the right is anchored to a cytoplasmic support site, such as a component of the cytoskeleton. Note that in reality the gates are not directly 'pulled' open or shut by the coupling molecule. Rather, the application of force biases the frequency at which the gate is opened and closed.

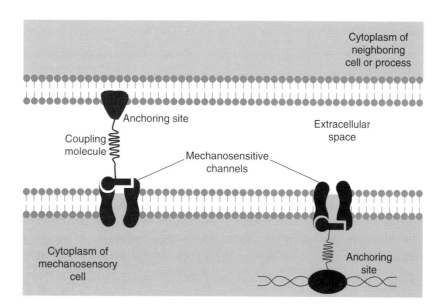

required to control the gate is delivered via allosteric and electrostatic forces generated by ligand binding or changes in transmembrane potential, respectively. In mechanosensitive channels, energy delivered to the gating apparatus appears to be derived from mechanical stimuli via direct physical links with the local environment.

12.3.1 Intrinsic and Extrinsic Forms of Mechanical Gating

Interestingly, some channels appear to be intrinsically capable of sensing changes in shape or tension within the lipid bilayer itself. For example, in 1990 Martinac and colleagues reported that the activity of mechanosensitive channels in liposomes reconstituted from *Escherichia coli* could be modulated by the addition of amphipathic molecules causing differential expansion of the inner or outer leaflets of the lipid bilayer. This observation suggests that interactions with local lipid structure may play a key role in the regulation of some mechanosensitive channels. In most other mechanosensitive channels, however, mechanical gating is modified or abolished by disrupting interactions with extracellular or intracellular elements. The nature of the molecular complex required for this extrinsic regulation of mechanosensitive channels is not yet known. Possible structure–function relations, however, can be inferred by considering the ways by which such channels might be coupled to their physical environment.

12.3.2 Channels Regulated by Coupling Molecules Oriented Orthogonally to the Membrane

Figure 12.1 illustrates hypothetical situations in which force is delivered to the channel gate via extracellular or cytoplasmic coupling molecules whose axes lie normal to the plasma membrane. In both cases, therefore, channel gating would be strongly influenced by orthogonal displacements of the plasma membrane relative to the site of anchoring. During cell-attached single channel recordings, axial tension within an orthogonal coupling molecule anchored intracellularly should increase in response to the application of negative pipette pressure and decrease in response

Figure 12.2   Relationship between orthogonal force and pipette pressure during cell-attached patch-clamp recordings. The patch of membrane isolated during a cell-attached recording is pulled away from the cell as pressure inside the pipette is made negative, and pushed toward the cell interior as the pipette pressure is made positive. Since the tension within an orthogonally directed coupling spring increases with length, orthogonal forces vary as monotonic functions of pipette pressure. However, as shown on the graph, the polarity of the force–pressure relationship depends on the site of anchoring of the coupling spring. The force–pressure relationship of a channel with extracellular anchoring is illustrated for completeness, but could not be measured in the recording configuration illustrated.

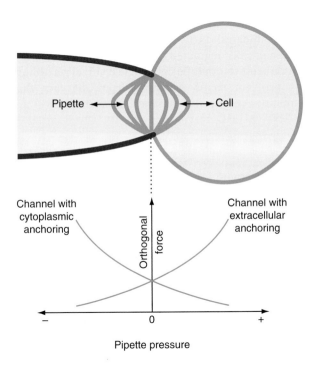

to positive pressure (Figure 12.2). Theoretically, axial tension in a coupling molecule anchored extracellularly would increase in response to positive pipette pressure and decrease in response to suction. Consequently, if an orthogonal coupling molecule regulates channel activity, the latter should vary as a monotonic function of pipette pressure, where the polarity of the response is determined by the site of anchoring. Ion channels with coupling molecules anchored orthogonally may be present in vertebrate hair cells, where extracellular filamentous 'tip-links'

Figure 12.3 Channels with gating springs oriented parallel to the cell membrane. In this diagram, the gating mechanisms of two channels are coupled to a common anchoring site. The anchoring site is illustrated as a membrane-bound protein but could have been replaced by another channel, or by a fixed cytoplasmic molecule located just beneath the plasma membrane. An important functional aspect is that for the channel's gating spring to impart changes in tangential force, the channel must move relative to the site anchoring the coupling molecule. The channels illustrated, therefore, are also attached via springs extending in opposite directions. The latter, which could be anchored to other proteins or channels, are simply placed to emphasize that for *relative* movements to occur, the channels must be stabilized to a component that is physically isolated from the anchoring point of the gating spring.

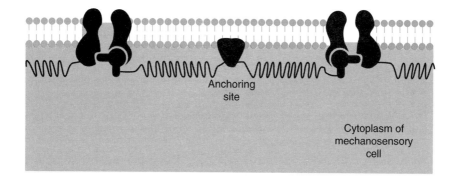

attached to adjacent stereocilia are thought to serve as gating springs for the mechanosensitive transduction channels involved in hearing and vestibular function.

12.3.3 Channels Regulated by Coupling Molecules Parallel to the Membrane

Figure 12.3 shows a different hypothetical architecture for mechanotransduction. In this case the long axes of the coupling molecules are oriented in a plane lying parallel to the plasma membrane. Regardless of how their coupling molecules are anchored (to each other or to other proteins or channels within or near the membrane), channels of this type would be most sensitive to changes in physical force applied in a plane tangential to the cell membrane. Under cell-attached patch-clamp recording conditions, increases in patch curvature evoked by applying either positive or negative pressure to a recording pipette would cause similar increases in tangential force or 'membrane tension' (Figure 12.4). Consequently, the activity of such channels should vary as approximately symmetric functions of positive and negative pipette pressures. Mechanosensitive channels of this type appear to be the ones most frequently encountered during single channel recordings in a variety of prepa-

rations. The apparent preponderance of such channels, however, may simply indicate that channels with a functional parallel coupling architecture are easier to isolate by patch-clamp methods.

12.3.4 Other Gating Configurations

The simplified orthogonal and parallel coupling architectures hypothesized in Figures 12.1 and 12.3 predict distinct functional properties for extrinsically regulated mechanosensitive channels during patch-clamp experiments (see Figures 12.2 and 12.4). While it is possible that these structural configurations may resemble those found in *real* channels, it must be emphasized that the molecular organization of mechanosensitive channels is presently unknown, and may be much more elaborate. Moreover, the presence of angled, or non-elastic, coupling molecules would introduce complicated vectorial bias to channel stretch-sensitivity. Indeed, it is likely that the evolution of multiple varieties of specialized mechanoreceptors has been paralleled by the appearance of varied architectural designs.

Figure 12.4 Relationship between tangential force and pipette pressure during cell-attached patch-clamp recordings. Relative to the cell interior, increases in pipette pressure cause the membrane patch to become concave, whereas suction provokes patch convexity. In both situations, however, the patch of membrane is effectively stretched, such that increased tangential forces are experienced by coupling molecules lying parallel to the plasma membrane.

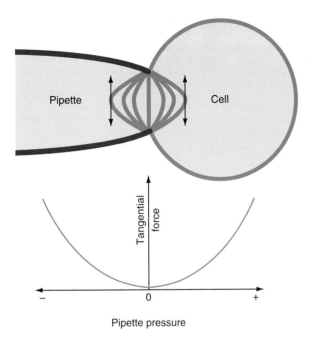

12.4 Classification of Stretch-Sensitive Ion Channels

In the absence of definitive structural information, the classification of mechanosensitive channels identified during patch-clamp experiments has been organized according to their ionic permeability and functional responses to modifications of pipette pressure.

12.4.1 Patch-Clamp Experiments Reveal the Existence of Stretch-Activated and Stretch-Inactivated Channels

As indicated above, the activity of many of the mechanosensitive channels characterized to date has been found to vary symmetrically in response to increases or decreases in pipette pressure. Such channels,

therefore, appear to be regulated by tangential membrane forces, as might result from the intrinsic monitoring of lateral tension within the bilayer, or from an extrinsic parallel coupling architecture (Figure 12.4). Functionally, two classes of symmetrically stretch-sensitive channels are recognized during patch-clamp recordings: those whose probability of opening increases with stretch, or *stretch-activated* channels; and those whose probability of opening decreases with stretch, or *stretch-inactivated* channels. Because tangential forces increase symmetrically as a function of positive and negative pressures (Figure 12.4), stretch-activated channels recorded during patch-clamp experiments display a U-shaped activation curve, whereas stretch-inactivated channels exhibit a characteristic bell-shaped activity profile (Figure 12.5).

12.4.2 Ionic Permeability of Stretch-Sensitive Channels

Stretch-sensitive ion channels have also been characterized according to their various relative permeabilities to different ions. Among the forms most commonly observed are the stretch-activated K^+ channels, which are K^+ selective, and the stretch-activated cationic channels, which are permeable to Ca^{2+}, Na^+ and K^+. Channels selective for either anions (including Cl^-) or Na^+ have also been reported. Through its effect on the equilibrium potential for transmembrane current flux, ionic permeability plays a key role in determining the functional role of mechanosensitive channels.

A wide diversity of mechanically gated channels are therefore recognized during patch-clamp experiments. In the absence of information concerning the molecular biology of defined subtypes of mechanosensitive ion channels, however, it is difficult to predict whether differences in mechanical gating and ionic permeability result from small differences in a common structural motif, or if completely distinct structural units explain the large diversity of mechanosensitive channel types.

12.5 Mechanosensitive Ion Channels and Mechanotransduction

As indicated earlier, many stretch-sensitive channels

Figure 12.5 Activity–pressure profiles of symmetrical stretch-activated and stretch-inactivated channels during patch-clamp experiments. Since tangential forces within a membrane patch increase symmetrically as a function of absolute pipette pressure (Figure 12.4), the activity of mechanosensitive channels having a parallel coupling architecture should also vary in a similar manner. During patch-clamp experiments, stretch-activated channels are distinguishable from stretch-inactivated channels by the opposite profiles of activity they show in response to changes in pipette pressure. The demonstration of U-shaped (stretch-activated) and bell shaped (stretch-inactivated) response profiles under experimental conditions provides strong support for the existence of a parallel coupling architecture in some mechanosensitive channels.

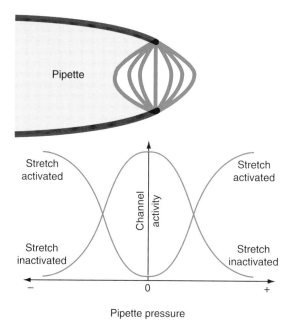

appear to require extrinsic molecules in order to display normal mechanosensitive gating. Since mechanosensory membranes are frequently embedded within cellular structures specialized for the detection of a particular type of stimulus, it has been difficult to obtain direct evidence that mechanosensitive channels function as physiological mechanotransducers using single channel recording. One exception has been the demonstration that stretch-inactivated cationic channels may serve as the molecular mechanoreceptors responsible for signal detection and transduction in *osmoreceptors*. In the remainder of this chapter we

briefly review the physiological role of these unique receptors and examine the biophysical basis for their operation in specialized neurons.

12.6 Osmoreceptors in the Central Nervous System

The existence of specific *osmoreceptors* in the central nervous system has been recognized for 50 years. In mammals, osmoreceptors are important for the coordination of behavioral, autonomic and neuroendocrine responses to perturbations in the volume and osmolality of the extracellular fluid. Thus, receptors of this type have been shown to control sensations such as thirst and appetite for salt, as well as sympathetic vascular tone and the secretion of hormones regulating blood pressure and body fluid balance. Perhaps the best example of osmoreceptor involvement concerns the regulation of the hypothalamo-neurohypophyseal system (Figure 12.6a). In mammals, circulating concentrations of the neurohypophyseal hormone vasopressin increase during hyperosmolality and decrease during hypoosmolality (Figure 12.6b). Because it is the body's chief antidiuretic hormone, increases in vasopressin secretion promote water reabsorption from the kidney and reduce the osmolality of extracellular fluids. Osmotically evoked changes in vasopressin release, therefore, play a fundamental role in systemic osmoregulation.

As illustrated in Figure 12.6a, the somata of the neurons that secrete the neurohypophyseal hormones vasopressin and oxytocin are located in the supraoptic and paraventricular nuclei of the hypothalamus, from where each cell sends an axon to the posterior pituitary. Collectively, these cells are referred to as magnocellular neurosecretory cells (MNCs) in order to distinguish them from the smaller 'parvocellular' hypothalamic neurons that do not project to the posterior pituitary. Hormone release from nerve terminals in the posterior pituitary has been shown to increase as a steep function of the frequency of action potential firing in the neurohypophyseal axons. Thus, hormone secretion into blood is primarily determined by the rate at which the somata of MNCs generate action potentials. The basis for the osmotic regulation of MNCs has been extensively studied in rats, where the release of both oxytocin and vasopressin is regulated in a similar manner by changes in plasma osmolality.

Figure 12.6   A classic example of osmoreceptor involvement: the osmotic regulation of the hypothalamo-neurohypophyseal system. (a) Sagittal view of the hypothalamo-neurohypophyseal system which comprises the somata of magnocellular neurosecretory cells (MNCs) in the supraoptic (SON) and paraventricular (PVN) nuclei of the hypothalamus, and their axon terminals in the posterior pituitary (PP). The axon terminals abut fenestrated capillaries which carry the secreted peptides into the systemic circulation. Individual cells secrete either oxytocin or vasopressin, and both types of MNCs are present in the PVN and SON. Anatomical landmarks illustrated include the optic chiasma (OC) and the anterior pituitary (AP). (b) Summarizes results of radioimmunoassay experiments, in rats, that have characterized how the concentration of vasopressin (VP) varies as a function of plasma osmolality. Note that physiologically significant hormone concentrations are present at the osmotic set point. (c) Summarizes results of electrophysiological experiments, in anesthetized rats, which have shown that the basal firing rate of MNCs is increased by hyperosmolality and decreased by hypoosmolality. (b: Threshold and slope values correspond to regression fits of data obtained in control rats: (From Robertson GL, 1985. Osmoregulation of thirst and vasopressin secretion: functional properties and their relationship to water balance, In Schrier RW, ed., *Vasopressin*, pp. 203–212, Raven Press, New York. Comparable data have been obtained for oxytocin release in rats: From Verbalis JG and Dohanics J, 1991. Vasopressin and oxytocin secretion in chronically hyposmolar rats, *Am. J. Physiol.* **261**, R1028–R1038. c: Threshold and slope values represent averages of data obtained from control rats reported by Walters JK and Hatton GI, 1974. Supraoptic neuronal activity in rats during five days of water deprivation, *Physiol. Behav.* **13**, 661–667 and by Wakerley JB, Poulain DA and Brown D, 1978. Comparison of firing patterns in oxytocin and vasopressin-releasing neurones during progressive dehydration, *Brain Res.* **148**, 425–440.)

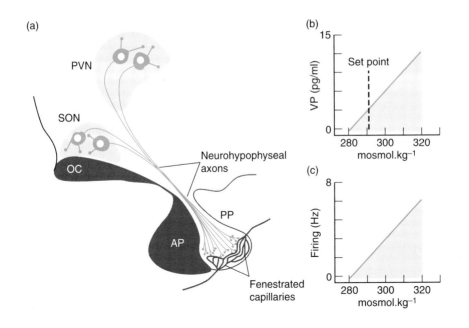

12.6.1 Electrical Activity and Neurohypophyseal Hormone Secretion

Electrophysiological recordings in rats have confirmed that the mean rate at which action potentials are discharged by MNCs *in vivo* varies as a positive function of plasma osmolality. Moreover, as shown in Figure 12.6b,c, the apparent osmotic threshold for neuro-

hypophyseal hormone secretion corresponds to the osmolality at which MNCs become electrically active. Osmoreceptor-mediated control of the hypothalamo-neurohypophyseal system, therefore, primarily reflects the mechanisms by which changes in osmolality modify the rate at which action potentials are discharged by the somata of MNCs.

12.6.2 Magnocellular Neurosecretory Cells in the Hypothalamus are Intrinsic Osmoreceptors

Osmoreceptor neurons located in a number of different brain regions contribute to the osmotic control of vasopressin secretion via synaptic mechanisms. For example, osmosensitive neurons in the *organum vasculosum lamina terminalis*, a midline circumventricular organ, have been found to regulate the firing rate of MNCs via the release of glutamate from axon terminals in the supraoptic nucleus. Osmotically evoked changes in firing rate, however, can also be recorded from MNCs in the absence of synaptic transmission, indicating that these cells behave as intrinsic osmoreceptors. Since they can be easily identified during physiological experiments, rat MNCs have been the focus of recent experiments examining the biophysical basis of osmoreception.

12.7 Osmoreception in Magnocellular Neurosecretory Cells

12.7.1 Osmoreceptor Potentials Reflect the Modulation of a Non-Selective Cationic Conductance

Increases in firing rate recorded from MNCs during hypertonic stimulation are accompanied by membrane depolarization, whereas decreases in firing frequency associated with hypotonicity result from hyperpolarization (Figure 12.7). Current–voltage analysis of MNCs under voltage clamp has revealed that the inward and outward currents generating these osmotic receptor potentials are associated with increases and decreases in membrane conductance, respectively (Figure 12.8). Under physiological conditions, the membrane currents evoked by both stimuli display a common reversal potential (–40 mV), suggesting that they may be mediated by the modulation of a single population of ionic channels. The reversal potential of these currents is not affected by changing the concentration of chloride ions in the external solution. In contrast, lowering the concentration of external Na⁺ shifts the reversal potential of the response toward E_K (Figure 12.8), whereas increasing the concentration of external K⁺ shifts the reversal potential toward E_{Na}. These findings indicate that the receptor poten-

Figure 12.7 Hypothalamic magnocellular neurosecretory cells (MNCs) are intrinsic osmoreceptors. Effects of osmotic stimulation on whole-cell membrane potential recorded from an MNC acutely dissociated from the rat supraoptic nucleus. Spike hyperpolarizing afterpotentials have been erased to highlight changes in membrane potential. Note that an individual cell responds to increased osmolality with membrane depolarization and to hypoosmolality with hyperpolarization. (Adapted from Oliet SHR and Bourque CW, 1993. Steady-state osmotic modulation of cationic conductance in neurons of the rat supraoptic nucleus, *Am. J. Physiol.* **265**; R1475–R1479, with permission).

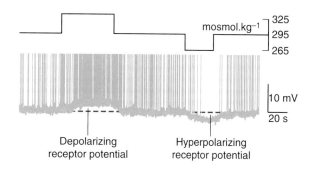

tials associated with osmoreception in vasopressin-releasing neurons result from the osmotic regulation of a macroscopic conductance permeable to both Na⁺ and K⁺.

12.7.2 Changes in Cell Volume Directly Regulate the Macroscopic Cationic Conductance in Magnocellular Neurosecretory Cells

Changes in fluid osmolality provoke inversely proportional changes in cell volume due to the obligatory flux of water across the semi-permeable cell membrane. Changes in cell volume, therefore, have long been assumed to be involved in the transduction mechanism responsible for osmoreception. In agreement with this hypothesis, osmotically evoked changes in cell volume have been found to mirror changes in macroscopic conductance in MNCs, but not in control neurons (Figure 12.9). The tight temporal coupling between changes in cell volume and membrane conductance suggests that the two events are intimately coupled, and may not require the generation of

Figure 12.8 Osmotic stimuli modulate a non-selective cationic conductance in osmoreceptor neurons. Current–voltage relations from isolated MNCs exposed to various osmotic conditions were recorded using the whole-cell configuration of the patch-clamp technique. The osmolality of the extracellular fluid was modified by addition or removal of mannitol in order to maintain constant concentrations of Na^+ and K^+ (upper panels). Traces in (a) show that in normal extracellular solution hypotonic stimuli increase membrane conductance (slope) whereas hypotonic stimuli reduce it. The reversal potential for both responses is approximately –40 mV. Part (b) shows that removing Na^+ ions from the external solution does not prevent osmotically evoked changes in slope conductance. but causes a shift of the reversal potential toward the equilibrium potential for K^+ ions ($\approx$ –98 mV in these recording conditions). (Adapted from Oliet SHR and Bourque CW, 1993. Steady-state osmotic modulation of cationic conductance in neurons of the rat supraoptic nucleus, *Am. J. Physiol.* **265**; R1475–R1479, with permission.)

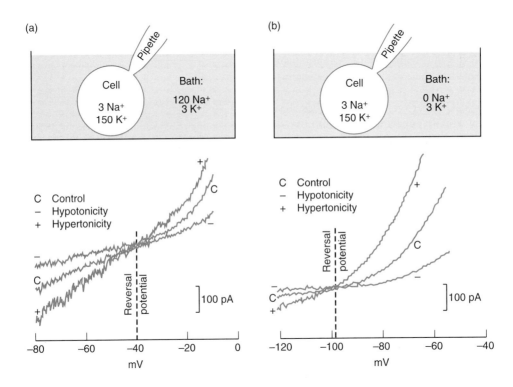

long-lived second messengers. However, transmembrane water fluxes associated with osmotic stimulation produce immediate and proportional changes in the concentration of cytoplasmic solutes (Figure 12.10a). It is possible, therefore, that the cationic membrane conductance of MNCs is regulated by changes in the concentration of one or more cytosolic constituents. This hypothesis was tested directly by examining the effects of eliciting changes in cell volume under constant osmotic conditions. As shown in Figure 12.10b, decreases in cell volume provoked by applying negative pressure to the recording pipette

cause increases in cationic conductance similar to those evoked by hypertonic stimulation (Figure 12.10a). Conversely, decreases in membrane conductance are evoked by increasing cell size either by blowing into the recording pipette, or by exposing the cell to a hypotonic solution. Interestingly, upon changing the concentration of external Na^+ or K^+, identical shifts in reversal potentials are observed for the responses evoked by osmotic stimuli (e.g. Figure 12.8) and those produced by changes in pipette pressure (not illustrated). The membrane conductance regulated by changes in pipette pressure, therefore,

Figure 12.9 Osmotically evoked changes in cationic conductance parallel changes in cell volume in osmoreceptor neurons. In response to the application of a hypertonic stimulus both MNCs (left) and control neurons (right) undergo a decrease in somatic volume (bottom panels). Only MNCs, however, display an accompanying change in membrane conductance (top panels). (Adapted from Oliet SHR and Bourque CW, 1993. Mechanosensitive channels transduce osmosensitivity in supraoptic neurons, *Nature* **364**, 341–343, with permission.)

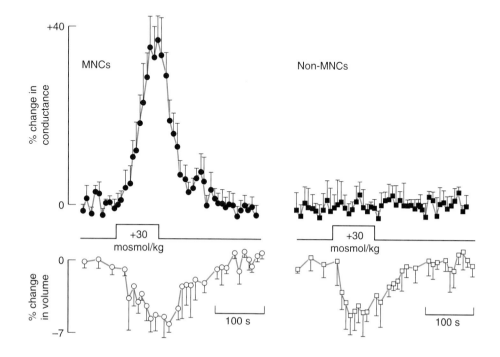

appears to be the same as that modulated by osmotic stimuli. Since the pressure-evoked changes in volume are not associated with changes in solute concentration, the cationic conductance of MNCs appears to be specifically regulated by variations in cell volume, rather than by the concentration, or dilution, of an internal solute.

12.7.3 Magnocellular Neurosecretory Cells Express Stretch-Inactivated Cationic Channels

The existence of a cationic conductance directly regulated by cell volume suggests that volume-regulated ion channels might transduce the effects of osmotic stimuli in MNCs. Cell-attached patch-clamp recordings (see Figure 12.11a) were therefore performed on these cells using pipettes containing various blockers of known voltage- and ligand-gated channels. These experiments revealed the presence of single channels exhibiting a reversal potential of –40 mV and an open channel conductance of 30 pS (Figure 12.11b,c). In individual membrane patches, comparable changes in channel activity could be evoked either by changing the osmolality of the extracellular fluid, or by modifying the pressure inside the recording pipette (Figure 12.11d). These findings suggest that mechanosensitive channels may be responsible for osmoreception in MNCs. Since an unknown amount of residual pipette pressure remains following the formation of a seal between the tip of the pipette and the cell membrane, the functional nature of mechanosensitive channels cannot be determined by examining their response to a single pulse of pressure (see Figure 12.5). As shown in Figure 12.12, the activity of the channels recorded on MNCs varied as a bell-shaped function of

Figure 12.10   Volume changes directly regulate the cationic conductance in magnocellular neurosecretory cells. Panel (a) shows that decreases in volume evoked by hypertonicity are associated with increases in cytoplasmic solute concentration. Panel (b) illustrates that an isotonic decrease in cell volume can be caused by applying suction to the inside of a recording pipette. Corresponding whole-cell current–voltage relations, recorded from a single acutely isolated MNC, reveal that decreases in cell volume evoked either by hypertonicity (a), or by the application of pipette suction (b), cause similar changes in cationic conductance. Note that the reversal potentials of both responses are similar (vertical dashed line drawn through –40 mV). (Adapted from Bourque CW and Oliet SHR, 1995. Mechanosensitive ion channels and osmoreception in magnocellular neurosecretory neurons. In *Neurohypophysis Recent Progress of Vasopressin and Oxytocin Research*. Saito T, Kurokawa K, Yoshida S, (eds). Elsevier Science, BV, Amsterdam, pp. 205–213.)

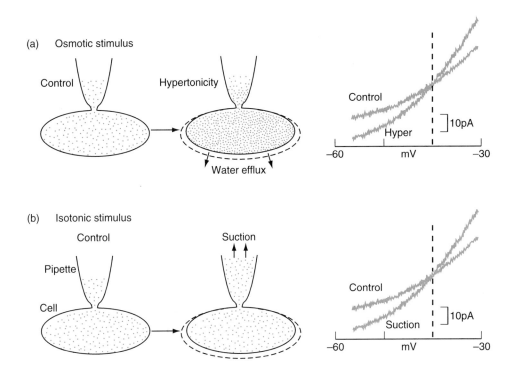

pipette pressure, indicating that they are of the stretch-inactivated variety.

12.7.4 Molecular Basis for Mechanotransduction in Osmoreceptors

Under hypotonic conditions cell swelling would increase tangential force, reducing the activity of the cationic channels and hyperpolarizing the cell (Figure 12.13). Conversely, hypertonic cell shrinking would reduce tangential force, increasing the opening probability of cationic channels and depolarizing the cell. The presence of stretch-inactivated cation channels in rat MNCs, therefore, is consistent with their role as intrinsic osmoreceptors. The involvement of these channels has functional implications concerning the osmotic regulation of the hypothalamo-neurohypophyseal system. Indeed, since channel activity can be virtually abolished by pressure-evoked membrane stretch (Figure 12.12), one should observe complete suppression of the macroscopic conductance under strong hypotonic conditions. The graphs shown in Figure 12.14 confirm this prediction by revealing that the inhibition of macroscopic conductance observed during progressive hypoosmolality saturates near 275 mosmol.kg^{-1}. Thus the osmolality at which the stretch-inactivated channels become active is strikingly similar to the osmotic pressure at which the electrical activity of MNCs and systemic neuro-

Figure 12.11 Osmoreceptor neurons express cationic channels modulated by osmotic stimuli and changes in pipette pressure. Single channel recordings were obtained from isolated MNCs using the cell-attached configuration of the patch clamp technique (a). (b) Shows single channel currents observed at the membrane potentials indicated. The graph in (c) reveals that the single channel has a slope conductance of $\approx$30 pS and a reversal potential near –40 mV. Traces in (d) illustrate recordings from a membrane patch containing at least three channels. Note that channel activity was increased either by applying a hypertonic stimulus (addition of mannitol to the bath), or by raising the pressure inside the recording pipette. Changes in pipette pressure were achieved by blowing or sucking into a tube connected to the patch pipette and were monitored using a water manometer. (Adapted from Bourque CW and Oliet SHR, 1995. Mechanosensitive ion channels and osmoreception in magnocellular neurosecretory neurons, In *Neurohypophysis Recent Progress of Vasopressin and Oxytocin Research*. Saito T, Kurokawa K, Yoshida S, (eds). Elsevier Science, BV, Amsterdam, pp. 205–213, with permission, and from Oliet SHR and Bourque CW, 1993. Mechanosensitive channels transduce osmosensitivity in supraoptic neurons, *Nature* **364**, 341–343, with permission.)

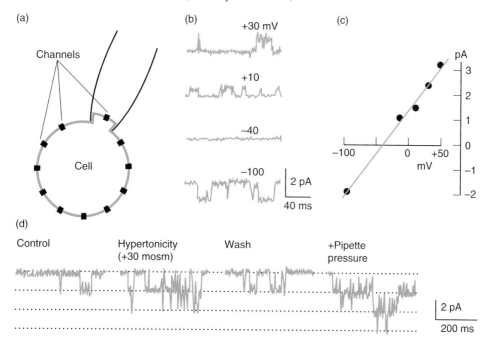

hypophyseal hormone secretion become detectable *in vivo* (Figure 12.6). This observation provides strong support for the involvement of stretch-inactivated cation channels in osmoreception.

12.8 Conclusions

Mechanosensitive ion channels represent obvious candidates as molecular mediators of mechanotransduction, the process by which local physical force is transformed into an electric current. Given the broad range of functions apparently regulated by mechano-receptors, it is not surprising that a large and diverse group of stretch-sensitive channels has been characterized during patch-clamp recording experiments. The observation of channels displaying symmetric or asymmetric forms of mechanosensitive gating implies the existence of a variety of different structural mechanisms by which the gating apparatus may receive physical force from the local environment. In addition to cloning the subunits comprising the pore region of mechanosensitive channels, therefore, it will be important to identify the structure of extrinsic molecules comprising the transduction apparatus regulating their function in specialized types of mechanoreceptors.

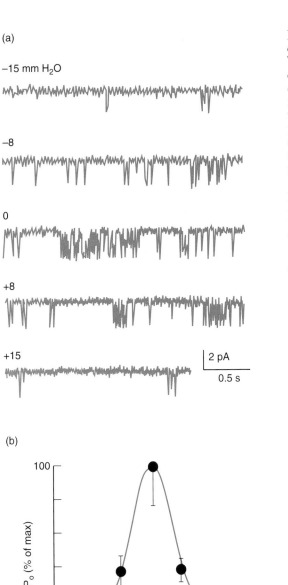

(a)

−15 mm H$_2$O

−8

0

+8

+15

2 pA

0.5 s

(b)

P$_o$ (% of max)

Pressure (mm H$_2$O)

Figure 12.12   Mechanosensitive channels in magnocellular neurosecretory cells are stretch-inactivated. The effects of exposing a single mechanosensitive channel to a wide range of pipette pressures were examined during cell-attached patch-clamp recording from an acutely isolated MNC. (a) Shows representative excerpts of channel activity recorded at the pressures indicated. (b) Shows mean changes in probability of opening (p_o) observed during recordings from many patches, expressed as percentage of the maximal activity recorded in individual patches. The bell-shaped relation between channel p_o and pipette pressure suggests that mechanosensitive channels in MNCs are inactivated by stretch. (b: From Bourque CW and Oliet SHR, 1995. Mechanosensitive ion channels and osmoreception in magnocellular neurosecretory neurons, In *Neurohypophysis Recent Progress of Vasopressin and Oxytocin Research*. Saito T, Kurokawa K, Yoshida S, (eds). Elsevier Science, BV, Amsterdam, pp. 205–213, with permission; and adapted from Oliet SHR and Bourque CW, 1993. Mechanosensitive channels transduce osmosensitivity in supraoptic neurons, *Nature* 364, 341–343, with permission.)

conditions. Whether the mechanosensitivity of such channels is an artifact, or is physiologically relevant, remains to be established. As indicated by Morris (1992), observations of this kind highlight the need for caution when considering the possible role of a mechanosensitive channel in a physiological process.

The biophysical characteristics of stretch-inactivated cation channels in magnocellular neurosecretory cells correspond well with the osmotic regulation of macroscopic conductance, membrane potential and action potential firing. The role of stretch-inactivated channels in osmoreception, therefore, provides one of the clearest demonstrations of the involvement of mechanosensitive channels in a mechanically regulated physiological process.

Further Reading

Guharay, F. and Sachs, F. (1984) Stretch-activated single ion channel currents in tissue-cultured embryonic chick skeletal muscle. *J. Physiol.* 352, 685–701.

Martinac, B., Adler, J. and Kung, C. (1990) Mechanosensitive ion channels of *E. coli* activated by amphipaths. *Nature* 348, 261–263.

Morris, C. E. (1992) Are stretch-sensitive channels in molluscan cells and elsewhere physiological mechanotransducers? *Experientia* 48, 852–858.

Mechanosensitive channels have been observed in a wide variety of cell types, suggesting that they may also perform functions unrelated to mechanosensory transduction. Moreover, recent experiments have revealed that ligand- or voltage-gated channels can display mechanosensitive gating under certain experimental

Figure 12.13   Osmotic modulation of stretch-inactivated channels. The diagram illustrates how cell swelling evoked by hypotonic stimuli may increase tangential force in parallel coupling molecules regulating the gating mechanism of mechanosensitive channels in magnocellular neurosecretory cells. Because channel activity is reduced by stretch, the associated decrease in macroscopic cationic conductance generates a hyperpolarizing receptor potential. Reversing the mechanism explains how a depolarizing receptor potential is generated in response to a hypertonic stimulus.

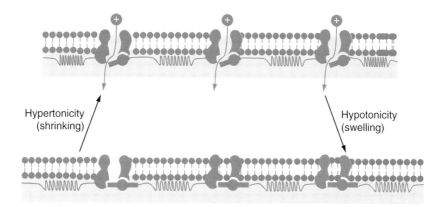

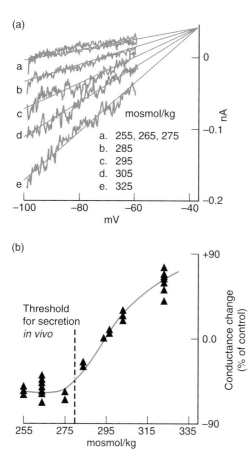

Figure 12.14   Osmotic modulation of macroscopic conductance shows saturation during strong hypotonicity. Traces in (a) show currents recorded in response to voltage ramps applied between −100 and −60 mV during exposure of a single cell to solutions of varying osmolalities. The solid lines extrapolate current–voltage relations to the reversal potential of the cationic conductance (−40 mV). (b) Changes in membrane conductance observed in 22 cells during osmotic stimulation from 295 mosmol.kg⁻¹. Note that decreases in conductance saturate under hypotonic conditions and that the resulting apparent threshold for the osmotically evoked conductance is similar to the threshold for hormone secretion observed *in vivo* (see Figure 12.6). (Adapted from Oliet SHR and Bourque CW, 1993. Steady-state osmotic modulation of cationic conductance in neurons of the rat supraoptic nucleus, *Am. J. Physiol.* **265**, R1475–R1479, with permission.)

Part IV

Metabotropic Receptors in Synaptic Transmission and Sensory Transduction

The GABA$_B$ Receptor

Gamma-aminobutyric acid (GABA) is the primary inhibitory neurotransmitter in the mammalian central nervous system. It is found in virtually every area of the brain. It exerts fast and powerful synaptic inhibition by acting on GABA$_A$ receptors. These receptors are directly coupled to an integral chloride channel and produce inhibition by increasing the membrane chloride conductance (see Chapter 10). This form of synaptic inhibition is critical for maintaining and shaping neuronal communication.

However, like other neurotransmitters that activate fast, ionotropic responses lasting for milliseconds, GABA can activate a second class of receptors which produce slow synaptic responses capable of lasting for seconds. The receptors producing these slow, metabotropic responses are called GABA$_B$ receptors. GABA$_B$ receptors are G-protein-coupled to a variety of different cellular effector mechanisms. These different effectors enable GABA$_B$ receptors to produce not only inhibition, but a variety of other effects on neuronal function as well. Thus, GABA$_B$ receptors enable GABA to modulate neuronal activity in a fashion that is not possible through GABA$_A$ receptors alone.

This chapter will focus on GABA$_B$ receptors and the different effects that these receptors can have on cellular function.

13.1 GABA$_B$ Receptors were Originally Discovered Because of their Insensitivity to Bicuculline and their Sensitivity to Baclofen

The discovery of GABA$_B$ receptors was made possible by the development in the early 1970s of the compound β-parachlorophenyl GABA (baclofen). Baclofen is a GABA analog that can be orally administered and will penetrate the blood–brain barrier (see Section 4.2). It was hoped that after gaining access to the brain this compound would act on GABA receptors and be an effective anticonvulsant.

Indeed, baclofen did mimic many of the actions of GABA and was found to reduce skeletal muscle tone and inhibit spinal reflex activity, making it a successful agent in treating spinal cord spasticity. Yet, despite these similarities with GABA, several important differences between the actions of GABA and baclofen were reported, the most notable of which was that the actions of baclofen were insensitive to the classical GABA antagonist, bicuculline.

It was at this time that Norman Bowery and his colleagues, while attempting to establish a peripheral model of receptors mediating synaptic inhibition, began to investigate the role of GABA in modulating transmitter release. They chose to study the effect of GABA on the release of norepinephrine from the rat isolated atrium. Norepinephrine release was measured using tritium-labeled norepinephrine as a tracer. They found, as predicted, that application of GABA decreased the release of ^{3}H-norepinephrine in a dose-dependent manner. Interestingly, this effect of GABA was insensitive to bicuculline as well as another GABA antagonist, picrotoxin, and was not mimicked by classical GABA agonists, such as isoguvacine and THIP (see Table 10.1). They found similar results when they measured the effect of GABA on the release of ^{3}H-norepinephrine in another peripheral preparation, the rat isolated anococcygeus muscle. In both of these preparations the GABA analog, baclofen, mimicked the action of GABA by depressing the release of ^{3}H-norepinephrine in a dose-dependent manner (Figure 13.1). Futhermore, neither the effect of GABA nor that of baclofen appeared to be mediated by an increase in chloride conductance, suggesting that a receptor other than the classical GABA receptor was responsible for the pre-synaptic inhibition of ^{3}H-norepinephrine release.

To determine whether this bicuculline-insensitive action of GABA was confined to the periphery, Bowery and co-workers tested the effect of GABA and baclofen on potassium-evoked ^{3}H-norepinephrine

Figure 13.1   GABA and baclofen suppress ^{3}H-norepinephrine release from the rat atria. The release of ^{3}H-norepinephrine was assessed by taking samples of the superfusate every 4 min and measuring the tritium content (in dpm) by liquid scintillation spectrometry. Electrical stimuli were delivered to the tissue at times indicated by the open circles. These stimuli caused the release of ^{3}H-norepinephrine and so increased the tritium content of the sample. GABA (filled triangles) and baclofen (filled squares) reduced the release of ^{3}H-norepinephrine by the stimulus. The effect of these drugs was insensitive to co-application of bicuculline methobromide. (From Bowery NG, Doble A, Hill DR, Hudson AL, Turnbull MJ and Warrington R, 1981. Structure/activity studies at a baclofen-sensitive, bicuculline-insensitive GABA receptor, In DeFeudis FV and Mandel P, eds, *Amino Acid Neurotransmitters* Raven Press, New York, with permission.)

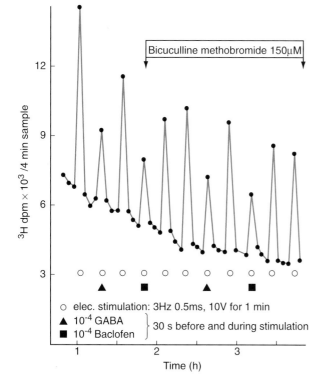

baclofen, but not by other known GABA agonists. Radioligand receptor binding in brain using ^{3}H-baclofen and ^{3}H-GABA demonstrated two distinct binding sites for GABA with different distributions. These results led Bowery and his co-workers in 1979 to propose the existence of a new class of GABA receptors, which they termed GABA_B receptors, while designating the classical GABA receptor as the GABA_A receptor.

13.2 GABA_B Receptors have Unique Properties that Distinguish them from GABA_A Receptors

Since the time of their discovery, many differences between GABA_B and GABA_A receptors have been reported. In particular, GABA_A receptors are ionotropic receptors (receptor channels) and GABA_B receptors are metabotropic receptors coupled through G-proteins to a variety of different intracellular effector systems. These effector systems include adenylyl cyclase, inositol triphosphate synthesis, voltage-dependent calcium channels and potassium channels. These will be discussed in greater detail later in this chapter. However, there are several other important properties of GABA_B receptors that distinguish them from GABA_A receptors. These are discussed below.

13.2.1 GABA_B Receptors are Bicuculline-Insensitive and Baclofen-Sensitive

GABA is the endogenous agonist at both GABA_A and GABA_B receptors. GABA_B receptors are distinguished pharmacologically from GABA_A receptors by their insensitivity to the antagonist bicuculline and their selective activation by the prototypic agonist baclofen (Figure 13.2). Baclofen activates GABA_B receptors in a stereospecific manner with the (–) isomer being about 100 times more potent than the (+) isomer. Baclofen binding to the GABA_B receptor induces a conformational change in the receptor that favors its interaction with G-proteins and the subsequent exchange of guanosine 5'-diphosphate (GDP) for guanosine 5'-triphosphate (GTP).

While they are activated by the selective agonist baclofen, GABA_B receptors are not activated by classical

release from brain slices. They found that, as in the periphery, GABA appeared to suppress ^{3}H-norepinephrine release by acting on a bicuculline-insensitive receptor that was separate from the classical bicuculline-sensitive GABA receptor. This action of GABA was mimicked by the GABA analogue

Figure 13.2   Structures of selected GABA$_B$ receptor agonists and antagonists. (Adapted from Mott DD and Lewis DV, 1994. The pharmacology and function of central GABA$_B$ receptors, *Int. Rev. Neurobiol.* **39**, 97–223, with permission.)

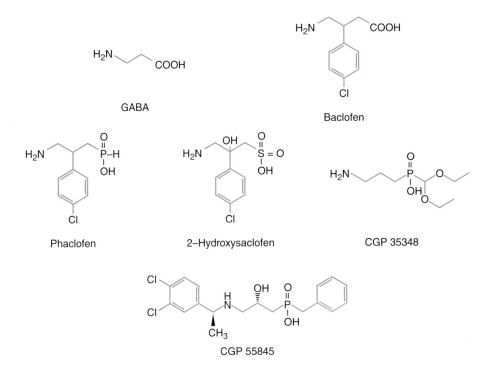

agonists at the GABA$_A$ receptor, such as muscimol and isoguvacine. Similarly, modulators of GABA$_A$ receptors such as benzodiazepines, barbiturates and neurosteroids are ineffective at GABA$_B$ receptors.

GABA$_B$ receptors are antagonized by a variety of agents, such as phaclofen, 2-hydroxysaclofen, CGP 35348 and CGP 55845. The most potent of these agents, CGP 55845, has an affinity for GABA$_B$ receptors ($IC_{50} = 7$ nM) that is higher than that of bicuculline for GABA$_A$ receptors ($IC_{50} = 68$ nM). The development of high affinity GABA$_B$ receptor antagonists has dramatically enhanced our knowledge of this receptor.

13.2.2 Ligand Binding to GABA$_B$ Receptors Requires the Presence of Divalent Cations

GABA$_B$ receptor binding assays using ^{3}H-baclofen or ^{3}H-GABA revealed that divalent cations were required for binding. This differs from GABA$_A$ receptors, which have no such requirement. Several different divalent cations were tested for their ability to increase GABA$_B$ binding and were found to have the following order of potency: $Mn^{2+} = Ni^{2+} > Mg^{2+} > Ca^{2+} > Sr^{2+} > Ba^{2+}$. Their effect was concentration dependent with physiological concentrations of calcium or magnesium being near optimal to promote GABA$_B$ receptor binding. Interestingly, other divalent cations, including Hg^{2+}, Pb^{2+}, Cd^{2+} and Zn^{2+}, were found to inhibit GABA$_B$ receptor binding. The ability of some divalent cations to enhance binding while others inhibit it suggests that the GABA$_B$ receptor is modulated by distinct excitatory and inhibitory cation binding sites.

13.2.3 GABA$_B$ Receptors are Located Throughout the Brain at both Pre-synaptic and Post-synaptic Sites

GABA$_A$ and GABA$_B$ receptors can be found in most regions of the brain. In most of these areas the number of GABA$_A$ receptors is either greater than or equal to the number of GABA$_B$ receptors. However, there are a few brain regions, such as the brainstem and certain thalamic nuclei, where GABA$_B$ receptors can account for up to 90% of the total GABA binding sites.

Electrophysiological recordings have revealed that at a subcellular level GABA$_B$ receptors are located on both pre-synaptic terminals, as Bowery first discovered, where they modulate the release of a variety of different neurotransmitters, as well as on post-synaptic membranes, where they produce post-synaptic inhibition. This subcellular distribution was confirmed using monoclonal antibodies targeted against baclofen (see Appendix 2.2). Following application of the antibody both immunostained terminals and dendrites were observed in several different brain areas, indicating the presence of GABA$_B$ receptors in both pre-synaptic and post-synaptic membranes. The role of these pre-synaptic and post-synaptic GABA$_B$ receptors will be discussed in greater detail later in this chapter (see Section 13.5).

13.2.4 GABA$_B$ Receptors are Thought to Belong to the Superfamily of Receptors with Seven Transmembrane Domains

Unlike the GABA$_A$ receptor, the GABA$_B$ receptor has not yet been cloned. However, it is likely that the molecular sequence of this receptor is more homologous to that of other G-protein linked receptors than with the sequence of the GABA$_A$ receptor. Functional homology of the GABA$_B$ receptor with other G-protein linked receptors, such as adenosine (A1) and serotonin (5HT$_{1A}$), which belong to the family of genes that encode seven transmembrane domain proteins, suggests that the GABA$_B$ receptor also belongs to this family. In fact, antisense oligodeoxynucleotides, targeted against the region of messenger RNA that encodes the homologous second transmembrane spanning region of this class of receptors, reduce the expression of GABA$_B$ receptors that inhibit adenylyl cyclase. Thus, it seems likely that over this highly conserved second transmembrane spanning region, GABA$_B$ receptors bear a strong similarity to members of the seven transmembrane superfamily of receptors. It will be interesting to determine whether other similarities exist when the molecular sequence of GABA$_B$ receptors is finally discovered.

13.2.5 The GABA$_B$ Receptor is an 80 kDa Protein

GABA$_B$ receptor purification is useful both in the effort to determine the molecular sequence of this receptor as well as for determining the exact mechanism by which it couples to effector mechanisms. Purification of the GABA$_B$ receptor from synaptic membranes of bovine brain was achieved through the use of a baclofen-coupled affinity column (see Figure 13.3). Repeated application of solubilized receptor to the column followed by elution with baclofen revealed a purified protein in the affinity eluate. This protein had a molecular weight of approximately 80 kDa. When tested in a GABA$_B$ receptor binding assay, the protein bound ^{3}H-GABA with high affinity. ^{3}H-GABA binding was specifically displaced by the addition of GABA, baclofen or 2-hydroxysaclofen, a GABA$_B$ receptor antagonist, indicating that the purified protein was a GABA$_B$ receptor (Figure 13.3).

13.3 GABA$_B$ Receptors are G-Protein-Coupled to a Variety of Different Effector Mechanisms

In contrast to GABA$_A$ receptors, GABA$_B$ receptors have the potential to produce a variety of different neuronal responses because they are coupled to several intracellular effectors (Figure 13.4). These different effectors enable GABA, acting through GABA$_B$ receptors, to have a broader range of effects than it could by acting on GABA$_A$ receptors alone. The primary actions of GABA$_B$ receptor activation include modulation of adenylyl cyclase activity, inhibition of voltage-dependent calcium channels and activation of potassium channels. In addition, GABA$_B$ receptors have been suggested to alter both inositol triphosphate synthesis and phospholipase A$_2$ activity. However, these latter two effects are controversial and so will not be discussed in this chapter. Instead, we will focus on the effector systems through which GABA$_B$ receptors mediate most of their known effects. GABA$_B$ receptors are coupled to each of these effectors through inhibitory G proteins. Therefore, we will first discuss the evidence linking GABA$_B$ receptors to G proteins and then the different cellular actions mediated by GABA$_B$ receptors.

Figure 13.3 The GABA$_B$ receptor is an 80 kDa protein. A receptor binding assay was used to assess the displacement by GABAergic compounds of GABA binding to a purified 80 kDa protein, thought to be the GABA$_B$ receptor. When added in increasing concentrations, baclofen (open squares), GABA (filled circles) and the GABA$_B$ receptor antagonist 2-hydroxy-saclofen (filled squares) bound to the purified GABA$_B$ receptor, whereas bicuculline (open circles) did not. These results indicated that the purified 80 kDa protein was the GABA$_B$ receptor. (Adapted from Nakayasu H, Nishikawa M, Mizutani H, Kimura H and Kuriyama K, 1993. Immunoaffinity purification and characterization of γ-aminobutyric acid (GABA)$_B$ receptor from bovine cerebral cortex, *J. Biol. Chem.* **268**, 8658–8664, with permission.)

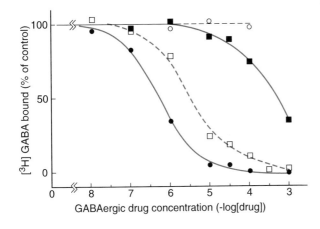

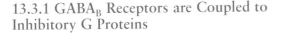

13.3.1 GABA$_B$ Receptors are Coupled to Inhibitory G Proteins

Guanyl nucleotide binding proteins (G proteins) carry signals from activated membrane receptors to effector enzymes and channels. These molecules enable a single receptor to be connected functionally to a variety of different effector mechanisms in a single cell or to different effectors in different cells. Several different G proteins have been identified and these can be divided into several families. In this chapter we will discuss only three classes of G proteins, G$_s$, G$_i$, and G$_o$. These G proteins have opposing effects on adenylyl cyclase with G$_s$ protein stimulating and G$_i$ and G$_o$ protein inhibiting the accumulation of cAMP.

All G proteins are composed of three subunits, termed α, β and γ. While it was thought for many years that the α subunit alone was able to stimulate the effector systems, it has now become apparent that

under certain circumstances, the βγ subunit can also carry a signal. The pathway by which the G protein carries the signal to an effector system begins when an agonist, in this case GABA or baclofen, binds to the GABA$_B$ receptor. This causes the receptor to undergo a conformational change which enhances the binding of the G protein. Binding of G protein with the receptor catalyzes the exchange of GDP for GTP on the α subunit of the G protein. The binding of GTP to the α subunit promotes the dissociation of the G protein from the receptor which causes the receptor to convert back to its low affinity conformation. The G protein further dissociates into its α and βγ subunits which are now free to act independently on an effector such as adenylyl cyclase. The signal ends when an endogenous GTPase in the α subunit converts the GTP back to GDP. This promotes dissociation from the effector and reassociation with the βγ subunit.

GABA$_B$ receptors are coupled to each of their effector systems through G proteins. Coupling of GABA$_B$ receptors and G proteins was originally deduced from binding studies of ^{3}H-GABA and ^{3}H-baclofen to crude synaptic membranes prepared using whole rat brain. In these studies it was hypothesized that if GABA$_B$ receptors were coupled to G proteins then the addition of GTP should promote the dissociation of G protein from the receptor and a corresponding decrease in receptor affinity. This hypothesis was proven correct. It was found that the addition of guanyl nucleotides, such as GTP, did not affect the binding of ^{3}H-GABA to GABA$_A$ receptors, but potently inhibited GABA$_B$ receptor binding (Figure 13.5). This effect was concentration dependent and was not mimicked by adenosine 5'-triphosphate (ATP), indicating that it was specific for guanyl nucleotides. The inhibition of ligand binding produced by GTP was caused by a decrease in GABA$_B$ receptor affinity and not a decrease in the number of available GABA$_B$ receptors. Thus, it was concluded that the addition of GTP promoted the dissociation of G protein from the GABA$_B$ receptor, causing the receptor to revert to its low affinity conformation.

The identity of the G proteins coupled to GABA$_B$ receptors was established through two different experiments. First, it was observed that inhibition of GABA$_B$ receptor binding by GTP was blocked by pertussis toxin. This demonstrated that GABA$_B$ receptors are coupled functionally to inhibitory G proteins, G$_i$ and/or G$_o$. Second, reconstitution experiments were

Figure 13.4   A schematic diagram depicting the major effector systems to which GABA$_B$ receptors are coupled. The dotted lines indicate that the mechanism of coupling to potassium channels has not been conclusively demonstrated. The question marks (?) indicate that GABA$_B$ receptors may also couple to other effectors.

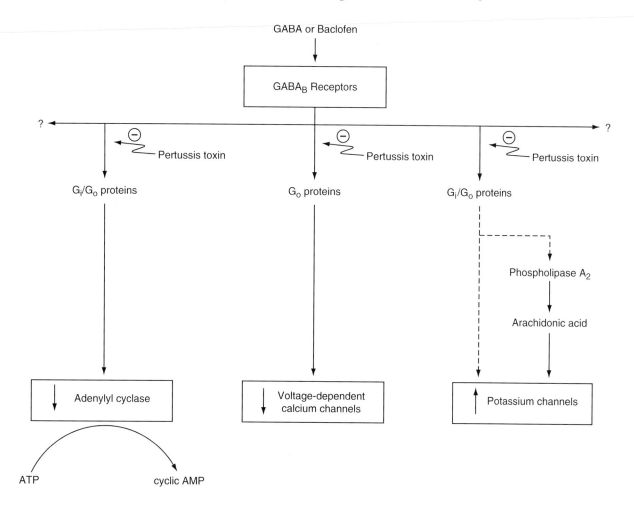

used to identify further the G protein. As mentioned above, agonist binding to G-protein-coupled receptors shows the high affinity state only when G protein is bound to the receptor. Treatment of the membrane with pertussis toxin or N-ethylmaleimide (NEM) ADP-ribosylates the α subunit of both the G$_i$ protein and G$_o$ protein, thereby preventing association of these subunits with the receptor. This causes the receptor to remain in the low affinity conformation. The addition of purified G protein to pertussis toxin- or NEM-treated membrane restores the high affinity binding. For GABA$_B$ receptors in membranes from bovine brain, ^{3}H-GABA binding was increased by the addition of purified G$_o$, G$^*_o$ (see footnote) or G$_{i1}$ but not by the addition of G$_{i2}$ (Figure 13.6). Alterations in the $\beta\gamma$ subunit of the G protein did not affect the ability of G$_o$, G$^*_o$ or G$_{i1}$ proteins to increase ^{3}H-GABA binding, nor did they enable G$_{i2}$ protein to increase ^{3}H-GABA binding. These data indicate that GABA$_B$ receptors are selectively coupled to G$_o$, G$^*_o$ or G$_{i1}$ proteins and that this selective coupling is determined by the α subunit. The ability of GABA$_B$ receptors to couple to a variety of different subtypes of G protein raises the possibility that these receptors are

G$^*_o$ is also named G$_{oB}$ or G$_{o2}$, which corresponds to a splice variant of G$_o$ protein (Goldsmith *et al.* 1988, *Biochemistry* **27**, 7085–7090).

Figure 13.5 The effect of GTP on ³H-GABA binding to GABA_A and GABA_B receptors. ³H-GABA binding to crude synaptic membranes from whole rat brain was measured in the presence of either isoguvacine or baclofen to saturate GABA_A and GABA_B receptors, respectively. The addition of increasing concentration of GTP had no effect on GABA_A receptor binding but produced a concentration-dependent inhibition of GABA_B receptor binding. (From Hill DR, Bowery NG and Hudson AL, 1984. Inhibition of GABA_B receptor binding by guanyl nucleotides, *J. Neurochem.* **42**, 652–657, with permission.)

Figure 13.6 The effect of purified G proteins on ³H-GABA binding to NEM-treated membranes. The ability of baclofen to displace ³H-GABA binding from NEM-treated membranes from bovine cerebral cortex was assessed. The addition of purified G proteins markedly increased baclofen binding. This effect was largest when G_o protein (open circles), $G_o{}^*$ protein (filled circles) or G_{i1} protein (open squares) were added. The addition of brain G_{i2} protein (open triangles) or lung G_{i2} protein (filled triangles) had much less effect. (From Morishita R, Kato K and Asano T, 1990. GABA_B receptors couple to G_o, $G_o{}^*$ and G_{i1} but not to G_{i2}, *FEBS Lett.* **271**, 231–235, with permission.)

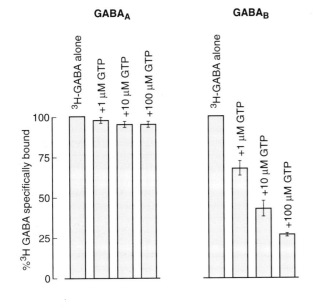

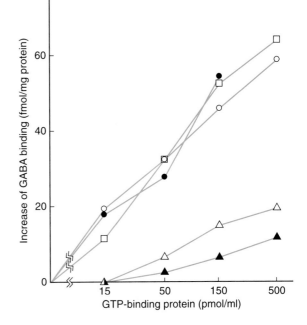

linked to their different effector mechanisms via different G proteins. This possibility will be discussed in subsequent sections as we examine the different effectors to which GABA_B receptors are coupled.

13.3.2 GABA_B Receptors Regulate the Activity of Adenylyl Cyclase

The first effector system we will discuss is adenylyl cyclase. Adenylyl cyclase is an enzyme responsible for converting ATP to cyclic AMP. Cyclic AMP, in turn, activates several different target molecules, such as cyclic AMP-dependent protein kinase, to regulate cellular functions including gene transcription, cellular metabolism and synaptic plasticity. Eight isoforms of adenylyl cyclase (types I to VIII) have so far been iden-

tified. This multiplicity of different isoforms enables cells to show a range of responses to regulatory factors, such as calcium, protein kinase C (PKC), and α and βγ subunits of G proteins.

GABA_B receptors are negatively coupled to adenylyl cyclase

The observation that GABA_B receptors were coupled to inhibitory G proteins raised the possibility that these receptors may be able to modulate adenylyl cyclase activity. To test this possibility adenylyl cyclase activity was measured by the enzymatic conversion of

[α-^{32}P]ATP to cyclic [^{32}P]AMP in crude synaptosomal preparations from a variety of regions of the rat brain. Application of baclofen or GABA caused a decrease in cAMP levels, reflecting a reduction in basal adenylyl cyclase activity (Figure 13.7 a). This decrease was even greater if forskolin was first applied to stimulate adenylyl cyclase activity. The inhibition of cAMP formation by baclofen was blocked by the GABA$_B$ receptor antagonist, CGP 35348, but not by the GABA$_A$ receptor antagonist, bicuculline (Figure 13.7b). Similarly, the GABA$_A$ agonist, isoguvacine, did not alter adenylyl cyclase activity. These results demonstrated a negative coupling between GABA$_B$ receptors and adenylyl cyclase.

GABA$_B$ receptors are negatively coupled to adenylyl cyclase through inhibitory G proteins

Receptor coupling to adenylyl cyclase is accomplished through G proteins. Negative coupling of GABA$_B$ receptors to adenylyl cyclase suggested that the G protein involved in the transduction mechanism was either G$_i$ or G$_o$ protein. To test this hypothesis the effect of baclofen on adenylyl cyclase activity was measured after application of pertussis toxin. Under these conditions, baclofen had no effect on cAMP accumulation. Since pertussis toxin selectively inactivates G$_i$ proteins and G$_o$ proteins, these results demonstrate that GABA$_B$ receptors are linked to adenylyl cyclase through one or both of these G proteins.

Reconstitution experiments have also been used to demonstrate that GABA$_B$ receptors are linked to adenylyl cyclase through inhibitory G proteins. Purified phospholipids were combined with purified GABA$_B$ receptors, partially purified G$_o$ protein/G$_i$ protein, partially purified adenylyl cyclase and GTP to form a reconstituted membrane preparation. This preparation was then incubated with forskolin, to activate the adenylyl cyclase, and either baclofen or GABA, to activate the GABA$_B$ receptors. In theory, during this incubation the baclofen or GABA should bind to the GABA$_B$ receptor, causing a decrease in the formation of cAMP by adenylyl cyclase as compared with the level of cAMP formation in the absence of baclofen or GABA. This was exactly what happened (Figure 13.7c). Furthermore, the inhibitory effect of baclofen and GABA on adenylyl cyclase was antagonized by the addition of the GABA$_B$ receptor

antagonist, 2-hydroxysaclofen, demonstrating that the inhibition was mediated by GABA$_B$ receptors.

To demonstrate the necessity of each element in the preparation, partially reconstituted membrane preparations were prepared. As predicted, inhibition of cAMP formation by baclofen or GABA was not observed if either the GABA$_B$ receptor or the G$_o$ protein/G$_i$ protein was omitted from the preparation. Furthermore, the omission of adenylyl cyclase resulted in the almost complete absence of cAMP formation. The inability of GABA$_B$ receptors to inhibit cAMP formation in the absence of G$_o$ protein and G$_i$ protein indicates that GABA$_B$ receptors are linked to adenylyl cyclase through either or both of these G proteins.

GABA$_B$ receptors facilitate neurotransmitter-mediated activation of adenylyl cyclase

In contrast to its direct inhibition of adenylyl cyclase through G$_o$ proteins and/or G$_i$ proteins, GABA$_B$ receptor activation can also have another seemingly opposite effect on cAMP accumulation. When adenylyl cyclase is stimulated to produce cAMP by a G$_s$-protein-coupled receptor, GABA$_B$ receptor activation will enhance this increase in cAMP accumulation. For example, addition of baclofen enhances by two- to three-fold the increase in cAMP accumulation produced by norepinephrine (β receptors), adenosine (A2 receptors) or vasoactive intestinal peptide (VIP) receptors (Figure 13.8). This effect is contrary to the inhibition of adenylyl cyclase discussed above.

The mechanism of this effect lies in the ability of the $\beta\gamma$ subunit from the G$_i$/G$_o$ protein, liberated by the activation of GABA$_B$ receptors, to synergize the interaction of the α_s subunit of the G$_s$ protein with certain types of adenylyl cyclase. For example, the activation of adenylyl cyclase type II by the α_s subunit is markedly potentiated by the subsequent binding of $\beta\gamma$ subunits. These $\beta\gamma$-subunits can come from either G$_s$ or G$_i$/G$_o$ proteins. In this way adenylyl cyclase type II can act as a molecular 'coincidence detector' by responding only minimally to activation by a single signal but synergistically to the coincident arrival of dual signals through separate pathways.

According to this mechanism, α and $\beta\gamma$ subunits liberated by the activation of GABA$_B$ receptors could produce opposing effects. The α_i/α_o subunits could directly inhibit one type of adenylyl cyclase while the βγ subunits could synergize the stimulation of adenylyl cyclase type II by α_s subunit. This α_s subunit was generated by the interaction of another neurotransmitter with a G_s-coupled receptor. Depending upon the overall balance between the inhibitory and stimulatory effect of these two processes on adenylyl cyclase activity, this could result in a net increase in cAMP accumulation. Thus, $GABA_B$ receptor activation has the potential to regulate the activity of a variety of G_s-protein-coupled neurotransmitters.

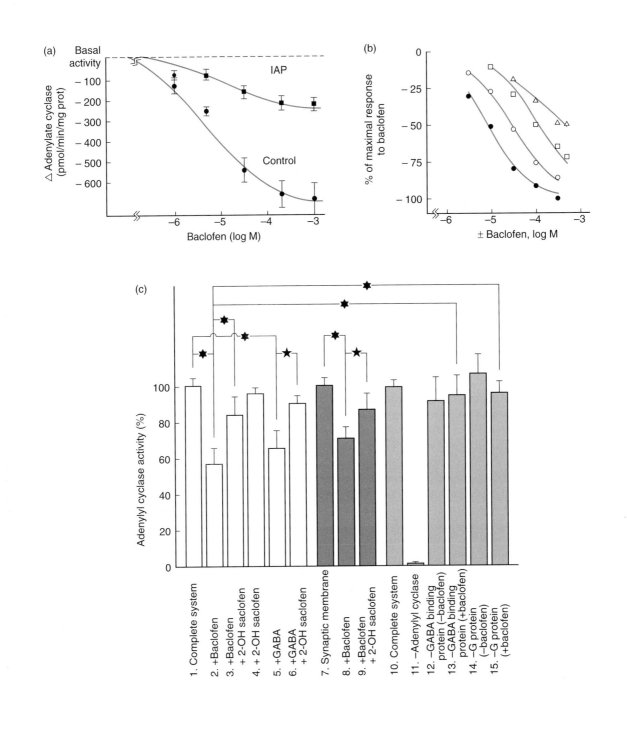

13.3.3 GABA$_B$ Receptor Activation Inhibits Voltage-Dependent Calcium Channels

The second effector system that is coupled to GABA$_B$ receptors that we will discuss is voltage-dependent calcium channels. These channels are one of the major elements controlling the entry of calcium into neurons. Multiple types of voltage-dependent calcium channels exist in neuronal membranes. These channels are termed voltage dependent because they are activated by depolarization of the neuronal membrane. Based on the level of depolarization required for activation, they have been divided into two groups, low voltage activated (LVA, see Appendix 17.4) and high voltage activated (HVA, see Section 7.5). Within each group the channels are further classified according to their electrophysiological and pharmacological characteristics. These different classes of calcium channels play different roles in neuronal function. For example, HVA N-type, P-type and Q-type channels have been implicated in the control of neurotransmitter release, whereas LVA T-type channels are thought to control neuronal oscillatory activity, including spontaneous and repetitive burst firing. HVA L-type channels participate in action potential generation and signal transduction.

Pioneering experiments

The entry of calcium through voltage-dependent cal-cium channels is modulated by a variety of different neurotransmitters, including GABA acting on GABA$_B$ receptors. This receptor is one of the most widespread receptors coupled to inhibition of calcium channels, with GABA$_B$ receptor-mediated inhibition of calcium currents reported in many different types of peripheral and central neurons.

Inhibition of calcium currents by GABA$_B$ receptor activation was first observed in electrophysiological recordings made from neurons in the dorsal root ganglion (DRG). In this preparation both GABA and baclofen were found to decrease the calcium-dependent plateau phase of the action potential (Figure 13.9a). This effect of baclofen was stereo-specific, with (−)baclofen being the active isomer, and was blocked by the GABA$_B$ antagonist, phaclofen, but not the GABA$_A$ antagonist, bicuculline. The inhibition was not mimicked by the GABA$_A$ agonist, isoguvacine.

While these results indicated that the reduction in the plateau phase of the action potential was produced by GABA$_B$ receptor activation, it was possible that the reduction was caused by an increase in an outward potassium current, rather than a decrease in a calcium current. To distinguish between these possibilities it was necessary to examine directly the effects of GABA$_B$ receptor activation on isolated calcium currents. This was accomplished through the use of voltage clamp recordings in DRG neurons. The calcium current was isolated pharmacologically by the appli-

Figure 13.7   GABA$_B$ receptors couple to adenylyl cyclase through inhibitory G proteins. (a) Adenylyl cyclase activity in membranes of cerebellar granule cells was measured by the conversion of [α-^{32}P]ATP to [^{32}P]AMP. In control preparations baclofen decreased the activity of adenylyl cyclase in a concentration dependent manner (filled circles). Treatment of the membranes with pertussis toxin (IAP) antagonized the effect of baclofen on adenylyl cyclase activity (filled squares). (b) The inhibition of adenylyl cyclase activity by baclofen was antagonized in a concentration-specific manner by the GABA$_B$ receptor antagonist, CGP 35348. The inhibition produced by increasing concentrations of baclofen alone (filled circles) was compared with that observed in the presence of baclofen plus either 0.6 mM (open circles), 1.5 mM (open squares) or 5 mM (open triangles) CGP 35348. (c) The effect of baclofen and GABA on adenylyl cyclase activity measured in reconstituted membranes (open bars), synaptic membranes (filled bars) and partially reconstituted membranes (striped bars). Note that the removal of the G protein from the reconstituted system (#15) blocked the inhibitory effect of baclofen (#2). See text for details. Significant differences are indicated by an asterisk (*) signifying $p < 0.05$ or a star (★) signifying $p < 0.01$. (a: From Xu J and Wojcik WJ, 1986. Gamma aminobutyric acid B receptor-mediated inhibition of adenylate cyclase in cultured cerebellar granule cells: blockade by islet-activating protein, *J. Pharmacol. Exp. Ther.* **239**, 568–573, with permission. b: Adapted from Holopainen I, Rau C and Wojcik WJ, 1992. Proposed antagonists at GABA$_B$ receptors that inhibit adenylyl cyclase in cerebellar granule cell cultures of rat, *Eur. J. Pharmacol. Mol. Pharmacol. Section* **227**, 225–228, with permission. c: From Nakayasu H, Nishikawa M, Mizutani H, Kimura H and Kuriyama K, 1993. Immunoaffinity purification and characterization of γ-aminobutyric acid (GABA)$_B$ receptor from bovine cerebral cortex, *J. Biol. Chem.* **268**, 8658–8664, with permission.)

Figure 13.8   The effect of GABA$_B$ receptor activation on norepinephrine stimulated cAMP accumulation. (a) The effect of different GABA$_B$ receptor agonists on the cAMP accumulation produced by 100 µM norepine-phrine in rat brain cerebellar slices is shown. Baclofen (open circles), kojic amine (open squares) and GABA (open triangles) were applied at increasing concentrations in the presence of norepinephrine. All of the GABA$_B$ ligands produced a marked potentiation of the cAMP formation produced by the norepinephrine. (b) Baclofen (100 µM) potentiates the cAMP formation induced by increasing concentrations of norepinephrine. The effect of norepinephrine alone (open circles) and norepinephrine plus baclofen (filled circles) is shown. (From Karbon EW, Duman RS and Enna SJ, 1984. GABA$_B$ receptors and norepinephrine-stimulated cAMP production in rat brain cortex, *Brain Res.* **306**, 327–332, with permission.)

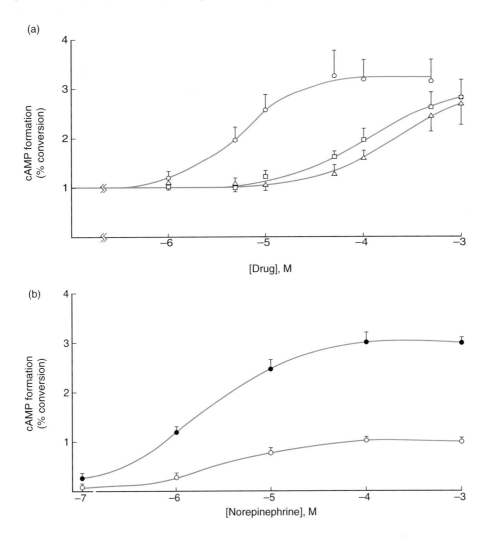

cation of blockers of sodium (tetrodotoxin) and potas-sium (cesium, tetraethylammonium) currents. Under these conditions a +80 mV depolarizing step in the membrane voltage from a holding potential of −80 mV evokes a large, sustained inward current. This current is a calcium current since it is blocked by the addition of cadmium, a calcium channel blocker, or by exchanging calcium in the external solution with the impermeant divalent cation manganese. Baclofen and GABA reversibly reduced the amplitude of this current (Figure 13.9b,c). In contrast, in the same preparation these drugs had no effect on the amplitude of a phar-

Figure 13.9   Baclofen suppresses voltage-dependent calcium currents in DRG neurons. (a) The effect of baclofen on the action potential in a DRG neuron. Baclofen (100 μM; bac) reversibly depressed the calcium-dependent plateau phase of the action potential compared with control (con) or wash (rec). (b) In the same preparation 50 μM baclofen depressed the pharmacologically isolated calcium current (bottom). This current was evoked by a depolarizing voltage step from −80 mV to 0 mV (top). See text for details. (c) The current–voltage relationship for the voltage-dependent calcium current in a DRG neuron is shown in control (con), in 100 μM baclofen (bac) and after 5 min of wash (rec). The current–voltage curve represents the amplitude of the calcium current evoked by a voltage step from the holding potential of −80 mV to a variety of test potentials. Baclofen markedly inhibited the calcium current. (From Dolphin AC, Huston E and Scott RH, 1990. GABA$_B$-mediated inhibition of calcium currents: a possible role in presynaptic inhibition, In Bowery NG, Bittiger H and Olpe H-R, eds. *GABA$_B$ Receptors in Mammalian Function*, Wiley, Chichester, with permission.)

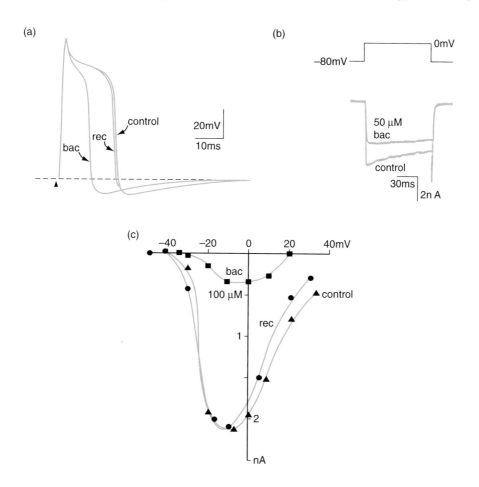

macologically isolated voltage-activated potassium current nor did they affect the holding current, suggesting no effect on the resting potassium conductance. This evidence indicated that GABA$_B$ receptor activation could depress voltage-dependent calcium currents in DRG neurons. Similar studies of pharma-cologically isolated calcium currents in several different cell types have confirmed subsequently that GABA$_B$ receptor activation can inhibit voltage-dependent calcium currents in many different types of both peripheral and central neurons.

GABA$_B$ receptors inhibit a variety of voltage-gated calcium channels

The voltage-dependent calcium current evoked in a given cell is typically produced by the activation of several different calcium channel types (see Figure 7.44). Thus, partial suppression of this current by GABA$_B$ receptor activation could be produced by a partial inhibition of several different channel types or the complete inhibition of only a single type. Because of the different physiological functions of the various voltage-dependent calcium channels, it is important to determine the type(s) of calcium channel inhibited by GABA$_B$ receptors. This can be accomplished through the use of calcium channel antagonists that are specific for different types of calcium channel. The ability of a selective antagonist to occlude further inhibition of a calcium current by baclofen indicates that the antagonist and baclofen are acting on the same subset of channels. Alternately, specific calcium channel antagonists can be used to isolate selectively a single type of calcium current and the effect of GABA$_B$ receptor activation assessed. Finally, kinetic analysis of the calcium current inhibited by GABA$_B$ receptors can be used to determine the electrophysiological characteristics of the inhibited current, which can then be compared with the known properties of identified calcium channels.

Using these techniques, GABA$_B$ receptors have been shown to inhibit a variety of different types of calcium channels, including N-type, L-type, T-type and P-type as well as a type of calcium channel (R-type) that is resistant to blockers of N-type, L-type and P-type (Figure 13.10). Inhibition of N-type calcium channels by GABA$_B$ receptors is the most common and has been seen in many different cell types. In comparison, GABA$_B$ receptor-mediated inhibition of L-type channels is dependent upon the cell type. For example, it is observed in cerebellar granule neurons and hippocampal pyramidal neurons, but not in cerebellar Purkinje neurons, spinal cord neurons or thalamocortical neurons. Similarly, GABA$_B$ receptor-mediated inhibition of T-type calcium channels showed a dependence upon cell type. Baclofen suppressed current through these channels in DRG neurons and interneurons in the *stratum lacunosum moleculare* of the hippocampus, but not in thalamocortical neurons or pyramidal neurons of the hippocampus. Thus, GABA$_B$ receptor activation can inhibit a variety of different types of voltage-dependent calcium channels and the type of calcium channel inhibited depends upon the cell type.

Figure 13.10   Baclofen suppresses the P-type calcium current in cerebellar Purkinje neurons. In the presence of 1 µM ω-conotoxin (CgTX) and 3 µM nimodipine (nimod.) to block N-type and L-type calcium channels a voltage step from −80 mV to +10 mV elicits an inward calcium current (top left). This current is partially inhibited by 50 µM baclofen. Application of the P-type calcium channel antagonist ω-agatoxin-IVA (ω-aga-IVA; 100 nM) partially blocks the current and occludes any further inhibition by baclofen (top right). The time course of the peak calcium channel current amplitude throughout the experiment is shown below. CgTX and nimod. are applied throughout the experiment (open bar), ω-aga-IVA is applied for the period of time indicated by the solid bar. Note that ω-aga-IVA suppressed the calcium current and completely occluded any further inhibition by baclofen, demonstrating that baclofen was acting on the P-type calcium current. In this experiment barium was exchanged for calcium so the currents that were measured represent barium currents through calcium channels. (From Mintz IM and Bean BP, 1993. GABA$_B$ receptor inhibition of P-type Ca^{2+} channels in central neurons, *Neuron* **10**, 889–898, with permission.)

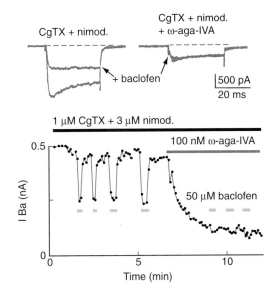

Inhibition of calcium channels is dependent upon G$_o$ proteins

GABA$_B$ receptors inhibit voltage-dependent calcium channels through inhibitory G proteins. The involvement of G proteins was demonstrated in several ways. First, simply omitting the GTP from the pipette solution during whole-cell recording will block the effect of baclofen on the calcium current (Figure 13.11a). This occurs because there is no GTP present to replace that which washes out into the pipette during the experiment. Alternately, loading the cell with guanosine 5'-O-(2-thiodiphosphate) (GDP-β-S), a GDP analog that inhibits the binding of GTP to G proteins, will antagonize the effect of baclofen on calcium currents. Conversely, an enhancement of the baclofen effect can be achieved if cells are loaded with guanosine 5'-O-(3-thiotriphosphate) (GTP-γ-S), a non-hydrolyzable GTP analog that irreversibly activates G proteins. When GTP-γ-S is applied alone it can mimic the effect of baclofen on calcium currents. Exposure of neurons to pertussis toxin blocked the inhibitory effect of baclofen (Figure 13.11a), demonstrating that GABA$_B$ receptors couple to calcium channels through inhibitory G proteins.

The identity of this inhibitory G protein was established through several lines of investigation.

First, cultured DRG neurons were treated with anti-G$_o$ antibodies or anti-G$_i$ antibodies, raised against the C-terminal decapeptide of the α$_o$ subunit of the G$_o$ protein and α$_i$ subunit of the G$_i$ protein, respectively (Figure 13.11b). The hypothesis was that by binding to the G protein one or both of these antibodies would prevent the association of the G protein with the GABA$_B$ receptor and thereby prevent inhibition of the calcium current by baclofen. To enable the incorporation of antibodies into the cells, DRG neurons were replated immediately before recording. Antibodies in the culture medium could then enter the cells as their neurites and attachment plaques were severed. The amount of inhibition of the N-type calcium current produced by baclofen was evaluated for each group of antibody-treated cells and compared with the level of baclofen-induced inhibition in untreated cells. The inhibition of the N-type calcium current produced by baclofen was reduced only in the group of neurons treated with the anti-G$_o$ antibodies, indicating that baclofen couples to N-type calcium channels through a G$_o$ protein.

Second, the ability of baclofen to inhibit calcium currents in cultured DRG neurons was evaluated after antisense oligonucleotides had been used to knock down the expression of G$_o$ or G$_i$ proteins. DRG neurons were injected with 20-mer phosphorothioate antisense oligonucleotides complementary to a unique sequence in either the α$_o$ subunit of the G$_o$ protein or the α$_i$ subunit of the G$_i$ protein or a nonsense sequence. Inhibition of calcium current by baclofen was unaffected in neurons injected with the nonsense oligonucleotide and with the oligonucleotide complementary to the α$_i$ subunit of the G$_i$ protein. However, baclofen-induced inhibition of the calcium current was reduced in neurons injected with the α$_o$ oligonucleotide. Immunocytochemical localization of the α$_o$ subunit of the G$_o$ protein using a confocal microscope demonstrated the presence of this protein in the plasma membrane of control cells as well as in cells treated with nonsense oligonucleotide and α$_i$ oligonucleotide. However, the level of this protein was markedly reduced in neurons treated with the α$_o$ oligonucleotide, indicating that this oligonucleotide specifically reduced the expression of the α$_o$ subunit of the G$_o$ protein. Similarly, the α$_i$ subunit of the G$_i$ protein was present in the membrane of control cells as well as in cells treated with nonsense oligonucleotide and α$_o$ oligonucleotide, but substantially reduced in cells treated with α$_i$ oligonucleotide. These findings indicate that both oligonucleotides were capable of specifically reducing the expression of the α subunit of the G protein for which they were targeted but that only the reduction in the α$_o$ subunit of the G$_o$ protein resulted in a suppression of the effects of baclofen.

G$_o$ proteins inhibit calcium currents through a direct interaction with the calcium channel

The mechanism by which GABA$_B$ receptor-activated G$_o$ proteins couple to calcium channels is also of importance. In theory, the α$_o$ subunit of the G$_o$ protein could inhibit the calcium channel by physically interacting with the channel itself or it could activate an enzyme that would produce a second messenger that would diffuse to the channel and cause the inhibition. However, the experimental evidence indicates that a direct interaction between the G$_o$ protein and the calcium channel is most likely. In these experiments, cell-attached patches in DRG neurons were used to determine whether the inhibition of calcium currents produced by baclofen involved a diffusible second messenger. It was hypothesized that if baclofen, applied outside the patch pipette, was able to inhibit calcium currents then a second messenger must be involved to relay the signal to calcium channels in the area of membrane under the patch pipette. This is not what happened. Baclofen applied outside the patch pipette did not affect the amplitude of calcium

Figure 13.11   GABA$_B$ receptors are coupled to calcium channels through G$_o$ protein. (a) Calcium currents in cerebellar granule cells were evoked by stepping from a holding voltage of –80 mV to a test voltage of +10 mV. Current was expressed as a percentage of the maximal current in the cell at the beginning of the experiment. Bath application of baclofen (100 µM; baclo) for the time indicated by the filled bar reduced the size of the calcium current (left). This inhibition was antagonized by removal of GTP from the internal pipette solution (center) and by pretreatment of the neurons 12–16 h earlier with pertussis toxin (PTX) (right). These observations indicate that GABA$_B$ receptors mediate inhibition of calcium channels through inhibitory G proteins. (b) The effect of anti-G protein antibodies on the inhibition of the calcium current by baclofen in dorsal root ganglion neurons. Calcium currents were evoked by a voltage step from –80 mV to 0 mV as shown (top recordings in A–C). **A**: In the presence of non-immune serum (ser) 50 µM baclofen (bac) markedly inhibited the calcium current from its control (con) level. This effect was reversible upon washout (rec) of the baclofen. **B**: In the presence of a 1:50 dilution of anti-G$_o$ antibodies (OC1) targeted to the C-terminal peptide of α$_o$ protein the effect of baclofen on the calcium current was antagonized. **C**: At the same dilution, the anti-G$_i$ protein antibodies (SG1) had no effect on the inhibition of the calcium current produced by baclofen. **D**: A bar chart showing the average maximal inhibition of the calcium current produced by baclofen in cells treated with either no serum (con; n=18), serum with no antibodies (ser; n=15), serum with anti-G$_o$ antibodies (OC1; n=4) or serum with anti-G$_i$ antibodies (SG1; n=20). (a: From Amico C, Marchetti C, Nobile M and Usai C, 1995. Pharmacological types of calcium channels and their modulation by baclofen in cerebellar granules, *J. Neurosci.* **15**, 2839–2848, with permission. b: Adapted from Menon-Johansson AS, Berrow N and Dolphin AC, 1993. G$_o$ transduces GABA$_B$-receptor modulation of N-type calcium channels in cultured dorsal root ganglion neurons, *Pflügers Arch.* **425**, 335–343, with permission.)

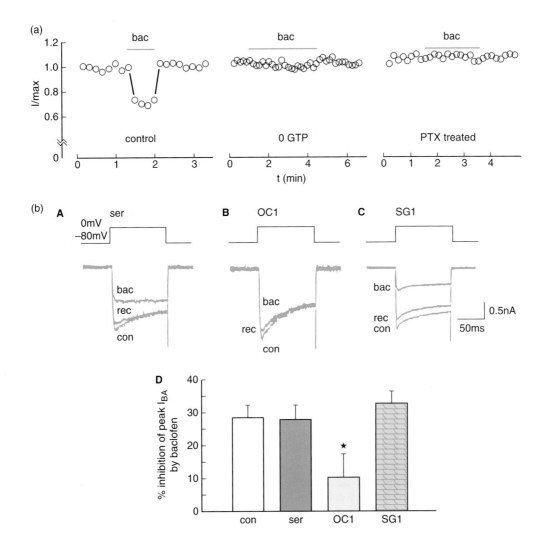

currents in cell-attached patches. However, in the same cell, baclofen applied inside the patch pipette produced clear inhibition of the calcium current, demonstrating that baclofen was able to inhibit calcium currents in these cells. The inability of baclofen, applied outside the patch pipette, to inhibit calcium channels under the patch indicates that a diffusible second messenger was not involved in the inhibition. Thus, GABA$_B$ receptor-activated G$_o$ protein appears to inhibit calcium currents through a direct interaction with the calcium channel.

However, it has also been reported that under some circumstances second messengers may contribute to the inhibition of calcium currents produced by GABA$_B$ receptors. These second messengers may produce inhibition by regulating the degree of phosphorylation of calcium channels. In particular, diacylglycerol and protein kinase A and C have been suggested to mediate this regulation. Thus, the G$_o$ protein that couples GABA$_B$ receptors to voltage-dependent calcium channels is capable of interacting directly with the calcium channel itself; however, under certain circumstances, second messenger systems may also contribute to the interaction.

GABA$_B$ receptors inhibit calcium channels by altering their voltage dependence

It was originally proposed that G-protein-coupled receptors, such as GABA$_B$ receptors, that inhibit calcium channels do so by reducing the number of functional calcium channels. However, subsequent experiments demonstrated that maximal depolarization of the neuronal membrane could overcome the transmitter-mediated inhibition of the calcium current, a result that cannot be explained by a mechanism that involves a reduction in the number of functional channels. Instead, it appears that receptor activation induces a large shift in the voltage dependence of channel activation. Thus, following exposure to the transmitter, almost all of the channels are still fully functional and can be opened by a maximal depolarization. However, a percentage of the channels undergo a shift in voltage dependence so that they are no longer opened by small to moderate depolarizations. In practice this means that a transmitter, such as GABA, is able to inhibit the calcium current during activation by low to moderate depolarization but the

inhibitory effect of the transmitter is lost during strong depolarizations (Figure 13.12). In light of this, calcium channels have been proposed to exist in two states termed 'willing' and 'reluctant' to describe their ease of activation. These two states exist in equilibrium and according to the following model where C$_{willing}$ is the closed channel in the absence of transmitter, C$_{reluctant}$ is the closed channel in the presence of transmitter, O is the open channel and T is the transmitter:

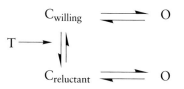

Calcium channels predominantly exist in the willing mode in the absence of transmitter and can be activated by small to moderate depolarizations. In contrast, activation of G$_o$-coupled receptors, such as GABA$_B$ receptors, shifts the balance of the equilibrium to favor the 'reluctant' state in which large depolarizations are required to open the channels.

13.3.4 GABA$_B$ Receptors Activate Potassium Channels

The final effector coupled to GABA$_B$ receptors that we will discuss is potassium channels. Through these potassium channels, GABA$_B$ receptors hyperpolarize the membrane and reduce the input resistance of neurons. For example, a voltage clamp recording from a neuron that is held at a potential of −61 mV will exhibit a strong outward current when baclofen or GABA are applied. In addition, if the neuron is repetitively given brief voltage steps through the recording electrode continuously before and during the application of agonist, the current deflection produced by these voltage steps will increase when agonist is applied (Figure 13.13a,b). This indicates that the input resistance of the membrane has decreased. The extent of the decrease can be calculated according to Ohm's Law which states that:

$$V = I \times R$$

where V is the amplitude of the applied voltage step,

Figure 13.12 Inhibition of the calcium current by baclofen is voltage dependent. (a) In cerebellar Purkinje neurons a voltage step from −80 mV to +20 mV (top) in the presence of 1 μM ω-conotoxin and 3 μM nimodipine evokes a P-type calcium current (bottom). This current is suppressed by the subsequent application of baclofen (50 μM) and recovers following washout of the baclofen. (b) The inhibition of this P-type calcium current by baclofen is voltage dependent. This graph shows the amplitude of the calcium current evoked by depolarizing steps to a variety of different test potentials in control (filled circles), 50 μM baclofen (open triangles) and after washout of the baclofen (open circles). The holding potential was −80 mV. Baclofen inhibited the current most effectively when it was evoked with voltage steps to potentials below +20 mV. Strong depolarizations were able to overcome the inhibition produced by baclofen. (Adapted from Mintz IM and Bean BP, 1993. GABA$_B$ receptor inhibition of P-type Ca^{2+} channels in central neurons, *Neuron* 10, 889–898, with permission.)

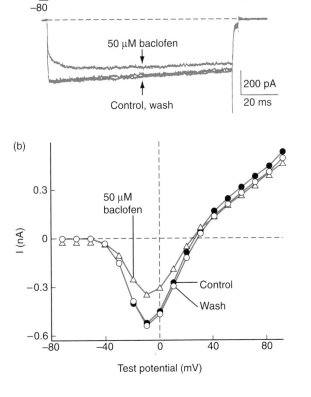

I is the recorded current produced by the voltage step and R is the resistance of the membrane. Rearrangement of this equation to solve for the membrane resistance gives us:

$$R = V/I$$

Thus, by simply dividing the amplitude of the hyperpolarizing voltage step by the amplitude of the current deflection during the pulse, it is possible to calculate the input resistance of the membrane before and during the application of agonist. Since conductance (g) is the inverse of resistance it is now possible to determine the membrane conductance before and during the application of the agonist using the following equation:

$$g = 1/R$$

A decrease in membrane input resistance or an increase in membrane conductance signifies that current can flow more easily through the membrane. In the presence of agonist this means that more ion channels in the membrane are open. This is exactly what happens in the presence of GABA or baclofen. Subsequent application of a GABA$_B$ receptor antagonist, such as 2-hydroxysaclofen or CGP 55845, blocks both the outward current and conductance increase produced by GABA or baclofen, confirming that these effects occur through GABA$_B$ receptors.

The GABA$_B$ receptor-mediated current reverses at the equilibrium potential for potassium ions

Varying the holding potential of the membrane from −41 mV to −121 mV causes the baclofen-evoked outward current to reverse and become inward at potentials below −80 mV. The relationship between the amplitude of the current (I) and the holding potential (V) is expressed in an I/V curve. For the GABA$_B$ receptor-mediated current this I/V curve shows inward rectification (Figure 13.13c). This indicates that over that range of potentials from −41 to −121 the channels pass inward current better than they pass outward current. The point on the I/V curve at which the current is zero is termed the reversal potential. For the GABA$_B$ current illustrated in Figure 13.13c this potential is about −80 mV. This reversal potential corresponds well with the calculated equilibrium potential for potassium ions using the ionic conditions in this experiment. However, in physiological ionic conditions both the reversal potential of the GABA$_B$ current and the equilibrium potential for potassium generally correspond to a potential somewhere between −90 and −95 mV.

The hyperpolarization is caused by the opening of potassium channels

The agreement between the equilibrium potential for potassium and the reversal potential of the GABA$_B$ receptor-mediated current suggested that this current was caused by an increase in the potassium conductance of the membrane. This was further confirmed by increasing the extracellular concentration of potassium ions from 5.8 mM to 17.4 mM (Figure 13.13c). According to the Nernst equation for potassium this should have caused a +29 mV depolarizing shift in the equilibrium potential for potassium. Measurement of the reversal potential of the GABA$_B$ receptor-mediated current indicated a shift of +26 mV, an amount close to that predicted by the Nernst equation. This indicated that the GABA$_B$ current was a potassium current. This conclusion was further confirmed when it was observed that compounds that are known to block potassium channels, such as extracellular barium or intracellular cesium, also blocked the response to baclofen and GABA.

GABA$_B$ receptor-activated potassium channels display flickering behavior

Single channel potassium currents can be recorded from cell-attached patches of cultured hippocampal neurons. These currents appear in response to the application of baclofen or GABA to the extracellular solution outside the pipette. Furthermore, these currents are blocked by the GABA$_B$ receptor antagonist, 2-hydroxysaclofen, but are not affected by the GABA$_A$ antagonist, bicuculline, indicating that they are GABA$_B$ receptor-dependent. As with the whole-cell current discussed above, GABA$_B$ receptor-mediated single channel currents are potassium selective as alterations in the concentration of potassium ions in the pipette cause a corresponding shift in the reversal potential of the single channel current. The single channel current amplitude that occurs with highest probability is about 4 pA (Figure 13.14). This corresponds to a conductance of 67 pS.

A prominent characteristic of these single channel currents is a rapid flickering between open and closed states. In addition to channel closings, this flickering appears to show a variety of different subconductance levels (Figure 13.15a). These different conductance levels are particularly prominent during wash-on and wash-out of the baclofen (Figure 13.15b). Indeed, histograms of the current amplitudes reveal many peaks, which appear to occur at multiples of the smallest peak. This smallest peak represents an elementary current amplitude of 0.36 pA (Figure 13.4), which corresponds to a conductance of 5–6 pS.

During most channel openings and closings, even during large events (> 4 pA), the turn-on and turn-off of the current is extremely rapid. Since the elementary current amplitude is only 0.36 pA, this means that to cause these rapid openings or closings many of these elementary channels would need to open or close synchronously. However, it is extremely unlikely that these channels would behave independently in such a synchronized fashion. Therefore, it has been suggested that these elementary channels function cooperatively. According to this hypothesis, these elementary co-channels would form oligomers of varying size which would function as a single unit. Activation of the oligomer would cause many of the channels to open simultaneously. The flickering behavior of the current would then represent the transient opening and closing of the elementary channels within the oligomer. However, this hypothesis remains to be conclusively demonstrated.

GABA$_B$ receptors are coupled to potassium channels by inhibitory G proteins

Just as they are linked to their other effector systems, GABA$_B$ receptors are coupled to potassium channels through G proteins. This conclusion is based on the observation that GDP-β-S, a hydrolysis-resistant GDP analog, reduced the potassium current produced by baclofen. In contrast, GTP-γ-S, a hydrolysis-resistant GTP analog, mimicked the effect of baclofen. Exposure to pertussis toxin blocked the activation of potassium channels by both baclofen and GABA, indicating that the effect of GABA$_B$ receptors on potassium channels is achieved through either one or both of the inhibitory G proteins, G_i and/or G_o.

The coupling of G proteins to potassium channels requires a second messenger

The exact mechanism by which $GABA_B$ receptors couple to potassium channels is not yet known. It is possible that the G proteins activated by $GABA_B$ receptors could couple directly to the potassium channel or they could activate an enzyme that would produce a diffusible second messenger capable of activating the channel. In support of a direct interaction, it has been demonstrated that the α_o subunit of G_o protein can directly activate potassium channels in cell-free membrane patches. This observation indicates that G_o protein is capable of directly activating

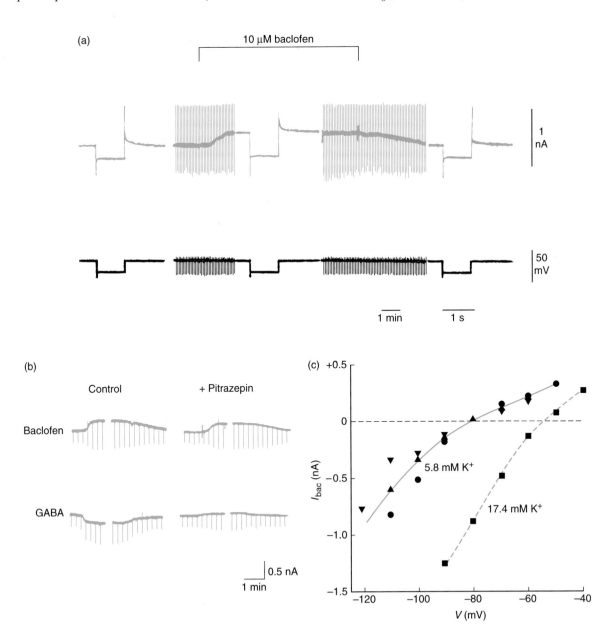

potassium channels but does not tell us whether GABA$_B$ receptors operate through this mechanism.

In contrast, two lines of evidence support a role for a diffusible second messenger capable of coupling the GABA$_B$ receptor-activated G proteins with potassium channels. First, cell-attached patch clamp recordings of GABA$_B$ receptor-activated potassium channels have demonstrated that application of GABA or baclofen to the extracellular solution outside the patch pipette will result in the activation of potassium channels in the area of membrane under the patch pipette. This observation suggests that activation of GABA$_B$ receptors results in the production of a second messenger capable of diffusing to potassium channels under the patch. The onset of potassium channel activity occurs with a delay of about 30–90 s after the exposure of the cell to the agonist, presumably because of the time needed for production and diffusion of a second messenger. Second, excised outside-out patches never exhibited potassium channel activity in response to the application of baclofen or GABA. This most likely occurred because the second messenger system was not available in the excised patch. Thus, unlike their regulation of calcium channels, which occurs through a direct interaction of the G protein with the calcium channel, GABA$_B$ receptors appear to couple to potassium channels through a G-protein-activated diffusible second messenger. However, this does not exclude the possibility that under certain circumstances a direct G-protein interaction with the channels may also occur.

Which second messenger couples GABA$_B$ receptors to potassium channels?

The ability of a GABA$_B$ receptor-coupled second messenger system to activate potassium channels raises the question of the identity of this second messenger. Unfortunately, its identity is, at present, still a matter of some debate. However, several different second messengers can be ruled out. For example, it seems unlikely that cAMP is involved in the interaction because exposure of neurons to 8-bromo-cAMP, a membrane-permeant cAMP analog, is unable to affect the baclofen-induced potassium current. Similarly, the direct intracellular injection of cAMP also fails to reduce the baclofen-activated potassium current. It also appears unlikely that second messengers produced by phospholipase C activation are involved. First, phorbol esters, which activate protein kinase C, do not activate the baclofen-induced current. Second, chelation of intracellular calcium does not inhibit the potassium current, making a role for 1,4,5-IP$_3$ unlikely.

In contrast, a role for phospholipase A$_2$ has been proposed based on the observation that arachidonic acid applied to the inner surface of excised inside-out

Figure 13.13   GABA$_B$ receptor activation produces an outward current that is mediated by potassium ions. (a) In a voltage clamped hippocampal pyramidal neuron baclofen (10 µM) produces an outward current. Both the current (top) and voltage (bottom) recordings are shown. The cell was held at a potential of −61 mV. Voltage steps lasting 1 s were delivered repetitively during the experiment to assess the membrane conductance. At three points in the experiment the recording was expanded to better show the response to the voltage step. Note that in the presence of baclofen the current response to the voltage step increases, indicating an increase in membrane conductance. See text for details. (b) Another voltage clamped pyramidal cell shows a similar outward current in response to baclofen (top left). Baclofen also increased the membrane conductance of this neuron as indicated by an increase in the amplitude of the current deflection in response to repetitive voltage steps (downward deflections). In this cell GABA evokes an inward current and conductance increase (bottom left), suggesting that it is primarily acting on GABA$_A$ receptors. Blockade of the GABA$_A$-linked chloride conductance with pitrazepin (10 µM) has no effect on the baclofen-evoked outward current (top right) but causes the GABA response to become an outward current (bottom right). This occurs because blockade of the chloride current enables us to see the outward current produced by GABA acting on GABA$_B$ receptors. (c) Current–voltage relationship for the baclofen-evoked current in a pyramidal cell when the extracellular concentration of potassium ions is 5.8 mM (circles, triangles) and 17.4 mM (squares). Altering the extracellular potassium concentration depolarized the reversal potential of the baclofen-evoked current, as predicted. See text for details. (Adapted from Gähwiler BH and Brown DA, 1985. GABA$_B$-receptor-activated K$^+$ current in voltage-clamped CA$_3$, pyramidal cells in hippocampal cultures, *Proc. Natl. Acad. Sci. USA* **82**, 1558–1562, with permission.)

Figure 13.14   Baclofen activates single channel currents with a mean amplitude of 4 pA. (a) Some examples of single channel currents evoked by GABA in cultured hippocampal neurons. Currents were recorded in the cell-attached patch configuration and GABA was applied through the bath to the membrane outside of the patch. Currents in the lower two rows were selected for this figure because of their small amplitude. (b) Current amplitude probability histograms of the GABA$_B$ receptor-mediated single channel current. These histograms were constructed from data collected from the same patch as in (a). The graph on the left shows two histograms (solid and dotted line) representing the current amplitudes taken from two unbroken segments of data in this patch. Note that in both cases a channel with an amplitude of about 4 pA occurred with the greatest probability. The histogram on the right was taken from sections of the data that had the smallest currents. The smaller peak corresponds to elementary channel current with an amplitude of 0.36 pA. (From Premkumar LS, Chung S-H and Gage PW, 1990. GABA-induced potassium channels in cultured neurons, *Proc. R. Soc. Lond. B* **241**, 153–158, with permission.)

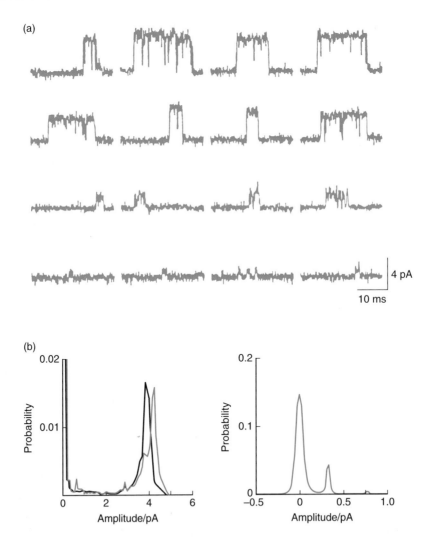

membrane patches mimics the effect of baclofen on single potassium channel currents. The potassium channels activated have similar properties to those activated by baclofen in cell-attached patches.

However, this observation only indicates that this second messenger is capable of mimicking the effect of baclofen and not that it mediates the baclofen response in the intact cell. Thus, the diffusible second messenger that couples GABA$_B$ receptors and potassium channels has yet to be conclusively demonstrated.

13.4 Conclusions

GABA$_B$ receptors differ in several ways from GABA$_A$ receptors. In particular, GABA$_B$ receptors are metabotropic receptors which are G-protein-coupled to several different effector systems. These systems include adenylyl cyclase, voltage-dependent calcium channels and potassium channels. Furthermore, as more information is discovered about these receptors it may become apparent that they couple to other effector systems as well. By coupling to so many different effector systems, GABA$_B$ receptors enable GABA to have a broader range of effects on neurons than it could by acting only on GABA$_A$ receptors. The discussion so far has focused on the intrinsic properties of the GABA$_B$ receptor and the effector systems to which they are coupled. We will now turn our attention to the role that these receptors play in synaptic activity.

13.5 The Functional Role of GABA$_B$ Receptors in Synaptic Activity

GABAergic synapses in the central nervous system contain both GABA$_A$ and GABA$_B$ receptors capable of responding to the synaptic release of GABA. A GABA$_B$ receptor-mediated response is produced by the release of GABA into the synaptic cleft from pre-synaptic terminals in response to action potential invasion of that terminal. This causes the concentration of GABA in the synaptic cleft to rise. The duration of the increase in GABA in the synaptic cleft is very brief (milliseconds) because the duration of the release is very short. In addition, the concentration rise is very brief because the GABA that is released quickly diffuses out of the synaptic cleft and there exists an avid uptake system to actively remove GABA from the synaptic cleft (see Section 10.5.1). These systems combine to tightly regulate GABA concentration in the synaptic cleft.

GABA that does reach the receptors has the ability to activate GABA$_A$ and GABA$_B$ receptors. Activation of GABA$_A$ receptors produces a rapid, synchronous opening of chloride channels, resulting in a fast inhibitory post-synaptic current. However, because of the rapid disappearance of GABA from the cleft, these channels have very little opportunity to reopen. Thus, whereas the activation rate of the fast inhibitory current is determined by the rate with which GABA binds to the GABA$_A$ receptors, the decay of this current is determined by the mean open time of the channels. In contrast, GABA binding to GABA$_B$ receptors initiates a second messenger-mediated process which is considerably slower. Because of the delay inherent in the second messenger system, GABA has disappeared from the cleft before the GABA$_B$ receptor-mediated response even begins. Thus, the kinetics of this response are determined not by the binding of GABA to the GABA$_B$ receptor but rather by the kinetics of the second messenger system involved.

In response to synaptically released GABA, GABA$_B$ receptors could activate any of the effectors to which they are coupled. The functional effects of GABA$_B$ receptors are exerted by both post-synaptic and pre-synaptic receptors. These GABA$_B$ receptors play very different roles in neuronal function. The primary functional effect of post-synaptic GABA$_B$ receptors is to hyperpolarize the post-synaptic membrane. In contrast, the primary functional effect of pre-synaptic receptors is to inhibit the release of neurotransmitter.

13.5.1 Post-synaptic GABA$_B$ Receptors Produce an Inhibitory Post-synaptic Current (IPSC)

When stimulated by synaptically released GABA, post-synaptic GABA$_B$ receptors can activate several different effector systems. However, their primary effect is to produce an increase in the potassium conductance of the post-synaptic membrane. For a neuron near its resting potential, this increase in potassium conductance produces a large hyperpolarization of the membrane in current clamp which is revealed in a whole-cell voltage clamp recording as an outward current. This outward current, termed an inhibitory post-synaptic current or IPSC, is produced by the summation of the unitary current flowing through each of the GABA$_B$ receptor-activated potassium channels (Figure 13.16a).

The kinetics of the GABA$_B$ receptor-mediated response are slow

Because it is coupled through a second messenger system, the GABA$_B$ receptor-mediated hyperpolarization has a time course that is very different from that produced by an ionotropic receptor channel, such as GABA$_A$ (Figure 13.16b). Measurements of the time required from stimulation of the pre-synaptic terminals to the initiation of the post-synaptic hyperpolarization have ranged from 12 to 35 ms. This onset latency is considerably longer than that of the GABA$_A$

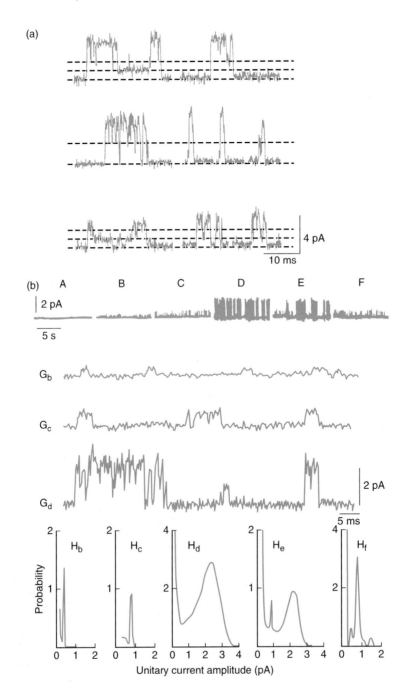

receptor-mediated response, which has an onset latency of less than 3 ms. Once the GABA$_B$ response begins, its rise time is also slow and it does not reach a peak for 130–300 ms. This slow rise time is thought to occur because of the asynchronous activation of potassium channels by the diffusing second messenger. Finally, the response decays back to baseline over the next 200–1300 ms. This slow rate of decay may reflect the rate of GTP hydrolysis, suggesting that it is the decline of activated G protein that ultimately terminates the response. The prolonged duration of the GABA$_B$ response (400–1500 ms) enables GABA to produce inhibition over a much broader time window than would GABA$_A$ receptors alone.

The GABA$_B$ IPSC produces inhibition by hyperpolarizing the neuronal membrane

When pre-synaptic fibers are electrically stimulated to release GABA from their terminals, both a GABA$_A$ IPSC and a GABA$_B$ IPSC are generated in the post-synaptic cell. These IPSCs are produced by the synchronous release of GABA from many pre-synaptic terminals and thus represent the collective response of many GABA receptors.

If the peak amplitude of each of these currents is measured at a variety of different holding potentials a current–voltage (I–V) curve can be generated for each response, relating the peak amplitude of the recorded current to the membrane holding potential. This I–V curve is useful because the slope of the curve indicates the membrane conductance at the peak of the response. By subtracting the resting membrane conductance from this value, the change in membrane conductance produced during the peak of the recorded current can be determined. By using this method it has been found that activation of both GABA$_A$ and GABA$_B$ receptors produces an increase in membrane conductance, reflecting the opening of chloride and potassium channels, respectively. However, the peak increase in membrane conductance produced by activation of GABA$_A$ receptors is much greater than that produced by activation of GABA$_B$ receptors. For example, in hippocampal pyramidal neurons the peak conductance measurements of the GABA$_A$ IPSC range from 90 to 140 nS. This compares with a range of 13 to 19 nS for the peak conductance of the GABA$_B$ IPSC in these same cells. Similar differences between the peak conductance values of GABA$_B$ and GABA$_A$ receptors have been reported in other areas of the brain.

Despite its small conductance, the GABA$_B$ response produces a relatively large hyperpolarization from resting membrane potential in most neurons. This occurs because in physiological ionic conditions the equilibrium potential for potassium is quite negative relative to the resting membrane potential of most cells. Therefore, even though the conductance of the GABA$_B$ IPSC is small, the driving force for potassium is quite large. In fact, because of this large driving force for potassium and the long duration of the GABA$_B$ response, the GABA$_B$ IPSC can move an amount of charge that is close to that carried by the GABA$_A$ IPSC. For example, in granule cells of the dentate gyrus about 8 pC of charge leave the cell during the GABA$_B$ IPSC. This compares favorably to the 9–35 pC that are carried by the GABA$_A$ response.

Figure 13.15   GABA$_B$ single channel currents have multiple subconductance states. (a) Some examples of single channel currents recorded from cell-attached patches of cultured hippocampal neurons. These currents were selected to emphasize different subconductance states of the channels. All currents were evoked by application of GABA except for the current in the panel on the upper right which was evoked by baclofen. Dotted lines indicate different conductance levels. (b) Exposure of a cell to GABA (100 µM) and bicuculline (100 µM) causes the slow development of single channel currents in a cell-attached patch. These currents appear to go through several different conductance states until finally reaching their maximal amplitude. The panel in A represents the baseline response of the patch before the addition of agonist. The panels in B–D show activity in the patch at 25 s (B), 1.5 min (C) and 4 min (D) after the addition of agonist. Panels E and F show patch activity after 5 and 10 min of wash, respectively. The recording in the middle three rows represent an expansion of a portion of the panels shown in B (G$_b$), C (G$_c$) and D (G$_d$). Finally, the current amplitude probability histograms (H$_b$–H$_f$) were produced from data collected at the same times as panels B–F. Note the progressive increase in the current amplitude following the application of GABA. (From Premkumar LS, Chung S-H and Gage PW, 1990. GABA-induced potassium channels in cultured neurons, *Proc. R. Soc. Lond. B* **241**, 153–158, with permission.)

Figure 13.16 Synaptically released GABA activates post-synaptic GABA$_B$ receptors to produce a slow IPSC. (a) Stimulation of inhibitory fibers evokes a stimulus artifact (arrow) followed by a GABA$_B$ receptor-mediated IPSC in a hippocampal neuron. The GABA$_B$ IPSC was pharmacologically isolated from the excitatory synaptic current using DNQX, which blocks AMPA receptors, and APV, which blocks NMDA receptors. It was also isolated from the GABA$_A$ inhibitory current using bicuculline which blocks GABA$_A$ receptors. The neuron was held at a potential of −60 mV in whole-cell voltage clamp. Note the slow onset of the IPSC and its long latency. (b) GABA$_A$ and GABA$_B$ inhibitory post-synaptic potentials (IPSPs) were recorded in current clamp from a dentate gyrus granule cell. These hyperpolarizing potentials were evoked by stimulating inhibitory fibers. They were isolated from glutamatergic excitatory potentials by application of DNQX and APV. GABA$_A$ and GABA$_B$ IPSPs are indicated by an arrow labelled 'A' and 'B', respectively. In control (top left) a stimulus evoked a stimulus artifact (upward deflection) followed by both a GABA$_A$ and GABA$_B$ IPSP, which can be seen as the fast and slow components of the hyperpolarizing response, respectively. Application of picrotoxin blocks the GABA$_A$ IPSP leaving only the slow GABA$_B$ IPSP (top center). The subsequent addition of 2-hydroxysaclofen blocks this GABA$_B$ IPSP. Similarly, in another cell application of 2-hydroxysaclofen to the control response (bottom left) blocks the GABA$_B$ IPSP, leaving an isolated GABA$_A$ IPSP (bottom center). The effect of this antagonist is reversible (bottom right). Note the difference in the time course of the isolated GABA$_B$ IPSP (top center) and the isolated GABA$_A$ IPSP (bottom center). (a: From Mott DD and Lewis DV, unpublished observations. b: From Mott DD and Lewis DV, 1992. GABA$_B$ receptors mediate disinhibition and facilitate long-term potentiation in the dentate gyrus, *Epilepsy Res.* **Suppl. 7**, 119–134, with permission.)

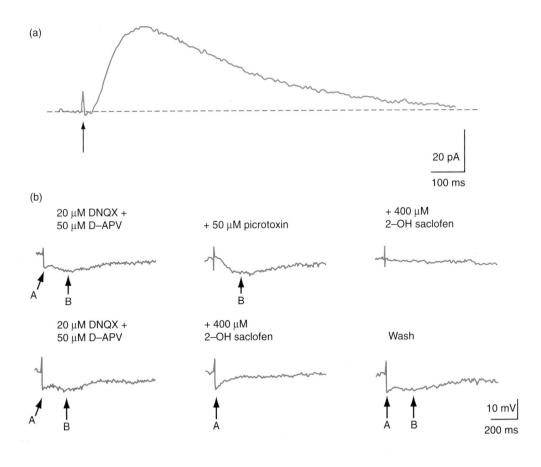

Because it produces a large hyperpolarization with a fairly small conductance increase, the GABA$_B$ IPSC inhibits neurons primarily through hyperpolarization. This type of hyperpolarizing inhibition is particularly effective at suppressing voltage-dependent currents, such as NMDA receptor-mediated responses. However, since it can be overcome by neuronal depolarization, it is not as effective at inhibiting voltage-independent currents. This type of inhibition differs from that produced by GABA$_A$ receptors. GABA$_A$ receptors are associated with a large conductance increase. In addition, the resting potential of most cells is close to the equilibrium potential for chloride, causing the driving force for chloride to be low (see Section 10.5.3). Thus, GABA$_A$ receptor-mediated inhibition is produced primarily by the conductance increase caused by the opening of the GABA$_A$ receptor– chloride channels. This type of inhibition shunts the post-synaptic membrane thereby short-circuiting excitatory responses. This inhibition powerfully suppresses both voltage-dependent and voltage-independent excitatory currents and cannot be overcome by depolarization. Thus, through their coupling to potassium channels GABA$_B$ receptors produce a unique type of neuronal inhibition that differs from that produced by GABA$_A$ receptors in both form and function.

13.5.2 Pre-synaptic GABA$_B$ Receptors Inhibit the Release of Many Different Transmitters

In addition to their presence post-synaptically, GABA$_B$ receptors are also located on pre-synaptic terminals where they can inhibit the release of neurotransmitter. These receptors have been identified on the terminals of GABAergic neurons as well as on the terminals of neurons that release a variety of other transmitters, including, in part, glutamate, dopamine, serotonin and norepinephrine. Indeed, GABA$_B$ receptors were discovered when Bowery and his colleagues observed that GABA or baclofen inhibited the release of norepinephrine from neurons in the rat isolated atrium, indicating the presence of GABA$_B$ receptors on the terminals of these neurons.

Most evidence demonstrating that GABA$_B$ receptors can inhibit transmitter release has been obtained using applied agonists. This begs the question of whether pre-synaptic GABA$_B$ receptors are synaptically activated. In theory, these receptors could be synaptically activated by the diffusion of GABA from its release site to the GABA$_B$ receptor on the terminal of interest. Indeed, this has been shown to be the case for both glutamate and GABA release. In particular, inhibition of GABA release by pre-synaptic GABA$_B$ receptors has been especially well examined. It has been demonstrated conclusively that synaptically released GABA can feedback onto GABA$_B$ receptors on pre-synaptic GABAergic terminals to suppress the subsequent release of GABA from that terminal.

Pre-synaptic GABA$_B$ autoreceptors inhibit the release of GABA

When GABA is released from the pre-synaptic terminal it not only diffuses to the post-synaptic membrane, but some fraction of the released GABA feeds back onto GABA$_B$ receptors located on the activated terminal or onto pre-synaptic GABA$_B$ receptors on other nearby GABAergic terminals. These pre-synaptic GABA$_B$ receptors, when activated, suppress the release of GABA from the terminal. Consequently, activation of the terminal a second time, during this GABA$_B$ response, results in a reduced release of GABA, causing both the GABA$_A$ IPSC and GABA$_B$ IPSC evoked by the second activation to be smaller.

This effect can be clearly observed if paired electrical stimuli are used to activate GABAergic axons that synapse onto a neuron which is recorded in whole-cell voltage clamp (Figure 13.17). The first stimulus evokes the release of GABA, resulting in the production of a GABA$_A$ IPSC (Figure 13.17a). However, a second identical stimulus delivered 300 ms later, during the peak of the GABA$_B$ suppression of GABA release, evokes a GABA$_A$ IPSC that is greatly reduced (Figure 13.17b). Application of the GABA$_B$ antagonist, 2-hydroxysaclofen, blocks the reduction in the second IPSCs, indicating that the suppression is mediated through GABA acting on GABA$_B$ receptors. The ability of pre-synaptic GABA$_B$ receptors to suppress both GABA$_A$ and GABA$_B$ IPSCs endows the GABAergic system with a powerful feedback mechanism capable of suppressing GABAergic inhibition in an activity-dependent manner.

Figure 13.17 Pre-synaptic GABA$_B$ receptors cause paired pulse depression of IPSCs. (a) The pharmacologically isolated GABA$_A$ IPSC in a neuron in the somatosensory cortex is reversibly blocked by bicuculline. This GABA$_A$ IPSC was evoked by electrical stimulation of inhibitory fibers and recorded in whole-cell voltage clamp. It was isolated from the excitatory synaptic current by applying CNQX, which blocks AMPA receptors, and APV, which blocks NMDA receptors. The neuron was held at a membrane potential of −70 mV, causing the GABA$_A$ IPSC to be an inward current. (b) Under these same conditions if paired stimuli are delivered 300 ms apart the GABA$_A$ IPSC evoked by the second stimulus of the pair is reduced (left). This reduction of the second IPSC is blocked by the GABA$_B$ antagonist, 2-hydroxysaclofen (center). This effect is reversible after washout of the antagonist (right). The cell recorded in this experiment was from a very young (postnatal day 10) rat. In animals of this young age the post-synaptic GABA$_B$ response is developmentally immature, whereas the pre-synaptic GABA$_B$ response is fully developed. This difference in development explains why no GABA$_B$ IPSC is evident in this figure and gives further confirmation that paired pulse depression of IPSCs is mediated by pre-synaptic GABA$_B$ receptors. In older animals both a GABA$_A$ and a GABA$_B$ IPSC are easily apparent and both are depressed by pre-synaptic GABA$_B$ receptors (see Figure 13.18). (Adapted from Fukuda A, Mody I and Prince DA, 1993. Differential ontogenesis of presynaptic and postsynaptic GABA$_B$ inhibition in rat somatosensory cortex, *J. Neurophysiol.* 70, 448–452, with permission.)

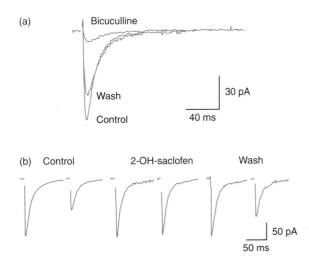

The time course of the depression of GABA release is similar to the time course of the post-synaptic GABA$_B$ IPSC.

Just like the post-synaptic effect of GABA$_B$ receptors, the time course of the inhibition of GABA release by GABA$_B$ receptors reflects a second messenger-coupled mechanism. Following the stimulation of an inhibitory pathway, the onset of the pre-synaptic inhibition is slow reaching a peak about 200 ms after the initial stimulus (Figure 13.18). The duration of the effect is also quite prolonged and can extend for up to several seconds. Thus, although GABA has a brief lifetime in the synaptic cleft, the activation of pre-synaptic GABA$_B$ receptors by this GABA enables it to modulate the subsequent release of transmitter for up to several seconds.

Do GABA$_B$ receptors suppress transmitter release by inhibiting voltage dependent calcium channels?

The mechanism underlying the inhibition of transmitter release by pre-synaptic GABA$_B$ receptors is unknown. The ability of GABA$_B$ receptors to inhibit voltage-dependent calcium currents appears to be the most likely explanation. However, it is important to understand that most studies that have demonstrated the inhibition of voltage-dependent calcium channels by GABA$_B$ receptors have used calcium channels on neuronal somata as a model for those on nerve terminals. This was done because the direct study of nerve terminals is hampered by their electrophysiological inaccessibility. Therefore, although these studies demonstrate that GABA$_B$ receptor activation can inhibit calcium currents, they do not directly indicate that this same action occurs on nerve terminals or that it is involved in modulating the release of neurotransmitter. Thus, we still await direct evidence supporting a role for GABA$_B$ receptor-mediated inhibition of calcium channels in regulating transmitter release.

13.6 Conclusions

GABA$_B$ receptors enable GABA to produce a variety of effects on neuronal function. These receptors are located both post- and pre-synaptically where they can be activated by synaptically released GABA. Post-

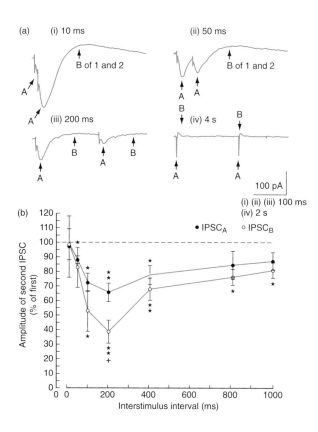

(a)

(i) 10 ms — B of 1 and 2, A, A

(ii) 50 ms — B of 1 and 2, A A, B

(iii) 200 ms — B, B, A, A

(iv) 4 s — B, A, A

100 pA

(i) (ii) (iii) 100 ms
(iv) 2 s

(b)

Amplitude of second IPSC (% of first)

● IPSC$_A$ ○ IPSC$_B$

Interstimulus interval (ms)

Figure 13.18 Paired pulse depression of IPSCs is maximal when stimuli are delivered 200 ms apart. (a) Isolated GABA$_A$ and GABA$_B$ IPSCs were recorded in whole-cell voltage clamp from dentate gyrus granule cells. Since the cell was held at a membrane potential of −80 mV, the GABA$_A$ IPSC is an inward current and the GABA$_B$ IPSC is an outward current. Inhibitory fibers were electrically stimulated to evoke IPSCs. Paired stimuli were delivered at increasing intervals to determine the time course of the inhibition of GABA release produced by pre-synaptic GABA$_B$ receptors. Responses to paired stimuli at four different intervals are shown. In this cell suppression of the second IPSC was greatest when the stimuli were delivered 200 ms apart. GABA$_A$ and GABA$_B$ IPSCs are indicated by an arrow labeled 'A' and 'B', respectively. (b) Graph of the averaged data obtained from six cells showing the time course of the suppression of the second IPSC. It can be clearly observed that for both the GABA$_A$ and GABA$_B$ IPSC the second response is maximally depressed when the stimuli are delivered about 200 ms apart. As can be seen in this graph, the time course of the pre-synaptic GABA$_B$ receptor-mediated response is very similar to that for the post-synaptic GABA$_B$ response. Asterisks indicate a significant depression of the IPSC (*$p < 0.05$, **$p<0.01$); (+) indicates that the GABA$_B$ IPSC was significantly more depressed than the GABA$_A$ IPSC. (From Mott DD, Xie CW, Wilson WA, Swartzwelder HS and Lewis DV, 1993. GABA$_B$ autoreceptors mediate activity-dependent disinhibition and enhance signal transmission in the dentate gyrus, *J. Neurophysiol.* **69**, 674–691, with permission.)

synaptic GABA$_B$ receptors generate a slow inhibitory current that is carried by potassium ions. This current produces a hyperpolarizing inhibition, which is important for inhibiting voltage-dependent conductances, such as NMDA receptor-mediated responses. Pre-synaptic GABA$_B$ receptors can inhibit the release of a variety of different neurotransmitters, including GABA. The ability of GABA$_B$ receptors to regulate GABA release provides an important mechanism for the feedback control of both GABA$_A$ and GABA$_B$ inhibition. Thus, by acting at both post- and pre-synaptic sites, GABA$_B$ receptors have the potential to produce profound changes in neuronal function.

Further Reading

Bowery, N.G., GABA$_B$ receptor pharmacology. *Annu Rev. Pharmacol. Toxicol.* **33**, 109–147, 1993.

Gage, P. W., Activation and modulation in neuronal K$^+$ channels by GABA. *Trends in Neurosci.* **15**, 46–51, 1992.

Lewis, D. V., Mott, D.D., Swartzwelder, H. S. and Xie, C.W., The role of presynaptic GABA$_B$ receptors in stimulus-dependent disinhibition and the induction of long-term potentiation. In *Presynaptic Receptors in the Mammalian Brain*, ed. T. V. Dunwiddie and D. M. Lovinger, Birkhaeuser, Boston, 1993, pp. 161–179.

Wojcik, W. J. and Holopainen, I., Role of central GABA$_B$ receptors in physiology and pathology. *Neuropharmacology* **6**, 201–214, 1992.

The Metabotropic Glutamate Receptors

The amino acid glutamate is the primary excitatory neurotransmitter in the mammalian central nervous system (CNS). In its role as a neurotransmitter, glutamate mediates its actions on cells by activation of two major classes of glutamate receptors: the ionotropic glutamate receptors and the metabotropic glutamate receptors. As discussed in Chapter 11, the ionotropic glutamate receptors are ligand-gated cation channels and these receptors mediate the fast excitatory synaptic responses to glutamate. In contrast, the metabotropic glutamate receptors (mGluRs) are coupled to various second messenger cascades through GTP-binding proteins, and these receptors mediate the slow, or neuromodulatory, actions of glutamate in the nervous system.

In this chapter, we will address what is currently known about the structure and function of the members of the mGluR family. The cloning, second messenger coupling, and some specific physiological roles of the mGluRs in regulation of neuronal excitability and synaptic transmission will be discussed.

14.1 The Discovery of Metabotropic Glutamate Receptors

The role for glutamate as the neurotransmitter mediating fast excitatory synaptic transmission in the CNS has been clearly established. Neuronal excitability and transmission within glutamatergic neuronal circuits can be modulated by several different neuroactive substances, including norepinephrine, serotonin adenosine, GABA, and many others. The neuromodulatory actions of these substances are mediated by activation of receptors that couple to second messenger systems via GTP binding proteins (G proteins). Until recently, it was believed that modulation of transmission through glutamatergic circuits occurred only through the actions of these extrinsic neuromodulatory inputs. However, the discovery by Sladezcek and co-workers in 1985 that glutamate can stimulate phosphoinositide (PI) hydrolysis in cultured striatal neurons suggested that glutamate receptors coupled to second messenger systems by G proteins might exist. At approximately the same time, a study by Nicoletti and co-workers showed that excitatory amino acids stimulate PI hydrolysis in slices of rat hippocampus. With the demonstration in 1987 that certain quisqualate-induced currents elicited in *Xenopus* oocytes injected with rat brain mRNA were sensitive to inhibition by pertussis toxin, which inactivates certain G proteins, the presence of a true 'metabotropic', or G-protein-coupled glutamate receptor in brain was confirmed.

The finding that G-protein-coupled glutamate receptors exist in brain suggests that glutamate not only mediates fast excitatory synaptic transmission in the CNS, but may also act to modulate transmission through the same neuronal circuits.

14.2 Cloning of a Family of Metabotropic Glutamate Receptors

14.2.1 The mGluR Family

In 1991, two independent groups successfully cloned the first metabotropic glutamate receptor (mGluR1) by expression cloning in *Xenopus* oocytes using a rat cerebellar cDNA library. mGluR1 was found to couple to activation of phospholipase C (PLC) and resultant stimulation of phosphoinositide hydrolysis. Hydrophobicity analysis of the deduced amino acid sequence of mGluR1 suggests that the protein may have seven transmembrane domains, similar to other G-protein-coupled receptors. Interestingly, however, mGluR1 shares no sequence homology with other G-protein-coupled receptors, suggesting that mGluR1 is a member of a distinct gene family.

Using the nucleotide sequence for mGluR1, several different groups have used homology strategies to pull out other mGluR clones. To date, eight distinct mGluR gene products have been cloned (mGluR1–mGluR8). Of these receptors, multiple splice variants have been found for mGluR1 (a,b,c), mGluR4 (a,b) and mGluR5 (a,b)

14.2.2 Subclassification of mGluRs

The eight mGluR subtypes can be placed into three main groups based on similarities in sequence, pharmacological profiles, and coupling to second messenger systems in expression systems (Figure 14.1). The group I mGluRs include mGluR1 and mGluR5, and the splice variants thereof. These receptors share approximately 60% sequence identity, and appear to couple primarily to the PLC/PI hydrolysis cascade when expressed in heterologous expression systems. The group I mGluRs are most potently activated by quisqualate, and are selectively activated by 3,5-dihydroxyphenylglycine (DHPG) relative to the other cloned mGluRs. The group II mGluRs, which couple to inhibition of adenylyl cyclase in expression systems, include mGluR2 and mGluR3. These receptors have 70% sequence identity with each other, but less than 50% homology with the six mGluR clones. The group II mGluRs are potently and selectively activated by (2S, 1'R, 2'R, 3'R)-2-(2',3'-dicarboxycyclopropyl) glycine (DCG-IV). The group III mGluRs (mGluR4,

Figure 14.1   mGluRs can be placed into three main pharmacological groups. Three mGluR groups showing the clones and second messenger coupling of each when expressed in heterologous expression systems, along with the most specific agonist for the clones in each group. Dendrogram shows the approximate sequence identity between the eight cloned mGluRs. AC, adenylyl cyclase; PLC phospholipase C.

	Group	Selective agonist	Transduction
mGluR1 / mGluR5 (63%)	I	DHPG	+PLC
mGluR2 / mGluR3 (68%)	II	DCG-IV	- AC
mGluR4 / mGluR7 (71%) / mGluR8 (74%) / mGluR6 (69%)	III	L-AP4	- AC

(43%, 46% nodes shown in dendrogram)

mGluR6, mGluR7 and mGluR8) also couple to inhibition of adenylyl cyclase when expressed in cell lines. The group III mGluRs share approximately 70% sequence identity within the group, and less than 50% identity with the other four mGluRs. L-2-amino-4-phosphonobutyric acid (L-AP4) is the most potent and selective agonist at the group III mGluRs. Pharmacological evidence obtained from brain slice studies indicates that additional mGluR clones exist that have not yet been cloned.

14.2.3 Structure–Function Relationships of mGluRs

General structure

Hydrophobicity analysis of the primary amino acid sequence suggests that the mGluRs may have seven transmembrane domains, similar to the structure of the other G-protein-coupled receptors (Figure 14.2). All of the cloned receptors have a signal peptide, suggesting that the N-terminal regions of these receptors are extracellular. This region is followed by the seven putative transmembrane domains and a presumably intracellular carboxy-terminal domain. The most highly conserved regions of the mGluR proteins are a hydrophobic domain in the large N-terminal region of the protein, and the C-terminal portions of the first and third putative intracellular loops. Although the mGluRs appear to share some overall structural similarities with other G-protein-coupled receptors, the primary amino acid sequence of the mGluRs shows no homology to these receptors, suggesting that the mGluRs represent a distinct family of G-protein-coupled receptors. Furthermore, analysis of the structure–function relationships of the mGluRs reveals that functional characteristics of these receptors are localized in very different regions of the protein as compared with the other G-protein-coupled receptors.

Agonist binding domains

The ligand binding domain for most G-protein-coupled receptors has been shown to be located in a pocket formed by the transmembrane regions. However, recent evidence suggests that the agonist

Figure 14.2   Construction of chimeric receptors between mGluR1 and mGluR2 indicate that the N-terminal extracellular domain determines the agonist specificity of the mGluRs. Chimeric receptors were constructed by exchanging the large N-terminal domain of mGluR1a (top left, thin line) with that of mGluR2 (top middle, thick line), resulting in a chimeric receptor consisting of the N-terminal domain of mGluR2 and the remainder of the receptor mGluR1a (top right). (Adapted from Takahashi K, Tsuchida K, Taneba Y *et al.*, 1993. Role of the large extracellular domain of metabotropic glutamate receptors in agonist selectivity determination, *J. Biol. Chem.* **258**, 19341–19345, with permission.)

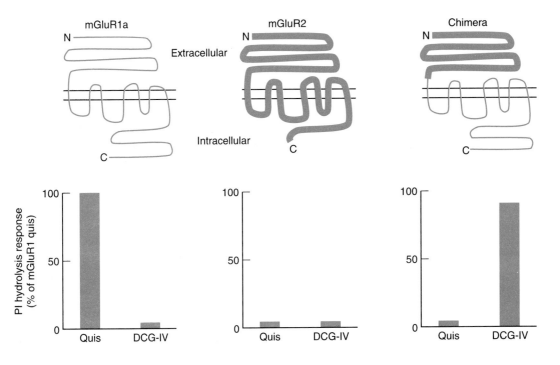

binding site for mGluR may be localized in the large N-terminal extracellular domain. Recall that the group II mGluRs (mGluR2 and 3) are selectively activated by DCG-IV, and are activated with very low potency by quisqualate, which is the most potent agonist known for the group I mGluRs (mGluR1 and 5). By constructing chimeric receptors between mGluR1 and mGluR2 in which the large N-terminal domains are exchanged, one can construct an mGluR that stimulates PI hydrolysis (a group I mGluR characteristic) and is potently activated by DCG-IV and poorly activated by quisqualate (group II mGluR characteristics) (Figure 14.2). These findings clearly implicate the large N-terminal domain of mGluRs in agonist binding. Consistent with this idea, the N-terminal domain of mGluRs shares some homology with bacterial amino acid binding proteins. Point mutations in mGluR1a at residues predicted from the bacterial amino acid binding proteins to be involved in glutamate binding

dramatically alter the affinity of the receptor for glutamate and quisqualate, suggesting that this homology is structurally important for glutamate binding. By comparing the known three-dimensional structure of these bacterial periplasmic binding proteins with the mGluRs, a model was developed in which the N-terminal domain of the mGluR protein forms two globular domains connected by a hinge region, with the glutamate binding domain localized inside the pocket formed by these domains (Figure 14.3). These results support the conclusions of the chimeric receptor studies that the large N-terminal region of the mGluRs contains the ligand binding domain.

G-protein coupling

The G-protein-coupling domains of the receptors for other small molecule transmitters have been studied

Figure 14.3 General structural properties of mGluRs. (a) Schematic diagram of the putative seven transmembrane domain topology of the mGluR family, indicating the regions involved in agonist binding and G-protein coupling. (b) Theoretical model of the structure of mGluRs showing the large globular hinged agonist binding domains. (From a model proposed in O'Hara PJ, Sheppard PO, Thogersen H *et al.*, 1993. The ligand binding domain in metabotropic glutamate receptors is related to bacterial periplasmic binding proteins, *Neuron* **11**, 41–52, with permission.)

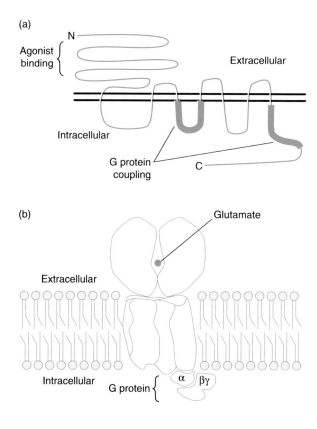

shown that the less conserved second intracellular loop and the proximal portion of the C-terminal tail are critical for the specificity of G-protein coupling in these receptors (see Figure 14.3). Interestingly, although the location within the protein of the G-protein-coupling domains is clearly distinct from that of the other G-protein-coupled receptors, these regions do share some structural similarity with the third intracellular loop of these other receptors. Specifically, the G-protein-coupling domains of the mGluRs are predicted to form amphipathic α-helical stretches similar to those seen in the third intracellular loop of some other G-protein-coupled-receptors. Thus, although the amino acid sequences are not conserved between the mGluRs and other G-protein-coupled receptors, some structural similarities are present in the G-protein-coupling domains.

14.3 mGluRs Couple to a Variety of Second Messenger Systems in Brain

G-protein-coupled receptors can activate many different second messenger cascades. The result of increases in intracellular second messengers is usually activation or inhibition of cellular enzymes that result in changes in cellular function. The second messenger system activated by a given receptor will depend on the structural characteristics of the receptor itself as well as the complement of G proteins and signal transduction molecules expressed in a given cell. Metabotropic glutamate receptors have been found to couple to a wide variety of second messenger systems in various brain regions. Among these second messenger systems are stimulation of phosphoinositide hydrolysis, inhibition of adenylyl cyclase, potentiation of cAMP formation, stimulation of cGMP formation, activation of phospholipase D and stimulation of arachidonic acid release, among others. In addition, evidence suggests that mGluRs can couple to ion channels independent of diffusible second messengers. It is important to note that the fact that a given receptor couples to a given second messenger system when expressed in heterologous expression systems (*Xenopus* oocytes, HEK293 cells, CHO cells, etc.) does not necessarily mean that the same receptor will couple to the same second messenger system *in vivo*.

extensively, and much evidence indicates that this function is localized primarily in the third intracellular loop of these receptors. However, the third intracellular loop of the mGluRs is one of the most highly conserved regions, making this an unlikely candidate for the domain responsible for defining the *specificity* of G-protein coupling for the mGluRs, although it still may be involved in general coupling to G proteins. Using chimeric receptors constructed with different regions of mGluR1c and mGluR3, Pin *et al.* have

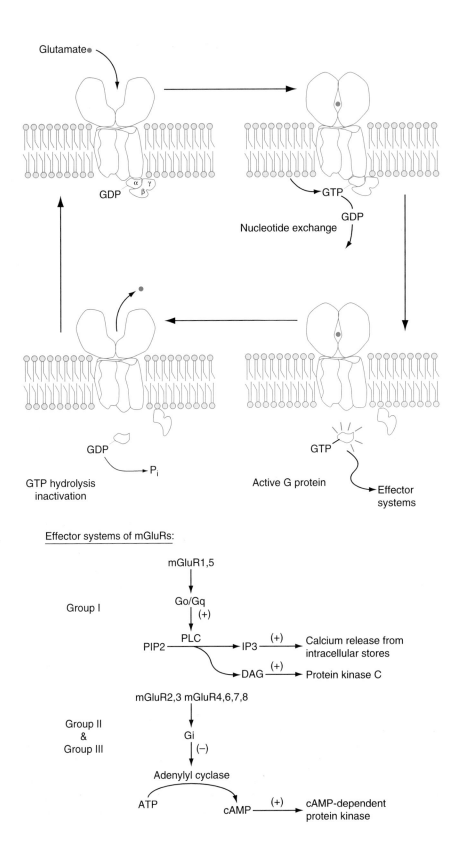

14.3.1 Stimulation of Phosphoinositide Hydrolysis

Activation of many G-protein-coupled receptors can result in activation of phospholipase C (PLC). PLC is a phosphoinositide-specific phosphodiesterase that catalyzes the hydrolysis of phosphatidylinositol-4,5-bisphosphate (PIP2) to yield diacylglycerol and free inositol-1,4,5-trisphosphate (IP3), both of which act as second messengers (Figure 14.4). Activation of PI hydrolysis also results in liberation of other intracellular messengers that alter cell function. For instance, arachidonic acid is released subsequent to the rise in diacylglycerol (DAG) levels due to the action of a DAG-specific phopholipase. Furthermore, the increased levels of arachidonic acid, coupled with the increased levels of intracellular calcium, may activate guanylyl cyclase and subsequent increases in the formation of cGMP. Excitatory amino acids have been shown to stimulate PI hydrolysis in the hippocampus, cerebral cortex, striatum and cerebellum, and in cultured astrocytes and neurons from various brain regions. Although subtle differences exist between different brain regions, the general agonist profile for stimulation of PI hydrolysis is very similar to that of the group I mGluRs. While this suggests that the group I mGluRs can couple to stimulation of PI hydrolysis *in vivo*, this does not rule out the possibility that these receptors can also couple to other second messenger systems in the brain.

14.3.2 Inhibition of Adenylyl Cyclase

Cyclic AMP is a soluble second messenger that activates a protein kinase which in turn phosphorylates and thereby alters the function of various cellular proteins. Some G-protein-coupled receptors can stimulate the production of cAMP by activation of adenylyl cyclase, which catalyzes the conversion of ATP to cAMP. These receptors couple to adenylyl cyclase via the stimulatory GTP binding protein, G_s. In contrast, other receptors can have cellular effects by decreasing the level of cAMP production. This is accomplished by coupling to the inhibitory G protein, G_i (Figure 14.4)

Many studies suggest that mGluRs can couple to a G_i-like protein and thus inhibit cAMP responses. The pharmacological profile for mGluR-mediated inhibition of cAMP formation varies widely depending on the preparation. Although there are other explanations for these discrepancies, one possibility is that several distinct mGluR subtypes exist in the brain that are negatively coupled to adenylyl cyclase, as is suggested by the fact that both the group II and group III mGluRs are negatively coupled to adenylyl cyclase in expression systems. Thus, the pharmacological profile of mGluR-mediated inhibition of cAMP responses for a given brain region will depend largely on the relative levels of expression of these different receptors.

14.3.3 Potentiation of Cyclic AMP Formation

It has long been known that glutamate stimulates cAMP formation in brain slices. However, this increase in cAMP levels was found to be dependent on the presence of endogenous adenosine. At that time, it was assumed that this was due to depolarization-evoked release of adenosine by iGluR activation. However, more recent data suggest that this response is due to activation of an mGluR which potentiates the cAMP response elicited by other receptors (including A2 adenosine receptors, β-adrenergic receptors, vasoactive intestinal peptide receptors, and others) that are directly coupled to adenylyl cyclase via G_s. This mGluR appears to belong to a large group of receptors, including the $GABA_A$ receptor, the α-adrenergic receptor, the H1 histaminergic receptor and others, that interact synergistically with G_s-coupled receptors to increase cAMP accumulation.

Figure 14.4   G-protein coupling of mGluRs. The G-protein cycle of agonist binding, G-protein interaction and nucleotide exchange leading to activation followed by GTP hydrolysis-inactivation is a general cycle that can be applied to all of the heterotrimeric G proteins. When the group I mGluRs activate G proteins of the G_o/G_q family, the activated α subunit stimulates phospholipase C, leading to hydrolysis of membrane phosphoinositides and subsequent production of the PKC activator diacylglycerol (DAG) and the calcium mobilizing molecule, inositol trisphosphate (IP3). In contrast, activation of G_i by the group II and group III mGluRs leads to an active α subunit which *inhibits* adenylyl cyclase function. Thus, the net result of activation of $G_{i\alpha}$ by group II and III mGluRs is a decrease in cAMP levels and a decrease in cAMP-dependent protein kinase activity.

The mechanism by which mGluR activation potentiates cAMP responses is not currently understood. However the pharmacological profile of this response suggests that it is distinct from mGluR-mediated stimulation of PI hydrolysis, and therefore not likely mediated by a group I mGluR. In fact, a thorough pharmacological analysis suggests that this response may be mediated by a group II mGluR.

A potential mechanism for receptor-mediated potentiation of cAMP responses was recently proposed by Tang and Gilman (1991), who showed that although G protein $\beta\gamma$ subunits inhibit type I adenylyl cyclase, they potentiate activation of type II adenylyl cyclase by the α subunit of G_s. Thus, it is possible that by activation of G_i and release of G protein $\beta\gamma$ subunits, group II mGluRs potentiate the cAMP response elicited by activation of G_s-coupled receptors.

14.3.4 Activation of Phospholipase D

Application of mGluR agonists results in a stimulation of phospholipase D (PLD) activity in rat hippocampal slices. Activation of PLD results in the metabolism of phosphatidylcholine (PC) and generation of phosphatidic acid and free choline. Subsequent degradation of phosphatidic acid (PA) by the action of phosphatidate phosphohydrolase results in the generation of DAG, which is a known activator of protein kinase C (PKC). Because PC is a much more abundant membrane constituent than is PI (PC is the major membrane phospholipid), activation of PLD could result in a much larger DAG response than that resulting from PI hydrolysis. Furthermore, the species of DAG produced by PLD activity are different from those generated by the actions of PLC. Thus, PLD-catalyzed breakdown of PC could preferentially activate different isoforms of PKC than PLC-catalyzed breakdown of PI.

The pharmacological profile of mGluR-mediated stimulation of PLD activity is distinct from that of any other known mGluR-mediated response. Interestingly, glutamate appears to be ineffective as an agonist at this response, whereas the putative excitatory amino acid transmitter, L-cystine sulfinic acid (L-CSA), is the most efficacious agonist at PLD stimulation. Taken together with evidence that L-CSA fits most of the criteria for a neurotransmitter in brain, these data suggest that L-CSA may be an endogenous agonist of the hippocampal PLD-coupled metabotropic excitatory amino acid receptor.

14.4 Modulation of Ion Channels and Synaptic Transmission by mGluRs

14.4.1 Calcium-Activated Potassium Current

Among the first experiments showing mGluR-mediated effects of excitatory amino acids on neuronal cells were those that demonstrated that application of excitatory amino acids could alter the firing properties of neurons. Application of glutamate or related agonists inhibited the accommodation of hippocampal pyramidal cell firing that occurred during a depolarizing stimulus (Stratton *et al.*, 1989; Charpak *et al*, 1990; Desai and Conn, 1991; Hu and Storm, 1991). This accommodation of spike frequency (spike frequency adaptation) is largely mediated by activation of the afterhyperpolarization (AHP) current, $I_{K,AHP}$ (Charpak *et al.*, 1990). The AHP current is a calcium-activated potassium current that is activated by the large increases in intracellular calcium that occur following a burst of action potentials (Figure 14.5). Activation of this channel produces a large potassium conductance increase, resulting in a membrane hyperpolarization and termination of repetitive action potential firing. Blockade of this channel by excitatory amino acids is independent of ionotropic glutamate receptor activation, based on its persistence in the presence of ionotropic glutamate receptor antagonists in response to glutamate and quisqualate and the fact that $I_{K,AHP}$ is reduced by agonists selective for mGluRs vs. the iGluRs. Inhibition of $I_{K,AHP}$ by mGluR agonists could be mediated by either a reduction in calcium influx or by inhibition of potassium efflux. Charpak *et al.* (1990) showed that the reduction of $I_{K,AHP}$ by quisqualate was not accompanied by a decrease in calcium influx that occurs during the depolarization. Thus, the likely mechanism for this effect is actual reduction in the activity of the potassium channel. $I_{K,AHP}$ is blocked by application of the group I mGluR agonists DHPG and quisqualate, but not by the group II agonist DCG-IV or the group III agonist, L-AP4. These findings suggest that activation of group I, but not group II or III mGluRs results in a depression of $I_{K,AHP}$ in hippocampal pyramidal cells. Interestingly, mGluR-mediated inhibition of the AHP is intact in mice genetically engineered to lack mGluR1 expression. Furthermore, immunocytochemistry studies show that mGluR5, but not mGluR1, is expressed in hippocampal pyramidal cells. Taken together, these results suggest that mGluR5 is the receptor that mediates excitatory amino acid-induced depression of $I_{K,AHP}$ in hippocampal pyramidal cells.

14.4.2 Leak Potassium Current

Several groups have shown that activation of mGluRs depolarizes various types of neurons including hippocampal pyramidal cells, neocortical pyramidal cells, sympathetic pre-ganglionic neurons and inhibitory interneurons in the hippocampus. This depolarization is associated with an increase in membrane resistance, suggesting that the underlying mechanism involves inhibition of some membrane conductance. The underlying conductance is a voltage-independent potassium conductance ($I_{K,leak}$). In neocortical pyramidal neurons, activation of mGluRs and resultant inhibition of the $I_{K,leak}$ converts these cells from a state of periodic burst-firing to a tonic, single-spike-firing mode. In hippocampal pyramidal cells, inhibition of the leak potassium current appears to underlie a slow synaptic response that occurs following brief tetanic afferent stimulation. In hippocampal pyramidal cells, mGluR-mediated inhibition of $I_{K,leak}$ is clearly mediated by G-protein activation, since this effect is blocked by intracellular GDPβS, and remains tonically active after agonist application in the presence of GTPγS. However, mGluR-mediated inhibition of $I_{K,leak}$ is not blocked by the general protein kinase inhibitor, staurosporine, at concentrations that block the effects of phorbol esters and cAMP analogs, suggesting that this effect is not mediated by activation of PKC or PKA. The mechanism of mGluR inhibition of $I_{K,leak}$ is therefore unclear. The pharmacological profile of mGluR-mediated inhibition of $I_{K,leak}$ in hippocampal pyramidal neurons suggests that this effect is mediated by a group I mGluR.

14.4.3 Voltage-Dependent Potassium Currents

In addition to $I_{K,AHP}$ and $I_{K,leak}$, activation of mGluRs by quisqualate inhibits a voltage-dependent potassium current, termed I_M (Charpak *et al.*, 1990) (Figure 14.6). The M current is activated at membrane potentials slightly depolarized to resting potential (approximately −60 mV) in hippocampal neurons.

Therefore, I_M serves to oppose small depolarizations (see Appendix 17.3). Because the M current is active near the resting potential, it is possible that inhibition of I_M may contribute to the depolarization of these cells induced by mGluR activation.

14.4.4 Calcium Currents

Several studies have shown that mGluR activation decreases high voltage-activated calcium currents in a variety of neurons. It is interesting to note that the effects of mGluR agonists on calcium channels in CA3 pyramidal cells were not observed in cell-attached patches when the agonist was applied outside the patch, suggesting that the depression of calcium channel function is not mediated by the actions of an easily diffusible second messenger (Figure 14.7). Other studies also implicate a more direct coupling in mGluR-mediated reduction of voltage-gated calcium channels. The agonist rank order of potency for modulation of calcium channels in dissociated CA3 pyramidal cells is quisqualate > glutamate > ibotenate > *trans*-ACPD. This agonist rank order of potency is very similar to that observed for mGluR-mediated stimulation of PI hydrolysis (group I mGluRs, see above). Because the pharmacological profile so closely resembles that of the group I mGluRs, but mGluR-mediated calcium channel inhibition is independent of diffusible second messengers, it is possible that group I mGluRs can also couple directly to calcium channels through a GTP-binding protein. However, this has not yet been clearly established.

There is also one report that activation of mGluRs can facilitate L-type calcium currents in cultured cerebellar granule cells. However, unlike the inhibition of calcium channel function described above, this enhancement of L-type currents occurs in cell-attached patches when the agonist is applied outside the patch, suggesting that this effect is mediated by a diffusible second messenger. Although the pharmacological profile of this response is consistent with group I mGluRs, the second messenger responsible for this effect has not been identified.

Figure 14.5   Group I mGluR modulation of $I_{K, AHP}$. At rest (a) voltage-sensitive sodium channels (VSSC), voltage-sensitive calcium channels (VSCC), and $I_{K, AHP}$ are inactive. Following a depolarization sufficient to fire multiple action potentials and multiple rounds of VSCC activation (b), there is sufficient elevation of intracellular Ca^{2+} to activate $I_{K, AHP}$ (c) resulting in membrane hyperpolarization and termination of repetitive firing. Traces at the bottom show a standard intracellular recording from a hippocampal pyramidal cell and the membrane potential response to 100 ms depolarizing current injection. The depolarization results in firing of several action potentials, followed by a prolonged period of hyperpolarization, the AHP. Application of the group I mGluR agonists DHPG or quisqualate (Quis) results in a blockade of the AHP and an increase in cell firing during prolonged depolarizations.

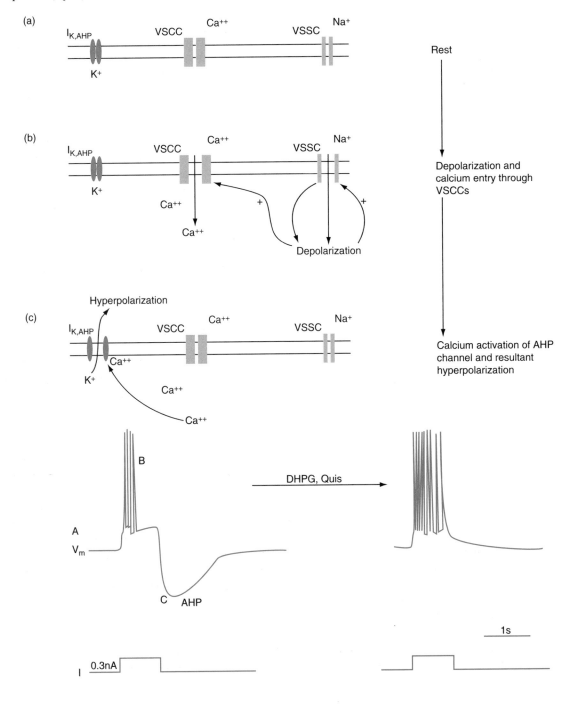

Figure 14.6 Inhibition of the M-type potassium current (I_M) by mGluR activation. Potassium currents recorded from rat hippocampal CA3 pyramidal cells recorded in the whole-cell configuration are shown. The cell was voltage clamped at −29 mV. At this potential, I_M is fully active. The cell was then stepped to various hyperpolarized potentials. The initial sag in the current traces represents the slow inactivation of I_M. The amplitude of I_M is determined by measuring the amplitude of this sag. Note that quisqualate reduces the amplitude of I_M (this experiment was performed in the presence of kynurenate to prevent activation of iGluRs by quisqualate). (Adapted from Charpak S, Gahwiler BH, Do KQ and Knopfel T, 1990. Potassium conductances in hippocampal neurons blocked by excitatory amino acid transmitters, *Nature* 347, 765–767, with permission.)

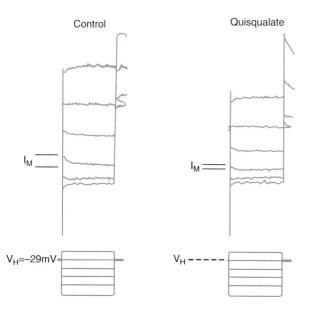

14.4.5 Multiple Metabotropic Glutamate Receptors Modulate Excitatory and Inhibitory Synaptic Transmission

One of the most consistent effects of mGluR activation between different brain regions is a modulation of synaptic transmission. mGluRs serve as glutamate autoreceptors, decreasing glutamate release from presynaptic terminals. This effect of mGluR activation has been observed in many different brain regions, including the cerebral cortex, hippocampus, striatum, amygdala, nucleus of the solitary tract, thalamus and spinal cord. In addition, mGluR heteroreceptors are localized on GABAergic nerve terminals where they regulate GABAergic synaptic inhibition. This effect has also been observed in the hippocampus, striatum and olfactory bulb among other areas. Evidence suggests that receptors from all of three major mGluR groups serve as both glutamate autoreceptors and heteroreceptors on GABAergic nerve terminals. The fact that these actions are so ubiquitous and given that receptors from all three mGluR groups are involved in modulating excitatory and inhibitory synaptic transmission speaks of the importance of these actions in brain function.

The mechanisms involved in mGluR-mediated depression of excitatory and inhibitory synaptic transmission are not well understood. However, it is clear that one potential mechanism involves the above-mentioned depression of voltage-gated calcium channel function. Because calcium entry through these channels is a critical step in neurotransmitter release, it is easy to see how blocking the function of voltage-gated calcium channels could block the vesicular release of neurotransmitters.

In addition to this mechanism, however, it appears that other mechanisms are also involved in the depression of synaptic transmission induced by mGluRs. If one blocks action potential-dependent glutamate release using tetrodotoxin (TTX), which blocks voltage-gated sodium channels, small periodic synaptic currents can still be recorded. The frequency of these TTX-insensitive events is not affected by blockade of voltage-gated calcium channels, although evoked synaptic transmission is completely eliminated by blockade of calcium channels. Because these TTX-insensitive release events (miniatures) are independent of action potential firing, the frequency of miniatures is a measure of the spontaneous transmitter release probability. Therefore, if an agonist reduces the frequency of occurrence of these miniature synaptic events, then this suggests that the agonist has reduced the probability of spontaneous neurotransmitter release at the synapses in question (see Chapter 8).

In the adult rat hippocampus, mGluRs of both group I and group III can reduce evoked excitatory synaptic transmission at the synapse between CA3 and CA1 pyramidal cells. Activation of group III mGluRs with L-AP4 reduces the frequency, but not the amplitude, of miniature EPSCs (mEPSCs) recorded from CA1 pyramidal cells in the hippocampus, suggesting that group III mGluR activation results in a decrease in the probability of glutamate release.

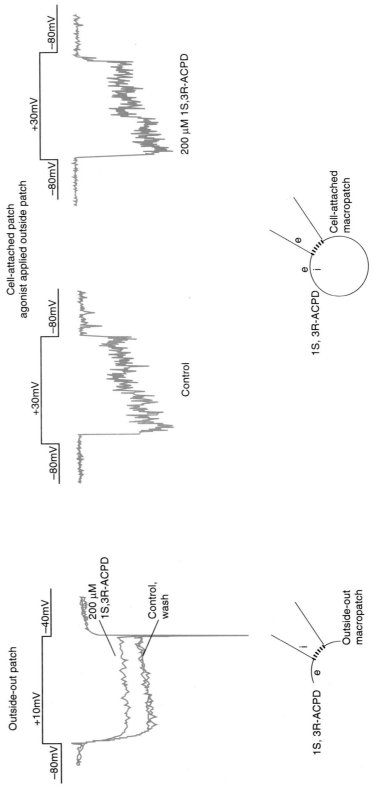

Figure 14.7 Inhibition of voltage-activated calcium currents in hippocampal pyramidal cells by mGluRs is not mediated by a readily diffusible second messenger. The left panel shows macroscopic calcium currents recorded from outside-out patches from a rat CA3 pyramidal cell. The membrane is held at –80 mV and stepped to + 10 mV, resulting in activation of voltage-sensitive calcium channels. 200 μM 1S,3R-ACPD applied to the surface of the patch results in a reversible reduction of the calcium current. However, when macroscopic calcium currents are recorded in the cell-attached mode and the agonist is applied outside the patch (thus, the agonist cannot reach the mGluRs that are located adjacent to the calcium channels being recorded), 1S,3R-ACPD has no effect. These findings suggest that the mGluR-mediated reduction in calcium currents is not mediated by a readily diffusible second messenger in these cells. i, intracellular; e, extracellular; ●, mGluR; ≈, Ca²⁺ channel; 1S, 3R-ACPD, 1S, 3R-1-aminocyclopentane-1,3-dicarboxylate. (Adapted from Swartz KJ and Bean BP 1992. Inhibition of calcium channels in rat CA3 pyramidal neurons by a metabotropic glutamate receptor, *J. Neurosci.* **12,** 4358–4371, with permission.)

Group I mGluR agonists such as DHPG, which also reduce evoked EPSCs, have no effect on mEPSC frequency. However, blockade of voltage-gated calcium channels has no effect on these action potential-independent release events, suggesting that group I mGluRs depress synaptic transmission at this synapse by inhibiting voltage-gated calcium channels whereas group III mGluRs decrease the probability of glutamate release.

Evidence suggests that the multiple physiological actions of mGluR activation in the nervous system are critical for normal function in several neuronal circuits and play important roles in a variety of CNS functions. Two circuits in which the roles of mGluRs have been particularly well characterized include the retina and the cerebellum. The functions of some specific mGluR subtypes in these circuits will be discussed in some detail below.

14.4.6 Synaptic Transmission in the Retina: A Critical Role for mGluR6

In the retina, information flows from photoreceptor cells to retinal interneurons, the bipolar cells, and finally to the output cells of the retina, the retinal ganglion cells. Neither photoreceptor cells nor bipolar cells are capable of producing action potentials, so information is passed on by passive spread of potentials in these cells. The retinal ganglion cells are capable of firing action potentials and send projections to the lateral geniculate nucleus and the superior colliculus. Photoreceptor cells are maintained in a depolarized state in the absence of light, and thus release their neurotransmitter, glutamate, in a constitutive manner. This depolarization is due to the constitutive activation of a cGMP-gated cation channel. Light striking the photoreceptor cell leads of a decrease in intracellular cGMP and resultant closure of the cGMP-gated channels. Closing these channels results in hyperpolarization of the photoreceptor cell and a consequent decrease in glutamate release from the terminals. The photoreceptor cells synapse onto two main classes of bipolar cells: ON and OFF. The OFF bipolar cells respond to glutamate with the stereotypical depolarization, whereas the ON bipolar cells respond to glutamate by hyperpolarizing. Thus, because light decreases the amount of glutamate released, the effect of light shining on a photoreceptor cell is hyperpolar-

ization of the OFF bipolar cell and depolarization of the ON bipolar cells. The primary receptor type localized on OFF-bipolar cells are of the AMPA/Kainate subtype, which is consistent with the finding that glutamate depolarizes these cells. In contrast, the receptor type localized on the ON-bipolar cells is an L-AP4-sensitive mGluR. Activation of this receptor by either glutamate or L-AP4 inhibits a cGMP-activated cation current in retinal bipolar cells that is similar to that found in photoreceptor cells described above. This effect is likely to be mediated by inhibition of guanylyl cyclase or by activation of a cGMP phosphodiesterase.

On examination of the distribution of mGluRs in the retina, one finds that mGluR6 is specifically localized in the ON bipolar cells. Because mGluR6 is a group III mGluR and is accordingly activated by L-AP4, it was hypothesized that the glutamate-induced hyperpolarization in the ON bipolar cells might be mediated by mGluR6. This hypothesis was tested using targeted disruption of the mGluR6 gene in mice. In the mice containing the disrupted mGluR6 gene (and thus no mGluR6 protein), the ON response was lost whereas the OFF response remained intact. This finding is consistent with the hypothesis that mGluR6 localized on retinal ON bipolar cells mediates this ON response (glutamate-induced hyperpolarization).

14.4.7 mGluR1 in Cerebellar Function (see also Section 19.3)

Activity-dependent persistent changes in synaptic strength are believed to represent a cellular basis for learning and memory. In the cerebellum, certain patterns of synaptic stimulation can result in a long-term depression (LTD) of synaptic transmission. The Purkinje cells receive two main types of excitatory inputs: a single strong input from a climbing fiber and many weak inputs from parallel fibers. LTD can be induced at the parallel fiber–Purkinje cell synapse by repetitive conjunctive activation of the climbing fiber and parallel fiber inputs to a Purkinje cell (see Figure 14.8). Based on a large body of work, it appears that LTD at the parallel fiber–Purkinje cell synapse requires activation of voltage-gated calcium channels in the Purkinje cells in conjunction with activation of both iGluRs and mGluRs in the Purkinje cells. The calcium channel activation is achieved in intact cerebellum by

Figure 14.8   mGluR1 is required for LTD at the parallel fiber–Purkinje cell synapse. Schematic representation of the Purkinje cell circuitry. Each Purkinje cell receives a single climbing fiber and many parallel fiber connections. Time course of the amplitude of EPSCs evoked by test stimuli to the parallel fibers, and the effect of conjunctive stimulation (CS) of parallel fibers and climbing fibers, or by pairing large depolarizations of the Purkinje cell (to induced calcium spikes) with stimulation of parallel fibers. Both protocols induce LTD. In the mGluR1 knockout mice, CS does not induce LTD. Inset shows traces taken at the points indicated by '1' and '2' on the time course showing the marked LTD of parallel fiber EPSCs induced by CS in cerebellar slices from wild-type but not mGluR1 knockout mice. (Adapted from Aiba A, Kano M, Chen C *et al.*, 1994. Deficient cerebellar long-term depression and impaired motor learning in mGluR1 mutant mice, *Cell* **79**, 377–378, with permission.)

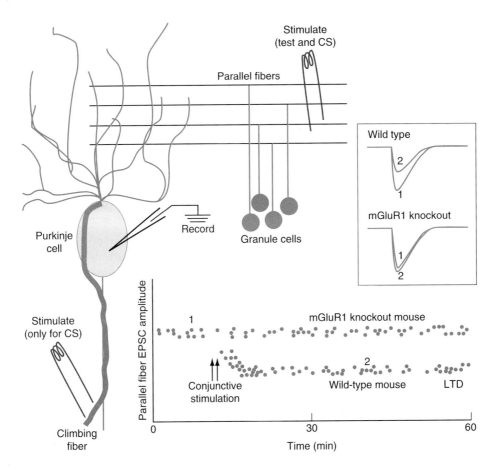

climbing fiber activation, whereas the iGluR and mGluR activation is a result of parallel fiber activation. LTD in the cerebellum is believed to be a basis for motor learning.

The predominant mGluR expressed in cerebellar Purkinje cells is mGluR1. In order to test the hypothesis that mGluR1 is involved in LTD at the parallel fiber–Purkinje cell synapse, several different approaches have been used. First, it was found that anti-

bodies directed against the N-terminal tail of mGluR1 (which is involved in agonist binding, see above) were able to block LTD in cultured cerebellar Purkinje cells. In addition, two separate groups have developed mutant mice in which the gene coding for mGluR1 has been disrupted. Both groups showed that LTD could not be induced in the cerebellum of the mGluR1 mutant mice using protocols that induce LTD in the wild-type mice. Furthermore, the mGluR1 knockout mice demonstrated profound impairment in several motor tasks and were also impaired in one test of motor learning: classical conditioning of the eyeblink responses. Interestingly, several spontaneously occurring mutant mouse strains that are ataxic show no expression of mGluR1 in the cerebellum. These results suggest that mGluR1 plays a critical role in cerebellar function.

14.5 Conclusions

In summary, the recent discovery of the mGluR family dramatically changes the traditional view of glutamatergic neurotransmission. Because activation of mGluRs can modulate activity in glutamatergic circuits in a manner previously associated only with extrinsic neuromodulators, the mGluRs provide a mechanism whereby glutamate can modulate or fine-tune activity at the same synapses at which it elicits fast synaptic responses. In addition, the mGluR-mediated actions of glutamate on circuits involving other neurotransmitters suggest that glutamate is not only an important fast neurotransmitter, but also the predominant neuromodulatory substance in the mammalian CNS. With at least eight distinct mGluR gene products cloned to date and multiple splice variants of several of these, the mGluR family is rather large compared with the G-protein-coupled receptor families for other neurotransmitters. In addition, these receptors share no sequence homology with the previously discovered G-protein-coupled receptors. Recent advances at the molecular level suggest that the mGluRs are both structurally and functionally distinct from any of the other G-protein-coupled receptors discovered to date.

Because of the ubiquitous distribution of mGluRs, these receptors have the potential of participating in virtually all known functions of the CNS. Indeed, although only recently discovered, these receptors have already been implicated in a variety of processes including motor control, learning and memory, developmental plasticity, vision, sensory processing, nociception, epileptogenesis, cardiovascular regulation, and responses to neuronal injury. In addition, because the mGluRs have very specific heterogeneous distribution patterns, the opportunity exists to develop pharmacological agents that selectively interact with specific mGluR subtypes and thereby target a subset of

receptors involved in specific CNS functions. Therefore, understanding the physiological roles of specific mGluR subtypes may well have a dramatic impact on the development of novel treatment strategies for a variety of neurological disorders.

Further Reading

Aiba, A., Kano, M., Chen, C. *et al.* (1994) Deficient cerebellar long-term depression and impaired motor learning in mGluR1 mutant mice. *Cell* **79**, 377–378.

Charpak, S., Gahwiler, B.H., Do, K. Q. and Knopfel, T. (1990) Potassium conductances in hippocampal neurons blocked by excitatory amino acid transmitters. *Nature* **347**, 765–767.

Chavis, P., Nooney, J.M., Bockaert, J., Fagni, L., Feltz, A. and Bossu, J.L. (1995) Facilitatory coupling between a glutamate metabotropic receptor and dihydropyridine-sensitive calcium channels in cultured cerebellar granule cells. *J. Neurosci.* **15**, 135–143.

Conquet, F., Bashir, Z., Davies, C. *et al.* (1994) Motor deficit and impairment of synaptic plasticity in mice lacking mGluR1. *Nature* **372**, 237–243.

Desai, M.A. and Conn, P.J. (1991) Excitatory effects of ACPD receptor activation in the hippocampus are mediated by direct effects on pyramidal cells and blockade of synaptic inhibition. *J. Neurophysiol.* **66**, 40–52.

Gerber, U., Sim, J.A. and Gahwiler, B.H. (1992) Reduction of potassium conductances mediated by metabotropic glutamate receptors in rat CA3 pyramidal cells does not require protein kinase C or protein kinase A. *Eur. J. Neurosci.* **4**, 792–797.

Gereau, R.W. and Conn, P.J. (1995) Roles of specific metabotropic glutamate receptors in regulating hippocampal CA1 pyramidal cell excitability. *J. Neurophysiol.* **74**, 122–129.

Gereau, R.W. and Conn, P.J. (1995) Multiple presynaptic metabotropic glutamate receptors modulate excitatory and inhibitory synaptic transmission in hippocampal area CA1. *J. Neurosci.* **15**, 6879–6889.

Guerineau, N.C., Gahwiler, B.H., and Gerber, U. (1994) Reduction of resting K^+ current by metabotropic glutamate and muscarinic receptors in rat CA3 cells: mediation by G-proteins. *J. Physiol.* **474**, 27–33.

Hu, G.-Y. and Storm, J.F. (1991) Excitatory amino acids acting on metabotropic glutamate receptors broaden the action potential in hippocampal neurons. *Brain Res.* **568**, 339–344.

Masu, M., Iwakabe, H., Tagawa, Y. *et al.* (1995) Specific deficit of the ON response in visual transmission by targeted disruption of the mGluR6 gene. *Cell* **80**, 757–765.

O'Hara, P.J., Sheppard, P.O., Thogersen, H. *et al.* (1993) The ligand binding domain in metabotropic glutamate receptors is related to bacterial periplasmic binding proteins. *Neuron* **11**, 41–52.

Pin, J.-P. and Duvoisin, R. (1995) The metabotropic glutamate receptors: structure and function. *Neuropharmacology* **34**, 1–26.

Pin, J.-P., Joly, C., Heinemann, S.F. and Bockaert, J. (1994) Domains involved in the specificity of G protein activation in phospholipase C-coupled metabotropic glutamate receptors. *EMBO J.* **13**, 342–348.

Sahara, Y. and Westbrook, G.L. (1993) Modulation of calcium currents by a metabotropic glutamate receptor involves fast and slow kinetic components in cultured hippocampal neurons. *J. Neurosci.* **13**, 3041–3050.

Shiells, R.A. and Falk, G. (1992) Properties of the cGMP-activated channel of retinal on-bipolar cells. *Proc. R. Soc. Lond.* **247**, 21–25.

Shiells, R.A. and Falk, G. (1992) The glutamate-receptor linked cGMP cascade of retinal on-bipolar cells is pertussis and cholera toxin-sensitive. *Proc. R. Soc. Lond.* **247**, 17–20.

Sladeczek, F., Pin, J.-P., Recasens, M., Bockaert, J. and Weiss, S. (1985) Glutamate stimulates inositol phosphate formation in striatal neurons. *Nature* **317**, 717–719.

Stratton, K.R., Worley, P.J. and Baraban, J.M. (1989) Excitation of hippocampal neurons by stimulation of glutamate Q_p receptors. *Eur. J. Pharmacol.* **173**, 235–237.

Swartz, K.J. and Bean, B.P. (1992) Inhibition of calcium channels in rat CA3 pyramidal neurons by a metabotropic glutamate receptor. *J. Neurosci.* **12**, 4358–4371.

Takahashi, K., Tsuchida, K., Taneba, Y., Masu, M. and Nakanishi, S. (1993) Role of the large extracellular domain of metabotropic glutamate receptors in agonist selectivity determination. *J. Biol. Chem.* **258**, 19 341–19 345.

Tang, W.-J. and Gilman. A.G. (1991) Type-specific regulation of adenylyl cyclase by G protein βγ subunits. *Science* **254**, 1500–1503.

Trombley, P.Q. and Westbrook, G.L. (1992) L-AP4 inhibits calcium currents and synaptic transmission via a G-protein-coupled glutamate receptor. *J. Neurosci.* **12**, 2043–2050.

15

The Olfactory Receptors

The olfactory systems of all organisms have the capacity to discriminate between different odorant stimuli. Humans, for example, are capable of distinguishing between thousands of distinct odors. A subtle alteration in the molecular structure of an odorant can lead to a change in the perceived odor. Perception of an odor by the brain can be divided into odorant recognition and neural processing. The first events include the transductory processes, which code the odor stimulation in the generation of propagated action potentials. The second events, the processing of sensory information, occur in the neuronal networks of the olfactory bulb and higher cortical centers.

This chapter focuses on odorant recognition, the initial events that take place in the olfactory neuroepithelium and more precisely in the olfactory receptor neurons.

15.1 The Olfactory Receptor Cells are Sensory Neurons Located in the Olfactory Neuroepithelium

15.1.1 The Olfactory Neurons are Bipolar Cells that Project to the Olfactory Bulb

The vertebrate olfactory mucosa contains several million sensory neurons that reside in a pseudostratified columnar epithelium 200 μm thick (Figure 15.1). Three cell types dominate this epithelium: the olfactory sensory neuron, the sustentacular or supporting cell and the basal cell (Figure 15.1). The supporting cell is a glia-like cell which secretes part of the mucus components and the basal cell is a stem cell that divides and differentiates throughout life to become functional olfactory sensory neurons.

The olfactory receptor cell is a sensory bipolar neuron that projects a single non-branching dendrite to the epithelial surface and a single unmyelinated axon to the olfactory bulb (Figure 15.1). Each dendrite terminates in a dendritic knob, which gives rise to 5–20 thin cilia into the nasal lumen. These cilia (0.1–0.2 μm in diameter and up to 200 μm in length) lie in the thin layer of mucus bathing the epithelial surface. They provide an extensive, receptive surface for the interaction of odors with the cell since they increase the receptive area of an olfactory knob

Figure 15.1   Olfactory receptors lie in the olfactory epithelium. The vertebrate olfactory epithelium is located in the dorsal recess of the nasal cavity, the nasopharynx. It contains olfactory receptor cells, supporting cells and basal cells. Ventilatory air currents bring the odorant molecules to the olfactory mucosa. (From Kandel ER, Schwartz JH and Jessel TM, 1991. *Principles of Neural Science*, 3rd edition, Elsevier, New York, with permission.)

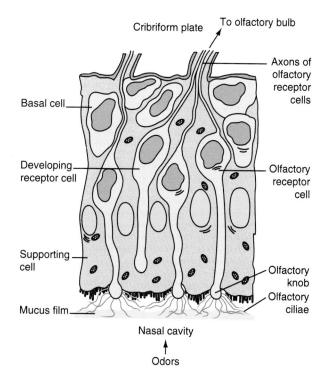

Figure 15.2   The olfactory receptor cells project to mitral cells in the olfactory bulb. (a) Lateral view of the nasopharynx. The cribriform plate of the ethnoid bone lies over the olfactory mucosa. (b) View from the bottom side of the encephalon to show the olfactory bulbs. (c) Drawing of the neuroepithelium and of a sagittal section through an olfactory bulb (enlargement of the section in (a). The olfactory epithelium is separated by a basement membrane from the 'lamina propria', a highly vascular and glandular tissue that lies adjacent to the nasal cartilage. The single axon of each olfactory receptor cell courses through the holes of the ethnoid bone, ramifies and synapses on the dendrites of the neurons of the olfactory bulb to form the olfactory glomeruli. As many as 1000 afferent fibers synapse on the dendrites of a single mitral cell. Local circuit neurons in the olfactory bulb are omitted. (a and c: From Berne RM and Levy MN, 1993. *Physiology*, 3rd edition, Mosby Year Book, St Louis, Missouri; House EL and Pansky B, 1967. A *Functional Approach to Neuroanatomy*, 2nd edition, McGraw Hill, New York, with permission. b: Drawing: Jérôme Yelnik.)

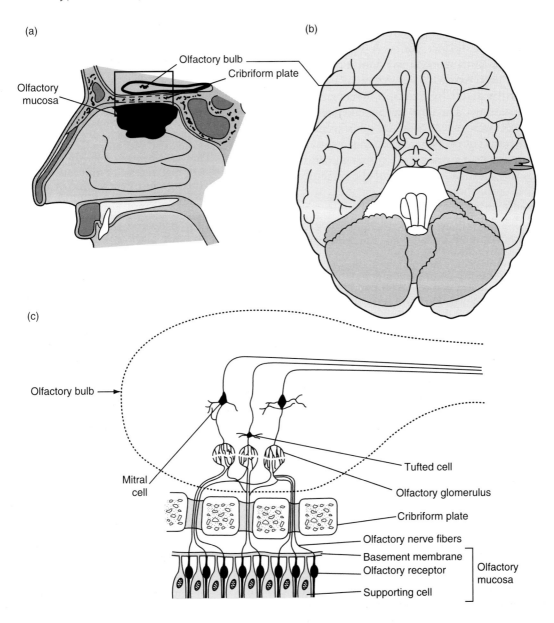

(5 µm^2) up to 100-fold. A small unmyelinated axon projects from the opposite pole of the cell, penetrates through the basement membrane and after making a 90° angle joins between 10 and 100 others to form a bundle of axons ensheathed with Schwann cells. These bundles penetrate across the cribriform plate (a porous region of the ethnoid bone), join to form the olfactory nerve (the first cranial nerve) and project to the ipsilateral olfactory bulb. Every axon synapses onto secondary neurons, the mitral cells located in the olfactory bulb where decoding of the odor message is initiated (Figure 15.2). This synapse is a complex structure known as a glomerule (see Figure. 2-2e) which consists of 100–1000 afferent olfactory axons converging upon the dendritic arbor of a single mitral cell. This allows mitral cells to sample chemosensory information from a wide area of the olfactory epithelium, increasing the chance of detecting small concentrations of odorants that may reach the chemosensory surface in a non-uniform manner.

15.1.2 Odorants Diffuse Through the Extracellular Mucous Matrix Before Interacting with the Chemosensory Membrane of Olfactory Receptor Neurons

The cilia and dendritic knob are the only parts of the sensory neuron exposed to the external environment. They were therefore candidates for the site of odor recognition and transmembrane signaling. The sense of smell is based on molecular recognition. The molecules of odorants are recognized by specialized receptors located in the cilia of olfactory cells which lie in a 30 µm thick viscous liquid medium, the mucus, which covers the olfactory epithelium (Figure 15.1). It is a structured extracellular matrix (see Section 4.1.4) which contains glycoproteins, mucopeptides, detoxification enzymes and immunoglobulins secreted by supporting cells and Bowman's glands. It protects the epithelium against microorganisms and biological toxins.

The mucus layer represents an aqueous environment into which primarily hydrophobic odorants must partition and gain access to odorant receptors in the cilia membrane. Using radioactively labeled odorants, odorant-binding proteins have been identified in the mucus. They belong to a family of hydrophobic ligand carrier proteins. They may trap odorants entering the nasal cavity and carry them to the nasal area.

Alternatively, they may provide a reservoir of binding sites for odorants, protecting olfactory neurons from exposure to high concentrations of odorants.

15.2 The Response of Olfactory Receptor Neurons to Odors is a Membrane Depolarization which Elicits Action Potential Generation

15.2.1 Pioneering Experiments

In order to define the membrane potential changes of olfactory receptor cells in response to an odor, cell activity is recorded with intracellular recording techniques in the salamander (*Ambystoma tigrinum*). The olfactory epithelium is exposed after surgery and cells are penetrated with an electrode filled with a dye. At the end of the recording session, the dye is injected into the cell, allowing the determination of recordings as being from a receptor cell or not on the basis of morphological examination of histological sections.

An example of recordings is shown in Figure 15.3. The odor stimulus, ethyl *n*-butyrate is delivered at the epithelial surface. It evokes a slow membrane depolarization, about 8 mV in amplitude, upon which are superimposed nine action potentials or spikes. A log dilution of the odorant evokes a smaller depolarization, 6 mV, upon which are superimposed four spikes. In the same cell, a different odorant, anisole, does not evoke a response. These observations suggest that both the amplitude of the membrane depolarization and the number of spikes code for the stimulus strength. However, only the action potentials will propagate to the olfactory bulb along the single axon of the olfactory neuron (see Figure 15.2).

15.2.2 Questions

Question 1: How is an odor recognized by the olfactory receptor neurons? (see Section 15.3).

Question 2: How does an odor give rise to a membrane depolarization?

- What underlies membrane depolarization: the generation of an inward current or the inhibition of an outward current?

Figure 15.3 The reponse of olfactory neurons to an odorant stimulation is a slow membrane depolarization which can evoke action potentials. Intracellular recordings from an olfactory receptor neuron in response to ethyl *n*-butyrate (a) and a log step dilution (b). (c) In contrast, in the same cell, anisole does not evoke a response. $V_m = -60$ mV. Calibrations: 20 mV, 500 ms. (Adapted from Getchell TV, 1977. Analysis of intracellular recordings from salamander olfactory epithelium, *Brain Res.* **123**, 275–286, with permission.)

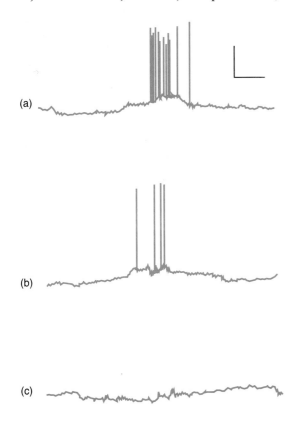

- What are the channels opened or closed and responsible for this current?
- Why do these channels open or close in response to odorant stimulation?

All these questions concern the transduction mechanisms and will be explained from the single channel properties to the membrane depolarization (see Section 15.4).

Question 3: How does the response of the olfactory neuron code for the characteristics of the odorant stimulation (nature of the odorant, its concentration, and the duration of the stimulus)? (see Section 15.5).

15.3 Odorants Bind to a Family of G-Protein-Linked Receptors which Activate Adenylate Cyclase

The different results presented in this section were not obtained in this order. The study of the mechanisms of olfactory transduction began with the development of a cilia-enriched, cell-free preparation of the olfactory epithelium. In this preparation, Doron Lancet and co-workers (1985) obtained evidence that cAMP and G proteins are involved in olfactory transduction since exposure of isolated cilia from rat olfactory epithelium to numerous odorants led to the rapid activation of adenylate cyclase and an elevation of intracellular cAMP concentration. Both effects being dependent on the presence of GTP, this suggested the involvement of a G protein. Then came the characterization of the olfactory receptors and the identification of the G protein linked to these receptors. For clarity, the results are presented in the order of the molecular events that take place from odorant recognition to cAMP formation.

15.3.1 Odorant Receptors are a Family of G-Protein-Linked Receptors

When the cilia of olfactory neurons are enzymatically removed by application of Triton X-100 to the olfactory mucosa in the frog, the response to odorants is lost and restored upon regeneration of the cilia. This observation that the selective removal of the cilia of olfactory cells results in the loss of olfactory responses led to the suggestion that the olfactory receptors are densely expressed in olfactory cilia. The other observation that the activation of adenylate cyclase by odorants is dependent on the presence of GTP led to the hypothesis that odorant receptors are G-protein-linked receptors. Based on this assumption, the authors tried to identify molecules in the olfactory epithelium that resemble members of the seven transmembrane domain superfamily (see Chapter 5).

The expected properties of the odorant receptors deduced from the responses of olfactory cells to odorants *in vivo* are:

- their diversity, making them capable of interacting with extremely diverse molecular structures since a high diversity of olfactory molecules are recognized;
- their ability to transduce odorant binding into intracellular signals that generate the membrane response;
- their specific expression in the olfactory epithelium, the tissue in which odorants are recognized.

Different members of a large multigene family that encodes seven transmembrane domain proteins (a characteristic of the superfamily of G-protein-linked receptors) have been cloned and characterized. Important differences between the olfactory protein family and the other G-protein-linked receptors are present within the third, fourth and fifth transmembrane domains. The olfactory receptors also exhibit between themselves considerable sequence diversity in these transmembrane domains (Figure 15.4). These domains are thought to contribute to the formation of the ligand-binding site in group Ia of G-protein-linked receptors. Group Ia contains the receptors for small ligands such as photons (rhodopsin), for catecholamines (α- and β-adrenergic receptors and dopamine receptors), opiates and enkephalins (opioid receptors). *In vitro* mutagenesis experiments showed that adrenergic ligands interact with β-adrenergic receptors by binding within the plane of the membrane such that the ligand contacts many, if not all, of the transmembrane domains. This divergence within transmembrane domains may explain the specific recognition of a large number of odorants of diverse molecular structures (benzene, phenols, camphor, isoamyl acetate, menthol, terpenes, etc.).

Receptors that belong to the superfamily of seven transmembrane domain proteins interact with G proteins to generate intracellular signals. *In vitro* mutagenesis experiments indicate that one site of association between the receptor of the group Ia and G proteins resides between the third cytoplasmic loop. As shown in Figure 15.4, this loop is relatively short and shows sequence diversity.

To examine the hypothesis that the cloned cDNA, if they express olfactory receptors, must hybridize preferentially with mRNA from olfactory epithelium, a Northern blot analysis is performed. Poly (A)⁺ RNA isolated from different tissues are hybridized with a ^{32}P-labeled mixture of segments of the cDNA cloned. No hybridizing RNA can be detected in brain or retina and in non-neural tissues including lung, liver,

Figure 15.4 Putative transmembrane organization of the olfactory receptor family and transmembrane organization of G-protein-coupled receptors of group I. (a) Schematic representation of a putative odorant receptor. The vertical cylinders delineate the seven putative membrane-spanning domains. The degree of shading of the transmembrane domains in the diagram is proportional to the degree of sequence variability found in these domains among different members of the putative odorant receptor family. The high degree of variability encountered in transmembrane domains III, IV and V is apparent. (b) Transmembrane organization of group I G-protein-coupled receptors. This group is characterized by the presence of a sequence DRY (aspartate-arginine-tryptophan) and a disulfide bond (S-S) between the extracellular loops 1 and 2. (c) The third intracellular loop i3 in most G-protein-coupled receptors participates in the coupling with G proteins (e.g. the β$_2$-adrenergic receptor). (a: Adapted from Buck L and Axel R, 1991. A novel multigene family may encode odorant receptors: a molecular basis for odor recognition, *Cell* 65, 175–187; and from Anholt RRH, 1993. Molecular biology of olfaction, *Crit. Rev. Neurobiol.* 7, 1–22, with permission. b, c: From Bockaert J, 1995, Les récepteurs à sept domaines transmembranaires: physiologie et pathologie de la transduction, *Médecine et Sciences* 11, 382–394, with permission.)

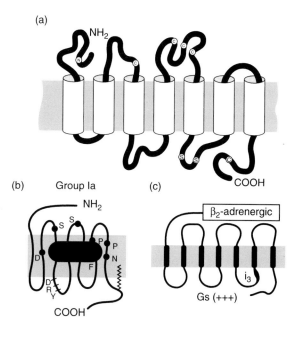

spleen and kidney. In contrast, hybridization is detected in olfactory epithelium, demonstrating that the expression of the family of olfactory proteins cloned is restricted to the olfactory epithelium.

15.3.2 The Activation of Odorant Receptors Leads to the Activation of Adenylate Cyclase and the Rapid Formation of cAMP via the Activation of a G_s-like Protein

Preparations of frog olfactory cilia contain a high concentration of substrate for ADP ribosylation by cholera toxin. This toxin specifically labels the α subunit of the G_s protein in other tissues. In the olfactory tissue it labels a G-type protein of slightly different motility. To characterize the candidate G protein mediating odorant transduction, cDNA clones homologous to a highly conserved region of the G_α subunit were isolated from a rat olfactory library.

The activation of odorant receptors leads to the activation of a $G_{olf\alpha}$ protein

By screening the rat olfactory cDNA library, a $G_{olf\alpha}$ subunit that is expressed abundantly and exclusively by olfactory neurons has been identified. This $G_{olf\alpha}$ subunit shares 88% amino acid identity with $G_{s\alpha}$ present in neurons. In order to play a role in olfaction, this G protein must be expressed preferentially in the olfactory neurons, be coupled to odorant receptors and be able to stimulate the formation of cAMP.

Immunocytochemical experiments demonstrate that $G_{olf\alpha}$ is abundant in crude olfactory cilia preparations where olfactory receptors are also densely expressed (see above), a localization appropriate for a G protein involved in odorant signal transduction. In order to test that $G_{olf\alpha}$ is able to stimulate adenylate cyclase, a murine lymphoma cell line, which is deficient in endogenous stimulatory G proteins, is infected with a recombinant retrovirus encoding $G_{olf\alpha}$. The expressed G proteins are activated by aluminum fluoride ions (AlF_4^-) known to activate G proteins in the absence of receptor activation (the olfactory receptors are of course absent in the cell line). In such conditions, membranes prepared from $G_{olf\alpha}$-expressing cells show an increase in adenylate cyclase activity in response to AlF_4^- though membranes prepared from non-$G_{olf\alpha}$-expressing cells do not. The coupling of $G_{olf\alpha}$ to olfactory receptors could not be tested in these experiments since they were performed before the molecular cloning of olfactory receptors.

An odorant-sensitive adenylate cyclase is present in membranes of olfactory cells

The enzyme adenylate cyclase is present in extraordinarily high amounts in crude olfactory cilia preparations (a cell-free preparation). Activation of adenylate cyclase in this preparation by non-hydrolyzable GTP analogs or the diterpene forskolin reveals a specific activity 10-fold higher than in brain membranes. The application of a mixture of odorants enhances the adenylate cyclase activity in a dose-dependent manner. This is observed only in the presence of GTP (Figure 15.5) or GTP-γ-S. The concentration of odorants required to activate adenylate cyclase *in vitro* correlates well with that known to give responses *in vivo*. Moreover, non-odorant compounds known to stimulate adenylate cyclase in other membranes such as isoprenaline, prostaglandins and histamine are ineffective. These results suggest that odor reception involves the binding of odor molecules to a family of receptors linked to a G_{olf} protein and the subsequent activation of adenylate cyclase by the α subunits of activated G_{olf}.

Figure 15.5 *Effects of odorants on olfactory cilia adenylate cyclase.* The adenylate cyclase activity of frog olfactory cilia membranes is assayed in the presence of 0.5 mM IBMX. The experiment is performed in the presence of 10 μM GTP. The results are normalized with respect to the activity elicited by GTP alone (G), which is about twice the basal activity level. AA: *n*-amyl acetate; CN: 1,8-cineole; CV: L-carvone; CT: citral (each at 1 mM); MX: a mixture of the preceding four components at a concentration of 0.25 mM each. (From Pace U, Hanski E, Salomon Y and Lancet D, 1985. Odorant-sensitive adenylate cyclase may mediate olfactory reception, *Nature* 316, 255–258, with permission.)

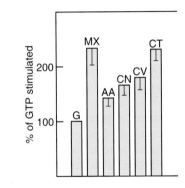

The adenylate cyclase activated by $G_{olf\alpha}$ is type III adenylate cyclase. Calmodulin is abundant in olfactory cilia, and on isolated dendritic cilia from frog olfactory tissue, the activity of the odorant-sensitive adenylate cyclase (type III) is stimulated by calmodulin. This effect is dose dependent and strictly Ca^{2+} dependent. Adenylate cyclase type III is a Ca^{2+}-calmodulin sensitive isoenzyme. Activation by calmodulin can generate concentrations of cAMP three to six times higher than those elicited by maximal concentrations of a mixture of odorants. Thus, enhanced production of cAMP can be evoked by the coincidence of two distinct activation signals, $G_{olf\alpha}$ and Ca^{2+} bound to calmodulin.

The formation of cAMP precedes the onset of the current

One important criterion for a candidate second messenger of chemo-electrical transduction is that its formation must precede the onset of the odorant-induced membrane permeability changes which proceed on a sub-second time scale (see Figure 15.11). In order to study the kinetics of cAMP formation in response to odorant stimulation, the basal level of cAMP is first estimated in a preparation of isolated olfactory cilia from rat. The application of the odorant isomenthone in the presence of GTP (to allow G-protein activation) evokes a rapid increase of cAMP, reaching a maximal level between 25 and 50 ms and declining thereafter to the basal level in 250–500 ms (Figure 15.6a). This cAMP increase clearly precedes the electrical response and is dependent on the dose of odorant (Figure 15.6b). In contrast, no variations in inositol trisphosphate (IP_3) concentration is observed. These observations favor the role of cAMP as a second messenger in rat olfactory transduction.

In antennal preparations from the cockroach, the application of an odorant induces the rapid (250–500 ms) formation of IP_3 and stimulates adenylate cyclase to a lesser extent. IP_3 seems to have a role in olfactory transduction in this preparation. In cells where IP_3 formation is observed in response to odorants, it could have the following role: IP_3 would bind to receptors linked to Ca^{2+} channels located in the ciliary plasma membrane and evoke Ca^{2+} influx; Ca^{2+} would bind to calmodulin and activate adenylate cyclase type III (see above); this pathway would

Figure 15.6 *Rapid kinetics of odorant-induced accumulation of cAMP in rat olfactory cilia.* (a) In a preparation of isolated olfactory cilia, the application of 1 µM isomenthone evokes a rapid increase of cAMP concentration which declines thereafter to the base line. The inositol trisphosphate concentration (IP_3) is not affected. (b) Odorant dose-dependence of the cAMP accumulation. Various doses of isomenthone, 0.1 µM, 1 µM, 10 µM and 100 µM (from bottom to top), induce a rise in cAMP accumulation with different onset and decay times. (From Breer H, Boekhoff I and Tareilus E, 1990. Rapid kinetics of second messenger formation in olfactory transduction, *Nature* 345, 65–68, with permission.)

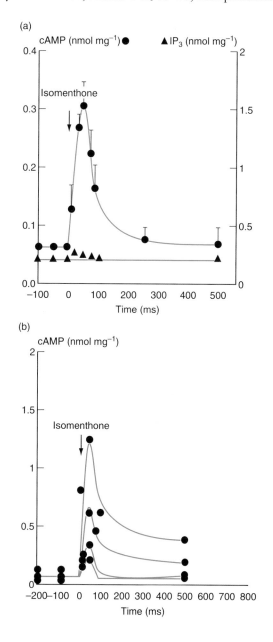

greatly enhance cAMP production when adenylate cyclase type III is at the same time activated by $G_{olf\alpha}$. The involvement of IP_3 or other second messenger pathways in olfactory transduction is still a matter of debate. In this chapter, we will focus on the olfactory transduction pathway via cAMP.

15.4 cAMP Opens a Cyclic Nucleotide-Gated Channel and Generates an Inward Current

15.4.1 The Olfactory Cyclic Nucleotide-Gated Channel is a Ligand-Gated Channel Composed of at Least Two Different Subunits

A protein similar to the cyclic nucleotide-gated channel from rods (visual cells) was looked for in olfactory epithelium. At present, cDNAs encoding two olfactory cyclic nucleotide-gated channel subunits have been cloned and characterized. Their expression is restricted to olfactory epithelium. The hydropathy plot of the sequence of the channel from rods and cone receptors (cGMP-gated channel) and olfactory receptor neurons led to a model of the secondary structure of the channel (Figure 15.7). This model presents six putative membrane-spanning regions. A region located on the C-terminal side of the sixth

Figure 15.7 *Hypothetical model of the two-dimensional architecture of cyclic nucleotide-gated channels.* From Bönigk W, Altenhofen W, Muller F *et al.*, 1993, Rod and cone photoreceptor cells express distinct genes for cGMP-gated channels, *Neuron* **10**, 865–877, and from Zufall F, Firestein S and Shepherd GM, 1995. Cyclic nucleotide-gated channels and sensory transduction in olfactory receptor neurons, *Ann. Rev. Biophys. Biomol. Struct.* **23**, 577–607, with permission.)

domain shows significant sequence similarity with cyclic nucleotide binding sites such as, for example, the cGMP-dependent protein kinase.

The first subunit cloned (named $rOCNC_1$) contains sequence motifs reminiscent of voltage-gated channels, in particular K^+ and Ca^{2+} channels. The two classes of channels share in fact a common putative transmembrane topology. The subunit $rCOCN_1$ can form functional homo-oligomeric channels activated by cAMP when expressed in *Xenopus laevis* oocytes and mammalian cell lines. It presents a cyclic nucleotide-binding domain, comprising 80–100 amino acids located near the carboxyl terminus.

The second subunit cloned ($rCOCN_2$) cannot form functional channels by itself when expressed alone. However, when co-expressed with the first subunit, the channel activity detected resembles more closely that of the native channel and particularly concerning its low sensitivity to cAMP (see Section 15.4.3). This suggests that the native channel is a hetero-oligomer composed of at least the first and second cloned subunits in an unknown ratio.

15.4.2 cAMP Directly Opens a Cyclic Nucleotide-Gated Channel

The olfactory receptor cells are dissociated from the olfactory epithelium of the toad (*Bufo marinus*) by the action of proteolytic enzymes. A gigaohm seal is formed between the patch pipette and the membrane of a cilium. Because of the small diameter (0.1–0.25 μm) of the cilia, small patch pipette tips are used. The membrane patch is then excised, exposing the cytoplasmic surface of the cilium membrane to the bath solution (inside-out configuration). Nakamura and Gold (1987) were the first to show that in the presence of cAMP in the bath, single channel events are recorded from inside-out patches. However, they could not resolve single channel activity because of high densities of the cAMP-gated channels in the cilia membrane and therefore in the patch of membrane.

An alternative strategy was offered by the finding that cyclic nucleotide-gated channels also occur at low density in the membrane of the olfactory knob, dendrite and soma of olfactory receptor neurons. In such preparations, the activity of a single channel activated by cAMP can be recorded. Olfactory receptor neurons are isolated from the nasal epithelium of tiger

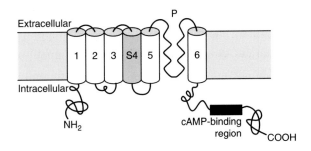

Figure 15.8 Single channel recordings of a cyclic AMP-gated channel. (a) The activity of a single cAMP-gated channel is recorded from inside-out patches of dendritic membrane of an isolated olfactory receptor neuron. Recordings without (A, E) and in the presence (B–D) of a continuous application of cAMP (10 µM) in the medium bathing the intracellular side of the membrane. $V_H = -60$ mV. (b) Amplitude histogram for the cAMP-induced unitary current. Each division on the ordinate scale is 20 counts, total of 2000 events. Peak = 2.9 pA, $V_H = -60$ mV. (c) Open time distribution for the cAMP-evoked channel activity. The single exponential fit has a time constant of $\tau_o = 1.89$ ms (bin width 0.2 ms, total of 2000 events). (From Zufall F, Firestein S and Shepherd GM, 1991. Analysis of single nucleotide-gated channels in olfactory receptor cells, *J. Neurosci.* **11**, 3573–3580, with permission.)

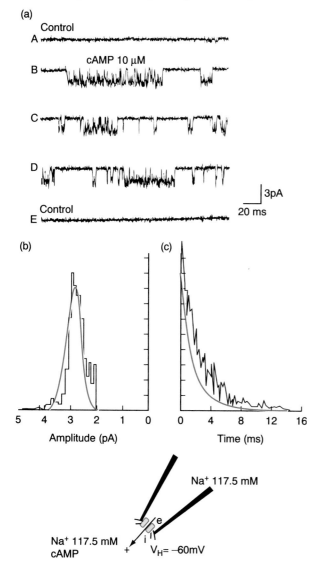

salamanders (*Ambystoma tigrinum*). The activity of the channel is recorded in patch clamp in the inside-out configuration, in the absence of divalent cations (see below). When the holding potential is –60 mV, the control recordings show no channel openings. In the presence of a continuous application of cAMP in the bath, single channel openings occur (Figure 15.8a). These effects are fully reversible upon returning to cAMP-free solution.

The inward current steps have a mean amplitude of –3 pA when the driving force is –60 mV (Figure 15.8b). This gives a unitary conductance of around 30–45 pS. The activity of the channel consists of single openings and bursts of openings (mean open time 1.9 ms, Figure 15.8c). As these results were obtained in inside-out configuration (the cytoplasmic surface of the cilium membrane faces the bath solution), where intracellular components are absent and particularly protein kinases, it is possible to conclude that cAMP directly gates the channel.

$$R+n(\text{cAMP}) \rightleftharpoons R-n(\text{cAMP}) \rightleftharpoons R^*-n(\text{cAMP}) \dashrightarrow \text{current}$$

where R is the cyclic nucleotide-gated channel in the closed state; R* is the cyclic nucleotide gated channel in the open state; cAMP is the ligand that gates the channel; and *n* is the number of cAMP molecules that bind to the channel.

cGMP also opens the olfactory cyclic nucleotide-gated channel

The results obtained with the application of cGMP are very similar. On the same patch of membrane cGMP evokes the same single channel openings as cAMP. Since the patches tested are always sensitive to both nucleotides, it is concluded that cAMP and cGMP act upon the same channel. The role of cGMP *in vivo*, if there is a role, is unclear since there is a very active odor-sensitive adenylate cyclase present in olfactory neurons and no detectable odor-sensitive guanylate cyclase activity.

Figure 15.9 *Voltage-dependence of the cAMP-induced unitary current.* The activity of a single channel is recorded in inside-out patches of dendritic membrane of an isolated olfactory receptor. A saturating concentration of cAMP (0.1 mM) is continuously present in the medium bathing the intracellular side of the membrane. (a) Examples of single-channel openings at different holding potentials as indicated for each trace. The closed state is marked by a broken line. (b) i_{cAMP}–V relation. Each point represents 3000 events from the recording shown in (a) (From Zufall F, Firestein S and Shepherd GM, 1991. Analysis of single nucleotide-gated channels in olfactory receptor cells, *J. Neurosci.* **11**, 3573–3580, with permission.)

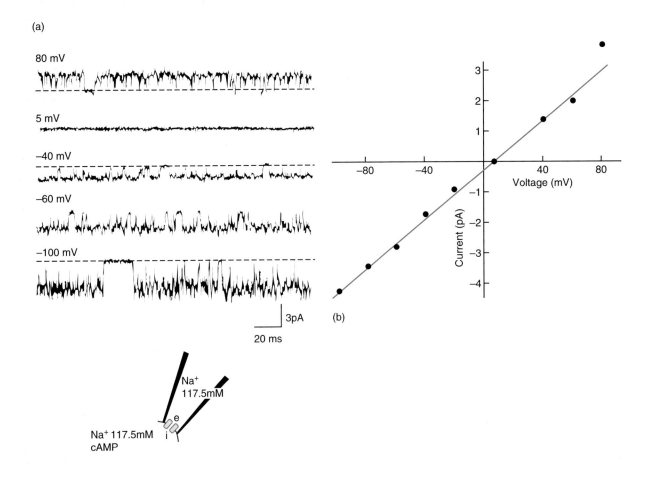

The unitary cAMP-induced current reverses around 0 mV

The voltage sensitivity of the channel is analyzed by exposing inside-out patches to saturating concentrations of cAMP while holding the membrane at different potentials. When measuring the unitary current amplitude, we obtain an i_{cAMP}/V plot (Figure 15.9b). This relation is approximately linear between −100 mV and +80 mV. The unitary current is inward for potentials more negative than +5 mV, reverses polarity at +5 mV and is outward for potentials more positive than +5 mV (Figure 15.9a, b). The reversal potential of i_{cAMP} varies slightly according to the experiment or the preparation studied.

The unitary conductance is constant in absence of divalent cations

The i/V relation of Figure 15.9b is described by the equation: $i_{cAMP} = \gamma_{cAMP} (V_m - E_{cAMP})$ where V_m is the membrane potential, E_{cAMP} is the reversal potential of the cAMP-induced current and γ_{cAMP} is the conductance of the cAMP-gated channel or unitary conductance. The value of γ_{cAMP} is the slope of the i/V plot. In the present experimental conditions (absence of divalent cations), it is equal to 45 pS and does not vary according to the membrane potential.

The cyclic nucleotide-gated channel is a non-specific cationic channel

The recorded value of the reversal potential of i_{cAMP} suggests that i_{cAMP} is either a cationic current or a current carried by Cl⁻ ions. A study of the ionic selectivity of the cAMP-gated channel was performed on macropatches of olfactory cell membrane from which only the macroscopic current is recorded. The results will therefore be explained in the next section.

The activity of the cyclic nucleotide-gated channel recorded in inside-out patches does not desensitize

Long exposures of single channels to even saturating concentrations of cAMP does not result in any detectable desensitization (see Figure 15.9a). In contrast, as we will see in the next section, recordings of the macroscopic cyclic nucleotide-gated current from intact olfactory neurons show strong desensitization to elevated intracellular cAMP concentration (see Fig. 15.11). This suggests that the mechanisms of desensitization require intracellular factors.

In the presence of increasing concentrations of external divalent cations the channel displays a flickering behavior

The effects of external divalent cations on cAMP-activated single channel currents are studied in inside-out membrane patches taken from the dendritic region of isolated olfactory receptor neurons of the tiger salamander (*Ambystoma tigrinum*). Since the effect of divalent cations was tested on the external side (i.e. in the pipette solution), each experiment with a different concentration of divalent cation corresponds to a new patch of membrane. A comparison of these experiments is reliable since single channel parameters such as amplitude, kinetics and open probability do not differ considerably among different patches. With

increasing concentrations of Ca²⁺, from 10 nM (control) to 1 mM, in the pipette solution (extracellular solution), in the presence of cAMP in the medium bathing the intracellular side of the membrane, a reduction of the apparent unitary current is observed (Figure 15.10a). At higher concentrations of Ca²⁺ ions, the transitions are in fact too rapid to be fully resolved and appear as a reduction of the mean unitary current.

The effect of Ca²⁺ ions also shows a strong voltage-dependence. The i_{cAMP}/V relation (Figure 15.10b) is 'S-shaped' in the presence of external Ca²⁺ ions. The same effect is observed in the presence of external Mg²⁺ ions (600 μM). These effects are explained by an open channel block by divalent cations. Therefore, at normal resting membrane potential, about −50 mV, and at physiological extracellular Ca²⁺ concentration (the Ca²⁺ concentration in the mucus is between 2 and 5 mM), single channel events are no longer resolvable. The block is partially relieved by depolarization. The physiological consequences are analyzed in Sections 15.4.3 and 15.5.

In the presence of increasing concentrations of cytoplasmic Ca²⁺ ions the mean open time of the channel is decreased

In inside-out patches of dendritic membrane of an isolated olfactory receptor, the activity of a single cyclic nucleotide-gated channel is first recorded in the continuous presence of a saturating intracellular concentration of cAMP (100 μM) and a control intracellular Ca²⁺ concentration (0.1 μM) (Figure 15.10c, upper traces). Single channel currents are recorded and the mean open probability is 0.6. Even during several second-long exposures to a saturating concentration of cAMP, the channel displays no obvious signs of desensitization. When the intracellular Ca²⁺ concentration is increased 30 times (to 3 μM, middle traces), the amplitude and kinetics of channel openings are unaffected but the recording contains longer intervals between bursts of openings. The channel mean open probability is strongly reduced (to 0.09). Returning to the control solution restored normal channel activity (lower traces). This effect suggests that intracellular Ca²⁺ ions act directly on an intracellular site of the channel and stabilize the channel in the closed state. It is very different from the open

Figure 15.10   Effect of extracellular and intracellular Ca²⁺ ions on single channel activity. Recording of the activity of a single cAMP-gated channel from inside-out patches of an isolated olfactory receptor cell. (a) The patches are exposed to increasing concentrations of external Ca²⁺ ions (in the pipette solution). The flickering behavior of the channel increases and the apparent i_{cAMP} amplitude is decreased. $V_H = -100$ mV. (b) i_{cAMP}–V relation for mean unitary current in different concentrations of external Ca²⁺ ions. (c) (Page 359) Modulation of single channel activity by intracellular Ca²⁺ ions. Top and lower traces are single channel currents elicited by application of 100 µM cAMP with Ca²⁺ at 0.1 µM. Middle traces are the same channel in the presence of 3 µM intracellular Ca²⁺. $V_H = -60$ mV. (a, b: From Zufall F and Firestein S, 1993. Divalent cations block the cyclic nucleotide-gated channel of olfactory receptor neurons, *J. Neurophysiol.* **69**, 1758–1768, with permission. c: From Zufall F, Shepherd GM and Firestein S, 1991. Inhibition of the olfactory cyclic nucleotide gated ion channel by intracellular calcium, *Proc. R. Soc. Lond. Ser. B* **246**, 225–230, with permission.)

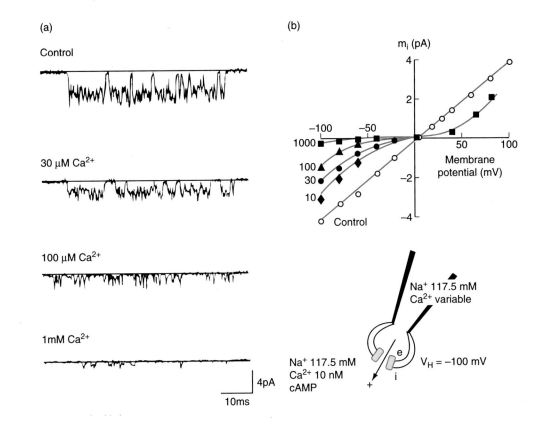

channel block by external divalent cations described above.

15.4.3 The Activation of N Cyclic Nucleotide-Gated Channels Evokes an Inward Depolarizing Current Carried by Cations

In a preparation containing N channels, cAMP induces a macroscopic current I such as $I_{cAMP} = N \times p_o \times i_{cAMP}$. To record this macroscopic current in isolation the activity of an isolated olfactory receptor cell (from the newt olfactory epithelium, *Cynops pyrrhogaster*) in response to a rise of intracellular cAMP is recorded in whole-cell patch clamp in the presence of blockers of all the voltage-gated currents. First a gigaohm seal is formed between the patch pipette and the membrane of the terminal swelling (cell-attached configuration, Figure 15.11a). The extracellular solution contains TEACl to block voltage-gated K⁺ conductances and CoCl₂ to block voltage-gated Ca²⁺ conductances. The pipette solution contains Cs⁺ and EGTA to block voltage- and Ca²⁺-activated K⁺ currents. cAMP (or cGMP) is added

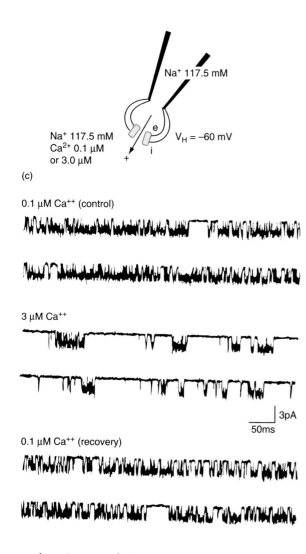

Na⁺ 117.5 mM

Na⁺ 117.5 mM
Ca²⁺ 0.1 μM
or 3.0 μM

$V_H = -60$ mV

(c)

0.1 μM Ca⁺⁺ (control)

3 μM Ca⁺⁺

3pA
50ms

0.1 μM Ca⁺⁺ (recovery)

The second subunit of the cyclic nucleotide-gated channel confers high sensitivity to cAMP

The olfactory cyclic nucleotide-gated channel subunit cloned first (named $rOCNC_1$), when functionally expressed in *Xenopus laevis* oocytes and mammalian cell lines, forms functional, presumably homo-oligomeric, channels. Although these channels share some characteristics with the native channels (they are selectively permeable to cations and activated by cAMP), their sensitivity to cAMP is 30-fold less than the native channels. The activity of the expressed channels is recorded in patch clamp in the inside-out configuration. These are macropatches which contain a high density of channels and the current recorded is therefore a macroscopic current. Bath application of low doses of cAMP (or cGMP) have no effect but high doses evoke a large inward current (like a whole cell inward current) (Figure 15.12a). One hypothesis could be that additional subunits are missing from the expression system.

A new cDNA cloned from the rat olfactory epithelium that encodes a second subunit of the olfactory cyclic nucleotide-gated channel, $rOCNC_2$, has been found (both these subunits present a structural homology with the voltage-gated K⁺ channel subunits). *Xenopus* oocytes are injected with *in vitro* transcribed $rOCNC_2$ RNA. Excised inside-out patches from these oocytes failed to respond to bath application of cAMP or cGMP, suggesting a failure of the protein to incorporate into the oocyte membrane or to form homo-oligomeric channels. When the oocytes are injected with equal amounts of $rOCNC_1$ and $rOCNC_2$ RNA, the excised inside-out patches now respond with a large current to bath application of low doses of cAMP (Figure 15.12b) and cGMP.

The cAMP-induced current is generated in olfactory cilia

The response amplitude and the time course differ markedly depending on the site of the seal, i.e. the site of cAMP introduction. The most effective site is the nearest to olfactory cilia. When cAMP is introduced to the terminal swelling (close to the cilia), it evokes a response of large amplitude, short latency and rapid rising time (Figure 15.13a). When cAMP is introduced to the cell body, the amplitude of the response is

to the pipette solution. At time zero the patch of membrane is ruptured to allow the pipette solution to diffuse into the olfactory cell from the tip of the opening of the recording pipette through the ruptured hole of the plasma membrane. When the intrapipette solution contains cAMP, an inward current is recorded approximately 100 ms after rupture of the patch membrane ($V_H = -50$ mV, Figure 15.11b). Since in the absence of cyclic nucleotide in the patch pipette, no current is recorded (Figure 15.11c), it is concluded that the inward current is induced by the intracellularly introduced cAMP. The amplitude of the cAMP-induced current is dose dependent (Figure 15.11d). The least effective dose is estimated to be in the order of 100 μM and the maximal reponse is observed for 1 mM intracellular cAMP.

Figure 15.11   A transient macroscopic inward current is induced in an olfactory neuron by the introduction of cAMP from the patch pipette. (a) First a gigaohm seal is formed on the dendritic knob. (b) A brief application of negative pressure ruptures the membrane at the pipette tip (arrowhead) and 0.5 mM cAMP is allowed to diffuse into the terminal knob. It induces a transient inward current. $V_H = -50$ mV. (c) When the pipette solution does not contain a cyclic nucleotide, no inward current is induced after the membrane rupture (arrowhead). (d) The dose-dependence is studied by measuring the inward current amplitude (pA) induced by different doses of cAMP (in mM). For each experiment, only one dose can be tested since cAMP is in the patch pipette solution (the number of cells tested for each point are in parentheses). (From Kurahashi T, 1990. The response induced by intracellular cyclic AMP in isolated olfactory receptor cells of the newt, *J. Physiol.* **430**: 355–371, with permission.)

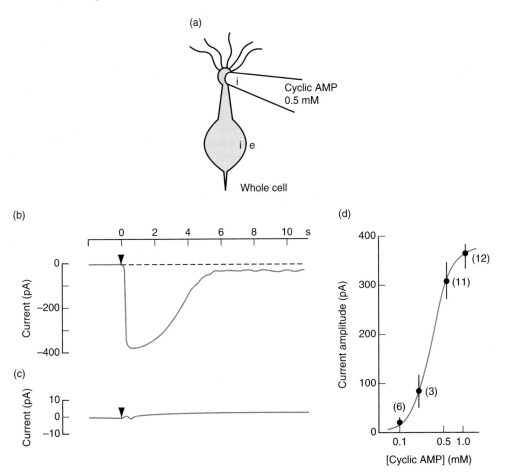

smaller, the latency longer and the rising time slower (Figure 15.13b). This agrees with the finding that excised patches from the ciliary membrane show a high sensitivity to cAMP. The density of cAMP-gated channels in the ciliary membrane is estimated to be about 2500–10 000 μm^{-2} (from a single channel conductance $\gamma = 30$ pS).

The cAMP-gated current is carried by cations

The whole cell current evoked by intracellular cAMP is recorded in the presence of blockers of voltage-gated channels. The cAMP-induced current–voltage relation is measured by rapidly changing the holding potential. A ramp voltage command varying from –50 to +46 mV is applied at a rate of 195 mV s^{-1} during the evoked current and after the end of the current

Figure 15.12 cAMP-induced currents in excised macropatches from oocytes injected with cloned rat olfactory cyclic nucleotide-gated channel RNA. (a) Inward currents recorded from inside-out macropatches from an oocyte injected with $rOCNC_1$ RNA in response to bath application of 10 µM or 500 µM cAMP. (b) Same experiment as in (a) for a patch excised from an oocyte injected with $rOCNC_1$ and $rOCNC_2$ RNA. (From Liman ER and Buck LB, 1994. A second subunit of the olfactory cyclic nucleotide-gated channel confers high sensitivity to cAMP, *Neuron* **13**, 611–621, with permission.)

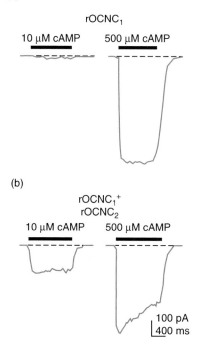

(a)

$rOCNC_1$

10 µM cAMP   500 µM cAMP

(b)

$rOCNC_1^+$
$rOCNC_2$

10 µM cAMP   500 µM cAMP

100 pA
400 ms

(Figure 15.14a). The curve obtained after the end of the current is subtracted from the one obtained at the peak of the current in order to eliminate the leak current. The *I–V* relation (Figure 15.14b) is almost linear, between –50 and +50 mV and the reversal potential of the cAMP-induced current is around –5 mV. This observed value can be accounted for by either a current carried by cations or by Cl⁻ ions.

To differentiate between these two possibilities, the *I–V* relations of the cAMP-induced current are measured under different ionic conditions. When K^+ ions replace all the Na^+ ions present in the extracellular medium, the *I–V* curve and the reversal potential are unchanged, suggesting that the channel is equally permeable to Na^+ and K^+. Changing the Na^+ extracellular concentration alone induced changes of the reversal potential of the response according to the Nernst equation for a cationic channel. In conclusion, the channel permeates all alkali metal ions such as Li^+, Rb^+ or Cs^+ ions but not Cl^- or choline ions.

The characteristics of I_{cAMP} are dependent on Ca^{2+} ions

In some olfactory receptor cells recorded in physiological solutions, the *I–V* relation shows significant outward rectification at potentials more negative than –50 mV in contrast to the linear behavior of the *I–V* relation in the absence of divalent cations. Based on the observations of open channel block in single channel recordings (see Figure 15.10a, b) it is proposed that extracellular Ca^{2+} ions bind to a site within the pore of the open cAMP-gated channel and block it. A membrane depolarization removes the block (as observed for Mg^{2+} ions and NMDA channels). The physiological consequence of such a block is that the generator current in these olfactory cells induced by odors depends simultaneously on cAMP concentration and membrane voltage.

Moreover, intracellular Ca^{2+} ions play a role. In control conditions we have seen that the macroscopic inward current evoked by a continuous application of cAMP is transient despite the fact that cAMP is continuously supplied from the pipette to the intracellular medium (see Figure 15.10c). When the extracellular solution is replaced by a Ca^{2+}-free solution, the cAMP-induced current is sustained during the recording (Figure 15.15a). Re-application of a standard extracellular medium containing 3 mM Ca^{2+} suppresses the maintained current. Conversely, after the end of the cAMP-induced current evoked in control external conditions, the application of a medium containing a low Ca^{2+} concentration (1 µM) re-induces an inward current after the response was once suppressed (Figure 15.15b). Finally, in the presence of control external Ca^{2+} concentration, the intracellular injection of the Ca^{2+} chelator EGTA prior to cAMP application slows down the decay time course of the cAMP-induced current.

In single channel recordings in the absence of a control intracellular Ca^{2+} concentration, the channel does not desensitize, but in the presence of a high intracellular Ca^{2+} concentration the channel mean open

Figure 15.13   Relation between the site of cAMP introduction and the response time course. (a) When 0.5 mM cAMP is introduced into the terminal knob, it evokes a response of large amplitude, short latency (0.20 ± 0.02 s) and rapid rising time (time from the onset to the peak = 0.9 ± 0.2s). (b) When 0.5 mM cAMP is introduced into the proximal part of the dendrite, which is about 20 μm long, it evokes a response of small amplitude (approximately half of that in (a)), long latency (1.4 ± 0.4 s) and slow rising time (2.8 ± 0.5 s). Arrowheads indicate the time when the patch membrane is ruptured. V_H = −50 mV. (From Kurahashi T, 1990. The response induced by intracellular cyclic AMP in isolated olfactory receptor cells of the newt, *J. Physiol.* **430**, 355–371, with permission.)

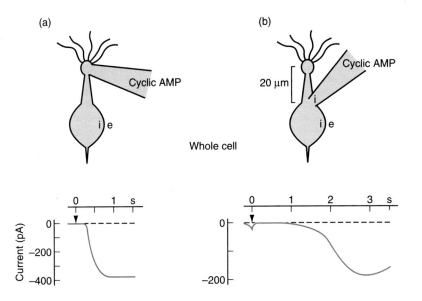

probability is strongly reduced (see Figure 15.10c). We know that the cAMP-gated channel is permeable to Ca^{2+} ions since Ca^{2+} influx during the odor response is observed in experiments using the Ca^{2+} indicator Fura-2 (see Appendix 11.1) in conditions where other pathways of Ca^{2+} entry are blocked. It is proposed that the main source of cytoplasmic Ca^{2+} ions is the Ca^{2+} influx as a constituent of the inward current. Cytoplasmic Ca^{2+} ions would act directly on an intracellular site on the channel and reduce the apparent affinity of the channel for cAMP. This would constitute a rapid and effective negative feedback loop, which could account for the short-term adaptation of the response to sustained cAMP or odor exposure recorded in intact neurons.

15.4.4 The Cyclic Nucleotide-Gated Conductance and the Odor-Gated Conductance are Identical

The unitary activity of a patch of olfactory dendritic membrane is recorded in patch clamp in the cell-attached configuration. A pulse of odor activates a channel present in the patch (Figure 15.16a). The external solution is then replaced by a solution containing IBMX (isobutylmethylxanthine), an inhibitor of phosphodiesterase, the enzyme that hydrolyses cAMP in 5'AMP (IBMX enhances the basal and evoked intracellular concentration of cAMP). In presence of IBMX in the bath the same channel activity is recorded from the same patch of membrane (Figure 15.16b). This suggests that the ion channels underlying the odor-induced unitary current and the cyclic nucleotide-induced unitary current are the same.

In whole-cell patch clamp recordings, the odorant-induced current has the same properties as the cAMP-induced current. Cilia are the most sensitive site both

Figure 15.14 Current–voltage relation of the cAMP-induced response. (a) Experimental design. Same experiment as in Figure 15.11b but a voltage ramp command from −50 to +46 mV at a rate of 195 mV s^{-1} is applied to the voltage clamped membrane before, at the peak of the response (A) and after the end of the response (B). Voltage-dependent K$^+$ currents are blocked by 35 mM TEACl and voltage-dependent Ca^{2+} currents by 3 mM CoCl$_2$ in the external solution. (b) I–V relation of the cAMP-induced response. This relation is obtained by subtracting the I–V curve recorded after the response (B) to the I–V curve recorded at the peak of the response (A) in order to subtract leak current. The current reverses at −5 mV. The external solution contains (in mM): 85 NaCl, 3 CaCl$_2$, 35 TEACl, 3 CoCl$_2$, 2 NaOH. The intrapipette solution contains (in mM): 122 K$^+$, 120 Cl$^-$, 0.5 cAMP. (From Kurahashi T, 1990. The response induced by intracellular cyclic AMP in isolated olfactory receptor cells of the newt, *J. Physiol.* **430**, 355–371, with permission.)

Figure 15.15 In the presence of a low external Ca^{2+} concentration, the cAMP-induced current is sustained. (a) Same experiment as in Figure 15.11a but in the presence of a Ca^{2+}-free external solution and 1 mM cAMP in the pipette. (b) The transient response induced by 1 mM cAMP is first recorded in the presence of 3 mM external Ca^{2+}. The subsequent application of a low external Ca^{2+} concentration after the end of the first response re-induces an inward current (cAMP is still present inside the patch pipette and freely diffuses inside the cell). V_H = −90 mV. (From Kurahashi T, 1990. The response induced by intracellular cyclic AMP in isolated olfactory receptor cells of the newt, *J. Physiol.* **430**, 355–371, with permission.)

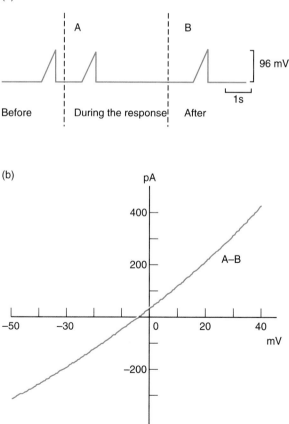

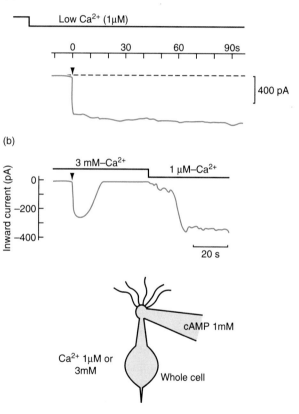

to intracellularly applied cAMP and to extracellularly applied odorants. Both responses reverse polarity near 0 mV and are carried by cations. To either stimulation of a long duration, responses show a rapid decay to a very low level, and the decay is strongly dependent on the influx of Ca^{2+} ions.

Figure 15.16   Odor and cyclic nucleotide-induced single channel activity in the same membrane patch. The activity of a single cyclic nucleotide-gated channel is recorded in cell-attached configuration from an isolated olfactory receptor neuron. A 150 ms pulse of odor stimulus is delivered at the arrow. It elicits a burst of single channel openings (a). A solution with 100 μM IBMX is then perfused into the bath. It elicits a similar activity in the same patch of membrane (b). Sample recordings at higher sweep speeds are shown below. Pipette potential: +40 mV. (From Firestein S, Zufall F and Shepherd GM, 1991. Single odor-sensitive channels in olfactory receptor neurons are also gated by cyclic nucleotides, *J. Neurosci.* **11**, 3565–3572, with permission.)

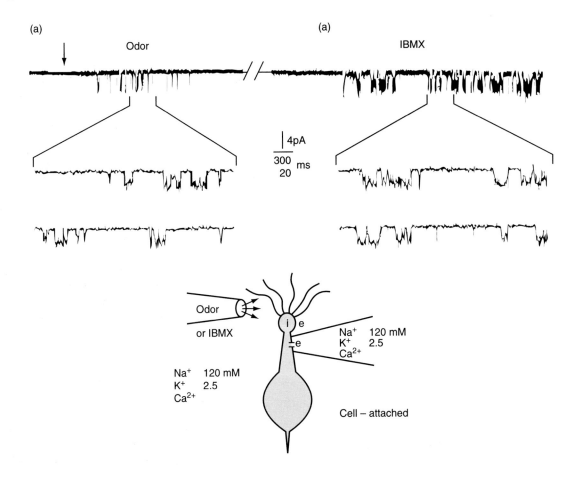

15.4.5 Conclusions (Figure 15.17)

These results, together with the preceding ones, demonstrate that the first event that initiates excitation of olfactory neurons is the binding of odorant to one or more receptors. These receptors are members of a diverse subfamily that itself belongs to the large superfamily of G-protein-linked receptors. Binding of the odorant on its receptor activates G_{olf}, a heterotrimeric protein closely related to the G_s protein. Binding of GTP to the activated α subunit of the G_{olf} protein triggers stimulation of adenylate cyclase type III. This leads to the formation of cAMP. When the intraciliary concentration of cAMP reaches a threshold level, cAMP opens directly cyclic nucleotide-gated channels present in the ciliary membrane. The cations Na^+ and Ca^{2+} flow into the cilia through the open channels and generate an inward depolarizing current. The cAMP concentration returns to its basal levels by the rapid degradation of cAMP by phosphodiesterase, which hydrolyses cAMP in 5'AMP. The increase of cytoplasmic Ca^{2+} concentration caused

Figure 15.17 The molecular cascade from odorant stimulation to activation of the cyclic nucleotide-gated channels. See text for explanations. OR, odorant receptor; ACIII, adenylate cyclase type III; CNG, cyclic-nucleotide-gated channel; PDE, phosphodiesterase. The open channel block by Ca^{2+} ions is not represented.

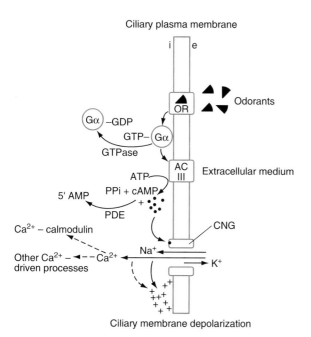

Ciliary plasma membrane

Odorants

$G\alpha$ –GDP

GTP–$G\alpha$

GTPase

ATP

AC III — Extracellular medium

PPi + cAMP

5' AMP

PDE

Ca^{2+} – calmodulin

CNG

Other Ca^{2+} – ◄– – Ca^{2+}

Na^+

driven processes

K^+

Ciliary membrane depolarization

by Ca^{2+} entry through cyclic nucleotide-gated channels, together with the action of the enzyme phosphodiesterase, contribute to stop the effect of cAMP and to make the cAMP-induced response transient. Such a system allows amplification of the signal: even a few molecules of the odorant that activates a few receptors induce the activation of many G proteins, the formation of many molecules of cAMP and the activation of many cationic channels.

15.5 The Odorant-Evoked Inward Current Evokes a Membrane Depolarization that Spreads Electronically to the Axon Hillock where it can Elicit Action Potentials

15.5.1 The Odorant-Induced Inward Current Depolarizes the Membrane of Olfactory Receptors: the Generator Potential

We showed in Section 15.2 that an odorant induces a depolarization of the membrane of olfactory receptor cells recorded *in vivo*. The same response is recorded *in vitro*. The *in vitro* preparation allows the analysis of the correspondence between the inward current and its consequence on membrane potential. Receptor cells are dissociated enzymatically from the olfactory epithelium of the newt, *Cynops pyrrhogaster*. Isolated olfactory cells are voltage-clamped by a patch pipette and their activity recorded in the whole-cell configuration. The odorant, *m*-amyl acetate, is dissolved in the external solution, placed in a pipette and ejected by pressure to the surface of the recorded cell. The cell interior is dialysed with the pipette solution. In such conditions, the resting membrane potential recorded is around –45 mV. When the membrane is clamped at resting level (I_H = 0 pA), a brief application of the odorant evokes an inward current of 300 pA (Figure 15.18a). Ejection of the vehicle solution alone does not induce any response, ruling out the possibility of a response to mechanical stimulation (pressure). If the recording is now switched to current clamp mode in order to record potential changes, the same brief application of the same odorant evokes at resting membrane potential a depolarization of 25–30 mV (Figure 15.18b). This depolarization is called the generator potential.

The membrane of the olfactory cells has a high input resistance in the order of 2–5 GΩ when measured in the isolated preparation with a patch pipette (this is estimated from the amplitude of the passive hyperpolarization evoked by a negative current pulse of known amplitude through the recording electrode). Thus the current required to depolarize the membrane by 10 mV from the resting potential can be as small as 10 pA. The synchronous opening of a few 45 pS channels at –50 mV would in theory be sufficient to drive the membrane potential to the threshold for spike initiation. At physiological Ca^{2+} concentrations,

Figure 15.18   Response to odorant in control conditions. The activity of an isolated receptor cell is recorded in patch clamp in the whole-cell configuration. Cells are bathed in a standard solution and pipettes are filled with a pseudo-intracellular medium. Upper traces indicate the timing of ejection of the odorant, *n*-amyl acetate (10 mM). (a) In voltage clamp mode, the odorant application induces an inward current ($V_H = -54$ mV). (b) In current clamp mode, the odorant application induces a depolarization. The (a) and (b) recordings are obtained from two different olfactory receptor cells and the differences in the latency of the responses are due to a different position of the pipette ejecting the odorant. (Adapted from Kurahashi T, 1989. Activation of a cation-selective conductance in the olfactory receptor cell isolated from the newt, *J. Physiol. (Lond.)* **419**, 177–192, with permission.)

however, the unitary conductance is so reduced that simultaneous activation of at least 100 channels could be required to generate a response.

The divalent cation block is relieved by depolarization. So, we can hypothesize that once a sufficient number of channels are activated, the membrane begins to depolarize. This relieves partly the cation block. Then more current flows through the open channels and the membrane further depolarizes. This hypothesis is based on the model of the glutamatergic NMDA receptor channel studied in Chapter 11. Consequently, the generator potential depends not only on the presence of cAMP but also on the membrane potential of the olfactory receptor neuron.

15.5.2 The Odorant-Induced Depolarization Takes Place in the Cilia – Spikes are Initiated in the Soma–Initial Axon Segment – The Pattern of Spike Discharge Propagated Along the Olfactory Cell Axon Codes for the Concentration and Duration of the Odorant Stimulus

The generator potential (the depolarization) is electrotonically conducted from the cilia to the axon initial segment where the voltage-gated Na+ channels are located and spikes are initiated in response to a membrane depolarization above threshold. In very few isolated olfactory cells (*in vitro* preparation), the depolarization evokes repetitive firing. Usually, depolarization causes only small spike-like events. Amputation of axons by the dissociation procedure may be responsible for the lack of spike initiation. In order to study the coupling between odorant-induced depolarization and the initiation of spikes and the coding of odorant concentration, the *in vivo* preparation is chosen.

Most olfactory neurons increase their firing rate with increasing odorant concentration. When the activity of an olfactory neuron is intracellularly recorded *in vivo* (see Section 15.2 and Figure 15.3), a slow (50 mV/s) depolarization and evoked action potentials are recorded in response to an odorant application (Figure 15.19). The depolarization amplitude increases with the stimulus intensity as well as the instantaneous frequency of firing. For the largest depolarizations, the maximal instantaneous frequency is about 25 s^{-1}. These observations suggest that the

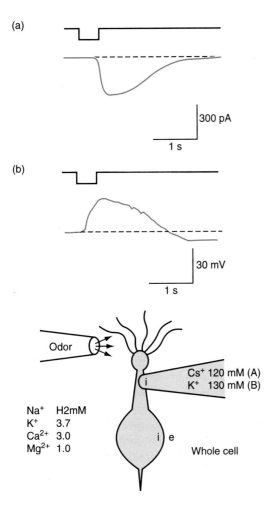

Figure 15.19 Dose–response relation recorded from an olfactory neuron stimulated with increasing concentrations of odorants. Olfactory stimuli consist of short puffs (200–300 ms) of isoamylacetate (ISO) or camphor (CAM). From A to D and from E to H the concentrations of isoamylacetate or camphor are increased. The activity of the neuron is recorded with an intracellular electrode, in current clamp mode (V_m = –62 mV). A: The lowest concentration of isoamylacetate evokes a succession of small depolarizations and an action potential is evoked when the membrane reaches –52 mV. B–D: A slow and graded depolarization appears when the concentration of isoamylacetate is increased. As the amplitude of the depolarization increases, the number of spikes generated also increases. Note the small amplitude of the spikes when the interval interspike is short. E–H: With camphor, the general features of the cell responses were the same. Calibrations: 60 mV, 500 ms. (Adapted from Trotier D and MacLeod P, 1983. Intracellular recordings from salamander olfactory receptor cells, *Brain Res.* **268**, 225–237, with permission.)

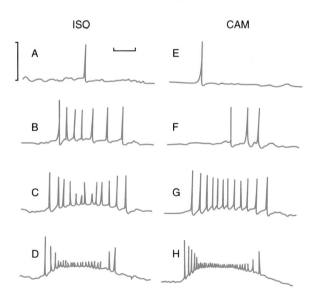

ISO   CAM

A   E

B   F

C   G

D   H

stimulus concentration is transduced by the cell into an increased frequency of firing.

15.5.3 The Nature of the Odorant would be Coded by the Nature of the Olfactory Neuron Stimulated and the Synaptic Arrangements in the Olfactory Bulb

It is hypothesized that each olfactory receptor cell expresses a single type of olfactory receptor. Thus, two odorants that are well discriminated would activate two different populations of olfactory neurons. This would hold true for all the odorants recognized. Now, how can the brain determine which type of neurons has been activated?

Specific recognition is conserved by the characteristic arrangements of the synaptic connections between the axons of olfactory cells and the second-order neurons in the olfactory bulb. There is a high convergence ratio 100–1000:1 of olfactory neurons to secondary neurons. It has been shown that the olfactory neurons expressing the same olfactory receptor project to the same region in the olfactory bulb on a small number of glomeruli, or even one. This was studied with *in situ* hybridization techniques (see Appendix 2.3). Taking advantage of the fact that copies of mRNA are transported in olfactory neurons to axon terminals, sections of the olfactory bulb are treated with a labeled probe which recognizes a known olfactory receptor mRNA: a single spot of labeled axons is observed in each olfactory bulb (left and right).

15.6 Conclusions

Olfactory receptor neurons amplify the odorant stimulus by a second messenger cascade that produces hundreds or more of effector molecules (G proteins, cAMP) in response to the capture of one odorant molecule. This mechanism of transduction of sensory information is slow. The delay between a threshold stimulus and the response is up to hundreds of milliseconds. The same type of mechanism underlies visual and gustatory transductions. If we compare with phototransduction, for example, the activation of rhodopsin by a single photon triggers a G protein (G_T) cascade which activates phosphodiesterase which hydrolyses cyclic GMP. In doing so, light causes closure of cGMP-gated cationic channels located in the plasma membrane of retinal rods and hyperpolarizes the membrane. The processes differ in that chemoreception involves an increase of cAMP concentration with a subsequent depolarization of the membrane whereas photoreception involves a decrease of cGMP concentration with a subsequent hyperpolarization of the membrane. It is striking that receptor cells use conventional G-protein-mediated mechanisms for transduction of the sensory stimulus, mechanisms also encountered in the transduction of neurotransmitter or hormone recognition.

Further Reading

Frings, S., Lynch, J.W. and Lindenman, B. (1992) Properties of cyclic nucleotide-gated channels mediating olfactory transduction. *J. Gen. Physiol.* **100**, 45–67.

Lancet, D. (1986) Vertebrate olfactory reception. *Ann. Rev. Neurosci.* **9**, 329–355.

Reed, R.R. (1990) How does the nose know? *Cell* **60**, 1–2.

Shepherd, G.M. (1994) Discrimination of molecular signals by the olfactory receptor neuron. *Neuron* **13**, 771–790.

Part V

Integration of Post-synaptic Currents and Synaptic Plasticity

The Integration of Synaptic Currents

Neurons of the mammalian central nervous system receive many afferents which contact different parts of their somato-dendritic arborization. When these afferents are activated, if their combined effect is depolarizing enough, they trigger the firing of sodium action potentials in the post-synaptic neuron. Classically, it is accepted that these action potentials are generated at a central point in the neuron, at the level of the initial segment of the axon (action potential generating zone, see Section 7.4.3 and Figure 16.1).

Action potentials are the response of the post-synaptic neuron. This response may be simple, consisting of a single action potential. In this case it can be described by a single characteristic: its latency. However, the post-synaptic response is generally more complex, consisting of several action potentials. It can then be described by several parameters: the latency of the first action potential, the duration of the response, the frequency of the action potentials that compose the response and the overall form – the pattern, or configuration – of the response (Figure 16.1b).

The events that lead to a post-synaptic response can be separated into several stages. When the afferent synapses are activated, an excitatory or inhibitory current is generated at the sub-synaptic membrane, as a result of activation of receptor channels by the neurotransmitter(s). These post-synaptic currents propagate through the dendrites to the soma and to the initial segment of the post-synaptic neuron. In the course of their propagation, the post-synaptic currents summate. If the sum of the post-synaptic currents is sufficient to depolarize the membrane of the initial segment as far as the threshold potential for activation of the voltage-sensitive sodium channels, a response is triggered in the post-synaptic neuron (Figure 16.1).

However, we will see in Chapter 17 that the presence of a post-synaptic response and the characteristics of this response are not only the result of the integration of different currents of synaptic origin over the somato-dendritic tree. In fact the response of the post-synaptic neuron is the result of two types of currents: currents across receptor channels in the post-synaptic membrane evoked by neurotransmitters and currents across voltage-sensitive channels present in the non-synaptic membrane. Currents of the first type are generated strictly at the post-synaptic membrane and their presence and duration is determined essentially by the interaction between the transmitter and the receptor channel and the intrinsic properties of the receptor channel. Currents of the second type are generated at the non-synaptic membrane (dendritic, somatic or at the initial segment) by voltage changes resulting from currents of synaptic origin, or from currents generated during the first action potential that is fired. The voltage-gated channels responsible for this second type of current are different from those of the sodium action potential and are generally activated in the subthreshold range of membrane potentials. The duration of these subliminal voltage-gated currents is determined by the gating properties of the corresponding channels. In this chapter, we will study the conduction and the summation of synaptic currents (first type of currents) over the dendritic tree. The characteristics of the diverse non-synaptic, subliminal currents (second type of currents) together with their role in the pattern of the post-synaptic discharge will be studied in Chapters 17 and 18.

16.1 Propagation of Excitatory and Inhibitory Post-synaptic Potentials Through the Dendritic Arborization

Excitatory and inhibitory post-synaptic potentials result, respectively, from depolarizing or hyperpolarizing currents through channels opened by neurotransmitters (receptor channels) in the post-synaptic membrane. These currents are generated over the somato-dendritic tree, at sites more or less distant from the soma (distal dendritic sites or proximal

Figure 16.1 Schematic representation of a neuron and some of its afferents. Examples of firing patterns. (a) Afferent fibers establish synaptic contacts on spines and dendritic branches which are situated at different distances from the soma of the post-synaptic neuron. When these afferents are activated, the depolarizing or hyperpolarizing post-synaptic currents are conducted towards the soma and initial segment of the axon. It is at this level that the response of the post-synaptic neuron is generated. The response is then conducted along the axon and its collateral branches. (b) Three examples of discharge configuration in response to the injection of a depolarizing current step. From top to bottom: regular discharge frequency (thalamic neurons, see Figure 18.2), a burst of action potentials followed by a silence (pyramidal neurons of the hippocampus, see Figure 17.6), and a long latency burst of action potentials (motoneurons innervating the ink gland of aplysia, see Figure 17.2).

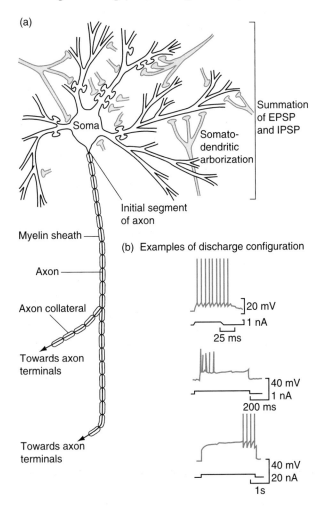

(a)

Soma

Summation of EPSP and IPSP

Somato-dendritic arborization

Initial segment of axon

Myelin sheath

Axon

Axon collateral

Towards axon terminals

Towards axon terminals

(b) Examples of discharge configuration

20 mV
1 nA
25 ms

40 mV
1 nA
200 ms

40 mV
20 nA
1 s

dendritic sites). Once generated, the post-synaptic currents propagate the length of the dendrites to the soma. For a long time it was thought that post-synaptic currents propagated passively and decrementally along the dendrites: passively because dendrites do not generate action potentials, the propagation of the signal depending only on the cable properties of the dendrite, and decrementally because the signal attenuates as it propagates, due to the leakage properties of the membrane. From this it would be expected that depolarizations evoked by distal excitatory synapses would be smaller in amplitude at the soma and would have a longer rise-time than depolarizations evoked by proximal synapses.

In fact, it seems that propagation is not always passive and not always decremental. There may be at least two types of propagation of post-synaptic currents through dendrites:

- a passive and decremental propagation, which implies an attenuation of distal post-synaptic currents; and
- a passive but only slightly decremental propagation, which occurs where the cable properties of the dendrite are very good and involve no attenuation, or a weak attenuation, of distal post-synaptic currents.

These two alternatives are treated in Sections 16.1.2 and 16.1.3.

Lastly, in certain neurons, the dendritic membrane contains voltage-sensitive Ca^{2+} channels and post-synaptic potentials can trigger dendritic calcium action potentials. Thus, for example, calcium action potentials propagate along the dendrites of the Purkinje cells of the cerebellar cortex (see Section 18.3).

16.1.1 The Complexity of Synaptic Organization (Figure 16.1)

Pre-synaptic complexity

A pre-synaptic afferent axon gives off many axon terminals (terminal boutons or en passant terminals). In this way, it generally establishes several synaptic contacts with the post-synaptic neuron. In addition, the post-synaptic neuron receives synapses coming from many other pre-synaptic axons. It is thus possible to distinguish several levels of complexity in post-synaptic potentials:

- the post-synaptic potential resulting from the activity of a single synaptic bouton: miniature potential;
- the post-synaptic potential representing the sum of post-synaptic potentials generated by synaptic boutons coming from the same pre-synaptic axon: unitary post-synaptic potential;
- the post-synaptic potential representing the sum of all the post-synaptic potentials generated at all the active synaptic boutons: composite post-synaptic potential.

Post-synaptic complexity

Different dendritic post-synaptic regions (spines, branches and main trunks) are not equivalent. The diameter of dendritic trunks is greater than that of branches, particularly distal branches. Thus different dendritic compartments have different resistances (note that $R = \rho l/s$, ρ being the resistivity, l the length and s the cross-section of the dendrite). This means that spines with a neck, or a very small diameter pedicle, have a high resistance. Consequently, synaptic currents generated at different points do not give the same potential change: for the same inward current I, the amplitude of the resulting post-synaptic depolarization (EPSP) will be greater for the dendritic regions where the resistance $r_m = 1/g_m$ is large ($V_{EPSP} = I_{EPSP}/g_m$).

Complexities of the propagation of post-synaptic action potentials

Post-synaptic potentials (EPSPs and IPSPs) propagate along the dendrites to the action potential initiation zone, which is generally situated in the initial region of the axon (initial segment). Depending on the cable properties of the dendrites, the post-synaptic potentials can change their characteristics (amplitude, rise-time) during their propagation.

16.1.2 Passive Decremental Propagation of Post-synaptic Potentials

'Decremental' means that the post-synaptic potentials attenuate as they propagate. This implies that the post-synaptic potentials are not regenerated at each point along the dendrites, as is the action potential as it travels along the axon. This passive propagation depends on the cable properties of the dendrite. In order to estimate quantitatively the modifications of post-synaptic potentials in the course of their conduction, a theoretical model of the passive properties of membrane potential changes (Rall, 1960) was established from data obtained on the squid giant axon. Thus a post-synaptic potential conducted with decrement (i) reduces in amplitude, and (ii) has a rise-time (rt) which gets longer as it is propagated along the dendrites (Figure 16.2a).

The reduction in amplitude of the post-synaptic current as it gets further from the generation site is due to the fact that the current does not only flow longitudinally along the dendrite but also transversely across the channels that are open in the dendritic membrane potential. This 'leak' of ions towards the extracellular medium results in a reduction in the post-synaptic current and in a consequent reduction in the amplitude of the post-synaptic potential. Thus, the fewer the number of channels open in the dendritic membrane, the higher will be the value of r_m, the better will be the cable properties of the dendrite and the less will be the reduction in amplitude of post-synaptic potentials of distal origin.

The increase in the rise-time of the post-synaptic potentials is due to the fact that part of the post-synaptic current serves to charge the capacity of each unit of membrane along the dendrite. The consequence of this is a change in the time course of the post-synaptic current: as it gets further from its point of generation, its rise-time becomes longer (it can also be said that the speed of rising becomes slower).

16.1.3 Passive and Non-decremental Propagation of Post-synaptic Potentials

This type of propagation means that post-synaptic potentials are conducted passively along the dendrites but, because of the good cable properties of the dendritic arborization, they are almost unattenuated as

Figure 16.2 Theoretical model of decremental conduction of excitatory post-synaptic potentials (EPSP) along dendrites. (a) Four EPSPs numbered 1 to 4 are generated at the instant t between $t = 0$ and $t = 0.25$ ms (black bar in simulation diagram on left), at different sites within the dendritic tree (schematic drawing on right). At the site of generation, these EPSPs are identical in amplitude and duration. After conduction along the dendrites, their shapes are different (theoretical recordings at the level of the soma, simulation diagram on left). It can be observed that the further away the site of generation of the EPSP (case 4), the smaller is its amplitude and the longer is its rise-time (rt) when it arrives at the level of the soma (compare the theoretical recordings 1 to 4). (b) Theoretical model of the linear summation of EPSP (see text for explanation). (From Rall W, 1977. *Handbook of Physiology, Vol. 1, Part 1. Cellular Biology of Neurons*, pp. 39–97, American Physiological Society, Bethesda, Maryland, with permission.)

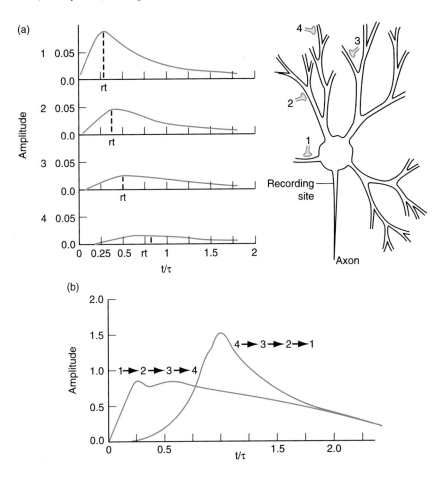

they propagate. Thus, in the model of the synapse of Ia afferent fibers with spinal motoneurons, it has been shown that the unitary EPSPs evoked by the activity of afferent fibers and recorded in the soma have very similar amplitudes even though their rise-times may be different, i.e. when they are generated at different distances from the soma. This implies that, in this model, there must be local dendritic mechanisms that allow an almost non-attenuating conduction of the distal post-synaptic potentials.

16.2 Summation of Excitatory and Inhibitory Post-synaptic Potentials

16.2.1 Linear and Non-linear Summation of Excitatory Post-synaptic Potentials

In general many excitatory synaptic afferents converge on a single neuron. At each excitatory synapse that is activated, there is an inward current of positive charges. When the membrane potential is not held at a fixed value, this inward current of positive charges depolarizes the post-synaptic membrane: this is the post-synaptic potential, or EPSP (see, for example, the current clamp recordings of the synaptic response to glutamate, Chapter 11).

A unitary EPSP (meaning one caused by the activation of a single afferent fiber, Section 16.1.1) cannot trigger action potentials. EPSPs generated in isolation are too small in amplitude to depolarize the membrane of the initial segment to the threshold potential for the opening of voltage-sensitive Na^+ channels. However, if many EPSPs generated at different sites in the dendritic arborization arrive more or less simultaneously at the level of the initial segment, the probability that they will generate action potentials becomes much greater. This is due to the fact that the EPSPs summate.

Linear summation of excitatory post-synaptic potentials

The term linear summation means that the composite EPSP (Section 16.1.1) resulting from the activity of several excitatory synapses has an amplitude that is equal to the geometric sum of the different EPSPs contributing to it. This is true when the EPSPs are generated at sites that are sufficiently far or isolated from one another to avoid interactions between them (on different dendritic branches, or on different dendritic spines, for instance).

A post-synaptic neuron generally receives many excitatory synapses at different points on its somatodendritic arborization (see Figures 16.1 and 16.2b). These EPSPs summate as they propagate, in a temporo-spatial manner. To grasp this phenomenon, it must be understood that the EPSPs generated at different sites in the dendritic arborization and conducted to the initial segment of the axon can arrive spread out in time. The offset between the EPSPs will depend on the distances between the generation sites and on the respective times at which they were generated. The examples demonstrated here are based on theoretical calculations of the cable properties of dendrites. These data give a qualitative understanding of the phenomena of summation but do not constitute a real experimental demonstration.

Let us consider the example of four EPSPs of the same amplitude, generated at different sites in the dendritic arborization, at times such that their arrivals at the initial segment are offset in time. Figure 16.2b shows the 'composite EPSP' obtained in two cases of arrival sequences. In the case: $1 \rightarrow 2 \rightarrow 3 \rightarrow 4$, the four EPSPs are generated at the same time t but since some are generated at more distal sites, their arrivals at the initial segment are staggered, the most proximal arriving first and the most distal, last. In the case $4 \rightarrow 3 \rightarrow 2 \rightarrow 1$, the most distal EPSPs are generated well before the proximal EPSPs, so that the distal EPSPs arrive before the proximal EPSPs. The theoretical results show that in the first case in which the proximal EPSPs occur first and are followed by the more distal EPSPs, the 'composite EPSP' has a short latency, a long duration and a small amplitude, while in the second case, in which the distal EPSPs arrive before the proximal EPSPs, the 'composite EPSP' has a long latency and a large amplitude (Figure 16.2b).

Non-linear summation of excitatory post-synaptic potentials

The term non-linear summation means that the 'composite EPSP' has an amplitude that is not equal to the geometric sum of the different EPSPs contributing to it. This occurs, for instance, when two EPSPs are generated at the same site or at sites that are close.

Let us take the example of two excitatory synapses whose neurotransmitter is glutamate and which are situated close together on the same dendritic segment (Figure 16.3), supposing that the membrane potential of the dendritic segment is V_m. When synapse 1 is active alone, $EPSP_1$ is recorded, due to the excitatory post-synaptic current I_1, such that $I_1 = g_{cations} (V_m - E_{cations})$, whose amplitude is $V_{EPSP1} = I_1/g_m$, where g_m is the membrane conductance (Figure 16.3a). When synapse 2 is active alone, $EPSP_2$ is recorded at level 2, due to the post-synaptic current I_2, such that $I_2 = g_{cations} (V_m - E_{cations})$, whose amplitude is $V_{EPSP2} = I_2/g_m$ (Figure 16.3b). If we suppose that when the two EPSPs are generated separately, $V_{EPSP1} = V_{EPSP2}$ (Figure 16.3a, b), what is the amplitude of the 'composite EPSP' when the two synapses are active at the same time?

When synapse 1 is activated first, $EPSP_1$ is recorded in the post-synaptic element and will be conducted passively to neighboring regions (Figure 16.3a). At time $t + \Delta t$, $EPSP_1$ arrives at the post-synaptic element

Figure 16.3   Non-linear summation of excitatory post-synaptic potentials. Suppose that there are two excitatory synapses situated close together on the same dendritic segment. (a) When afferent 1 is activated at time t, a depolarization of the post-synaptic membrane 1 is recorded at time t (EPSP$_1$ alone). This depolarization propagates in the two directions away from 1. (b) When afferent 2 is activated, at time $t + \Delta t$, a depolarization of the post-synaptic membrane 2 is recorded at time $t + \Delta t$ (EPSP$_2$ alone). (c) When the two afferents 1 and 2 are activated as before, but together, one at time t and the other at time $t + \Delta t$, a depolarization of the post-synaptic membrane 2 (ΣEPSP) is recorded at time $t + \Delta t$, which does not correspond to the geometric sum EPSP$_1$ alone + EPSP$_2$ alone, since EPSP'$_2$ has an amplitude which is smaller than EPSP$_2$ (see text for explanation).

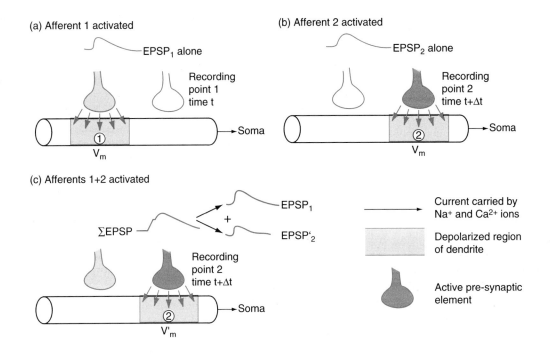

2. The membrane of the post-synaptic element 2 is then at a potential V'_m which is more positive than V_m (Figure 16.3c). If at this moment ($t + \Delta t$) synapse 2 is active, the post-synaptic current I'_2 will be smaller than if it had taken place independently from I_1 because the electrochemical gradient of Na$^+$ and Ca^{2+} ions is reduced. $I'_2 = g_{cations} (V'_m - E_{cations})$ and $I'_2 < I_2$ because $(V'_m - E_{cations}) < (V_m - E_{cations})$. The 'composite EPSP' will have an amplitude less than the geometric sum EPSP$_1$ + EPSP$_2$ (Figure 16.3c).

This is also the case when a single excitatory synapse is activated repetitively by the arrival of high frequency pre-synaptic action potentials. When an excitatory post-synaptic current is generated before the preceding current has ended, it has a smaller amplitude because the post-synaptic membrane is depolarized. Thus, during high frequency activation,

successive excitatory post-synaptic potentials have amplitudes that are smaller and smaller.

16.2.2 Linear and Non-linear Summation of Inhibitory Post-synaptic Potentials

When inhibitory synapses are active they cause, in the post-synaptic membrane, an outward post-synaptic current of positive charges (carried by K$^+$ ions) or an inward current of negative charges (carried by Cl$^-$ ions) which hyperpolarizes the membrane: this is the inhibitory post-synaptic potential, or IPSP.

Linear summation of IPSPs is symmetrically the same as linear summation of EPSPs. Non-linear summation of IPSPs is symmetrically the same as non-linear summation of EPSPs.

16.2.3 The Integration of Excitatory and Inhibitory Post-synaptic Potentials Partly Determines the Configuration of the Post-synaptic Discharge

Situation of the problem

In order for an action potential to be triggered at the initial segment, the membrane of the initial segment must be depolarized to the threshold potential for the opening of voltage-sensitive Na^+ channels. It is also necessary for this depolarization to have a relatively rapid rise-time so that the Na^+ channels do not inactivate during the depolarization. The characteristics of depolarization of the initial segment (amplitude, duration, rise-time) result partly from the summation of excitatory and inhibitory post-synaptic potentials.

Integration of depolarizing (excitatory) post-synaptic potential with hyperpolarizing (inhibitory) post-synaptic potential

A hyperpolarizing post-synaptic potential is due to a current whose reversal potential is more negative than the resting membrane potential of the cell. This type of inhibition is generally due to the opening of K^+ channels ($GABA_B$ type inhibition). Since the equilibrium potential of K^+ ions is more negative than the resting membrane potential, the opening of K^+ channels gives rise to an outward current (an exit of positive charges) and to a hyperpolarization of the membrane, i.e. an IPSP. If this IPSP is concomitant with an EPSP, it will reduce the amplitude of the EPSP. This type of summation of EPSP and IPSP is summarized in Figure 16.4.

Integration of depolarizing (excitatory) post-synaptic potential and silent (inhibitory) post-synaptic potential

A silent post-synaptic potential is due to a current whose reversal potential is close to the resting potential of the cell. Generally, this is caused by a current of Cl^- ions through $GABA_A$ channels (see Chapter 10). When the equilibrium potential of Cl^- ions is close to the membrane resting potential, the opening of Cl^- channels does not reveal a hyperpolarizing current at the resting potential (from which comes the term 'silent' for this inhibition). However, when the membrane is depolarized by an EPSP, the inhibition is no longer silent, but becomes hyperpolarizing and results in a reduction or even a complete suppression of the EPSP (Figure 16.5).

Integration of depolarizing (excitatory) post-synaptic potential and depolarizing inhibitory post-synaptic potential

A depolarizing inhibitory post-synaptic potential is due to a synaptic current whose reversal potential is more positive than the resting potential of the membrane but more negative than the threshold for the opening of the Na^+ channels of the action potential. This is generally due to the opening of Cl^- channels in cells in which the reversal potential for Cl^- ions is situated between the resting potential and the threshold potential for the opening of the Na^+ channels of the action potential. Thus, when the membrane is at its resting potential, this Cl^- current causes a slight depolarization of the membrane, but does not trigger action potentials. When the membrane is depolarized (by an EPSP) above the inversion potential of Cl^+ ions, this current causes a hyperpolarization of the membrane and an inhibition of the EPSP.

In summary, several types of inhibition appear over the length of the somato-dendritic arborization and these limit the effect of excitatory synapses. The opening or non-opening of the Na^+ channels of the action potential, and in consequence the generation of action potentials which will constitute the response of the post-synaptic neuron, are the result of this summation of excitatory and inhibitory post-synaptic potentials. However, the characteristics of the response of the post-synaptic neuron are determined not only by the amplitude and duration of the depolarization of synaptic origin but also by the characteristics of the membrane of the initial segment, also known as 'input-output' characteristics.

Figure 16.4   Integration of excitatory (EPSP) and inhibitory (IPSP) post-synaptic potentials. (a) Suppose that on a dendritic tree, there are glutaminergic excitatory synapses which are situated distally, and $GABA_B$ type inhibitory synapses which are situated proximally, and that all of these are active at the same instant t. (b) If only the excitatory synapses are active, a depolarization, a composite EPSP (ΣEPSP) will be recorded at the soma which corresponds to the linear and non-linear summation of all the different EPSPs (top trace). We will suppose that the ΣEPSP has an amplitude that is sufficient to trigger an action potential (upper trace). If only the inhibitory synapses are active, a hyperpolarization, a composite IPSP (ΣIPSP) will be recorded at the soma which corresponds to the linear and non-linear summation of all the different IPSPs (middle trace). When all these different synapses are activated at the same time t, a depolarization preceded by a hyperpolarization, a composite PSP, will be recorded at the soma, corresponding to the sum of the different synaptic potentials (ΣEPSP + ΣIPSP) (bottom trace). In this case the amplitude of the depolarization is no longer sufficient to trigger an action potential. (c) Electrical equivalent of the membrane at the level of the initial segment, for an EPSP alone. (d) Electrical equivalent for the membrane when an EPSP and an IPSP summate. The currents I_{EPSP} and I_{IPSP} are opposite and subtract from one another. By comparing with (c), it is observed that I_{EPSP} in (c) > I_{EPSP} + I_{IPSP} in (d) and $\Delta V_1 > \Delta V_2$.

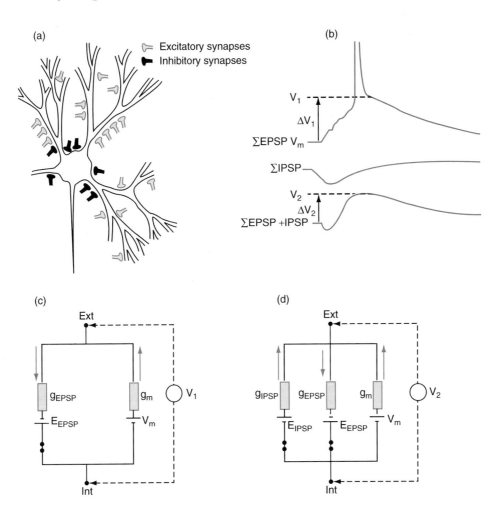

Figure 16.5   Role of silent inhibition. (a) This diagram shows two synapses, one glutamatergic with post-synaptic AMPA receptors (E_1) and the other GABAergic with $GABA_A$ post-synaptic receptors (I_1), situated close to one another on the same dendritic segment, such that the inhibitory synapse is closer to the soma than the excitatory synapse. (b) When the excitatory synapse is excited alone, an EPSP of ΔV_1 in amplitude is recorded (b_1). When the inhibitory synapse is activated alone, no change in potential is recorded because $V_m = E_{Cl}$ (B_2). When both synapses are activated, the EPSP which propagates towards the soma is reduced in amplitude (amplitude ΔV_3), or even canceled out. This type of inhibition is selective because it only acts on excitatory synapses that are situated distally. (c) Electrical equivalent of the membrane at the dendritic segment. If this is compared with Figure 16.4c, it can be seen that $\Delta V_3 < \Delta V_1$ because $g_m + g_{IPSP} > g_m$.

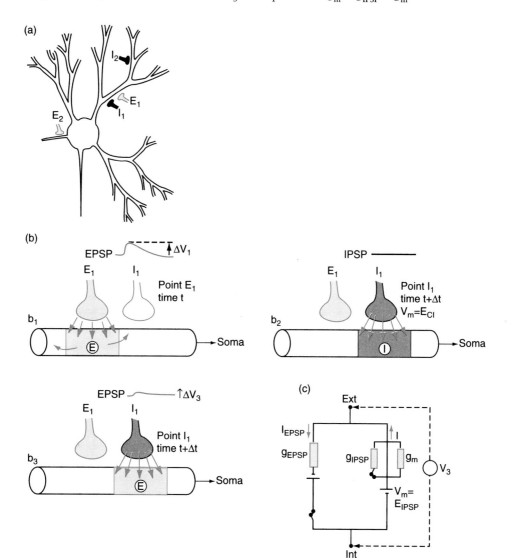

Further Reading

Buhl, E.H., Halasy, K. and Somogyi, P. (1994) Diverse sources of hippocampal unitary inhibitory post-synaptic potentials and the number of release sites. *Nature* **368**, 823–828.

Cauller, L.J. and Connors, B.W. (1992) Functions of very distal dendrites. In: McKenna, T.M., Davis, J. and Zornetzer, S.E. (Eds), *Single Neuron Computation*, pp. 199–229, Academic Press, New York.

Rall, W. (1977) Core conductor theory and cable properties of neurons. In: Brookhart, J.M., Mountcastle, V.B., Kandel, E.R. and Geiger, S.R. (Eds), *Handbook of Physiology*, vol. 1, part 1, pp. 39–97, American Physiological Society, Bethesda, MD.

Shepherd, G.M. (1994) The significance of real neuro-architectures for neural network simulations. In: Schwartz, E.L. (Ed.) *Computational Neuroscience*, pp. 82–96, New York: Oxford University Press.

Spruston, N., Jaffe, D.B. and Johnston, D. (1994) Dendritic attenuation of synaptic potentials and currents: the role of passive membrane properties. *Trends Neurosci.* **17**, 161–166.

Subliminal Voltage-Gated Currents

Not all neurons respond in the same way to a depolarization of the same amplitude and duration: it can be said that they do not have the same pattern of firing. Spinal motoneurons may respond with a low frequency regular discharge, oculomotoneurons discharge with a more sustained rhythm, certain pyramidal neurons of the hippocampus respond with a burst of action potentials followed by a long silence, and the neurons of the inferior olive respond with an irregular sustained activity forming bursts of action potentials (Figure 16.1b). It should be noted that the term firing pattern is not equivalent to the term discharge frequency, except in cases where the response consists of action potentials generated at a regular frequency. In this case only, the mean value of the discharge frequency is sufficient to describe the response of the neuron. In other cases, the mean frequency value has no significance.

Neurons, as pointed out by Llinas (1988), are not interchangeable, i.e. a neuron cannot be functionally replaced by one of another type even if their synaptic connectivity, type of afferent neurotransmitters and receptors to these neurotransmitters are identical. The electrical activity observed in a network is not only related to the *excitatory and inhibitory interactions* among neurons but also to their *intrinsic electrical properties* as well.

The nature of a neuron is defined by its 'input–output' characteristics, i.e. its firing pattern (output) in response to a depolarization of synaptic origin (input). Input–output characteristics are the result of currents other than those of the action potential. These currents, outward or inward, are activated by a depolarization of synaptic origin or by the depolarizing Na^+ current of the first action potential generated. Among these currents, we will distinguish those that tend to reduce the probability of the neuronal discharge (outward K^+ currents), and those that tend to increase it (inward Na^+, Ca^{2+} or cationic currents).

17.1 Principle of the Study of the Input–Output Characteristics of a Neuron

The firing pattern (configuration of the discharge) of a neuron is studied by simulating a depolarization of synaptic origin with intracellular injection of a depolarizing current whose different parameters (amplitude, duration, rise-time) can be perfectly controlled. In parallel, currents other than those of the action potential, present in the membrane and activated during the response, are studied under voltage clamp. Different blocking procedures are used (voltage changes or pharmacological blockade) in order to study only one current at a time. The aim of this type of study is to define the characteristics of each of these currents: activation and inactivation characteristics, pharmacological properties, etc. These currents are generally subliminal, i.e. they are activated at a potential more negative than the threshold potential of the action potential.

The role of the currents thus identified on the firing pattern of a neuron can then be demonstrated in several ways:

- By selectively blocking each of the studied currents and analyzing the consequences of this blockade on the configuration of the neuronal discharge recorded in current clamp mode. However, this is not always possible, either because selective pharmacological blocking agents do not exist, or because it is not possible to inactivate the current by voltage changes without inactivating other currents.

- By establishing on the basis of simulated currents a theoretical model of the behavior of the membrane in response to a depolarization. The simulated currents are those activated by the depolarization, i.e. the currents of the action potential as well as subliminal currents. Current characteristics obtained from voltage-clamp recordings are used for this simulation (the same type of model as that of Hodgkin–Huxley for the squid giant axon). Since this is a theoretical model of the neuronal response to depolarization, it is necessary to check that theoretical and experimental results agree.

In many experiments, recordings of the activity of vertebrate central neurons are made at the level of the soma and the question may remain as to where these currents are generated: at the level of the dendrites, the soma or the initial segment?

17.2 Ionic Currents that Slow the Approach to Spike Threshold: They Delay the Onset of the Discharge and Increase the Interspike Interval

Among the subliminal currents that tend to reduce the probability of the discharge, we will deal with two types of outward potassium currents: the early outward K$^+$ currents, I_A and I_D, and the outward K$^+$ currents sensitive to intracellular Ca^{2+} ions, $I_{K(Ca)}$.

17.2.1 The Early K$^+$ Currents: I_A and I_D

The I_A and I_D currents are early transient outward currents carried by K$^+$ ions (Appendixes 17.1 and 17.2). The threshold potential for activation of these K$^+$ currents is situated between –60 and –45 mV, i.e. at a value slightly more negative than the threshold potential for the inward Na$^+$ current of the action potential.

I_A and I_D will both be fully activated by a depolarization only if the membrane potential was previously at a potential more negative than –60 mV (they are inactivated at resting membrane potential). When these conditions are fulfilled, I_A and I_D oppose the depolarizing inward current of synaptic origin and thus delay the onset of the discharge and/or increase the duration of the interspike interval. These two early currents differ mainly by their kinetics of inactivation when the membrane potential is maintained at a value more positive than –60 to –50 mV: I_A is a fast-inactivating current (in the order of milliseconds) and I_D is a slowly inactivating current (in the order of seconds). Owing to these different inactivation kinetics, I_A will mainly control maintained repetitive firing and I_D will

mediate temporal integration of afferent depolarizing inputs. These roles will be explained using three examples: marine gastropod neurons, motoneurons that innervate the ink gland of aplysia, and pyramidal neurons of the rat hippocampus.

The I_A *current reduces the discharge frequency of the response: example of marine gastropod neurons*

Marine gastropod neurons have a relatively positive resting potential, of about –40 mV. When the membrane is depolarized, a response is recorded that consists of action potentials generated at a slow regular frequency (about 1.7 Hz) for the entire duration of the depolarization. Voltage clamp studies have shown the presence of an outward K$^+$ current called A current, I_A, with the same characteristics as those presented in Appendix 17.1. At the resting potential of the cell (around –40 mV), I_A is inactivated and cannot be activated (remember that it is necessary for the membrane potential to be more negative than –50 mV for I_A to be activated). Thus when a depolarizing current is injected into these neurons at rest, the membrane depolarizes linearly up to about –25 mV, the threshold for the opening of action potential Na$^+$ channels. A first action potential is then generated whose duration is about 25 ms (Figure 17.1a). The repolarization of the action potential is due to the exit of K$^+$ ions through the delayed rectification channels (I_K). This outward K$^+$ current hyperpolarizes the membrane transiently after each action potential. This is important because this after-hyperpolarization phase makes it possible to suppress the inactivation of I_A. Thus I_A will intervene only after emission of the first action potential.

In order to describe the role of I_A in the pattern of firing, the following theoretical model has been established (Figure 17.1b): the transient hyperpolarization that follows the first action potential decays with time, reflecting progressive closing of the K$^+$ channels of the delayed rectification. With the decay of I_K, the membrane repolarizes and approaches the threshold of activation of the action potential Na$^+$ current (I_{Na}) but also that of I_A (since I_A had previously been de-inactivated by the transient after-hyperpolarization). I_A, which is an outward (hyperpolarizing) current, opposes the injected or synaptic inward (depolarizing) current and delays the moment at

Figure 17.1 Comparison between the experimental response and the simulated response of marine gastropod neurons. (a) In response to a depolarizing current pulse (not shown), these neurons fire a low frequency (1.7 Hz) regular train of action potentials (e), lasting for the duration of the stimulation. (b) The currents thought to be active during neuronal activity are simulated, based on results from voltage-clamp recordings. These currents are the inward sodium current of the action potential (I_{Na}) and the outward potassium currents of the late rectification I_K and the early transient potassium current I_A. The inward and outward currents are represented without regard to their sign and the currents of the action potential are shown only partially because of their large amplitude. It can be seen in (a) that the simulated response (*) obtained from compilation of the kinetic values of the simulated currents is comparable to the experimental response (e). These results demonstrate that the presence of the I_A current is sufficient to explain the discharge pattern of these neurons. (From Connor JA and Stevens CF 1971. Prediction of repetitive firing behaviour from voltage clamp data on an isolated neurone soma, *J. Physiol. (Lond.)* **213**, 31–53, with permission.)

(a)

20mV

100ms

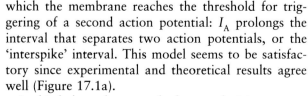

(b)

1.0
nA
0.5

I_A

I_{Na}

I_K

I_A

I_{Na}

which the membrane reaches the threshold for triggering of a second action potential: I_A prolongs the interval that separates two action potentials, or the 'interspike' interval. This model seems to be satisfactory since experimental and theoretical results agree well (Figure 17.1a).

In this balance between the hyperpolarizing current (I_A) and the depolarizing current (injected or synaptic), the depolarizing current will carry the most

weight when I_A begins to inactivate under the influence of the prolonged depolarization (Figure 17.1b). Thus I_A reduces the speed with which the membrane approaches the threshold for action potential firing (the activation threshold of the Na$^+$ channels). In summary, for a depolarizing synaptic current to generate action potentials in these cells, its amplitude must be great enough to depolarize the membrane to the threshold for action potentials, and it must also last longer than the period during which I_A is activated.

It follows that I_A can only play a role within a restricted range of discharge frequency. For example, if the frequency of the discharge increases, the membrane does not repolarize to a value sufficiently negative to de-inactivate I_A between each action potential and I_A will then not be activated by the next membrane depolarization. Furthermore I_A will play a role only when the membrane potential is not more negative than −50 or −60 mV before being depolarized.

I_D determines the latency and the response threshold of motoneurons innervating the ink gland of aplysia

When a relatively intense and long duration tactile stimulus is applied to aplysia an avoidance reflex of the head, mantle and bronchi is triggered, followed by a massive jet of violet ink which allows the aplysia to disappear from the view of its predators. Although weaker tactile stimuli may cause graded avoidance reflexes they are not effective in triggering the ink jet behavior. This ink is secreted by a gland situated on the edge of the mantle and innervated by motoneurons that have been identified and named L$_{14}$. The ink jet behavior can be reproduced by the application of a high intensity, long duration (more than 2 s) electrical stimulus to the head and neck. Its characteristics have been identified in this way and include: an activation threshold that is high in comparison with those of aplysia's other defense reflexes, and a long delay before it occurs. In addition, once the threshold has been reached, the response is immediately maximal: it is an all-or-none response (Figure 17.2a, b).

If a long duration depolarizing current is now injected directly into the motoneurons, mimicking the effective tactile stimulus, the same response as before is recorded: a burst of action potentials occurring with a long delay of about 2 seconds (Figure 17.2c). This shows that the long delay of the response depends only on the intrinsic properties of the membrane of the motoneurons and not on the synaptic delays in the circuit. Analysis of the membrane behavior during this delay, showed that there is a first rapid phase of depolarization (a) followed by a much slower phase of depolarization (b), which eventually brings the membrane to the threshold for triggering action potentials. What is the mechanism responsible for the slowing of the depolarization (phase B)? In order to answer this question, the motoneurons were recorded under two-electrode voltage clamp and the kinetics of the different currents activated by a depolarization were studied. A quantitative Hodgkin–Huxley type model based on the data obtained under voltage

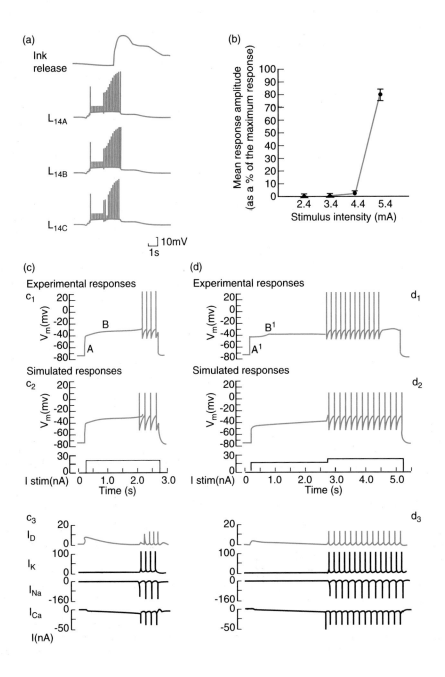

clamp was then established to verify the kinetics of the different currents activated which could account for the pattern of firing.

The suggested model is as follows: when the animal is not stimulated, the L_{14} motoneurons are silent, and their resting potential is about −70 mV. At this relatively negative potential value, I_D is not inactivated (Appendix 17.2). It can thus be activated by any depolarization which brings the membrane to a potential equal to or more positive than −60 or −50 mV. In fact, once I_D is activated, it opposes the depolarization of the membrane, i.e. slows it down. The balance between the hyperpolarizing I_D current and the depolarizing (synaptic or injected) current will lean in favor of depolarization if the depolarizing current lasts for a sufficiently long time. As I_D gradually inactivates (because V_m is more positive than −50 mV), its decay will allow the injected current to be more effective and thus to depolarize the membrane to the threshold of Na$^+$ channel activation (Figure 17.2c_2, c_3). The delay before the burst of action potentials occurs will depend on the mean time of inactivation of I_D.

This hypothesis of the role of I_D has been verified by the following experiment (Figure 17.2d_1): the motoneurons are first depolarized by injecting a subthreshold current pulse for 2.5 s, and then depolarized further for 2.5 s by injecting the same current pulse as in c_1. The first depolarizing current pulse provokes a rapid depolarization (A') followed by a slow depolarization (B'), without the generation of action potentials. The second current pulse provokes the immediate generation of a burst of action potentials.

The first pulse, or conditioning pulse, had caused the inactivation of I_D, and thus the second current pulse, which was no longer being opposed by I_D could then rapidly depolarize the membrane to the threshold for the generation of action potentials. These experimental results confirm the validity of the theoretical model (Figure 17.2d_2, d_3).

The high threshold of activation of the motoneurons (and in consequence, of the ink jet reflex) is the first consequence of the presence of I_D: a strong depolarizing current is necessary to oppose the hyperpolarizing I_D current. The second consequence is that only *long duration* depolarizing stimuli can provoke the occurrence of a burst of action potentials since it is necessary for the depolarization to last long enough to be still present when I_D has been largely inactivated (we have previously seen that short stimuli do not give rise to the ink jet reflex).

I_D delays the response of the pyramidal neurons of the hippocampus to excitatory afferent inputs

I_A co-exists with I_D in the pyramidal neurons of the rat hippocampus. They have characteristics (Appendixes 17.1 and 17.2) very similar to those of the invertebrate. I_A inactives at potentials more positive than −40/−50 mV with a time constant in the order of 10–50 ms (it is half inactivated at −60 mV), it is de-inactivated by hyperpolarizing pulses to potentials more negative than −50 mV and is subsequently activated by depolarizations to around −50 mV. I_D

Figure 17.2   Role of the I_A current in the pattern of discharge of motoneurons innervating the ink gland (ink sac) of aplysia. (a) Correlation between ink release (measured by spectrophotometry) and the configuration of the discharge of L_{14} motoneurons (recorded under current clamp) in response to a long duration stimulus (pulses of 1.5 ms, 6/s, for 3 s, not shown). This stimulus evokes a burst of action potentials in the three L_{14} motoneurons (three lower traces) with a long latency (1.5 s). Ink release begins towards the end of the motoneuron responses (top trace). The differences in amplitude between the action potentials within the burst are due to the recording system and the small vertical deflections are stimulus artifacts. (b) Quantitative analysis of ink release (as a percentage of the total quantity) by aplysia (n=20) as a function of stimulus intensity. (c, d) Demonstration of the role of I_D. The kinetics of the different inward and outward currents (c_3 and d_3) are simulated in response to either (c) a long duration (2.5 s) depolarizing current step, or (d) a subthreshold current step followed by a current step identical to that in (c). It can be seen that the simulated responses (c_2 and d_2) obtained from the simulated currents (c_3 and d_3) are similar to the experimental responses (c_1 and d_1). I_D, transient K$^+$ current; I_{Na}, inward Na$^+$ current of the action potential; I_K, K$^+$ current of late rectification; I_{Ca}, Ca^{2+} current. (a, b: From Carew TJ and Kandel ER, 1977. Inking in *Aplysia Californica*. Neural circuit of an all-or-none behavioral response, *J. Neurophysiol.* **40**, 692–707, with permission. c, d: From Byrne JH, 1980. Quantitative aspects of ionic conductance mechanisms contributing to firing pattern of motor cells mediating inking behaviour in *Aplysia Californica, J. Neurophysiol.* **43**, 651–668, with permission.)

inactivates at potentials more positive than $-60/-70$ mV with a time constant in the order of tens of seconds (it is half inactivated at -88 mV), it is de-inactivated by hyperpolarizing pulses to potentials more negative than -70 mV and is subsequently activated by depolarizations to around -60 mV. Therefore, the thresholds for both activation and inactivation of I_A lie 15–20 mV positive to those of I_D. Finally, I_D is fully blocked in the presence of low external concentrations of 4-aminopyridine (4-AP, 40 μM) although at this concentration I_A (Appendix 17.1) and other K$^+$ currents are not affected.

In order to test the role of I_D on the firing pattern of pyramidal neurons, the response of these neurons to the injection of a depolarizing current was recorded under current clamp ($V_m = -74$ mV). In control extracellular medium, the recorded response consists of a single or multiple action potentials with a latency of several hundreds of milliseconds (Figure 17.3a). In the presence of 40 μM 4-aminopyridine (4-AP), this latency is reduced to 50 ms (this remaining latency may be due to I_A, Figure 17.3b). The lengthening of the delay of the response in control conditions only occurs when the membrane potential has been previously hyperpolarized. The other K$^+$ currents do not contribute to this aspect of firing since neither TEA to block the delayed rectifier (see Chapter 7) nor external Cs$^+$ to block I_Q (Appendix 17.5), nor muscarine to block I_M (Appendix 17.3) have an effect on the initial delay of firing.

Figure 17.3   The activation of I_D delays the response to a depolarizing current step. The activity of hippocampal pyramidal neurons is recorded intracellularly in *in vitro* brain slices in current clamp mode. (a) Three depolarizing current steps of increasing amplitude (bottom I traces) evoke (or not) a discharge with a delay superior to 500 ms (three top V_m traces) ($V_{rest} = -74$ mV). (b) In the presence of 40 μM 4-aminopyridine (4-AP) in the extracellular medium, which blocks I_D (but not I_A), the same depolarizing current steps evoke firing without the initial long delay. The remaining short delay may be due to I_A. (c) (Left) A single depolarizing current pulse (bottom I trace) which fails to depolarize the membrane to the spike threshold (top trace, horizontal line) is chosen ($V_{rest} = -68$ mV); (right) when the same current pulse is repetitively injected, the depolarizing response gradually increases until the cell fires a spike (truncated). (From Storm JF, 1988, Temporal integration by a slowly inactivating K$^+$ current in hippocampal neurons, *Nature* 336, 379–381, with permission.)

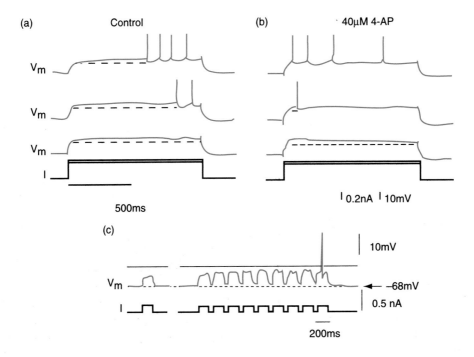

These results show that, as in the case of the invertebrate neurons, activation of I_D delays the generation of action potentials. Thus I_D may enable the cell to integrate excitatory synaptic inputs over very long times. When a series of identical pulses are given to mimic excitatory synaptic inputs (Figure 17.3c), the response (depolarization) gradually increases until the cell fires. In conclusion, as I_D activates in the subthreshold range (i.e. at potentials more negative than I_{Na}, the Na^+ current of the action potential) and takes tens of seconds to recover from inactivation, only *long duration* or *repetitive* depolarizing afferent inputs will provoke the occurrence of action potentials (it is necessary for the depolarization to last long enough to still be present when I_D has been largely inactivated).

In order to test the role of I_A on the discharge configuration of pyramidal neurons, the response of these neurons to the injection of depolarizing current was recorded under current clamp at a potential where I_D is mostly inactivated. In control extracellular medium, the recorded response consists of a single action potential with a latency of about 15 ms (Figure 17.4b, control). In the presence of a high concentration of 4-aminopyridine (5 mM) in the extracellular medium, this latency is reduced and the neuron fires repetitively (Figure 17.4b, 4-AP). The same current clamp recording made in the presence of TTX shows that the rise-time of the electrotonic potential, in response to a depolarizing current pulse, is about 50 ms slower in the absence than in the presence of 4-aminopyridine. This lengthening of the delay of the response and the interspike interval only occurs when the membrane potential reaches values at which the I_A current is activated. These results show that, as in the case of invertebrate neurons, activation of I_A delays the generation of action potentials and reduces the frequency of the discharge by lengthening the interspike interval.

17.2.2 The K^+ Currents Activated by Intracellular Ca^{2+} Ions: $I_{K(Ca)}$

$I_{K(Ca)}$ currents are outward K^+ currents sensitive to the concentration of Ca^{2+} ions in the intracellular medium (see Section 7.5.3). In vertebrate neurons, these currents may be more or less sensitive to voltage but for all of them an increase in the intracellular Ca^{2+}

Figure 17.4   The I_A current reduces the discharge frequency of hippocampal pyramidal neurons. (a) Patch clamp recording (whole-cell configuration) of the total outward current evoked by a voltage step from -70 mV to -30 mV, in the presence of TTX and Cd^{2+} ions to block, respectively, the inward Na^+ and Ca^{2+} currents. The late component of the total outward current (I_K) disappears in the presence of TEA (25 mM), while 80% of the early component (I_A) is blocked by 4-aminopyridine (4-AP, 5 mM). (b) Current clamp record ($V_m = -60$ mV) of the activity of a pyramidal neuron. Injection of a depolarizing current step evokes an action potential with a latency of 13.5 ms (control). In the presence of 4-AP (5 mM), the latency of the first action potential is reduced to 8 ms and a second action potential is generated. (From Segal M, Rogawski M and Barker J, 1984. A transient potassium conductance regulates the excitability of cultured hippocampal and spinal neurons, *J. Neurosci.* 4, 604–609, with permission.)

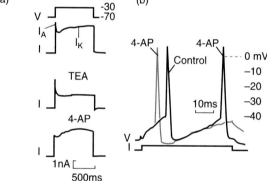

concentration is a necessary prerequisite to the activation of these currents. This increase may be the result of the entry of Ca^{2+} ions through voltage-dependent Ca^{2+} channels opened by depolarization, or the entry of Ca^{2+} ions through cationic receptor channels largely permeable to Ca^{2+} ions such as the NMDA-type glutamate receptors, or the release of Ca^{2+} ions from intracellular stores. The $I_{K(Ca)}$ currents hyperpolarize the membrane after each action potential (Ca^{2+}-sensitive after-hyperpolarizations) in a more lasting way than the outward K^+ current of the late rectification (see Chapter 7). These Ca^{2+}-sensitive after-hyperpolarizations have several roles in the mode of neuron discharge, roles that we will study taking the example of pyramidal neurons of the rat hippocampus.

$I_{K(Ca)}$ *tend to reduce the discharge frequency of* neurons

Action potentials recorded in pyramidal neurons of the rat hippocampus in response to a depolarizing current pulse (or in response to excitatory synaptic inputs) are followed by several transient phases of hyperpolarization called after-hyperpolarizations (AHP) or post-hyperpolarizations. Several phases of

after-hyperpolarization can be distinguished among which we will cite the fast phase (fAHP) (Figure 17.5a), which lasts about 2–3 ms, and the slow after-hyperpolarization (sAHP), which lasts more than 1 s (Figure 17.6a). The fAHP and sAHP disappear in the presence of a low extracellular Ca^{2+} concentration, or when the extracellular medium contains blocking agents that prevent the entry of Ca^{2+} ions (Co^{2+}, Mn^{2+}, Cd^{2+}) (Figure 17.5a and 17.6a) or after intracellular

Figure 17.5   Role of the rapid after-hyperpolarization in the discharge frequency of pyramidal neurons of the hippocampus. The activity of pyramidal neurons is recorded under current clamp, in brain slices maintained *in vitro*. Application of a depolarizing current step (bottom I traces) evokes an action potential followed by a period of after-hyperpolarization (AHP) which has at least two components. This figure illustrates the properties and the role of the fast component (fAHP; a, b, c, control V_m traces). The fAHP is reversibly blocked by Cd^{2+} ions (100 μM) (a) and by charybdotoxin (CTX, 10 nM for 25 min) (b). Thus charybdotoxin shortens the duration of the interspike interval (compare 1 and 2 in (c)) and increases the discharge frequency of pyramidal neurons. Trace 3 in (c) shows the superimposed recordings of 1 and 2, where the first action potentials in the two traces have been aligned. (From Lancaster B and Nicoll RA, 1987. Properties of two calcium activated hyperpolarizations in rat hippocampal neurones, *J. Physiol. (Lond.)* **389**, 187–203, with permission.)

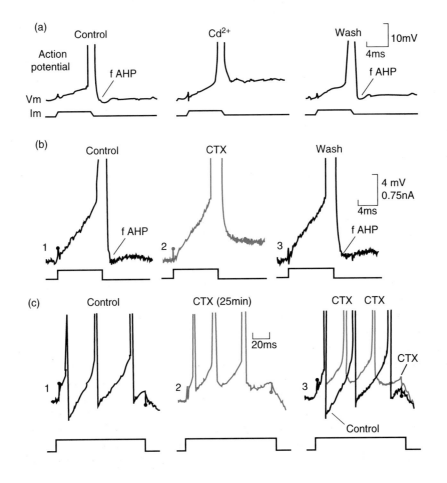

injection of Ca^{2+} chelators (EGTA or BAPTA), substances that form complexes with Ca^{2+} ions. In addition, these hyperpolarizations are associated with an increase in membrane conductance (and thus with channel opening), they have an amplitude that changes when the extracellular K^+ concentration is increased (although intracellular injection of Cl^- ions has no effect), and they have a reversal potential value that corresponds to the theoretical value of the reversal potential of K^+ ions. These results strongly suggest that the fAHP and sAHP are due to outward K^+ currents activated by Ca^{2+}: $I_{K(Ca)}$. Different Ca^{2+} sensitive K^+ currents have been described in hippocampal neurons such as the voltage- and Ca^{2+}-dependent I_C current (maxi-K current) and the voltage-independent and Ca^{2+}-dependent I_{AHP} (small-K current). The first may be responsible for the fAHP while the second is thought to be responsible for the sAHP.

The pharmacology of these two Ca^{2+}-sensitive hyperpolarizations (and underlying currents) is different: the fAHP is blocked by the application of TEA (tetraethylammonium) or charybdotoxin (CTX) in the extracellular medium (Figure 17.5b, c), while the sAHP is clearly reduced in the presence of noradrenaline or carbachol (Figure 17.6c, e). The fAHP and sAHP can thus be separated by their pharmacological properties, making it possible to study their respective roles in the configuration of the discharge of hippocampal pyramidal neurons. We will study only the current underlying the sAHP.

When hippocampal pyramidal neurons are stimulated by a long duration (600–800 ms) intracellular injection of depolarizing current at a potential where I_D is inactivated, the following current clamp recording is obtained: an initial burst of action potentials followed by a period of silence lasting to the end of the current pulse (Figure 17.6b, d, control). This period of silence, known as accommodation, is observed whatever the intensity of the injected current. By increasing the amplitude of the depolarizing current, the number of action potentials present in the initial burst is increased up to 6 or 8, but the period of silence is always present. If these neurons are depolarized by iontophoretic application of glutamate, the same phenomenon of accommodation is observed.

In order to identify the role of fAHP and sAHP in the mode of discharge of pyramidal neurons, selective blockers of one or the other have been used. In the presence of charybdotoxin, a fAHP blocker (Figure 17.5b), recordings show an increase in the frequency of occurrence of first action potentials (Figure 17.5c); without any change in the accommodation phase. In the presence of noradrenaline or carbamylcholine (agonist of acetylcholine) the accommodation of the discharge of pyramidal neurons disappears and action potentials are then emitted throughout the duration of the depolarization (Figure 17.6b, noradrenaline and Figure 17.6d, carbachol). These substances block the sAHP (Figure 17.6c, noradrenaline and Figure 17.6e, carbachol) without modification of the fAHP, which implies that they do not prevent the entry of Ca^{2+} ions into the pyramidal cells. Therefore, the effects of noradrenaline and acetylcholine are not due to inhibition of Ca^{2+} influx but instead may be attributed to closure of the Ca^{2+}-activated K^+ channels themselves.

How is I_{AHP}, the current underlying the sAHP, activated during the generation of action potentials and how does it act on the pattern of firing? I_{AHP} is activated by an increase in intracellular Ca^{2+} concentration and slowly inactivates. *In vivo*, it is activated after each action potential as a result of the entry of Ca^{2+} ions occurring during the depolarization phase. Since this current does not inactivate rapidly, it summates over the course of successive action potentials, increasing the interspike interval until the membrane is so strongly hyperpolarized that the occurrence of action potentials is completely inhibited. I_{AHP} limits the cell's firing frequency inside a burst of spikes (Figure 17.6b, d). It is also present after a burst of spikes and limits the interburst interval (Figure 17.6a, c, e).

17.2.3 The Voltage-Dependent K^+ Current Sensitive to Muscarine, I_M

I_M is a voltage-dependent K^+ current (Appendix 17.3). It was originally identified in frog sympathetic neurons and has been studied since in a variety of other vertebrate neurons. It is activated at voltages more positive than −60 mV with slow first-order kinetics and does not inactivate with time. I_M was so-called because it is inhibited by muscarinic acetylcholine receptor agonists such as the alkaloid muscarine (M for **m**uscarinic inhibition). It is therefore under muscarinic cholinergic synaptic control. I_M differs from the delayed rectifier current I_K involved in spike repolarization (Chapter 7) by having a 40 mV more negative activation threshold and has slower

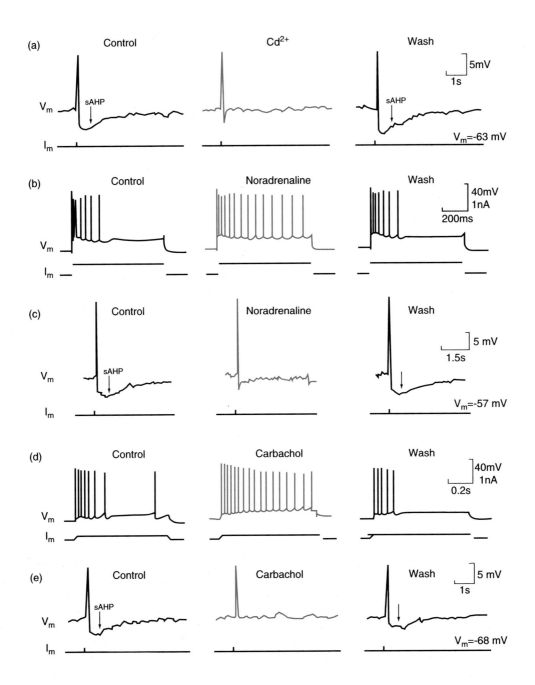

kinetics (Figure 17.7). It differs from I_A and I_D transient currents because it does not inactivate (Figure 17.7).

When a depolarizing current pulse is injected into a rat sympathetic neuron at resting membrane potential, the immediate effect is to start the cell depolarizing and to evoke a spike train which terminates after one or a few spikes (Figure 17.8A, left). In contrast, in the presence of muscarine, the same depolarizing pulse evokes a sustained firing of the cell. This is explained by the fact that in control conditions, the initial depolarization causes more M channels to open (since I_M is partly activated at rest and is a voltage-gated current). This results in a large increase in outward current

Figure 17.6   The role of slow after-hyperpolarization in the pattern of discharge of pyramidal neurons of the hippocampus. The activity of pyramidal neurons is recorded under current clamp (V_m traces) in *in vitro* brain slices. The neurons are stimulated by application of a depolarizing current step of variable duration (I_m traces). The recordings shown in (a), (c) and (e) are the same as those in (b) and (d), but with a different time scale and voltage calibration. In (a), (c) and (e) the burst of spikes shown in (b) and (d) appears as a large and short depolarization with truncated spikes. The response obtained is a burst of action potentials followed by a silence, although the stimulation is still present (b and d, control traces). At the end of the depolarizing step, the response is followed by a period of after-hyperpolarization, which has at least two components. This figure shows the characteristics and the role of *slow* after-hyperpolarization, sAHP (a, c and e, control traces). sAHP is blocked reversibly by Cd^{2+} ions (100 µM), which shows that it depends on the entry of Ca^{2+} ions (a). Noradrenaline (10 µM) and carbachol (2 µM) reversibly block the sAHP (c and e) and also remove the accommodation phase (b and d). (a, d, e: From Lancaster B and Nicoll RA, 1987. Properties of two calcium activated hyperpolarizations in rat hippocampal neurones, *J. Physiol. (Lond.)* **389**, 187–203, with permission. b, c: From Madison DV and Nicoll RA, 1982. Noradrenaline blocks accommodation of pyramidal cell discharge in hippocampus, *Nature* **299**, 636–638, with permission.)

Figure 17.7   Comparison between voltage-dependent K^+ currents. Drawings of idealized K^+ currents recorded in hippocampal pyramidal cells, indicating the kinetics, voltage range of activation and inactivation (shaded areas) and the typical voltage steps used to elicit the currents (solid lines). The effective blocking agents are indicated below. 4-AP, 4-aminopyridine; TEA, tetraethylammonium chloride. (From Storm JF, 1988. Temporal integration by a slowly inactivating K^+ current in hippocampal neurons, *Nature* **336**, 379–381, with permission.)

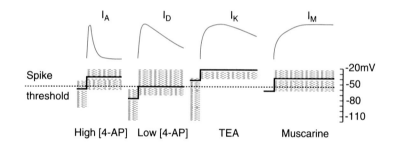

which partially restores the resting membrane potential (Figure 17.8b, left). Because of this, sustained current injection does not generate a maintained train of spikes. When the I_M current present at rest is depressed by muscarine application, the membrane now responds passively to the current pulse injection (since I_M cannot be activated) (Figure 17.8b, right) and the cell discharges continuously during the current pulse.

The sympathetic ganglionic neurons express both nicotinic and muscarinic cholinergic receptors which are activated by acetylcholine released from pre-ganglionic neuron terminals (see Figure 9.1c). A single shock (▲) to the pre-ganglionic trunk evokes two excitatory potentials, a fast (nicotinic) EPSP and a slow (muscarinic) EPSP (Figure 17.8c). The slow EPSP

results from a decrease in membrane conductance and reverses at E_K. It disappears in the presence of atropine, a muscarinic receptor antagonist. This K^+ current depressed by acetylcholine was identified as the I_M current. In the presence of muscarinic agonists, the I_M (outward) current present at rest (because I_M is partly activated at rest and does not inactivate) is reduced and the membrane depolarizes.

The crucial feature of I_M is that, because it increases as the membrane is depolarized, it clamps the membrane at potentials subthreshold to excitation. Conversely, when it is depressed during cholinergic synaptic transmission, it permits the cell to respond to a train of inputs by evoking fast nicotinic EPSPs of larger amplitudes.

Figure 17.8 Membrane potential changes evoked in the presence or absence of the outward K⁺ current I_M; (a) A rat sympathetic neuron is intracellularly recorded under current clamp. (Left) The injection of a 500 ms duration hyperpolarizing current pulse (I, top trace) evokes a passive membrane hyperpolarizing response (V, bottom trace). The symmetrical depolarizing current pulse evokes the firing of a single spike and a depolarization that is not symmetrical to the passive hyperpolarization. This shows the presence of a current activated by the depolarization which tends to oppose membrane depolarization. (Right) In the presence of extracellular muscarine, which depresses I_M, the same depolarizing current pulse now evokes a sustained firing of the cell. (b) Reconstruction of the membrane potential changes (V) induced by a 100 ms duration current pulse (I) in control conditions (left) and when the M conductance (G_M) is depressed by muscarine (right). (c) The fast (nicotinic) and slow (muscarinic) excitatory post-synaptic potentials (EPSP) evoked in a post-ganglionic neuron by a single shock to the pre-ganglionic trunk. (a: From Brown DA and Constanti A, 1980. Intracellular observations on the effects of muscarinic agonists on sympathetic neurones, *Br. J. Pharmacol.* **70**, 593–608, with permission. b: From Adams PR, Brown DA and Constanti A, 1982. Pharmacological inhibition of the M-current, *J. Physiol. (Lond.)* **332**, 223–262, with permission. c: From Adams PR and Brown DA, 1982. Synaptic inhibition of the M-current: slow excitatory post-synaptic potential mechanism in bullfrog sympathetic neurones, *J. Physiol. (Lond.)* **332**, 263–272, with permission.)

17.3 Ionic Currents that Speed the Approach to Spike Threshold: They Decrease the Delay of Onset of the Discharge and Reduce the Interspike Interval

These currents favor depolarization of the membrane up to the activation threshold for the voltage-gated Na⁺ channels of the action potential and thus tend to increase the probability of discharge. These inward currents are activated at potentials more negative than the threshold for opening Na⁺ channels of the action potential; their time course is also slower.

17.3.1 The Persistent Inward Na⁺ Current, I_{NaP}

I_{NaP} is an inward Na⁺ current present in many vertebrate central neurons (pyramidal neurons of the cerebral cortex or the hippocampus, for example). I_{NaP} is activated at potentials 10–20 mV more positive than the resting membrane potential, i.e. at subthreshold potentials, and is sensitive to TTX. It is called P for persistent (non-inactivating). In current clamp records, I_{NaP} is masked by the large outward currents present during the interspike interval.

When pyramidal neurons of the cerebral cortex are recorded under voltage clamp, the total I/V relation shows an inward rectification observed at membrane potentials 5–15 mV more positive than the resting membrane potential (Figure 17.9a, c, control). In the presence of TTX in the extracellular medium, this inward rectification disappears (Figure 17.9b, c, TTX). This observation, together with the lack of effect of extracellular Co^{2+} ions on this current, suggests that it is an inward current that uses Na⁺ as the charge carrier.

I_{Nap} has a fast activation time of 2–4 ms and once it is evoked, it is present for several hundreds of milliseconds: it is persistent. This phenomenon of persistence has been demonstrated by evoking EPSPs in a pyramidal neuron at different membrane potentials (Figure 17.10a, left):

- When the membrane is at the resting potential, the evoked EPSP has a rapid rise-time and a slow decay over about 70 ms (trace 1) and it sometimes generates an action potential (trace 2).

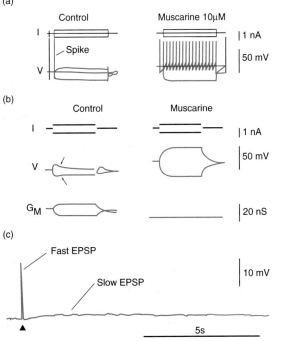

(a)

Control   Muscarine 10μM

I | 1 nA

  Spike | 50 mV

V

(b)

Control   Muscarine

I | 1 nA

                                               | 50 mV

V

G_M | 20 nS

(c)

  Fast EPSP

                                               | 10 mV

    Slow EPSP

▲

                        5s

Figure 17.9   Activation of I_{NaP} causes an inward rectification of the I/V curve at subthreshold potentials. The activity of a pyramidal neuron of the cerebral cortex is recorded under voltage clamp ($V_H = -70$ mV). (a) When a subthreshold depolarizing voltage step is applied (lower traces), an inward membrane current is recorded (arrow, upper trace). The symmetrical hyperpolarizing voltage step evokes a passive response. (b) In the presence of TTX (1 µM), the inward current in response to depolarizing step changes of potential (lower traces) disappears (TTX, three upper traces). (c) I/V curves obtained in the absence (control) and presence (TTX) of TTX. The value of I is measured 50 ms after the beginning of the potential step. In the absence of TTX an inward rectification of the I/V curve is observed, for potential steps of 5 to 15 mV, more positive than the resting potential. From Audinat E, Hermel JM and Crépel F, 1989. Neurotensin-induced excitation of the rat's frontal cortex studied intracellularly *in vitro*, *Exp. Brain Res.* 78, 358–368, with permission.)

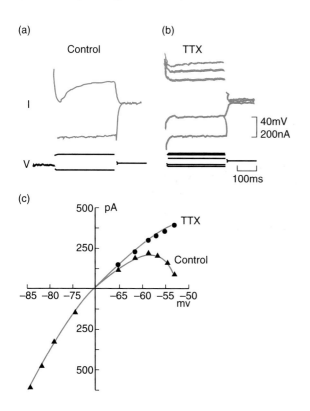

• When the membrane has been hyperpolarized, the evoked EPSP has a similar rise-time but a much faster decay, over about 30 ms (trace 3).

Membrane hyperpolarization prevents the EPSP from depolarizing the membrane up to the activation potential for I_{NaP}. The I/V relation plotted for this same neuron shows that only when an EPSP is evoked in the neuron at the resting potential does the membrane reach a level of depolarization sufficient to activate I_{NaP} (Figure 17.10a, right, arrow). Because of its persistent depolarizing action, I_{NaP} prolongs the synaptic depolarization well beyond that observed in a passive system. In addition, I_{NaP} contributes to the membrane depolarization and brings it more rapidly to the threshold of action potential generation (Figure 17.10a, left, trace 2).

The role of I_{NaP} on the pattern of discharge is difficult to study since this current cannot be selectively blocked. The pharmacological substances that block it, for instance TTX in the extracellular medium or QX-314 (a derivative of lidocaine) injected into the intracellular medium, are also blockers of the action potential Na$^+$ current, I_{Na}. The authors then posed the question of the role of I_{NaP} in the following way: during the interspike interval, does the membrane reach a level of depolarization sufficient for this current to be activated? Recordings of the activity of pyramidal neurons have shown that even when discharging at low frequency, during the interspike interval the membrane potential crosses the level at which I_{NaP} begins to be activated (Figure 17.10b). Furthermore, when discharging at high frequency, during the interspike interval, the membrane potential is entirely in the range in which I_{NaP} is totally activated. The presence of I_{NaP} causes a reduction of the interspike interval and thus an increase in the neuron discharge frequency. I_{NaP}, which has a rapid activation, counterbalances the outward currents which intervene during the interspike interval. As already shown, the duration of the interspike interval depends on this balance between the outward and inward currents activated at subthreshold potential levels.

17.3.2 The Low Threshold, Transient Ca^{2+} Current (I_{CaT})

The low activation threshold Ca^{2+} current is an inward current carried by Ca^{2+} ions and activated by a subthreshold depolarization to $-60/-50$ mV. It inactivates at potentials close to the resting potential. It is de-inactivated by a transient hyperpolarization of the membrane (Appendix 17.4). The low threshold

Figure 17.10   Activation of I_{NaP} prolongs the duration of the EPSP and accelerates neuronal firing frequency. The pyramidal neurons of the cerebral cortex are recorded in *in vitro* brain slices. (a) Current clamp recordings of EPSPs evoked by stimulation of afferent fibers at the resting potential (traces 1 and 2, $V_m = -70$ mV) or at a more hyperpolarized membrane potential (trace 3, $V_m = -80$ mV). It can be observed that the falling phase of the EPSP is much slower in trace 1 than in trace 3. In trace 2, the EPSP triggers action potentials. The I/V relation (right) obtained for this same cell shows the membrane potential at which I_{NaP} is activated in this preparation (vertical arrow). At this point there is an inflexion in the I/V relation. (b) Similarity between the potential value at which I_{NaP} is activated and the potential value through which the membrane passes during the interspike interval. Membrane current I (b_1) in response to a slow change in membrane potential V, starting from the resting potential (b_2). (b_3) Low and high frequency activity of pyramidal neurons recorded under current clamp. If the point at which current I starts to become non-linear is noted on curve b_1 and this is transposed to curve b_2 (arrows), the potential threshold value for activation of I_{NaP} is obtained. It can be seen that for high frequency discharge, the membrane potential during the interspike interval is in the range in which I_{NaP} is activated. Note the difference in time base between b_1 and b_2, and b_3. (a: From Stafström CE, Schwindt PC, Chubb MC and Crill WR, 1985. Properties of persistent sodium conductance and calcium conductance of layer V neurons from cat sensorimotor cortex *in vitro*, *J. Neurophysiol.* **53**, 153–170, with permission. b: From Stafström CE, Schwindt PC and Crill WR, 1984. Repetitive firing in layer V neurons from cat neocortex *in vitro*, *J. Neurophysiol.* **52**, 264–277, with permission.)

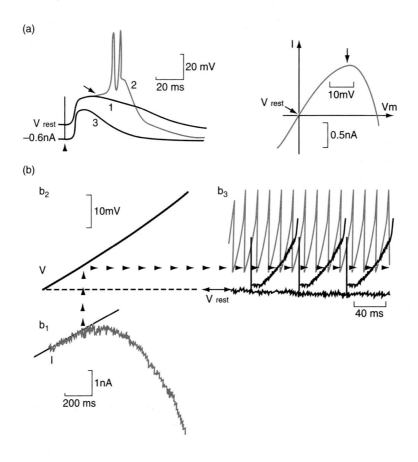

current I_{CaT} results from the activation of the T-type Ca^{2+} channels. Its activation and inactivation characteristics are similar to those of the outward K^+ current, I_A. However, its role is opposite since it is an *inward* current whose function is to depolarize the membrane. This Ca^{2+} current is called low threshold by comparison with the high threshold L-type, N-type and P-type Ca^{2+} currents (see Section 7.5).

The low threshold I_{CaT} was first discovered in the central nervous system, in the inferior olive. The inferior olive is a brainstem structure (see Figure 4.3b) which contains neurons whose axons, called climbing fibers, project to the Purkinje cells of the cerebellar cortex (see Figures 2.6 and 2.7a,b). When these neurons are stimulated directly by injection of a depolarizing current, they generate a complex response consisting of an initial fast-rising action potential (a somatic sodium spike) prolonged to 10–15 ms by a calcium plateau (a Ca^{2+}-dependent dendritic spike) and followed by a long phase of hyperpolarization. This hyperpolarization is typically terminated by a rebound depolarization (Figure 17.11a). Only this depolarizing rebound will interest us here; a complete analysis of the configuration of the discharge of inferior olive neurons will be presented in Section 18.1.

In an extracellular medium containing no Ca^{2+} ions, or containing Ca^{2+} channel blockers (Mn^{2+}, Cd^{2+}), the calcium plateau, the after-hyperpolarization and the depolarizing rebound disappear (Figures 17.11b and 17.12B$_1$). In contrast, in the presence of TTX, only the peak of the action potential disappears (Figure 17.12C$_1$). We observe that the rebound depolarization arises only after a hyperpolarization of the membrane potential. This suggests that the rebound depolarization results from an inward Ca^{2+} current, inactivated at resting membrane potential and de-inactivated by a hyperpolarization. The identification of the rebound current as I_{CaT} and the study of its properties were first carried out under current clamp.

The membrane excitability of inferior olive neurons is increased in two cases: when the membrane is

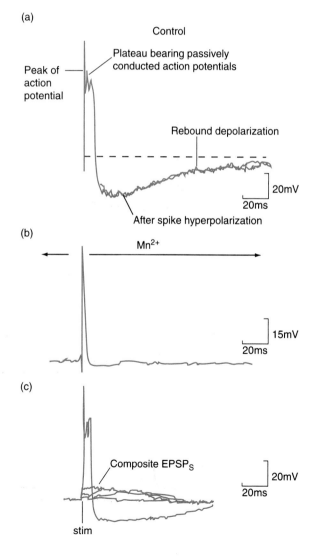

(a)

Control

Peak of action potential

Plateau bearing passively conducted action potentials

Rebound depolarization

20mV

20ms

After spike hyperpolarization

(b)

Mn^{2+}

15mV

20ms

(c)

Composite EPSP$_S$

20mV

20ms

stim

Figure 17.11 Responses of neurons of the inferior olive. Neuronal activity is recorded under current clamp, in *in vitro* brain slices. (a,b) Intracellular recordings of the response to direct stimulation (injection of a depolarizing current pulse, not shown). (c) Intracellular recordings of the synaptic response (stim: stimulation of afferent fibers). (a) In the presence of a control extracellular medium, an action potential with a calcium plateau (ADP or after-depolarization) is recorded. It is followed by a period of after-hyperpolarization (AHP) and a rebound depolarization. (b) In the presence of Ca^{2+} channel blockers (Mn^{2+}) in the extracellular medium, only the peak of the action potential is present; the other components are blocked, which suggests that they depend on the entry of Ca^{2+} ions. (c) Subthreshold stimulation of the afferent fibers to inferior olive neurons evokes an excitatory post-synaptic potential ('composite EPSP') the amplitude of which increases with the amplitude of the stimulus. Once the threshold for the sodium (or peak) action potential has been reached, the response is immediately maximal. It consists, as in (a), of a sequence: Na^+ action potential → Ca^{2+} plateau (after depolarization) → after-hyperpolarization → rebound depolarization. (From Llinas R and Yarom Y, 1981. Electrophysiology of mammalian inferior olive neurons *in vitro*. Different types of voltage-dependent ionic conductances, *J. Physiol. (Lond.)* 315, 549–567, with permission.)

slightly depolarized or when it is slightly hyperpolarized. Thus a subthreshold depolarizing current step does not evoke any activity when the membrane is at the resting potential (Figure 17.12A$_2$) but does evoke

activity when the membrane is depolarized (Figure 17.12A$_1$), which is classical, and also when it is slightly hyperpolarized, which is more surprising (Figure 17.12A$_3$). In the presence of Co^{2+} ions in the

Figure 17.12   Depolarization and hyperpolarization of the membrane both increase the excitability of inferior olive neurons. Neuronal activity (V_m traces) is recorded under current clamp, in *in vitro* brain slices. (a) Application of a subthreshold depolarizing current step (I traces), from resting potential (continuous line) does not evoke any response (A$_2$, only the passive response is present), whereas if the membrane is depolarized (A$_1$) or hyperpolarized (A$_3$), the same subthreshold current step leads to a response. In A$_3$, the calcium plateau and the after-hyperpolarization are of smaller amplitude than in A$_1$ because the number of Ca^{2+} channels activated is smaller and consequently the entry of Ca^{2+} ions is reduced. (b,c) The effect of Co^{2+} ions (b) and of TTX (c) on the response, when the membrane is at the resting potential (B$_2$ and C$_2$), when the membrane is depolarized (B$_1$ and C$_2$), or hyperpolarized (B$_3$ and C$_3$). It is observed that in the presence of Co^{2+}, the effect of hyperpolarization on the excitability of the neurons has disappeared (compare A$_3$ with B$_3$); this indicates that the initial depolarizing current which triggers the action potential from a hyperpolarized membrane potential is a Ca^{2+} current. When the membrane is depolarized, the action potential can be triggered even in the presence of Co^{2+} ions because the membrane is sufficiently depolarized to allow the current pulse to activate directly the Na$^+$ channels of the action potential (compare A$_1$ and B$_1$). In the presence of TTX, a low threshold calcium action potential is recorded when the membrane is hyperpolarized (C$_3$). (From Llinas R and Yarom Y, 1981. Electrophysiolosy of mammalian olive neurons *in vitro*. Different types of voltage-dependent ionic conductances, *J. Physiol. (Lond.)* 315, 549–567, with permission.)

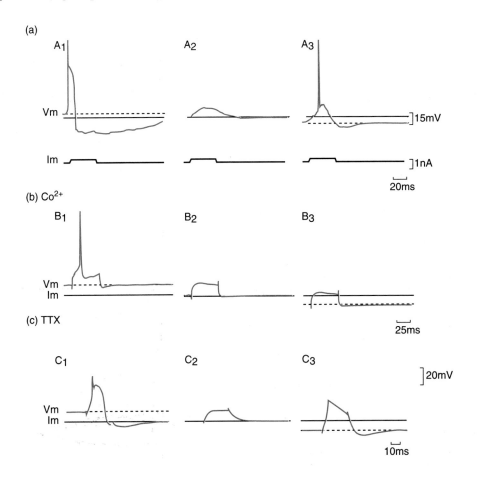

extracellular medium this property disappears (Figure 17.12b), while in the presence of TTX, it remains unchanged (Figure 17.12c). This suggests that a depolarizing current, blocked by Co^{2+} ions and therefore carried by Ca^{2+} ions, inactivated at the resting membrane potential and de-inactivated by a hyperpolarization, is responsible for the rebound depolarization.

I_{CaT} (which is probably here a somatic Ca^{2+} current) is de-inactivated by the Ca^{2+}-sensitive afterhyperpolarization which follows the calcium plateau of the action potential. It then allows a more rapid repolarization of the membrane and a depolarization, called a 'low threshold Ca^{2+} spike' (Figure 17.12A$_3$, C$_3$), up to the activation threshold for the voltage-sensitive Na^+ channels. I_{CaT} thus makes it possible for inferior olive neurons to respond with repetitive activity to a single stimulation (see Section 18.1).

17.3.3 The Cationic Anomalous Inward Rectifier Current (I_h, I_Q)

We will study here the current of the inward rectification which uses both K^+ and Na^+ as charge carriers. The time-course of its activation is slow and it is reversibly blocked by external Cs^+ ions (3 mM) although not affected by Ba^{2+} ions (Appendix 17.5). This current, which has been described in different neurons of the vertebrate central nervous system, is known as I_Q or I_h, according to the preparation. We will take the example of the Purkinje cells of the cerebellar cortex (see Figures 2.6 and 4.3b).

In current clamp recordings, when a long-lasting hyperpolarizing current pulse is applied, a membrane hyperpolarization is recorded that slowly decays even though the step current is maintained (Figure 17.13a). This rebound depolarization is still more clear when the membrane hyperpolarization is large. It results from the activation of a slow inward current (Figure 17.13b) which increases non-linearly as the membrane is hyperpolarized, as shown by the presence of rectification in the I/V relation. A decrease in membrane resistance is thus observed with membrane hyperpolarization. This paradoxical change in membrane resistance has been called anomalous rectification because it occurs in the opposite direction from delayed rectification. The anomalous rectification current is carried by both K^+ and Na^+ ions (since it is modified by changes in the extracellular concentration

of either of these ions) and reverses polarity around −50/−30 mV, depending on the preparation. It is thus an inward current at potentials more negative than −50 or −30 mV.

I_h activates around −55 mV. Since the resting potential of neurons is generally more negative than this value, I_h is partially activated at the resting membrane potential, where it is an inward current. The consequence of the activation of I_h at the resting membrane potential is to buffer hyperpolarizations and to maintain the resting membrane potential at a value more

Figure 17.13   The inward rectification current I_h of Purkinje cells of the cerebellar cortex. Neuronal activity is recorded in *in vitro* brain slices. (a) Recordings under current clamp. Application of hyperpolarizing current steps, away from the resting potential (lower I traces), evoke a hyperpolarization followed by a depolarizing rebound 50–70 ms after the beginning of the current step (upper V traces). Note that the further the membrane is hyperpolarized, the more the depolarizing rebound becomes visible (arrow). (b) Voltage clamp recordings. Application of hyperpolarizing current steps away from the resting potential maintained at −65 mV (lower V traces) evokes an inward current which appears about 50–70 ms after the beginning of the current step. Its amplitude increases with the amplitude of the hyperpolarizing voltage step (upper traces). (From Crépel F and Pénit-Soria J, 1986. Inward rectification and low threshold calcium conductance in rat cerebellar Purkinje cells. An *in vitro* study, *J. Physiol. (Lond.)* **372**, 1–23, with permission.)

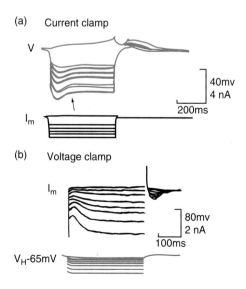

(a)   Current clamp

40mv
4 nA
200ms

(b)   Voltage clamp

80mv
2 nA
100ms

V_H−65mV

positive than E_K (E_K around -100 mV). I_h thus helps other currents to depolarize the membrane potential to a value close to the threshold for the generation of action potentials. This depolarizing behavior is so effective that it may be responsible for the spontaneous pacemaker activity of cells (see Chapter 18). I_h is a pacemaker current because, once activated by the hyperpolarization present during the interspike interval, it depolarizes the membrane up to a potential value at which other more effective depolarizing currents are activated.

A quantitative model of I_h has been established from its different characteristics in order to test this hypothesis. Since there are no known specific blocking agents for this current, one of the ways to understand its role in cellular activity is to establish a theoretical

Figure 17.14   Quantitative theoretical model of the inward rectification current and its role in the configuration of the discharge. (a) Comparison of the experimental (left) and simulated (right) responses to the injection of hyperpolarizing current steps (duration 540 ms, intensity -0.6, -1.2, -1.6 and -2.2 nA in 1 to 4 respectively; I traces are not shown). The simulated response is based on the parameters obtained from voltage clamp recordings. (b) Theoretical model of the variations of the inward rectification current I_h, and the conductance G_h during sustained activity of the neuron recorded under current clamp (V traces). It can be seen that I_h and G_h diminish progressively during the neuronal activity, which leads to an increase in the length of the interspike interval. (From Spain WJ, Schwindt PC and Crill WE, 1987. Anomalous rectification in neurons from the rat sensorimotor cortex *in vitro*, *J. Neurophysiol.* 57, 1555–1576, with permission.)

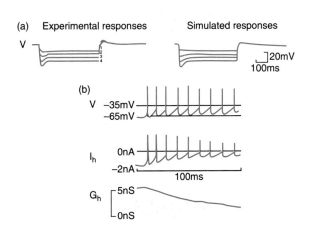

model. Figure 17.14a shows a comparison between the hyperpolarization recorded in response to a hyperpolarizing pulse applied at the resting membrane potential and that modeled under the same conditions. The amplitudes and the time courses of these two responses are similar. Knowing that this model gives a good description of the neuronal response to a hyperpolarization, the authors then made use of this same model in order to describe the behavior of I_h during sustained activity of the neuron (Figure 17.14b). I_h tends to follow Ohm's law during each action potential and each interspike interval (as described before, during the interspike interval, I_h is an inward depolarizing current). However, I_h decays with time since the membrane remains depolarized at potential values more positive than the resting potential throughout the period of repetitive activity. The progressive disappearance of I_h during the interspike interval contributes to the lengthening of this interval and to the appearance of the phenomenon of accommodation described previously in hippocampal pyramidal neurons (see Figure 17.6).

In summary, I_h is activated by the afterhyperpolarizations or synaptic hyperpolarizations and allows repolarization of the membrane. During sustained activity, however, as the membrane becomes more and more depolarized during the interspike interval, I_h is less and less activated and gradually reduces, causing a progressive lengthening of the interspike interval and a reduction of the frequency of the discharge. The reduction of I_h thus participates in the phenomenon of adaptation of the discharge.

Appendix 17.1
The Transient K⁺ Current, I_A

A K⁺ current which is rapidly activated by depolarizing steps from holding potentials negative to the resting membrane potential was originally described in molluscan neurons and termed A current, I_A, by Connor and Stevens (1971). I_A is a transient K⁺ current. Its characteristics distinguish it from the K⁺ currents of delayed rectification: it is a rapidly activating and inactivating K⁺ current and has pharmacological properties different from those of delayed rectifier currents.

Demonstration

The activity of medullary or hippocampal neurons in culture is recorded in voltage clamp mode in a medium containing TTX (to block Na^+ currents) and TEA (to block the K^+ currents of delayed rectification). When the membrane potential is maintained at –70 mV, depolarizing voltage steps (V_{step}, jumps of 10 to 58 mV in amplitude) evoke an outward current whose amplitude increases with the amplitude of the depolarization (Figure A17.1a). This current activates rapidly (within milliseconds) and then inactivates, rapidly and exponentially, during the step depolarization. It is termed the A current, I_A. Inactivation of I_A appears after a few milliseconds, which makes it short-lasting. In this respect I_A resembles more the I_{Na}, of the action potential than the current of the delayed rectification, I_K. The current plateau that follows the peak of the I_A current represents the sum of the leakage current and of the outward currents that are not blocked by TEA. If a hyperpolarizing voltage step ($V_{hyperpol}$) of varying amplitude is now applied for 50 ms before a depolarizing voltage step (V_{step}) to –20 mV (Figure A17.1b), it can be seen that I_A is totally inactivated at a membrane potential of –50 mV. When the membrane potential is more hyperpolarized than –60 mV, I_A can be activated and its amplitude increases with the difference $V_{hyperpol}$–V_{step}. Activation and inactivation curves have been constructed from the data in Figures A17.1a and A17.1b, respectively. The peak value of the amplitude of the I_A current is normalized relative to its maximum value. The membrane potential values given in abscissae for the activation curve are V_{step}, and $V_{hyperpol}$ for the inactivation curve.

Properties of Activation and Inactivation of I_A

I_A is inactivated when the membrane potential is maintained at a value more positive than –50 mV; at these membrane potentials I_A cannot be activated by a depolarization.

I_A is de-inactivated when the membrane potential is maintained at a value more negative than –50 mV; it can then be activated by depolarizations to membrane potentials positive to –50 mV.

Figure A17.1   Activation–inactivation properties of the I_A current. (From Segal M, Rogawski MA and Barker JL, 1984. A transient potassium conductance regulates the excitability of cultured hippocampal and spinal neurons, *J. Neurosci* **4**, 604–609, with permission.)

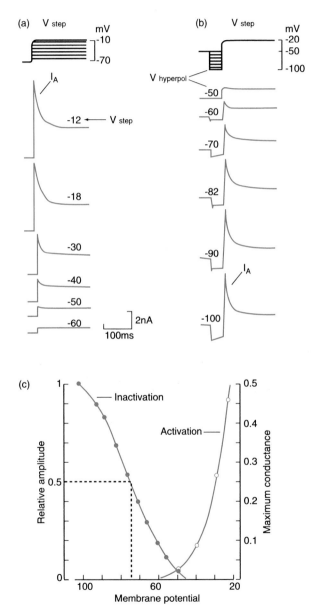

Pharmacology of I_A

The current is blocked by application of 4-amino-pyridine (4-AP, 3 mmol/l) in the extracellular medium. It is insensitive to TEA, Cs^+ and Ba^{2+} ions. Thus there are two ways of blocking I_A, either by depolarizing the membrane above −50 mV, or by applying 4-aminopy-ridine.

Functional Significance

The role of I_A is to delay the triggering of action potentials but only when the neuron has experienced a prior hyperpolarization (to remove the inactivation of I_A at resting membrane potential) and is then depolarized to the threshold voltage for I_A activation (−50 mV). I_A increases the interspike interval.

Appendix 17.2
The Slowly Inactivating K^+ Current, I_D

In addition to I_A, a K^+ current that activates rapidly (within milliseconds) but slowly inactivates (over seconds) was first described by Storm (1988) in hippo-campal pyramidal cells. It was termed D current because it **d**elays the cell firing. I_D has characteristics that distinguish it from the other K^+ currents: it inac-tivates more slowly than the transient A current I_A and activates more rapidly and at more negative potentials than the currents of the delayed rectification I_K; it has also different pharmacological properties.

Demonstration

The activity of pyramidal cells of the hippocampus are recorded intracellularly in *in vitro* brain slices. Voltage clamp experiments are performed in the presence of external 200 μM Cd^{2+} ions to depress Ca^{2+} dependent currents, 50 μM carbachol to block I_M (see Appendix 17.3) and 1–3 mM Cs^+ ions to block I_Q (see Appendix 17.5). When, in such conditions, a depolarizing volt-age step to −26 mV is applied from a holding poten-tial V_H = −80 mV, an outward current consisting of two components is recorded: a fast inactivating com-ponent, insensitive to low doses of 4-aminopyridine (4-AP), and a slowly inactivating component sensitive

Figure A17.2 Activation–inactivation properties of the I_D current. (From Storm JF, 1988. Temporal integration by a slowly inactivating K^+ current in hippocampal neurons, *Nature* **336**, 379–381, with permission.)

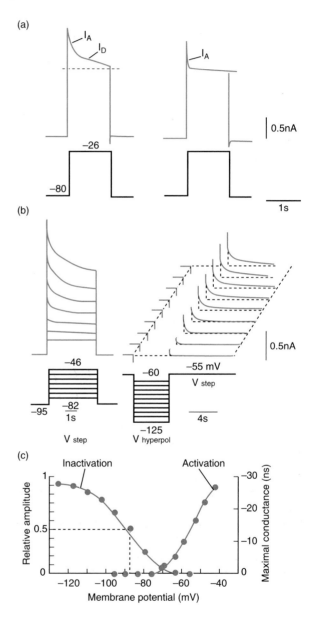

to 40 μM 4-AP (Figure A17.2a). The first component corresponds to I_A and the second one is termed I_D. In order to construct the activation and inactivation curves of I_D, the same protocol as explained in

Appendix 17.1 is applied (Figure A17.2b, c). It appears that I_D is half-inactivated at -88 mV.

Properties of Activation and Inactivation of I_D

I_D is inactivated when the membrane potential is maintained at a value more positive than -50 mV; at these membrane potentials I_D cannot be activated by a depolarization.

I_D is de-inactivated when the membrane potential is maintained at a value more negative than -60 mV; it can then be activated by depolarizations to membrane potentials positive to -70 mV.

Therefore, I_D contrasts with I_A in having a threshold for both activation and inactivation 10–20 mV more negative (compare Figures A17.1c and A17.2c).

Pharmacology of I_D

I_D is much more sensitive to 4-aminopyridine than I_A, the latter requiring 1–5 mM for a block and the former 30–40 µM. It is insensitive to TEA and Cs$^+$ ions. Thus there are two ways of blocking I_D, either by depolarizing the membrane above -70 mV or by applying 40 µM 4-aminopyridine to the extracellular medium.

Functional Significance of I_D

The role of I_D is to delay the triggering of action potentials but only when the neuron has experienced a prior hyperpolarization of large amplitude (to remove the inactivation of I_D) and is then depolarized to the threshold voltage for I_D activation (-60 mV). I_D delays neuronal firing in cells having a negative resting membrane potential or when the membrane has experienced a prior hyperpolarization resulting from an inhibitory post-synaptic current (IPSC).

Appendix 17.3
The M Current, I_M

The M current is a K$^+$ current originally described in sympathetic ganglionic cells (Brown and Adams, 1980). It is termed M because it is reduced by acetyl-choline acting at **M**uscarinic receptors.

Demonstration

I_M may be demonstrated in voltage clamp experiments in the presence of TTX by two protocols:

- by stepping the membrane potential from -60 mV to -30 mV. At -60 mV, most of the M channels are closed. A step to -30 mV reveals, superimposed on the leak current (measured from the response to a symmetrical hyperpolarizing step to -90 mV), a slowly developing outward current due to the slow opening of M channels in response to membrane depolarization (Figure A17.3a).

- by relaxation experiments: the membrane is held at $V_H = -30$ mV, a potential at which M channels remain open and contribute a steady outward current (Figure A17.3b). A negative step to -60 mV causes an instantaneous or transient inward current (I_t) followed by an inward current which slowly develops (slow inward relaxation, $I_{M(60)}$). When the membrane is repolarized to -30 mV, at the end of the voltage step, an instantaneous or transient current (I'_t) is recorded followed by an outward current which slowly develops (outward relaxation, $I_{M(30)}$).

When the membrane is stepped from -30 mV to -60 mV, all the M channels open at -30 mV do not close immediately nor at the same time. There is an instantaneous diminution of the outward current (recorded as a fast inward current). I_t represents the current through channels which are open at V_H (-30 mV), i.e. M channels and 'leak channels'. It therefore depends on the number of channels open at -30 mV and on the electrochemical gradient ($V_m - E_K$) which diminishes from -30 to -60 mV. An exponential diminution of outward current or slow inward relaxation ($I_{M(60)}$) then appears which reflects the kinetics of M channel closure in response to the hyperpolarizing step to -60 mV. When the membrane is stepped back to -30 mV, the M channels do not open instantaneously. There is a first instantaneous outward current (I'_t) which represents the current through channels open at -60 mV ('leak channels' only since M channels are closed). This instantaneous outward current is smaller than the fast inward one recorded

Figure A17.3   Characteristics of the M current in frog sympathetic ganglion cells. Currents are recorded from a bullfrog sympathetic neuron in voltage clamp mode. (a and b) See text. (c) Effect of muscarine on I_M. The membrane is held at −30 mV and stepped to −50 mV. Muscarine evokes an inward current (the current trace is lower): it reduces the steady outward current through M channels open at −30 mV. In contrast, the baseline level attained at −50 mV, at the end of the command step, remains the same: muscarine does not produce an inward current at voltages where the M channels are normally shut. Inward and outward relaxations are largely depressed. See also text. (a, b: Adapted from Brown D and Adams PR, 1980. Muscarinic suppression of a novel voltage sensitive K^+ current in a vertebrate neuron, *Nature* **283**, 673–676; and Adams PR, Brown DA and Constanti A, 1982. M-currents and other potassium currents in bullfrog sympathetic neurones, *J. Physiol.* **330**, 537–572, with permission. c: Adapted from Adams PR, Brown DA and Constanti A, 1982. Pharmacological inhibition of the M-current, *J. Physiol.* **332**, 223–262, with permission.)

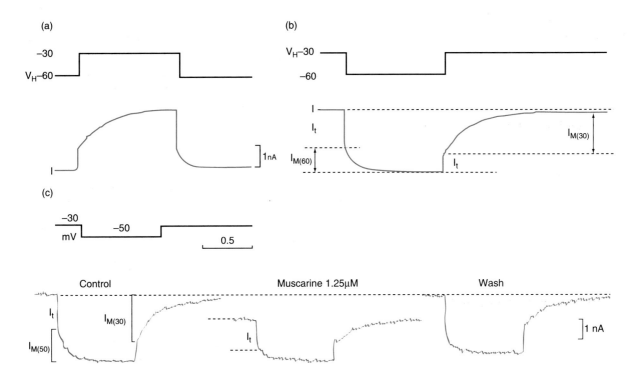

from −30 to −60 mV. It clearly indicates that M channels had closed in response to the preceding step from −30 to −60 mV (when the ohmic current is smaller in response to the same ΔV, it means that the membrane conductance is smaller). An outward current ($I_{M(30)}$) then appears through the M channels, which slowly open again in response to the depolarization. The form of the outward current evoked by the return to the steady holding potential can be distorted by the presence of other K^+ currents activated by this protocol (I_K, I_A, I_D and $I_{K(Ca)}$), particularly when the

membrane is stepped back to V_H from a potential more negative than −70 mV. The M channels seem to be fully closed at membrane potentials more negative than −60 mV as in response to hyperpolarizing commands from −60 mV ($V_H = -60$ mV) only ohmic (passive) current is recorded.

With increasing step commands the inward relaxation reverses in direction at step potentials between −70 and −100 mV. This reversal potential shifts to a more positive value on raising external K^+ concentration. Thus I_M is largely a K^+ current.

Properties of Activation and Inactivation of I_M

The M current is activated by depolarizations to membrane potentials positive to –60 mV. It activates slowly (within hundreds of milliseconds) and does not inactivate.

Pharmacology

A large dose of a muscarinic agonist shuts the M channels: the consequent loss of the steady outward current generates a steady inward current at –30 mV (difference between baseline control and muscarine) and a step to –50 mV now reveals mostly the leak current (I_l) since the M channels are already closed (Figure A17.3c).

Functional Significance of I_M

The M current contributes a steady-state component of outward K+ flux over a range of potentials positive to rest. At these potentials, it opposes depolarizing inputs to a neuron. It may serve to limit firing frequency by reducing the rate of depolarization near the threshold for spike generation in the face of a steady or phasic inward current. The removal of I_M by muscarinic cholinergic inputs leads to a slow depolarization which can enhance other depolarizing synaptic currents. The increased tendency to repetitive spike discharge in cells treated with muscarine would accord with this.

Appendix 17.4
The Low Threshold Transient Ca²⁺ Current, I_{CaT}

The T-type Ca²⁺ current is activated by small amplitude depolarizing steps from holding potentials negative to the resting membrane potential. It inactivates rapidly and slowly de-inactivates. It is named T for transient. It has voltage properties similar to that of the transient K+ current I_A (see Appendix 17.1) but opposite functions. It was originally described by Carbone and Lux in 1984.

Demonstration

The activity of chick dorsal root ganglion cells in culture is recorded in patch clamp (cell-attached patch). The patch pipette contains 110 mM BaCl₂ and the membrane is held at a hyperpolarized potential (V_H = –80 mV). When depolarizing voltage steps of small amplitude (to –50/–20 mV) are applied to the patch, unitary inward Ba²⁺ currents are recorded. These unitary inward currents have a small amplitude (Figure A17.4a) and the unitary conductance γ_T is equal to 8 pS in 110 mM Ba²⁺. Single-channel T currents are present at the beginning of the depolarizing step and then disappear though the membrane is still depolarized, which suggests a rapid inactivation of T channels. T channels are more resistant to 'run down' of activity following patch excision or whole-cell recording than L-type Ca²⁺ channels.

Figure A17.4 Unitary T-type Ca²⁺ current (i_{CaT}). The activity of a single T channel is recorded from dorsal root ganglion cell bodies in patch clamp (cell-attached patch). Mean i_{CaT} amplitude at –20 mV = –0.62 ± 0.03 pA. (Adapted from Nowycky MC, Fox AP and Tsien RW, 1985. Three types of neuronal calcium channel with different calcium agonist sensitivity, *Nature* **316**, 440–443, with permission.)

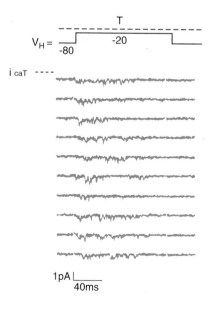

Activation and Inactivation Properties

The voltage dependence of the T current is studied in whole-cell recordings. In order to study the I–V

Figure A17.5 I–V relation of the whole cell T current from a freshly plated (5 h) dissociated rat hippocampal neuron recorded in 10 mM external $CaCl_2$. (Adapted from Yaari Y, Hamon B and Lux HD, 1987. Development of two types of calcium channels in cultured mammalian hippocampal neurons, *Science* **235**, 680–682, with permission.)

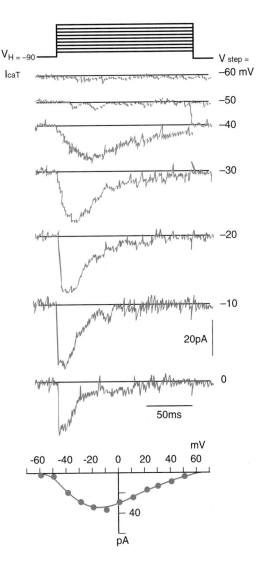

relation of the T current in isolation, the other Ca^{2+} currents present in the cell, such as the high threshold L-, N- and P-types Ca^{2+} currents (see Section 7.5), are pharmacologically blocked. However, in some preparations, T channels predominate and can be studied in the absence of blockers. For example, during development, embryonic hippocampal neurons in culture first express T-type Ca^{2+} channels and then, with neurite extension, also express high-threshold Ca^{2+} channels. To study the activation properties of I_{CaT}, the membrane potential is held at –90 mV. I_{CaT} activates in response to depolarizations positive to –50 mV and present a peak amplitude around –10 mV (Figure A17.5). The voltage dependence of activation is determined by applying different voltage steps from a holding potential V_H = –105 mV. The normalized peak current amplitude is plotted against the test potential (Figure A17.6b, c, ■). In chick sensory neurons, I_{CaT} is half-activated at –51 mV (in 10 mM external Ca^{2+}).

During a 150 ms depolarizing pulse to –10 mV, I_{CaT} rapidly inactivates (in 50 ms): it is transient (Figure A17.5). To study the inactivation properties of I_{CaT}, the membrane is clamped at different holding potentials and the current in response to a depolarizing step to –35 mV is recorded. A plot of peak current amplitude against holding potential (Figure A17.6a, c, ▼) gives a measure of the voltage dependence of inactivation. In chick sensory neurons, I_{CaT} is half inactivated at –78 mV (in 10 mM external Ca^{2+}).

The removal of inactivation (de-inactivation) of the T current is time-dependent. This is studied in lateral geniculate cells *in vitro* (in single electrode voltage clamp) with the following protocol: the membrane is held at –55 mV to inactivate completely the T current. A voltage step to –95 mV of variable duration is then applied. On stepping back to –55 mV, the peak amplitude of the T current is measured (I) and compared with its maximum amplitude (I_{max}). At 35°C, 500–600 ms at –95 mV are needed to totally remove inactivation (Figure A17.7). The removal of inactivation of the T current is also voltage-dependent: at potentials close to –55 mV the de-inactivation is less complete than at more hyperpolarized potentials.

T-type Ca^{2+} channels are selectively blocked in some preparations by low concentrations of the inorganic cation Ni^{2+} (40 μM). They are less sensitive to Cd^{2+} and Co^{2+} than the high threshold Ca^{2+} channels.

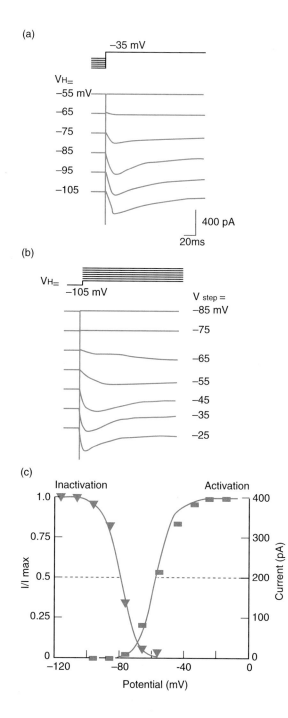

Figure A17.6 Voltage dependence of activation (b) and inactivation (a) of the whole cell T current recorded in 5–10 mM external $CaCl_2$. (c, left) I_{max} is the maximal peak current amplitude obtained at $V_H = -105$ mV. (c, right) I_{max} is the maximal peak current amplitude obtained at $V_{step} = -35/-20$ mV. (Adapted from Fox AP, Nowycky MC and Tsien RW, 1987. Kinetic and pharmacological properties distinguishing three types of calcium currents in chick sensory neurones, *J. Physiol.* **394**, 149–172, with permission.)

enced a prior hyperpolarization (to remove the inactivation of I_{CaT} at resting membrane potential) and is then depolarized to the threshold voltage for I_{CaT} activation (–50 mV). For example, after a hyperpolarization of the membrane due to Ca^{2+}-activated K^+ currents or synaptic hyperpolarizing currents ($GABA_A$ or $GABA_B$ currents), a small depolarization can activate the T current. The *low threshold* of activation of the T current makes it well suited for participating in pacemaking (see Section 18.1). Since it is particularly prominent in embryonic cells, it could also have a developmental role.

Appendix 17.5
The Anomalous Rectification and Inward Rectification Currents

Sir B. Katz was the first to observe in skeletal muscle fibers an increase of membrane conductance when the membrane is hyperpolarized. This rectification is called anomalous since it appears for variations in potential (hyperpolarizations) opposite to those that trigger delayed rectification (depolarizations). Later, this form of rectification was demonstrated in many different preparations.

Two types of anomalous rectification can be distinguished: one type of rectification is due to a current carried by K^+ ions (I_{AR}) (marine eggs, muscles and neurons of the olfactory cortex) and illustrates anomalous rectification in the strictest sense. A second type of rectification is due to a current carried by both K^+ and Na^+ ions (cardiac muscle fibers, photoreceptor sensory ganglion neurons, neurons of the cerebral cortex and of the hippocampus), and is called the inward rectification. The major characteristic of these currents is their activation by hyperpolarizations: the inward rectification.

Functional Significance

Owing to its activation–inactivation properties, the T current is negligible at resting membrane potential. It can be activated only when the neuron has experi-

Figure A17.7   Relative size of the T current (I/I_{max}) against the duration of the hyperpolarizing pulse to –95 mV (see text). (Adapted from Crunelli V, Lightowler S and Pollard CE, 1989. A T-type Ca^{2+} current underlies low-threshold Ca^{2+} potentials in cells of the cat and rat lateral geniculate nucleus, *J. Physiol.* **413**, 543–561, with permission.)

Figure A17.8   The anomalous rectification current is activated by hyperpolarization. The activity of mouse sensory ganglion cells in culture is recorded under current clamp. Hyperpolarizing current steps of 100 ms duration are applied to the membrane, starting from the resting membrane potential (about –55 mV). The rebound depolarization (arrow) appears after some time for step amplitudes which are greater than 15–20 mV. The extracellular medium contains 1 µmol/l TTX.

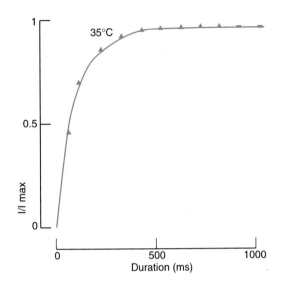

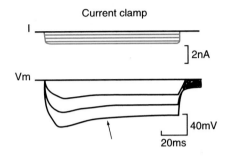

Figure A17.9   Relaxation experiment. The extracellular medium contains 14.5 mM K^+ and 116 mM Na^+.

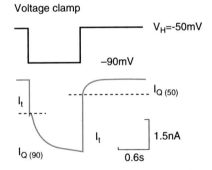

Demonstration

The activity of dorsal ganglionic neurons (sensory neurons) in culture is recorded under current clamp. When the membrane is hyperpolarized beyond the resting potential by hyperpolarizing current pulses, an electrotonic (passive) hyperpolarization is recorded, but in the process of time there appears a depolarizing rebound or sag (Figure A17.8, V_m traces, arrow). This phenomenon is the inward rectification.

Relaxation Experiments

Under two-electrode voltage clamp, a negative voltage step to –90 mV from a membrane potential maintained at V_H = –50 mV causes an instantaneous or transient inward current (I_t), followed by a slow inward relaxation current. When the membrane is repolarized to –60 mV at the end of the voltage step, an instantaneous or transient current (I'_t) is recorded, followed by an inward tail current (Figure A17.9). I_t corresponds to the leak current through channels

which are open at V_H, a current directly proportional to $V_m - E_K$. $I_{Q(90)}$ is the inward current through channels that have been opened by the hyperpolarizing voltage jump (the current of the anomalous rectification). When the membrane is repolarized, I'_t is the current that crosses the channels open at V_{-90}. I'_t is larger than I_t indicating that the anomalous rectification channels had opened in response to the preceding step from –50 to –90 mV (when the ohmic current is larger in response to the same ΔV, it means that the membrane conductance is larger). $I_{Q(50)}$ is the current that crosses the channels of the anomalous rectification, channels sensitive to potential that close gradually. This current reflects the kinetics of the closure of the anomalous rectification channels.

Properties

Anomalous rectification is a current activated by membrane hyperpolarization over the range −60 mV up to −120 mV and does not inactivate. Its reversal potential ranges from −30 to −60 mV. It is carried by K+ and Na+ ions (Figure A17.10) and it is blocked, reversibly, by 1–3 mM extracellular Cs+ ions (Figure A17.11).

Functional Significance of the Inward Rectification Current

The role of the inward rectification cationic current is to maintain the resting potential more positive than E_K. In addition, during the interspike interval, when the membrane is hyperpolarized (during the period known as the AHP), I_Q/I_h is activated and depolarizes the membrane. The depolarizing action of the inward rectification current helps to counterbalance the hyperpolarizing currents of the AHP. Thus its presence reduces the amplitude and duration of the AHP.

Figure A17.10   Ionic selectivity. A hyperpolarizing voltage step of 1.5 s duration and 30 mV amplitude is applied to the membrane from a potential held at V_H = −60 mV (upper traces). The current (lower traces) evoked by these hyperpolarizing steps is recorded under voltage clamp in a control medium (control and wash) or in a medium in which the Na+ ions have been replaced by choline ions (0Na+-choline). In the absence of Na+ ions the anomalous rectification current disappears almost completely. This shows that Na+ ions participate in the anomalous rectification current. It should be noted that the presence of choline ions does not lead to a change in the baseline current. Under these experimental conditions, E_K equals about −90 mV.

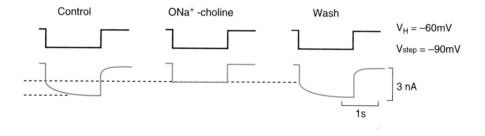

Figure A17.11   Pharmacology. A hyperpolarizing potential step of 1.5 ms duration and 40 mV amplitude is applied to the membrane from a holding potential V_H = −50 mV (upper traces). The current evoked by this jump in potential is recorded under voltage clamp in the absence (lower traces, left and right) and in the presence (lower trace, middle) of 10 mM external Cs+. Cs+ ions reversibly block the anomalous rectification current but do not cause any variation in the baseline current.

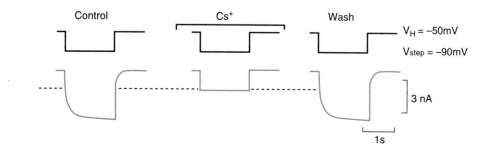

Further Reading

Crill, W. and Schwindt, P.C. (1983) Active currents in mammalian central neurons. *Trends Neurosci.* **6**, 236–240.

Llinas, R. (1988) The intrinsic electrophysiological properties of mammalian neurons: insights into central nervous system. *Science* **242**, 1654–1664.

Rudy, B. (1988) Diversity and ubiquity of K channels. *Neuroscience* **25**, 729–749.

Surmeier, D.J., Wilson, C.J. and Eberwine, J. (1994) Patch clamp techniques for studying potassium currents in mammalian brain neurons. In: Narahashi, T. (Ed), *Methods in Neuroscience: Ion Channels in Excitable Cells*, vol. 19, pp. 39–67.

See also references of Chapter 7.

Firing Patterns of Neurons

The electrical activity of a neuron is not only related to the excitatory or inhibitory synaptic inputs that it receives but to its intrinsic electrophysiological membrane properties as well, i.e. the conductances present in its dendritic, somatic and initial segment membranes, activated by synaptic currents in the near threshold range of membrane potential. As a result, the same post-synaptic depolarizing current will trigger different firing patterns according to the neuronal cell type recorded (see Figure 16.1b). In summary, the firing pattern(s) of a neuron result(s) from the integration of synaptic currents and subliminal voltage-gated currents or intrinsic currents. This is called the input–output characteristics of a neuron. We shall take examples in the mammalian central nervous system to explain the study of input–output characteristics of a neuron and to demonstrate how these characteristics determine the firing pattern.

18.1 Inferior Olivary Cells

The inferior olive is a brainstem nucleus containing neurons whose axons, known as climbing fibers, project to the Purkinje cells of the cerebellar cortex (see Figures 2.6 and 4.3b). When they are activated by synaptic stimulation (stimulation of afferents) or antidromic stimulation (stimulation of the axons belonging to the inferior olive neurons themselves) or direct stimulation (intrasomatic injection of a depolarizing current), the neurons of the inferior olive show a complex discharge configuration (see Figures 17.11a and 18.1a) characterized by an initial fast-rising spike (1 ms duration) which is prolonged to 10–15 ms by an after-depolarization plateau (ADP: after-spike depolarization) on which small action potentials are superimposed. It is followed by a large amplitude, long-lasting (150–200 ms) after-hyperpolarization which silences the spike generating activity and terminates in a rebound depolarization.

Figure 18.1 Analysis of the discharge configuration of inferior olive neurons. The activity of an olivar neuron is recorded intracellularly under current clamp in cerebellar slices. (a) Direct stimulation of the neuron by injecting a depolarizing current step evokes a sequence previously described in Figures 17.11 and 17.12, consisting of an action potential, followed by a plateau (ADP), a period of after-hyperpolarization (AHP) and a depolarizing rebound of variable amplitude (four superimposed traces). (b) Schematic representation of this discharge configuration and indication of the different currents that are activated (see text for explanation). (Adapted from Llinas R and Yarom Y, 1981. Properties and distribution of ionic conductances generating electroresponsiveness of mammalian inferior olive neurons *in vitro*, *J. Physiol. (Lond)* **315**; 569–584, with permission.)

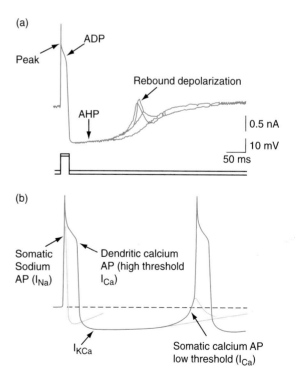

The rebound depolarization evokes another complex action potential: these cells have oscillatory membrane properties.

The analysis of the currents responsible for this discharge configuration (see Figures 17.11 and 17.12) gives the following description.

- The peak of the action potential is sensitive to TTX and is thus the result of the activation of the somatic voltage-dependent I_{Na}.
- The after-depolarization (ADP) and the small superimposed action potentials are sensitive to Ca^{2+} channel blockers. This represents the summation of Ca^{2+} action potentials which are the result of the activation of a high threshold Ca^{2+} current localized in the dendrites. This current is activated by the fast depolarization phase of the action potential.
- The after-hyperpolarization (AHP) is dependent on the amplitude of the ADP and is blocked by external Ba^{2+} ions. It results from the activation of the Ca^{2+}-sensitive K^+ currents $I_{K(Ca)}$.
- The rebound depolarization is due to the activation of a low threshold Ca^{2+} current (I_{CaT}, probably localized at the level of the soma, Appendix 17.4). This current is de-inactivated during the period of after-hyperpolarization and activated when the hyperpolarization decreases.

When the depolarizing current injected at the level of the soma allows activation of the voltage-sensitive Na^+ channels, a sodium action potential (spike) is generated in the soma–initial segment region and the dendritic membrane is depolarized up to the level of activation of the high threshold Ca^{2+} channels. The entry of Ca^{2+} ions through these channels causes a dendritic calcium plateau (ADP) and then the activation of Ca^{2+}-sensitive K^+ channels. The resulting $I_{K(Ca)}$ hyperpolarizes the membrane (AHP). This after-spike hyperpolarization allows the de-inactivation of T-type Ca^{2+} channels. As the amplitude of the AHP diminishes and the membrane potentials return to baseline, the low threshold Ca^{2+} current (I_{CaT}) is activated, generates a 'low threshold' Ca^{2+}-dependent spike and allows the sodium action potential–ADP–AHP sequence to be triggered once again. The cycle can thus repeat itself without any external intervention (Figure 18.1b).

18.2 Thalamic Cells

The thalamus relays and integrates information destined for the cerebral cortex (see Figures 1.14 and 4.3a). It is formed from many nuclei which are classically separated into two groups: the specific nuclei and the non-specific nuclei, according to whether they project to a localized area of the cerebral cortex or to several functionally different areas. When recorded in brain slices *in vitro*, the different thalamic neurons have similar properties. They have complex intrinsic properties that allow them to function either as relay systems or as oscillators: when they are stimulated they show either one of two totally different discharge configurations, according to the value of the membrane potential at the moment at which they were activated.

In Figure 18.2a, an identical depolarizing current pulse is delivered from two membrane potentials. From a slightly depolarized membrane potential, a depolarizing current pulse elicits a tonic, regular discharge, the frequency of which varies linearly with the amplitude of the injected current (Figure $18.2a_1$). When the membrane is at the resting potential, the same current pulse elicits only a subthreshold depolarization (Figure $18.2a_2$). Now, when the membrane is hyperpolarized (by the injection of a constant current pulse for at least 150 ms), a similar depolarizing current pulse triggers an all-or-none burst of spikes (Figure $18.2a_3$). This last response comprises two distinct parts, a slowly rising depolarization (low-threshold spike) and a rapid succession of two to seven fast action potentials (burst of spikes). The transition between one mode of discharge and the other occurs at a potential near −60 mV (Figure 18.2b). Modulation of the membrane potential by the activity of different afferents plays an important role in the triggering of either one or the other of the discharge configurations. Thus, an EPSP may trigger single spikes (repetitive firing) and an IPSP–EPSP sequence may trigger a burst of spikes.

The different currents present in the thalamic membrane were analyzed in order to establish hypotheses for the ionic mechanisms responsible for the two discharge configurations. In addition to the classical voltage-dependent Na^+ and K^+ currents that underlie the fast sodium action potential, different currents activated by a depolarization or hyperpolarization are present in thalamic neurons. Among these are:

Figure 18.2   The two discharge configurations of thalamic neurons. Neuronal activity is recorded intracellularly under current clamp in brain slices. (a) A subthreshold depolarizing current pulse when applied at the resting potential (dotted line, V_{rest}) evokes no response (a_2). In contrast, when the membrane is depolarized (a_1) or hyperpolarized (a_3) by injecting a continuous current, the same subthreshold current pulse now evokes a response. However, these two responses are very different: repetitive firing of the cell during the current pulse (a_1) or a slow depolarization which triggers action potentials (i.e. a single burst of high frequency spikes, a_3). (b) Responses of a thalamic cell to short duration current pulses. An abrupt switch in the configuration of the discharge is recorded when the membrane is depolarized by a constant current of increasing intensity (a slow rising ramp depolarization between A and C), and then hyperpolarized (between C and D). The recordings obtained at a higher sweep speed shows that the cell switches from a burst response (A, B) to tonic firing (C) and returns to a burst response (D). (Adapted from Llinas R and Jahnsen H, 1982. Electrophysiology of mammalian thalamic neurons *in vitro*, *Nature* **297**, 406–408, with permission.)

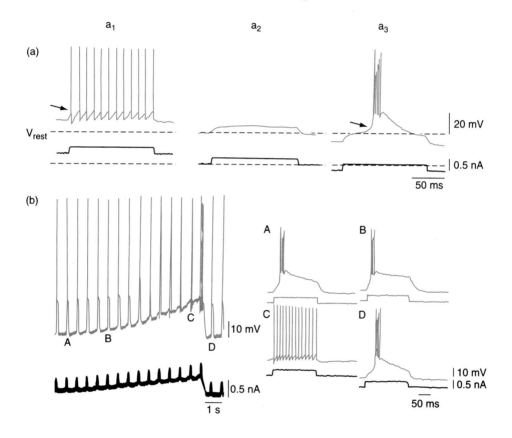

- a low threshold transient Ca^{2+} current (I_{CaT});
- a high threshold dendritic Ca^{2+} current;
- Ca^{2+}-sensitive K^+ currents ($I_{K(Ca)}$);
- an early voltage-sensitive, fast inactivating K^+ current (I_A).

Analysis of the regular frequency discharge pattern

This activity disappears completely in the presence of TTX or in a medium in which external Na^+ ions have been replaced by choline ions; this indicates that the regular discharge consists of sodium action potentials. These action potentials are followed by an after-hyperpolarization which is strongly reduced in the presence of Ca^{2+} channel blockers (Co^{2+}, Cd^{2+}, Mn^{2+}) in the external medium. As a consequence, in the presence of these blockers an increase of the frequency of discharge is observed (compare Figures $18.3a_2$ and b_2). In summary, a depolarizing current pulse applied at a membrane potential more positive than –60 mV activates the voltage-sensitive Na^+ current and triggers sodium action potentials. During each action potential, a high threshold Ca^{2+} current (probably localized at the dendritic level) is activated. In contrast to the inferior olivary cells, this Ca^{2+} current is not strong in thalamic cells. Because of this difference, thalamic spikes are not prolonged by a Ca^{2+} plateau (the number of Ca^{2+} channels in thalamic dendrites would be smaller, per unit area, than that in inferior olivary cells). However, the Ca^{2+} entry activates Ca^{2+}-sensitive K^+ currents and thus triggers the development of an

after-hyperpolarization of about 10 mV following each action potential (Figure 18.3c_2). In the interspike interval, if the after-hyperpolarization is of sufficient amplitude, it causes the de-inactivation of the early K^+ current I_A, which in turn slows the rhythm of the discharge (Figure 18.3a_2). As long as the membrane is depolarized by current injection, this regular activity will be maintained; I_{Na} is reactivated when $I_{K(Ca)}$ diminishes and I_A begins to inactivate. The disappearance of the AHP (by the application of Ca^{2+} channel

Figure 18.3   Analysis of the two discharge configurations of thalamic neurons. (a) Control responses. At the end of the injection of a hyperpolarizing current pulse, a slow depolarization which triggers action potentials is recorded (a_1), whereas when the membrane is depolarized slightly more, a low intensity current pulse evokes a regular tonic discharge (a_2). (b) The application of a Ca^{2+} channel blocker (Co^{2+}) in the presence of a reduced concentration of Ca^{2+} ions prevents the slow depolarization and the burst of action potentials (b_1) although the regular discharge is still present (b_2). Note that in these conditions the duration of the interspike interval is reduced and the after-hyperpolarization that follows each action potential is weaker (compare a_2 and b_2). (c) & (d) The same recording as in a_1 (c_1) and a_2 (c_2) indicating the currents that are activated in each of these two discharge configurations. (Adapted from Jahnsen H and Llinas R, 1984. Ionic basis for electroresponsiveness and oscillatory properties of guinea pig thalamic neurones *in vitro*. *J. Physiol.* **349**, 227–247, with permission.)

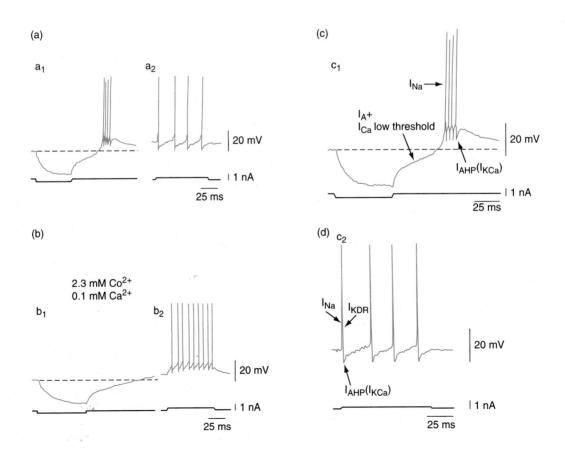

blockers, Figure 18.3b$_2$) suppresses the activation of I_A after each action potential (since I_A will stay inactivated due to the depolarized membrane potential in the interspike interval), and results in a higher frequency discharge.

Analysis of the bursting pattern of action potential discharge

Action potentials that rise from the peak of the slow depolarization disappear in the presence of TTX. In contrast, the slow depolarization is not affected by TTX but disappears in the presence of Ca^{2+} channel blockers (compare Figures 18.3a$_1$ and b$_1$). This demonstrates that the fast action potentials are sodium spikes and that the slow depolarization or low threshold spike results from a Ca^{2+} current. Since this slow depolarization only appears when the membrane has been previously hyperpolarized for at least 150 ms, this suggests that it is due to a low threshold Ca^{2+} current (I_{CaT}), normally inactivated at the membrane resting potential (or at potentials more positive than the membrane resting potential) and de-inactivated by a transient hyperpolarization of the membrane (the amplitude of the slow depolarization is related to the hyperpolarization of the membrane before its generation). The low threshold spike leads to the activation of a high threshold Ca^{2+} current, the entry of Ca^{2+} ions (probably in the dendrites) and the activation of Ca^{2+}-sensitive K$^+$ currents ($I_{K(Ca)}$). Each action potential is followed by a phase of after-hyperpolarization. The early K$^+$ current I_A also plays a role in the apparition of this pattern of discharge. When the membrane has been hyperpolarized for a short time, for instance during a short hyperpolarizing current step, or by an inhibitory afferent, and then stimulated with a long depolarizing current, the I_A current is activated and will prolong the duration of the hyperpolarization, thus permitting the de-inactivation of the low threshold I_{CaT} and the triggering of the response in the form of a burst of action potentials (Figure 18.3c$_1$).

Transposition from one discharge pattern to the other

When the membrane is at a potential more negative than the resting potential, the low threshold Ca^{2+} current is de-inactivated and thus may be activated. In this case, small depolarizations of the membrane evoke a response in the form of a burst of action potentials. In contrast, when the membrane potential is maintained at a value that is more positive than the resting membrane potential, the low threshold Ca^{2+} current is inactivated and the regular frequency firing pattern can thus occur. In conclusion, the responses of thalamic neurons to excitatory afferents depend on the value of the resting membrane potential, i.e. on the activity of the inhibitory afferent pathways.

It should be noted that the after-hyperpolarization which follows each action potential in thalamic neurons is much weaker than that which follows action potentials in neurons of the inferior olive (this is probably the result of a weaker influx of Ca^{2+} ions during the thalamic action potential). For this reason, the thalamic neurons can fire bursts of action potentials at higher frequencies.

18.3 Purkinje Cells

Purkinje cells are located in the cerebellar cortex in the so-called Purkinje cell layer (see Figures 2.6 and 4.3b).

The regular discharge pattern recorded in the soma of Purkinje cells

In response to the injection of a small amplitude depolarizing current pulse at the level of the soma, Purkinje cells respond, after a certain latency, with a regular discharge composed of short duration (1.5 ms) action potentials whose minimum mean frequency is 10–30 action potentials per second (Figure 18.4a$_1$, bottom trace). The amplitude of these action potentials is maximal in recordings made in the soma and diminishes progressively as the recordings are performed towards the distal dendrites (Figure 18.4a$_1$, b, from bottom to top). These action potentials disappear completely in the presence of TTX (1 μM) (Figure 18.5b). Together these results suggest that these are sodium action potentials generated in the axo-somatic region which then propagate passively towards the dendrites (but are concomitantly actively propagated along the axon, not shown).

More precise analysis of the discharge pattern of Purkinje cells in response to the application of a

Figure 18.4   Configuration of the discharge of Purkinje cells as a function of the intensity of the applied depolarizing current and the recording site. The activity of Purkinje cells is recorded intracellularly under current clamp in cerebellar slices. A continuous depolarizing current of low amplitude (column a_1) or of higher amplitude (columns a_2 and b) is injected into the soma. The response is recorded at several points, further and further away from the soma (columns a and b from bottom to top). A regular discharge of somatic action potentials is recorded in response to application of low-intensity current (column a_1) and an irregular discharge composed of somatic and dendritic action potentials is recorded in response to the application of higher intensity current (columns a_2 and b). (a: Adapted from Hounsgaard J and Mitgaard J, 1988. Intrinsic determinants of firing pattern in Purkinje cells of the turtle cerebellum *in vitro*. *J. Physiol. (Lond.)* **402**, 731–749, with permission. b: Adapted from Llinas R and Sugimori M, 1980. Electrophysiological properties of *in vitro* Purkinje cell dendrites in mammalian cerebellar slices, *J. Physiol. (Lond.)* **305**, 197–213, with permission.)

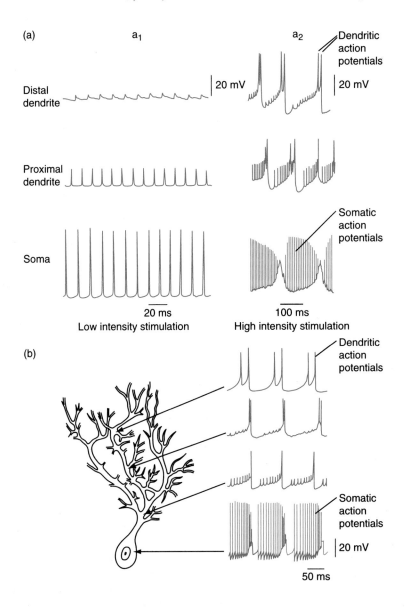

Figure 18.5 Sodium and calcium dependent action potentials in Purkinje cells. (a) Current clamp recording from proximal dendrites of the control discharge in response to a high intensity depolarizing current step (compare with Figure 18.4a$_2$, upper traces). (b) In the presence of TTX, the short duration action potentials disappear although the long duration action potentials are unchanged; this indicates that the short action potentials recorded in (a) are sodium-dependent action potentials. (c) In the presence of TTX and a Ca^{2+} channel blocker, Co^{2+}, both types of action potentials disappear, indicating that the long duration action potentials are calcium-dependent action potentials. (From Hounsgaard J and Mitgaard J, 1988. Intrinsic determinants of firing pattern in Purkinje cells of the turtle cerebellum *in vitro, J. Physiol. (Lond.)* **402**, 731–749, with permission.)

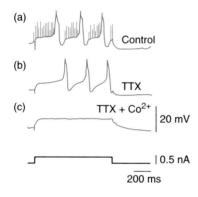

depolarizing current has shown that the regular discharge appears after a certain latency whose value depends on the intensity of the injected current. In addition, the duration of the discharge can outlast the duration of the depolarizing current pulse. Analysis of the ionic currents responsible for this discharge pattern has revealed, in particular, the activation and role of a current activated at subthreshold potentials, the persistent inward Na$^+$ current, I_{NaP}. In current clamp recordings, the presence of this current leads to a nonlinearity of membrane potential changes in response to subthreshold depolarizing current steps: an inward rectification of the I/V curve is seen for subthreshold depolarizing potentials. This rectification is sensitive to the presence of TTX and to changes in the external Na$^+$ concentration but is not sensitive to Ca^{2+} channel blockers. As seen in Section 17.3.1, I_{NaP} generates a slow, TTX-sensitive depolarizing response, which, once activated, may generate prolonged plateau

potentials that may last for tens to hundreds of milliseconds. It allows the membrane to be brought to the threshold for action potential generation when it is slightly depolarized.

In summary, the injection of a small amplitude depolarizing current pulse leads to the activation of the persistent inward current I_{NaP}, which depolarizes the membrane up to the threshold potential for activation of the voltage-gated Na$^+$ channels of the action potential. As long as the membrane is depolarized, the regular discharge is maintained by means of I_{NaP}. This discharge can continue beyond the duration of the depolarizing current step. This is also due to I_{NaP} which, by causing a depolarizing plateau, allows the activity of these neurons to be maintained.

The irregular discharge pattern recorded in the dendrites and composed of somatic and dendritic action potentials

When the intensity of the depolarizing current pulse injected into the Purkinje cell soma is increased, another discharge pattern is recorded in the soma: high frequency trains of sodium action potentials, interspersed with bursts of action potentials of long duration (> 5 ms) and small amplitude (Figure 18.4a$_2$, b). Recorded in the dendrites, the long duration action potentials have a much greater amplitude (Figure 18.4a$_2$,b, top traces). They disappear in the presence of Ca^{2+} channel blockers but remain unchanged in the presence of TTX (Figure 18.5). These results suggest that the slow action potentials are high threshold calcium action potentials, generated in the dendrites and conducted to the soma. They result from the activation of high threshold Ca^{2+} channels termed P channels as they were first described in Purkinje cells (see Section 7.5).

The other currents that are activated are:

- The K$^+$ currents sensitive to Ca^{2+} ions, $I_{K(Ca)}$, activated by the entry of Ca^{2+} ions during the dendritic calcium spikes. They cause an after-hyperpolarization (AHP) of the membrane after the burst of calcium action potentials.
- The rectifying inward current, I_h (see Figure 17.13), activated by the hyperpolarization of the membrane during the AHP. It allows repolarization of the membrane and makes it possible to maintain a

membrane potential more positive than the equilibrium potential for K+ ions (see Appendix 17.5).

In summary, when Purkinje cells are strongly depolarized by current injection into the soma, this causes a high frequency discharge of sodium action potentials in the soma and of calcium action potentials in the dendrites. The calcium action potentials are followed by a period of after-hyperpolarization (AHP) caused by the activation of Ca^{2+}-sensitive K^+ currents. The end of the after-hyperpolarization and the return to the resting membrane potential are due to activation of an I_h current.

Activation of Purkinje cells by stimulation of their afferents (e.g. stimulation of climbing fibers)

Purkinje cells are normally activated by numerous afferent fibers and among these are the climbing fibers, which are the axons of neurons of the inferior olive. In the adult, a single climbing fiber innervates each Purkinje cell. This innervation has the following characteristic: the climbing fiber winds itself around the dendrites making a great number of 'en passant' boutons along its course (see Figure 2.7a,b). These synapses are excitatory and the neurotransmitter is an excitatory amino acid. The activation of a climbing fiber thus causes a massive depolarization of the dendritic arborization and an activation of the high threshold Ca^{2+} channels present at different points along the dendrites. Thus in response to the activation of a climbing fiber, several Ca^{2+} action potentials are recorded in the dendrites. The Ca^{2+} action potentials propagate along the dendrites, and depolarize the axon initial segment to the threshold for triggering sodium action potentials. Ca^{2+} spikes force the cell to respond with a high frequency burst of Na^+ spikes at the level of the soma and axon. Afferent information coming from the inferior olive is thus amplified.

Further Reading

Connors, B.W. and Gutnick, M.J. (1990) Intrinsic firing patterns of diverse neocortical neurons. *Trends Neurosci* **13**, 99–104.

Häusser, M., Stuart, G., Racca, C. and Sakman, B. (1995) Axonal initiation and active dendritic propagation of action potentials in substantia nigra neurons. *Neuron* **15**, 637–647.

McCormick, D.A. and Pape, H.C. (1990) Properties of a hyperpolarization-activated cation current and its role in rhythmic oscillation in thalamic relay neurons. *J. Physiol. (Lond.)*; **431**, 291–318.

Schwindt, P.C., Spain, W.I., Foehring, R.C. et al. (1988) Multiple conductances and their functions in neurons from cat sensorimotor cortex *in vitro*. *J. Neurophysiol.* **59**, 424–449.

Stuart, G. and Häusser, M. (1994) Initiation and spread of sodium action potentials in cerebellar Purkinje neurons. *Neuron* **13**, 703–712.

Stuart, G. and Sakmann, B. (1994) Active propagation of somatic action potentials into neocortical pyramidal cell dendrites. *Nature* **367**, 69–72.

19

Synaptic Plasticity

Synaptic responses undergo short- and long-term modifications. We shall examine in this chapter the mechanisms underlying plasticity in adult synapses. Developmental forms of plasticity have been excluded.

19.1 Short-Term Potentiation of a Cholinergic Response as an Example of Short-Term Plasticity: The Cholinergic Response of Muscle Cells to Motoneuron Stimulation

Repetitive high frequency (> 15 Hz) stimulation of the pre-synaptic element (motoneuron) leads to short-term potentiation (STP) of the post-synaptic response of the muscle cell. As shown in Figure 19.1, successive pre-synaptic spikes produce in these conditions excitatory post-synaptic currents (EPSC) of greater and greater amplitudes. This phenomenon, first discovered at the neuromuscular junction, is also observed at the squid giant synapse and in mammalian afferent synapses to motoneurons.

In the squid giant synapse, synaptic facilitation has the following characteristics: when the pre-synaptic element repeatedly fires, an increase of the post-synaptic response amplitude is observed. This increase diminishes with a time constant in the order of tens of milliseconds. Simultaneous recordings of pre-synaptic action potentials, pre-synaptic Ca^{2+} current (I_{Ca}), variations of the intracellular Ca^{2+} concentration and post-synaptic depolarization show that the post-synaptic response amplitude increases when:

- the amplitude and length of pre-synaptic spikes are unchanged;
- the amplitude of the pre-synaptic I_{Ca} evoked by each pre-synaptic depolarizing pulse or action potential is constant;
- the increase of the pre-synaptic intracellular Ca^{2+}

concentration is identical in response to each depolarizing pulse or action potential.

The increase of intracellular Ca^{2+} concentration ($[Ca^{2+}]_i$, see Figures 8.3 and 8.4) in the pre-synaptic element slowly disappears, in about 1 s, whereas the Ca^{2+} current and the release of the neurotransmitter both last about 1 ms. Katz and Miledi, in 1965, were the first to propose that STP is due to residual Ca^{2+} ions still present in the active zone when the second pre-synaptic spike occurs. The following hypothesis was proposed: Ca^{2+} ions enter into the pre-synaptic element through voltage-gated Ca^{2+} channels opened by the depolarization; the intracellular Ca^{2+} concentration is very high at active zones at the end of the

Figure 19.1 Pre-synaptic facilitation at the frog neuromuscular junction. The activity of a frog sartorius muscle cell is recorded in normal Ringer's solution ($V_m = -90$ mV). The motor end plate currents are evoked by repetitive stimulations of the motor nerve (2 µA intensity, 5 ms duration). The average current intensity in response to the first stimulation is 0.5 µA. This amplitude gradually rises following second and third stimulations. The inward currents are represented upwardly, which is unusual. (Adapted from Katz B and Miledi R, 1979. Estimates of quantal content during chemical potentialization of transmitter release, *Proc. R. Soc. Lond. B* **205**, 369–378, with permission.)

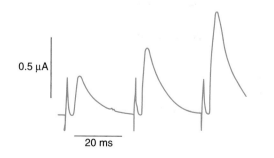

0.5 µA

20 ms

Figure 19.2 Rapid reduction of residual Ca²⁺ ions quickly eliminates STP. The activity of the crayfish dactyl opener muscle cell is recorded intracellularly in current clamp mode in response to the stimulation of an axonal branch of the pre-synaptic motoneuron. The electrode positioned inside the pre-synaptic axon is filled with diazo-2 (50 mM) and fluorescein (10 mM) in KCl (3 M) in order to both stimulate the pre-synaptic axon and fill it with the Ca²⁺ chelator. A conditioning tetanus (10 stimuli at 50 Hz) followed by a single stimulus at 2 Hz is applied to the axon. (a) Action potentials recorded from the preterminal axon branch. (b) The response (EPSP) of the post-synaptic muscle cell is recorded in control conditions (1), after the intracellular injection of diazo-2 (2) and after photolysis of diazo-2 by a UV flash given after the tetanus (3). See text for further explanations. (Adapted from Kamiya H and Zucker RS, 1994. Residual Ca²⁺ and short term synaptic plasticity, *Nature* **371**, 603–606, with permission.)

(a) Pre-synaptic recordings

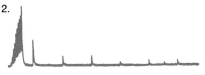

Pre-synaptic action potential

(b) Post-synaptic recordings

Before injection

1.

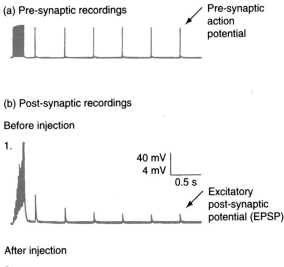

40 mV
4 mV
0.5 s

Excitatory post-synaptic potential (EPSP)

After injection

2.

UV flash (10 ms before 1st test)

3.

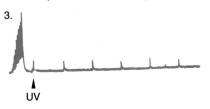

UV

action potential. These Ca²⁺ ions act rapidly and locally on target molecules to trigger the exocytosis of synaptic vesicles with a probability *p*. At the same time, the Ca²⁺ ions are also buffered in the cytoplasm and are expelled to the extracellular medium or inside the organelles. However, a residual, quite high $[Ca^{2+}]_i$ is still present close to the pre-synaptic membrane for some period of time. This $[Ca^{2+}]_i$ value is not high enough to trigger neurotransmitter release, but added to the incoming increase of $[Ca^{2+}]_i$ accompanying the arrival of the second action potential (when the delay between the two action potentials is short), it increases neurotransmitter release probability to the second action potential and thus causes potentiation of the post-synaptic response.

STP can also be induced by high frequency stimulation (conditioning tetanus) of the afferent motoneuron (model of the crayfish neuromuscular junction, Figure 19.2a). In that case, the post-synaptic response (EPSP) recorded at regular intervals after the tetanus is potentiated and then decays to control amplitude within 1.5 s (Figure 19.2b, 1). In order to test the hypothesis of Katz and Miledi, a photolabile Ca²⁺ chelator, diazo-2, is injected into the pre-synaptic terminals. The motoneuron is penetrated at the level of an axon branch with a microelectrode containing KCl (to record pre-synaptic activity), the photolabile Ca²⁺ chelator diazo-2 (to chelate Ca²⁺ ions with an affinity of 150 nM after photolysis) and fluorescein (to monitor progress of injection). First, the control STP is recorded (Figure 19.2b, 1). Then diazo-2 is injected into the pre-synaptic axon in order to test that before photolysis diazo-2 has little effect on STP since the unphotolysed chelator has a low power to chelate Ca²⁺ ions (Figure 19.2b, 2). A UV flash is given after the tetanus in order to produce a chelator with 150 nM Ca²⁺ affinity: the STP of the post-synaptic response is prevented (Figure 19.2b, 3).

These results show that STP is due to residual free Ca²⁺ ions following pre-synaptic activity. What are the molecular targets of Ca²⁺ action in short-term plasticity? Many candidates exist among vesicular, plasma membrane and cytoplasmic proteins of the pre-synaptic element (see Chapter 8). This identification awaits further experiments.

19.2 Long-Term Potentiation of a Glutamatergic Response: Example of the Glutamatergic Synaptic Response of Pyramidal Neurons of the CA1 Region of the Hippocampus to Schaffer Collateral Activation

19.2.1 The Schaffer Collaterals are Axon Collaterals of CA3 Pyramidal Neurons which Form Glutamatergic Excitatory Synapses with Dendrites of CA1 Pyramidal Neurons

The hippocampus is a telencephalic structure with a rostrocaudal extension in the rat (Figures 4.4 and 19.3a). It is composed of two closely interconnected crescent-like regions, Ammon's horn and the dentate gyrus. Ammon's horn is formed by a layer of principal neurons, the pyramidal neurons, and is subdivided in three regions called CA1, CA2 and CA3 (CA for Cornu Ammonis). The dentate gyrus is formed by a layer of principal neurons called granular cells. Numerous interneurons are present in each region.

The pyramidal cells of CA3 have branched axons. One branch leaves the hippocampus and projects to other structures. The other branches are recurrent collaterals that form synapses with dendrites of CA1 pyramidal neurons. These collaterals run in bundles and form the Schaffer collateral pathway. Axon terminals form asymmetrical synapses with the numerous spines of CA1 dendrites. These synapses are excitatory and the neurotransmitter is glutamate. Owing to the laminar organization of the hippocampal structure, it is possible to stimulate selectively the Schaffer collateral pathway and to record the evoked excitatory post-synaptic potential (EPSP) in a CA1 pyramidal soma either *in vivo* or *in vitro* (Figure 19.3a).

19.2.2 Long-Term Potentiation of the Glutamatergic EPSP Recorded in CA1 Pyramidal Neurons Results from an Increase of Synaptic Efficacy

Bliss and Lomo demonstrated in 1973 that a brief high frequency train of stimulation of either one of the three pathways in the hippocampus produces an increase of the amplitude of the EPSP recorded in a post-synaptic pyramidal neuron (Figure 19.3b). We

shall restrict our study of long-term potentiation (LTP) to the synaptic response of CA1 pyramidal neurons to Schaffer collateral stimulation, recorded in hippocampal slices, in the presence of bicuculline (an antagonist at $GABA_A$ receptors) in order to prevent the participation of GABAergic inhibitory responses resulting from interneuron activation.

A single stimulus applied repeatedly at a low frequency (0.02–0.03 Hz) to the Schaffer collaterals evokes a stable 'control' field EPSP recorded by an extracellular electrode placed in the dendritic field of CA1 pyramidal neurons (Figure 19.4a, b, d, EPSP1). This 'control' field EPSP is mediated predominantly by non-NMDA receptors since it is almost completely abolished by the bath application of CNQX, a selective antagonist of AMPA receptors. A tetanic stimulation (one train of 1 s duration, composed of 50–100 stimuli at 100 Hz) is then applied to the Schaffer collateral pathway through the same stimulating electrode. After this tetanus, the same single stimulus, again through the same stimulating electrode, now evokes a 'post-tetanic' field EPSP of larger amplitude and with a steeper initial slope than the control one: the field EPSP is potentiated (LTP, Figures 19.3b and 19.4b, d, EPSP1). This potentiation (by 30–50%) is persistent: it lasts hours when recorded in the *in vitro* hippocampal slice preparation and days when induced in the freely moving animal. The value of the initial slope of a field EPSP (or of an intracellular EPSP) is an accurate index of the changes of the *monosynaptically* evoked post-synaptic excitatory response since the field EPSP and the intracellular EPSP can be composed of monosynaptic as well as polysynaptic unitary EPSPs.

Principal features of LTP

(1) LTP is a long-lasting phenomenon: it persists for hours *in vitro* and days or weeks in the intact animal. (2) LTP results from an increase in the synaptic response without changes in the number of stimulated axons. This is readily shown in extracellular recordings, i.e. recordings with an electrode placed in the region of CA1 pyramidal dendrites (extracellular means outside the neurons and their processes) (Figure 19.4a). Stimulation of the Schaffer collateral evokes (Figure 19.4a):

Figure 19.3   Tetanic LTP in the hippocampus is induced by high frequency stimulation of afferent fibres. (a) Coronal section of the rat hippocampus showing the major excitatory connections. CA1, CA3, pyramidal layer of the regions CA1 and CA3 of the hippocampus; DG, dentate gyrus layer composed of granular cells (g) which send their axons (mossy fibers, mf) to CA3 pyramidal dendrites. CA3 pyramidal cells send axon collaterals, called Schaffer collaterals (Sch), to CA1 pyramidal apical dendrites. The tetanic stimulation (for example 1–4 trains of 10 stimulations at 100 Hz applied every 1 s) is applied to Schaffer collaterals and the AMPA-mediated post-synaptic response is recorded intracellularly in the soma of a pyramidal cell (EPSP or EPSC) and/or extracellularly (field EPSP) in the layer of CA1 pyramidal dendrites. comm, commissural fibers; pp, perforant path. (b) A CA1 pyramidal neuron represented upside down compared with its position in the coronal section and the afferent Schaffer collaterals. The AMPA-mediated EPSP evoked by a single stimulation of Schaffer collateral (one vertical bar) is recorded intracellularly (in the presence of bicuculline, a GABA$_A$ receptor antagonist). After a tetanic stimulation of the Schaffer collaterals (shown as high frequency bars), a potentiation of the glutamatergic EPSP evoked by a single stimulation is recorded. This potentiation lasts several minutes to hours. (Adapted from Kauer JA, Malenka RC and Nicoll R, 1988. A persistent postsynaptic modification mediates long term potentiation in the hippocampus, *Neuron*, **1**, 911–917, with permission.)

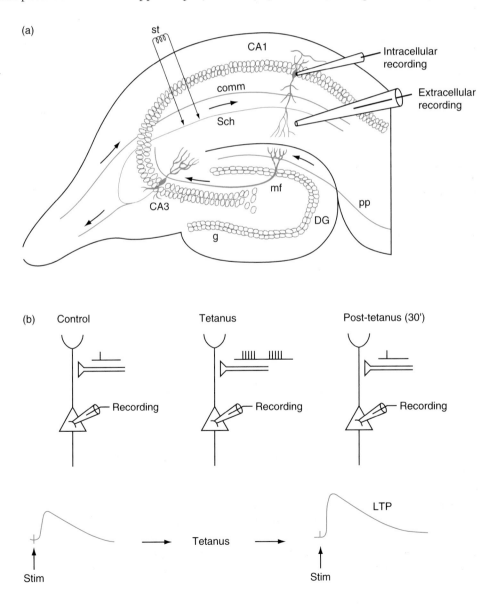

Figure 19.4   Tetanic LTP is synapse specific. (a) Extracellular recording of the response of a population of CA1 pyramidal neurons to stimulation (S_1) of afferent Schaffer collaterals. The stimulation S_1 evokes an afferent volley (the extracellular recording of pre-synaptic action potentials in all stimulated afferent axons) and a field EPSP (the extracellular recording of the post-synaptic response of pyramidal neurons). Sixty minutes after a tetanus applied through the same stimulating electrode, the field EPSP in response to S_1 stimulation is now persistently increased (LTP). (b) Input/output curves depicting the amplitude of the afferent volley vs. the initial slope of the field EPSP. Note the increased slope 60 min after the tetanus. (c) The post-synaptic responses (control $EPSP_1$ and $EPSP_2$) of a single pyramidal neuron are recorded intracellularly in current clamp mode (whole-cell patch) in response to stimulations S_1 and S_2. Then, stimulus S_1 is tetanized but not stimulus S_2. Sixty minutes after the tetanus on S_1, $EPSP_1$ is persistently potentiated (LTP) and $EPSP_2$ is not. (d) Diagram illustrating the time course of the initial slope of $EPSP_1$ and $EPSP_2$ before and after the tetanus on S_1. (From Aniksztejn L, personal communication.)

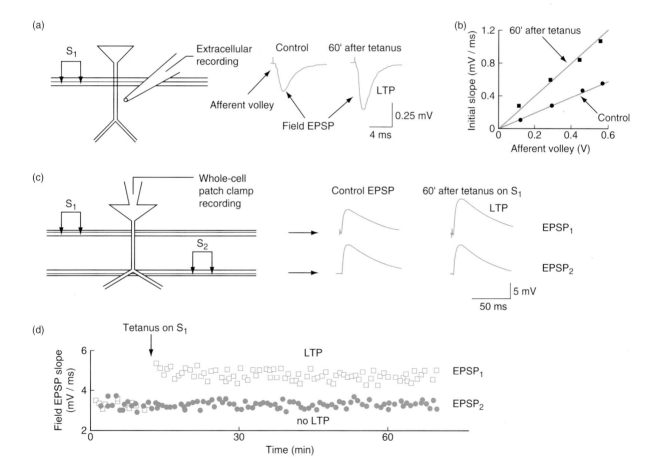

- *an afferent volley*, i.e. a pre-synaptic component corresponding to the response of the stimulated axons. Its amplitude is proportional to the number of axons activated by the stimulus. It is not affected by blockers of the synaptic transmission (cadmium, 0 calcium, etc.);
- *a field EPSP*, i.e. a post-synaptic component corresponding to the response of the population of pyra-

midal neurons connected to the stimulated axons. Its slope is proportional to the amplitude of the currents generated in the post-synaptic neurons.

Following a tetanic stimulation, the pre-synaptic component (the afferent volley) is unchanged whereas the peak amplitude and the initial slope of the post-synaptic one (field EPSPs) are both potentiated (by

30–200%). The input/output curves depicting the initial slope of the field EPSPs versus afferent volley amplitude have different slopes before (control) and 60 min after the tetanus (Figure 19.4b). This result shows that potentiation of the post-synaptic response does not result from an increase of the number of stimulated axons but from a genuine increase in synaptic efficacy: the same input evokes an enhanced output.

(3) LTP does not result from a persistent change of post-synaptic cell excitability since the response to a pulse of depolarizing current injected directly into the pyramidal cell is the same before and after the tetanus, at all potentials tested. It is also not due to a persistent reduction of the inhibitory GABAergic responses since it is still observed in the presence of bicuculline, a GABA$_A$ receptor antagonist.

(4) LTP is restricted to the synapses that have been tetanized. This is shown by recording intracellularly the EPSP evoked in one pyramidal neuron in response to the stimulation of two different Schaffer collaterals inputs (Figure 19.4c). When only one stimulation is tetanized (S_1), the response (EPSP$_2$) evoked by the other stimulation (S_2) is not potentiated: LTP is synapse specific.

(5) LTP can also be generated by a pairing diagram in which low frequency stimulation of the synaptic inputs is combined with intracellular depolarization of the post-synaptic neuron. This paradigm confirms the 'Hebbian theory', i.e. the concomitant activation of pre- and post-synaptic elements is a prerequisite for memory processes.

(6) LTP generating mechanisms are classically separated into two phases: a brief induction phase (1–20 s) followed by the expression phase, i.e. the mechanisms sustaining the persistent enhancement of synaptic efficacy. The demonstration of the presence of these two phases is described in the following section.

19.2.3 Induction of LTP Results from a Transient Enhancement of Glutamate Release and a Rise in Post-synaptic Intracellular Ca^{2+} Concentration

Tetanic stimulation evokes a large release of glutamate from Schaffer collateral terminals (in analogy to the enhanced release of neurotransmitter seen in most neurons following repetitive stimulation, see STP above). Glutamate present in synaptic clefts binds to the non-NMDA and NMDA receptor channels but also to the metabotropic glutamate receptors (receptors linked to G proteins) present in the post-synaptic membrane (see Figure 19.7).

Several observations led to the conclusion that in CA1, induction of LTP is voltage- and NMDA receptor-dependent. When the post-synaptic potential is hyperpolarized during tetanic stimulation, LTP is not induced. The application of APV, the selective antagonist of NMDA receptors, prevents the induction of LTP (Figure 19.5). In contrast, antagonists of non-NMDA receptors such as CNQX do not prevent the induction of LTP. These results indicate that, in the CA1 region of the hippocampus, post-synaptic depolarization generated by the enhancement of glutamate release *and* NMDA receptor activation are necessary for LTP induction.

The increase in glutamate release evokes an accumulation of Ca^{2+} in the dendrites of post-synaptic pyramidal cells as visualized with a fluorescent calcium-sensitive dye. When this transient elevation of [Ca^{2+}]$_i$ is prevented by the intracellular injection of a Ca^{2+} chelator agent (BAPTA) in the recorded pyramidal cell before the tetanus or by a strong post-synaptic depolarization which decreases the driving force for Ca^{2+} entry, LTP is not observed nor is it reduced. A simultaneous extracellular recording of the field EPSP shows that LTP, however, is generated in the other stimulated cells (which were not injected with BAPTA or depolarized). These results indicate that an increase of [Ca^{2+}]$_i$ is essential for the induction of LTP.

The duration for which [Ca^{2+}]$_i$ must remain elevated to induce LTP was tested by injecting into the recorded neuron a photosensitive Ca^{2+} chelator. This compound, diazo-4, has a low affinity for Ca^{2+} (K_D = 89 µM) which can be suddenly (in 100–400 µs) increased (K_D = 0.55 µM) when a UV flash inducing photolysis in its diazoacetyl groups is applied to the cell (Figure 19.6a). Thus introduction of diazo-4 into a cell does not affect ambient Ca^{2+} levels before UV light application. Manipulation of the delay between the LTP-inducing tetanus and photolysis of diazo-4 determines the minimum duration of post-synaptic [Ca^{2+}]$_i$ increase necessary to induce LTP. If a UV flash follows the 1 s duration tetanus without delay, the induction of LTP is prevented (Figure 19.6c). In contrast, when Ca^{2+} is chelated by diazo-4 photolysis occurring 2.5 s or more after the tetanus, LTP is

Figure 19.5 NMDA receptor activation is required for LTP induction. An intracellular glutamatergic EPSP is evoked by Schaffer collateral stimulation (a). When APV, an antagonist of NMDA receptors (20 μM, black bar), is applied before and during the tetanus (T_1, b), LTP is not induced since the EPSP recorded 1 h after wash of APV (c) has the same peak amplitude as the control one (a). When a second tetanus (T_2, d) is then applied in the absence of APV, it induces LTP (e). Note that APV evokes only a small change of the depolarization of the membrane evoked by the tetanus (compare b and d). T_1 and T_2 are identical periods of tetanic stimulation composed of 10–12 high frequency trains presented at 30 s intervals. Each train comprised 20 stimulations at 100 Hz. (Adapted from Collingridge GL, Herron CE and Lester RAJ, 1988. Frequency-dependent N-methyl-D-aspartate receptor-mediated synaptic transmission in rat hippocampus, *J. Physiol.* **399**, 301–312, with permission.)

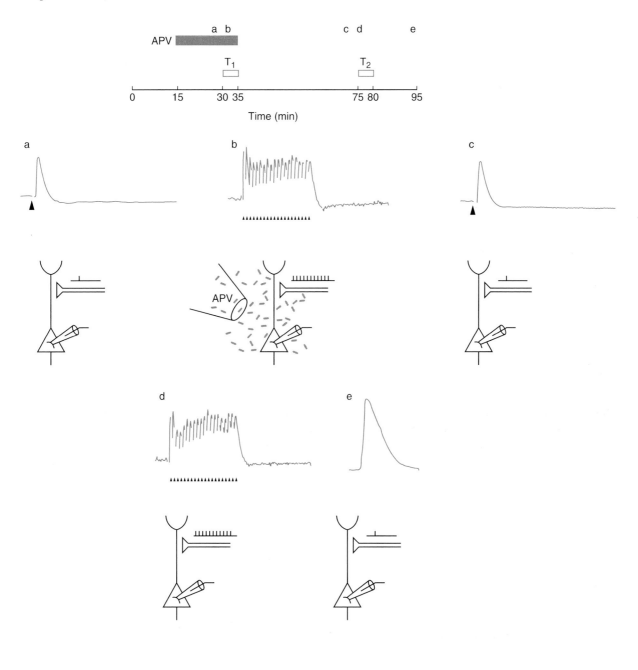

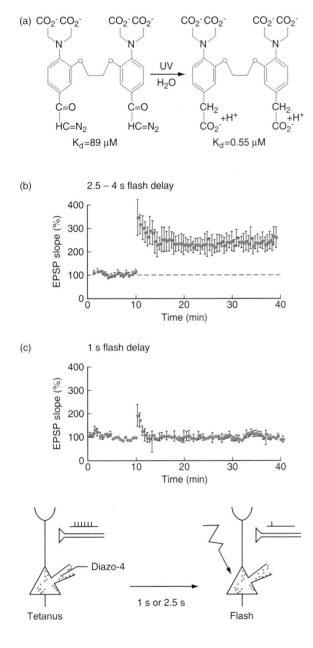

Figure 19.6 Photolysis of diazo-4 1 s after the start of the tetanus prevents LTP. The activity of CA1 pyramidal cells is recorded in current clamp mode (whole-cell configuration) in hippocampal slices. The whole-cell electrode contains diazo-4, a Ca^{2+} chelator (1–2.5 mM). (a) Structure of diazo-4 before and after photolysis. (b) Diazo-4 is photolyzed 2.5 s or 4 s after the start of the tetanus (stimuli given at 100–200 Hz during 1 s beginning at time 10 min). Even after this short delay, LTP of the glutamatergic EPSP is induced (n = 8). (c) Photolysis of diazo-4 immediately at the end of the 1 s duration tetanus (given at time 10 min) prevents the induction of LTP of the glutamatergic EPSP (n = 5). In the same experiments, LTP of the field (extracellular) EPSP is observed (not shown). (Adapted from Malenka RC, Lancaster B and Zucker RS, 1992, Temporal limits on the rise in postsynaptic calcium required for the induction of long term potentiation, *Neuron* 9, 121–128, with permission.)

from their terminals thus evoking a post-synaptic depolarization due to the activation of post-synaptic non-NMDA receptors and probably also the activation of metabotropic glutamate receptors. Activation of non-NMDA receptors depolarizes the spines to the point where the Mg^{2+} blockade of the NMDA receptors is removed, thus allowing the influx of Ca^{2+} ions into the spines through NMDA channels and a further

Figure 19.7 Schematic diagram of the role of NMDA receptors and intracellular Ca^{2+} ions in the induction of LTP. (a) The control stimulation (single shock) of Schaffer collaterals evokes the release of glutamate which activates post-synaptic AMPA ionotropic receptors and glutamatergic metabotropic receptors. In these conditions, NMDA receptors are blocked by Mg^{2+} ions and are not opened by glutamate. The activation of AMPA receptors evokes a post-synaptic control AMPA-mediated EPSP (bottom trace). (b) During the tetanic stimulation of Schaffer collaterals, the Mg^{2+} block of NMDA receptors is relieved (probably due to the depolarization generated by the accumulation of glutamate in the synaptic cleft) allowing Ca^{2+} to flow through the NMDA receptors into the post-synaptic element. It also depolarizes the membrane to the threshold for voltage-gated Ca^{2+} channel opening. The rise in intracellular Ca^{2+} concentration thus produced in the post-synaptic element triggers the subsequent events leading to the induction of LTP of the AMPA-mediated EPSP. The activation of metabotropic receptors would upregulate NMDA receptors.

induced (Figure 19.6b). Therefore an increase of $[Ca^{2+}]_i$ lasting at most 2.5 s (1 s during the tetanus + 1.5 s after) is sufficient for LTP induction.

The following model (Figure 19.7) is proposed to explain the induction of LTP in the CA1 region of the hippocampus: the high frequency stimulation (the tetanic stimulation) activates a certain number of afferent axons. This enhances the release of glutamate

depolarization of the membrane. The depolarization of synaptic origin can also bring the post-synaptic membrane to the threshold for voltage-gated Ca^{2+} channel activation allowing an additional Ca^{2+} entry.

The short-lasting (few seconds) rise in $[Ca^{2+}]_i$ that results from NMDA channels or NMDA and Ca^{2+} channel activation provides the necessary trigger for the subsequent events, activation of Ca^{2+}-dependent

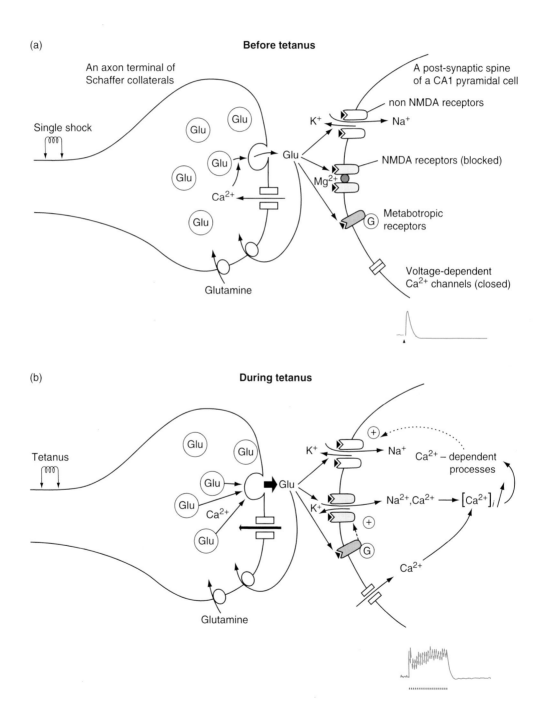

protein kinases and other Ca^{2+} dependent processes, which lead to the expression of LTP, i.e. a persistent increase in synaptic efficacy. Amongst the kinases involved in this cascade, the Ca^{2+} and phospholipid-dependent protein kinase C (PKC) plays a crucial role since its selective inhibition by intracellular injection of a PKC inhibitory peptide (PKCI) prevents LTP induction.

In conclusion, the initial induction of events leading to the expression of LTP involves an essential post-synaptic component: the combination of depolarization and activation of NMDA receptors which lead to Ca^{2+} entry into the post-synaptic spine (Figure 19.7b). This triggers a cascade of events leading to the persistent enhancement of the synaptic glutamatergic response (LTP).

19.2.4 The Expression of LTP Involves a Persistent Enhancement of the AMPA Component of the EPSP

Owing to the Mg^{2+} block of NMDA receptors, the control glutamatergic EPSP recorded in CA1 pyramidal neurons (in the presence of physiological concentrations of Mg^{2+}) is mainly mediated by non-NMDA receptors (Figure 19.7a) since it is negligibly affected by APV (the selective antagonist at NMDA receptors) and almost completely blocked by CNQX (see Figure 11.1). The same analysis of the relative contribution of NMDA and non-NMDA receptors was applied to the potentiated EPSP after a tetanus.

The EPSC (post-synaptic excitatory current) evoked in CA1 pyramidal neurons in response to Schaffer collateral stimulation is recorded with patch clamp techniques (whole-cell patch) at two different holding potentials. At $V_H = -80$ mV, the EPSC is mainly mediated by AMPA receptors because of the Mg^{2+} block of NMDA receptors at this hyperpolarized potential. In contrast, at $V_H = +30$ mV the control EPSC (which is inverted since the reversal potential of the glutamate response is 0 mV) is mixed and mainly mediated by NMDA receptors, as shown by the small effect of CNQX (Figure 19.8a). The early rising phase of the EPSC is mainly mediated by AMPA receptors while the current measured 100 ms after stimulation is mainly mediated by NMDA receptors.

The recorded cell is subjected to a procedure that induces LTP. After the tetanus, the membrane poten-

tial is returned to -80 mV and the test stimulation of Schaffer collaterals is regularly applied to verify that the EPSC is now potentiated (LTP has been induced) (Figure 19.8b). This potentiated EPSC is also recorded at $+30$ mV, in order to evaluate the amplitudes of the early AMPA and late NMDA components. The early component (AMPA-mediated) has approximately doubled while the late component (NMDA-mediated) remained stable (Figure 19.8c). Therefore LTP of the glutamatergic response, in this experiment, is primarily mediated by an enhancement of the AMPA component of the synaptic current.

This differential effect of the tetanus can be explained by:

- an increase in the density of AMPA receptors in the synaptic cleft (clustering);
- a change in the properties of AMPA receptors (affinity, unitary current amplitude);
- an increase in the effective spread of synaptic current from dendritic spines into dendrites (a change of diameter of the neck of the spines, for example).

This differential enhancement of the two components of the EPSC favors the hypothesis that *expression* of LTP requires post-synaptic mechanisms and does not result exclusively from a pre-synaptic mechanism, the persistent enhancement of glutamate release. If the expression of LTP resulted only from a pre-synaptic mechanism, a similar increase of both components of the EPSC should have been observed (assuming that AMPA and NMDA receptors are co-localized in the same post-synaptic membrane). Not all investigators agree on the mechanisms of LTP expression, since some of them recorded a parallel enhancement of the AMPA and NMDA components, or recorded an increased frequency of miniature EPSCs (reflecting an increased probability of transmitter release, see Chapter 8). As shown in Section 19.2.3, LTP *induction* clearly requires post-synaptic events (activation of NMDA receptors, increase of post-synaptic $[Ca^{2+}]_i$). Therefore, if LTP expression were pre-synaptic, it implies that some message must be sent from the post-synaptic spines to the pre-synaptic elements. This retrograde messenger would be generated post-synaptically and would trigger a sustained enhanced release of glutamate by the pre-synaptic element. Several such factors have been suggested but at present data are still controversial.

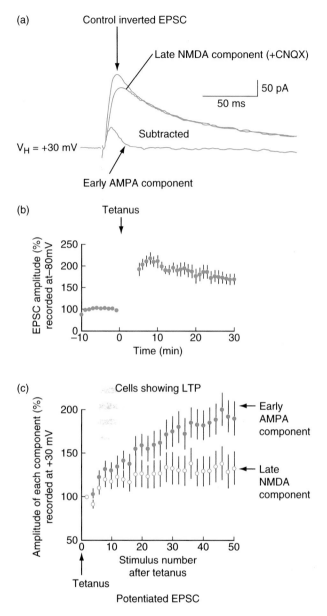

(a) Control inverted EPSC

Late NMDA component (+CNQX)

50 pA

50 ms

Subtracted

V_H = +30 mV

Early AMPA component

(b) Tetanus

Potentiated EPSC

(c) Cells showing LTP

Early AMPA component

Late NMDA component

Tetanus

Potentiated EPSC

Figure 19.8 Differential enhancement of the non-NMDA and NMDA components in LTP. The excitatory postsynaptic current (EPSC) evoked by Schaffer collateral stimulation is recorded in a CA1 pyramidal neuron in hippocampal slices with patch clamp techniques (whole-cell patch). (a) At V_H = + 30 mV, the EPSC is inverted (Control). Application of the non-NMDA selective antagonist (CNQX) selectively reduces the early portion of the current, leaving the late component (NMDA receptor-mediated) unaffected. The subtracted recording (Control − CNQX insensitive) illustrates the time course of the AMPA receptor-mediated component (CNQX-sensitive). (b) The EPSC peak amplitude (expressed as a percentage of control amplitude) is plotted against time, before and after the tetanus was applied to evoke LTP (V_H = −80 mV, except during the tetanus). The total EPSC is clearly potentiated by the procedure. (c) The EPSC peak amplitude, expressed as a percentage of the control amplitude, is measured from just after the induction of LTP to 30 min after (V_H = +30 mV). The early (CNQX-sensitive) AMPA receptor-mediated component is clearly potentiated while the late (CNQX-insensitive) NMDA receptor-mediated component is not significantly potentiated. The recordings in (b) and (c) are from the same cell; the membrane potential is continuously shifted from −80 to +30 mV. (Adapted from Perkel DJ and Nicoll RA, 1993. Evidence for all or none regulation of neurotransmitter release: implications for long term potentiation, *J. Physiol.* **471**, 481–500, with permission.)

19.2.5 Metabotropic Glutamate Receptors Regulate the Threshold of LTP Induction

In the presence of t-ACPD, a selective agonist of metabotropic glutamate receptors (mGluRs), a sub-threshold tetanus (that applied alone only triggers short-term potentiation) now generates an LTP (Figure 19.9a). This effect is blocked by APV, a selective antagonist of NMDA receptors and by protein kinase C (PKC) inhibitors. It indicates that activation of metabotropic glutamate receptors reduces the threshold of LTP induction, an effect mediated by NMDA receptors and PKC.

This effect is specific to mGluRs since application in similar conditions of agonists of iGluRs, AMPA or NMDA, in addition to the subthreshold tetanus, fails to trigger LTP. In control situations (in the absence of tetanus) a link between mGluRs, PKC and NMDA receptors is suggested by numerous experiments: (i) in intracellular recordings of pyramidal neurons of the CA1 region of the hippocampus in the presence of TTX (to block action potentials and therefore network activity) and K⁺ channels blockers, the mGluR agonist t-ACPD enhances the current generated by NMDA but not by AMPA applications; (ii) this effect is blocked by the intracellular injection of a PKC inhibitor; (iii) the intracellular injection of PKC enhances the NMDA receptor-mediated current; (iv) PKC phosphorylation sites are present on NMDA

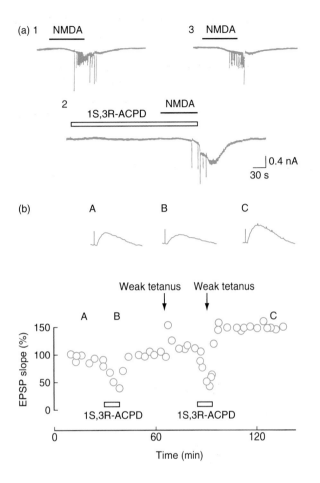

Figure 19.9 mGluR activation potentiates NMDA-mediated currents and facilitates LTP induction of AMPA-mediated EPSP. (a) The activity of a CA1 pyramidal neuron is recorded intracellularly in single electrode voltage clamp mode in slices. The external solution contains TTX to block synaptic activity and K+ channel blockers and the intracellular electrode is filled with CsCl. Bath application of NMDA (10 µM, 90 s) evokes an inward current (1) with rapid inward voltage-gated Ca^{2+} currents evoked in unclamped regions of the neuronal membrane. Bath application of 1S,3R-ACPD (50 µM, 4 min), a mGluR agonist, before and during NMDA application (10 µM, 90 s) potentiates the NMDA-evoked current (2). This effect is reversible since 5 min after washing, NMDA (10 µM, 90 s) evokes an inward current (3) of similar amplitude to that observed in the control (1). (b) The activity of a CA1 pyramidal neuron in recorded intracellularly in current clamp mode in slices. The diagram shows the amplitude of the initial slope of the AMPA-mediated EPSP recorded in response to Schaffer collateral stimulation. Bath application of 1S,3R-ACPD (50 µM, 2 min) reversibly depresses the EPSP (compare B to A). A subthreshold tetanic stimulation of Schaffer collaterals (weak tetanus: stimuli at 50 Hz during 0.5 s) induces a short-term potentiation of the EPSP (trace not shown). The same weak tetanus given during bath application of 1S,3R-ACPD (50 µM, 2 min) now induces a long-term potentiation of the EPSP (c). (a: Adapted from Ben Ari Y and Aniksztejn L, 1995. Role of glutamate metabotropic receptors in long term potentiation in the hippocampus. *Sem. Neurosci.* **7**; 127–135, with permission. b: Adapted from Aniksztejn L, Otani S and Ben Ari Y, 1992. Quisqualate metabotropic receptors modulate NMDA currents and facilitates induction of LTP through protein kinase C, *Eur. J. Neurosci.* **4**; 500–505, with permission.)

receptors; (v) in oocytes transfected with cDNAs coding for mGlu and NMDA receptors, the mGluR agonist t-ACPD increases NMDA currents, an effect blocked by PKC inhibitors; and (vi) in a wide range of cell types, kinases and phosphatases modulate NMDA receptor activity rapidly and reversibly.

These results suggest that the activation of postsynaptic mGluRs enhances (via PKC) the postsynaptic NMDA receptor-mediated current (activated by the release of glutamate evoked by a subthreshold tetanus applied to the afferents). This enhancement of NMDA receptor-mediated response together with the activation of AMPA receptors induce LTP of the glutamatergic AMPA receptor-mediated response.

19.2.6 The Multiple Ways to Induce LTP, the Multiple Forms of LTP

Although synchronous activation of several presynaptic fibers by high frequency stimulation is the most reliable way to evoke LTP (Figure 19.10a), LTP can be also evoked *in vitro* by (2) the combination of low frequency stimulation of pre-synaptic afferents and the post-synaptic injection of a depolarizing current pulse to activate voltage-gated Ca^{2+} channels (Figure 19.10b) and by (3) the combination of low frequency stimulation of pre-synaptic afferents and bath application of a selective agonist at metabotropic glutamate receptors (Figure 19.10c). All these forms of LTP induction are blocked by bath application of

APV, an antagonist at NMDA receptors, the intra-cellular injection of a Ca^{2+} chelator (BAPTA) or PKC inhibitors or the intracellular injection of a hyper-polarizing current pulse during tetanic stimulation (Figure 19.10d).

Another form of LTP is induced by the bath application of K^+ channel blockers such as tetraethyl-ammonium chloride (TEA) that depolarizes the pre-synaptic elements and enhances transmitter release (Figure 19.10e). This form of LTP also requires a rise of the post-synaptic intracellular Ca^{2+} concentration. This rise is produced by the entry of Ca^{2+} ions through voltage-gated Ca^{2+} channels activated by the depolar-ization resulting from the closure of K^+ channels by

Figure 19.10 (a–d) Tetanic LTP and (e,f) TEA-induced LTP: the multiple ways of induction (a–c, e) and blockade of induction (d, f).

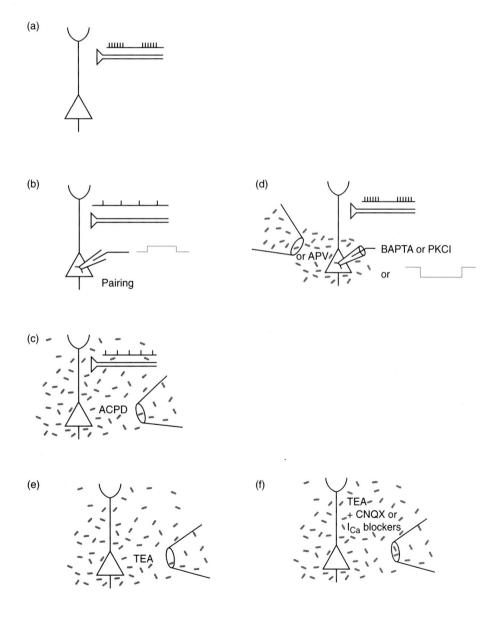

TEA. In contrast to tetanus LTP, TEA-induced LTP is not synapse specific since all the synapses are activated by bath application of TEA. Moreover, TEA-induced LTP is NMDA receptor-independent. It is blocked by bath application of CNQX (an antagonist at AMPA receptors), of Ca^{2+} channel blockers or by intracellular injection of a Ca^{2+} chelator (Figure 19.10f).

The observation that a rise of the intracellular Ca^{2+} concentration is a necessary prerequisite for LTP induction raises the possibility that a wide range of physiological or pathological processes known to evoke a rise of $[Ca^{2+}]_i$ would trigger long-lasting changes of synaptic efficacy. Both seizures, which generate synchronized giant paroxysmal activity and anoxic-ischemic episodes that generate LTP of *NMDA receptor*-mediated EPSPs (anoxic LTP), are in fact associated with long-lasting changes of synaptic efficacy. In such cases, LTP of excitatory synaptic transmission may participate in the pathological consequences of these insults.

19.3 The Long-Term Depression of a Glutamatergic Response: Example of the Response of Purkinje Cells of the Cerebellum to Parallel Fiber Stimulation

Purkinje cells represent the single-output neurons of the cerebellar cortex. Each Purkinje cell receives two distinct excitatory inputs, one from parallel fibers (axons of granule cells) and the other from a climbing fiber (axons of the contralateral inferior olive cells). These two types of input display distinct characteristics. A single climbing fiber terminates on each Purkinje cell. This powerful one-to-one excitatory input makes multiple synapses on the soma and proximal dendrites of the Purkinje cell (see Figures 2.6, 2.7 and 19.11). In contrast, many parallel fibers converge on each Purkinje cell (around 80 000) but each fiber makes few synapses on each Purkinje cell. The putative neurotransmitter at parallel fiber synapses is glutamate, which activates ionotropic AMPA and metabotropic glutamatergic post-synaptic receptors. The climbing fiber synapse uses as a transmitter an excitatory amino acid not yet identified. Both synapses lack NMDA receptors in the adult.

The dual arrangement of the two excitatory synaptic inputs raises the question of the role of the powerful input (climbing fiber) on the weaker input (parallel

Figure 19.11 Simplified neural circuit in the cerebellar cortex. Inset shows a more detailed view of the synaptic contacts between a parallel or a climbing fiber terminal and the Purkinje cell dendrite. AMPA-R, AMPA receptor; mGluR, metabotropic glutamate receptors; VDCC, voltage-dependent calcium channels; CF, climbing fiber; PF, parallel fiber; Pc, Purkinje cell. (Adapted from Daniel H, Blond O, Jaillard D *et al*. 1996. Synaptic plasticity in the cerebellum in cortical plasticity: LTP and LTD, In Fazeli S and Collingridge GL, eds, in press.)

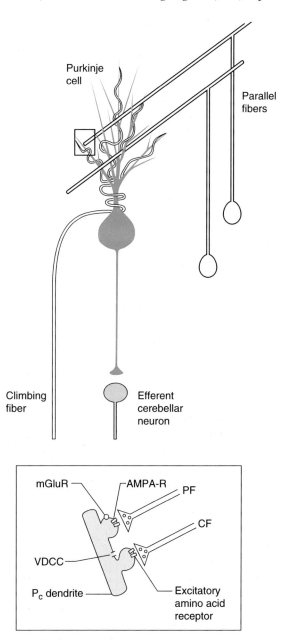

fibers). The coactivation of climbing fiber and parallel fiber inputs induces a persistent decrease in the efficacy of the parallel fiber–Purkinje neuron synapse or long-term depression (LTD).

19.3.1 LTD of a Post-synaptic Response (EPSC or EPSP) is a Decrease of Synaptic Efficacy

Ito and co-workers (1982) were the first to demonstrate in the rabbit cerebellum *in vivo* that conjunctive stimulation of the afferent climbing and parallel fibers leads to an LTD of synaptic transmission at parallel fiber–Purkinje cell synapses (Appendix 19.1). In other terms, LTD is attenuation of the Purkinje cell response to parallel fibers after conjunctive stimulation of parallel and climbing fibers. It is also observed in *in vitro* preparations such as slices of the rat cerebellum (Figure 19.12).

The activity of a Purkinje cell is recorded intracellularly in current clamp mode in rat cerebellar slices. The stimulation of parallel fibers evokes an EPSP resulting from the activation of post-synaptic AMPA receptors by glutamate released from the stimulated terminals (inset, Figure 19.11) since it is totally blocked by CNQX, a selective AMPA receptor antagonist (see Figure 11.1). After recording this control parallel fiber-mediated EPSP (Figure 19.12a, 1) during several minutes, parallel fibers are now stimulated in conjunction with intracellular depolarization (see Figure 19.20b). After this pairing stimulation, the same stimulation of parallel fibers as in the control now evokes a smaller EPSP (Figure 19.12a, 3, 4). The parallel fiber-mediated EPSP stays attenuated for the rest of the recording session (Figure 19.12a). It is a long-term depression.

This persistent decrease of the parallel fiber-mediated synaptic response is also observed in another type of *in vitro* preparation, a culture of Purkinje cells, granule cells and an inferior olivary explant. After repetitive conjunctive stimulation of a single granule cell (whose axon is a parallel fiber) and the inferior olivary explant (which sends an axon, the climbing fiber, to the recorded Purkinje cell) (Figure 19.13a), the EPSC recorded in the Purkinje cell in response to the granule cell activation is persistently decreased (Figure 19.13b). This *in vitro* preparation allows the stimulation of a single pre-synaptic granule cell before and after LTD induction. Therefore, it can be demon-

strated that LTD is observed though the number of parallel fibers stimulated before and after the conditioning stimulation is identical (a depressed EPSC or EPSP could in fact result from a decrease in the number of stimulated axons).

19.3.2 Induction of LTD Requires a Rise in Post-synaptic Intracellular Ca^{2+} Concentration and the Activation of Post-synaptic Non-NMDA Receptors

As already discussed in Chapter 18, the response of a Purkinje cell to the activation of its afferent climbing fiber is an all-or-none response composed of an initial depolarization and overshooting action potential with following depolarizing humps. Since activation of the afferent climbing fiber potently activates the voltage-gated Ca^{2+} channels present in the membrane of Purkinje dendrites, the consequent rise in intradendritic Ca^{2+} concentration was supposed to play a role in LTD. In order to record simultaneously the synaptic responses and the intracellular Ca^{2+} concentration, the activity of a Purkinje cell is recorded in patch clamp (whole-cell patch) in the presence of a fluorescent calcium dye, fura-2, injected into the cell (Figure 19.14 and Appendix 11.1). First, the control excitatory post-synaptic current (EPSC) in response to parallel fiber stimulation is recorded in the Purkinje cell (control, Figure 19.14a). Then, parallel fibers and climbing fibers are stimulated in phase at a low frequency (1–4 Hz). Five minutes after this conditioning stimulation, the response to the same parallel fiber stimulation recorded from the same Purkinje cell begins to decrease and stays attenuated thereafter (20 min, Figure 19.14a; EPSC, Figure 19.14b). Cerebellar LTD is associated with a large increase of Ca^{2+} concentration in Purkinje cell dendrites during the conditioning stimulation ($[Ca^{2+}]_i$, Figure 19.14b).

LTD of the response to parallel fibers is not observed when the parallel fibers are stimulated alone: what adds the climbing fiber stimulation?

Climbing fiber stimulation causes a sufficient depolarization to activate strongly voltage-dependent Ca^{2+} channels located in the membrane of Purkinje cell dendrites. It was thus suggested that the resulting increase

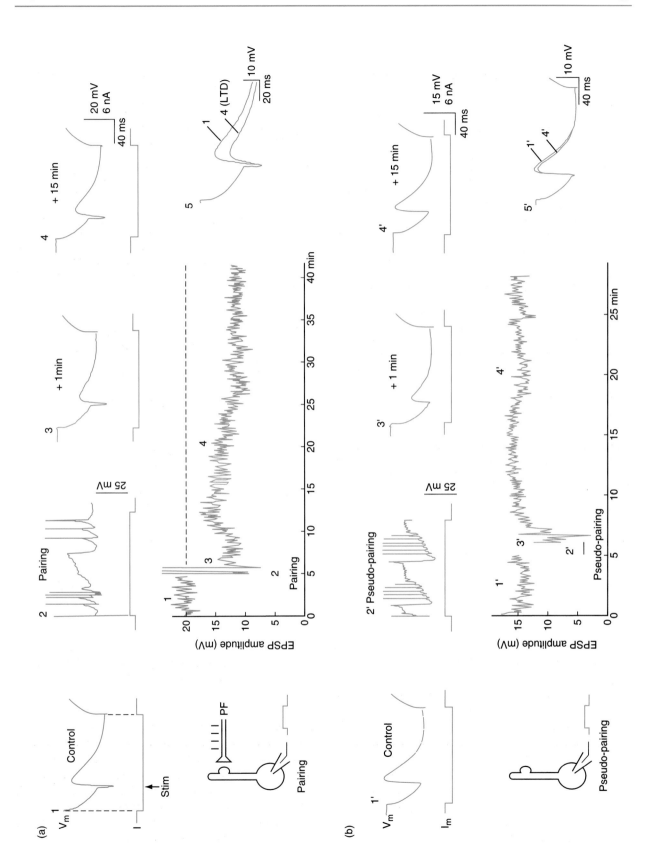

Figure 19.12 Cerebellar LTD. The activity of a Purkinje cell is recorded intracellularly in current clamp mode in slices. The response to parallel fiber stimulation is an AMPA-mediated EPSP. For each recording a hyperpolarizing current pulse is applied before and during the stimulation in order to test changes of membrane resistance during the course of the experiment. (a) After recording the control EPSP (1) during 5 min, a pairing procedure is given (2), i.e. low frequency (2–4 Hz) stimulation of parallel fibers (PF) and direct intracellular depolarization of the recorded Purkinje cell (PC). During the pairing procedure Na^+ and Ca^{2+} spikes are recorded (2). The pairing induces a long-term depression of the EPSP (4). The diagram of EPSP amplitude vs. time shows that LTD is observed at least during 35 min. In (5), traces (1) and (4) are superimposed in order to show the depression of amplitude and the slowing of the initial slope of the EPSP after pairing. (b) Same experiment as in (a) but a pseudo-pairing is applied instead of pairing, i.e. the direct intracellular depolarization only. Only a short-term depression of the EPSP is observed (3). Fifteen minutes after the end of the pseudo-pairing the EPSP is back to its control amplitude (5'). Insets: experimental designs for pairing and pseudo-pairing procedures. (Adapted from Daniel H, Hémart N, Jaillard D and Crépel F, 1992. Co-activation of metabotropic glutamate receptors and of voltage-gated calcium channels induces LTD in the cerebellar Purkinje cells *in vitro*, *Exp. Brain Res.* **90**, 327–331, with permission. Inset and all following ones: Adapted from Linden DJ, 1994. Long-term synaptic depression in the mammalian brain, *Neuron* **12**, 457–472, with permission.)

Figure 19.13 Cerebellar LTD is observed when a single parallel fiber is stimulated. (a) Co-cultures of rat cerebellar Purkinje cells (PC), granule cells and an explant of inferior olivary neurons are performed. The activity of a Purkinje cell is recorded in patch clamp (whole-cell patch) to record the evoked post-synaptic current (EPSC). The conditioning stimulation consists of the conjunctive stimulation of a single granule cell and the inferior olivary explant (2 Hz, 20s). (b) The Purkinje cell membrane is held at $V_H = -50$ mV, and the response (EPSC) to the activation of a granule cell is recorded before and 1, 5, 10 and 25 min after the conditioning stimulation. (From Hirano T, 1990. Depression and potentiation of the synaptic transmission between a granule cell and a Purkinje cell in rat cerebellar culture, *Neurosci. Lett.* **119**, 141–144, with permission.)

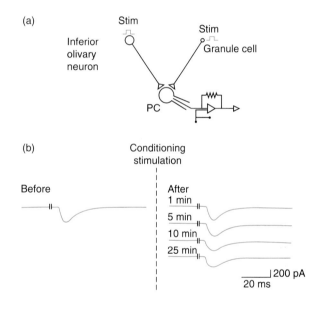

of intradendritic Ca^{2+} concentration would be a necessary prerequisite for LTD induction. This hypothesis is tested by hyperpolarizing the Purkinje cell membrane during conditioning stimulation or by injecting of a Ca^{2+} chelator into the Purkinje cell before the conditioning stimulus (Figure 19.15) or by removing the external Ca^{2+} ions, in order to prevent the rise of intradendritic Ca^{2+} concentration: all these procedures block LTD induction. Along the same line, climbing fiber stimulation can be replaced by direct intracellular depolarization of the Purkinje cell which evokes Ca^{2+} spikes (Figure 19.20b). In conclusion, LTD of synaptic transmission at parallel fiber–Purkinje cell synapses is triggered by a rise of intracellular Ca^{2+} concentration resulting from the entry of Ca^{2+} into Purkinje cell dendrites through voltage-gated Ca^{2+} channels opened by membrane depolarization.

LTD of the response to parallel fibers is not observed when the climbing fiber is stimulated alone: what adds to parallel fiber stimulation?

The glutamate released from parallel fiber terminals activates the non-NMDA receptors present in the post-synaptic membrane (ionotropic AMPA receptors and metabotropic glutamate receptors, mGluR1; see inset, Figure 19.11). AMPA receptors mediate the excitatory response (EPSP or EPSC) evoked by parallel fiber stimulation since it is totally blocked by the application of CNQX, a selective antagonist of this class of receptors. In order to test the role of AMPA

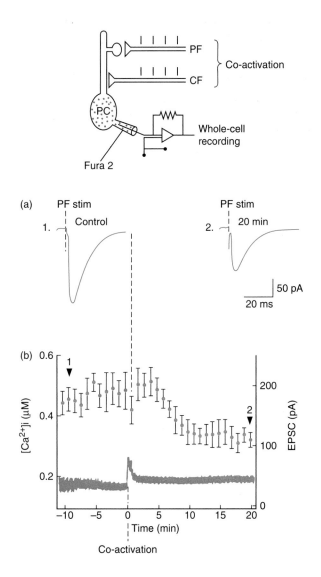

Figure 19.14 An increase of intracellular Ca²⁺ concentration is observed during LTD induction. The activity of a Purkinje cell is recorded in patch clamp (whole-cell patch) in a thin slice of rat cerebellum. The patch pipette also contains Fura-2 in order to record on-line the intracellular Ca²⁺ concentration. (a) The excitatory post-synaptic current (EPSC) recorded in response to parallel fiber stimulation (PF stim, 1 Hz) is recorded before (control) and 20 min after the conditioning stimulation (coactivation: conjunctive stimulation of parallel and climbing fibres). (b) Time course of changes in parallel fiber-mediated EPSC amplitude and in $[Ca^{2+}]_i$. The conditioning stimulation (given at time 0) induces an LTD of the EPSC (with a delay) and an immediate transient rise of $[Ca^{2+}]_i$. Note that the stimulation of parallel fibers before the conditioning stimulation does not induce significant changes of $[Ca^{2+}]_i$. (From Konnerth A, Dreessen J and Augustine GJ, 1992. Brief dendritic calcium signals initiate long lasting synaptic depression in cerebellar Purkinje cells, *Proc. Natl. Acad. Sci.* **89**, 7051–7055, with permission.)

mate or quisqualate (agonists on *both* AMPA and metabotropic receptors, or a solution containing *both* AMPA and an agonist of metabotropic receptors, Figure 19.20c, d). The activation of AMPA receptors alone by AMPA or kainate and the application of NMDA are ineffective. This is in keeping with the recent demonstration that antibodies directed against the mGluR1 subunit block LTD induction in cultured Purkinje cells. The final demonstration of the participation of mGlu receptors in LTD induction in acute cerebellar slices has been given recently by showing that LTD of the parallel fiber-mediated EPSP is markedly impaired in knock-out mice lacking mGluR1 (Figure 19.20f and Section 14.4.7).

In conclusion, activation of parallel fibers during conjunctive or pairing stimulation allows the release of glutamate and the activation of both AMPA and metabotropic glutamatergic post-synaptic receptors. This, with the concomitant rise in intracellular calcium concentration, are possibly the necessary and sufficient processes for LTD induction since the conditioning stimulation can be replaced by a direct depolarization of the Purkinje cell membrane to activate voltage-dependent Ca²⁺ channels (to mimic climbing fiber stimulation) and the concomitant application of agonists of AMPA and metabotropic receptors (to mimic parallel fiber stimulation) (Figure 19.20d).

receptors in LTD induction, CNQX is bath applied during or after a pairing protocol (direct Purkinje cell depolarization with parallel fiber stimulation). The blockade of AMPA receptors during the pairing protocol prevents LTD induction while it has no effect after the pairing protocol (once LTD is induced) (Figure 19.16).

In order to test the role of the non-NMDA receptors in LTD induction, parallel fiber stimulation can also be replaced by external application of agonists at non-NMDA receptors. Parallel fiber stimulation during the conditioning stimulus can be replaced by the application on the Purkinje cell dendrites of gluta-

Figure 19.15   The induction of cerebellar LTD requires an increase of intracellular Ca^{2+} concentration. The activity of a Purkinje cell is recorded intracellularly (current clamp mode) in a guinea pig cerebellar slice. The amplitude of the response (EPSP) to parallel fiber stimulation is recorded before and after the conditioning stimulation (conjunctive stimulation of PF and CF at 4 Hz during 25 s) in control cells (open circles). The same experiment performed after intracellular injection of the Ca^{2+} chelator EGTA into the recorded Purkinje cells shows that in such conditions LTD is not induced (solid circles). The respective averaged EPSPs are shown in the insets. The time 0 represents the end of conjunctive stimulation. The values at each plotted point represent the number of cells recorded. (From Kano M and Kato M, 1987. Quisqualate receptors are specifically involved in cerebellar synaptic plasticity, *Nature* **325**, 276–279, with permission.)

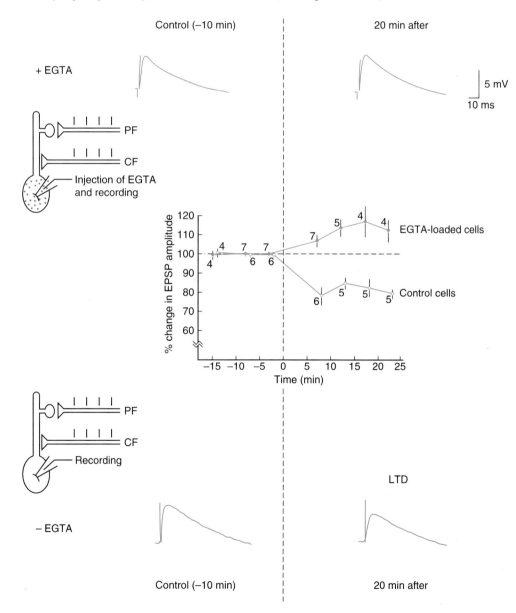

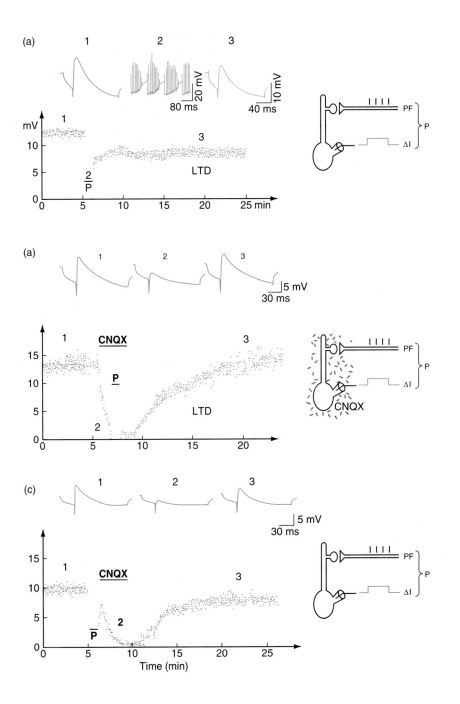

19.3.3 The Expression of LTD Involves a Persistent Desensitization of Post-synaptic AMPA Receptors

The fact that co-activation of Purkinje cells by climbing fibre stimulation and iontophoretic application of glutamate to Purkinje cell dendrites induces a long-lasting decrease of the response to this agonist led Ito to postulate that LTD of parallel fiber-mediated EPSP or EPSC is due to a long-term desensitization of ionotropic glutamate receptors of Purkinje cells (a desensitized state is a state where the probability of

Figure 19.16   The induction of cerebellar LTD requires the activation of post-synaptic AMPA receptors. The activity of a Purkinje cell is recorded in patch clamp (whole-cell patch, current clamp mode) in cerebellar thin slices. A hyperpolarizing current pulse (see Figure 19.12) is given before and during the stimulation in order to test that the membrane resistance does not vary during the experiment. (a) (top traces) A control EPSP is recorded in response to parallel fibre stimulation (1). After the conditioning stimulation (P for pairing: intracellular depolarizing pulses to evoke Ca^{2+} spikes in conjunction with parallel fibre stimulation (2)) an LTD of the parallel fibre-mediated EPSP is observed (3). Note the change in calibrations between 1, 3 and 2. (Bottom trace) Plot of the EPSP amplitude against time. (b) same experiment as in (a) but in the presence of CNQX (4 µM) in the bath before, during and after the conditioning stimulation (P). During CNQX application the parallel fibre-mediated EPSP (2) is completely blocked since it is mediated by AMPA receptors. (c) Same experiment as in (b) but CNQX is bath-applied after the conditioning stimulation (P). (a: Adapted from Hémart N, Daniel H, Jaillard D *et al.*, 1995. Receptors and second messengers involved in long term depression in rat cerebellar slices *in vitro*: a reappraisal, *Eur. J. Neurosci.* 7, 45–53, with permission.) From Daniel H, Blond O, Jaillard D *et al.*, 1996. Synaptic plasticity in the cerebellum in cortical plasticity: LTP and LTD, In Fazeli S and Collingridge GL, eds, in press.)

Figure 19.17   The post-synaptic glutamate response is selectively depressed. The reponse of a Purkinje cell to iontophoretic application of glutamate (glu) or aspartate (asp) is recorded intracellularly (current clamp mode, $V_m = -65$ mV) in cerebellar slices. (a) Glutamate or aspartate are alternatively ejected in the dendritic field of the recorded Purkinje cell. They both evoke a transient membrane depolarization which reaches the firing level. (b) The conditioning stimulation used to induce LTD consists of climbing fibre stimulation (2–4 Hz) paired for 1 min with the ejections of glutamate and aspartate at 2 min intervals. (c) Twenty minutes after the pairing procedure, the response to glutamate is selectively depressed (the response to aspartate is left unaffected). (Adapted from Crépel F and Krupa M, 1988, Activation of protein kinase C induces a long term depression of glutamate sensitivity of cerebellar Purkinje cells. An *in vitro* study, *Brain Res.* 458, 397–401, with permission.)

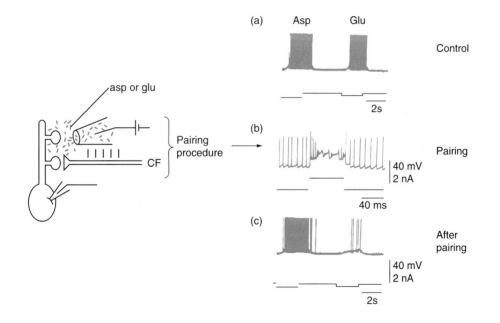

the channel opening is very low). This in fact would explain the decrease in synaptic efficacy.

In Purkinje cells in cerebellar slices, a pairing procedure known to induce LTD of the synaptic response induces a long-lasting decrease of the response to iontophoretic application of glutamate (or quisqualate, not shown) but not of aspartate (Figure 19.17). This suggests that LTD of synaptic transmission between parallel fibers and Purkinje cells is accompanied by LTD of the responsiveness of Purkinje cells to glutamate or quisqualate whereas that to aspartate is unaffected. The observed decrease in efficacy of glutamate or quisqualate in activating Purkinje cells could involve a desensitization of AMPA receptors. What are the mediators between Ca^{2+} entry and the long-term changes of AMPA receptors?

19.3.4 Second Messengers are Required for LTD Induction: Examples of PKC and Nitric Oxide

Activation of PKC

The metabotropic receptors mGluR1 are abundantly expressed in Purkinje cells. These receptors are coupled to phospholipase C and their activation leads to the formation of inositol trisphosphate (IP_3) and diacylglycerol (DAG). Therefore, during the conditioning stimulus, the Ca^{2+}-dependent kinases such as PKC can be activated by both the increase of intracellular Ca^{2+} concentration resulting from climbing fiber activation (see Figure 19.14b) and the activation of mGluR1 by glutamate released from parallel fibers. The role of PKC in LTD is tested by injecting into the recorded Purkinje cell a selective inhibitor of PKC (PKC 19–36) before the conditioning stimulus (Figure 19.18). In such conditions, LTD is not induced.

The hypothesis is as follows: during the conditioning stimulus, the formation of diacylglycerol (DAG) following activation of mGluRs, together with the cytosolic Ca^{2+} increase resulting from the activation of voltage-gated channels (and perhaps the release of Ca^{2+} ions from internal stores as a result of the formation of IP_3) leads to the activation of PKC. This with other second messenger cascades would phosphorylate AMPA receptors and activate their transition to a stable desensitized state (Figure 19.19).

Nitric oxide formation and cGMP

Nitric oxide (NO) is a highly diffusible messenger formed from arginine in the presence of NO synthase (NOS). This enzyme is not present in Purkinje cells but only in neighbouring cells. The target of NO is probably the soluble (cytoplasmic) guanylate cyclase

Figure 19.18 Protein kinase C inhibition prevents LTD induction. The activity of a Purkinje cell is recorded in patch clamp (whole-cell patch) in the presence of the selective PKC inhibitor, PKC 19–36 (●), a non-inhibitory control peptide (△) or the intracellular solution only (□) in the patch pipette. The control EPSC evoked by parallel fibre stimulation is recorded over 10 min and the conditioning stimulation is applied at $t = 0$. It consists of the conjunctive application of glutamate and intracellular depolarization. LTD of the EPSC is not observed in cells dialyzed with PKC 19–36. Scale bars: 100 pA, 2 s. P, pairing procedure. (Adapted from Linden DJ and Connor JA, 1991. Participation of postsynaptic PKC in cerebellar long term depression in culture, *Science* **254**, 1656–1659, with permission.)

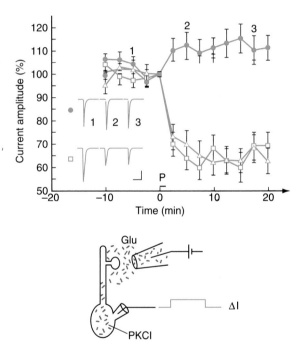

in cells where it is produced, as well as in neighboring cells. NO, by activating guanylate cyclase, would lead to the formation of cGMP.

In order to test a possible role of NO in LTD induction in cerebellar slices, a potent NO synthase inhibitor, *N*-methylarginine, is bath-applied during the experiment. It totally prevents LTD induction by a pairing protocol. This result, together with the observations that bath application of an NO donor (sodium nitroprusside) and the intracellular injection of cGMP both durably depress the parallel fiber-mediated EPSP,

Figure 19.19 Schematic drawing of some of the putative mechanisms of cerebellar LTD induction.

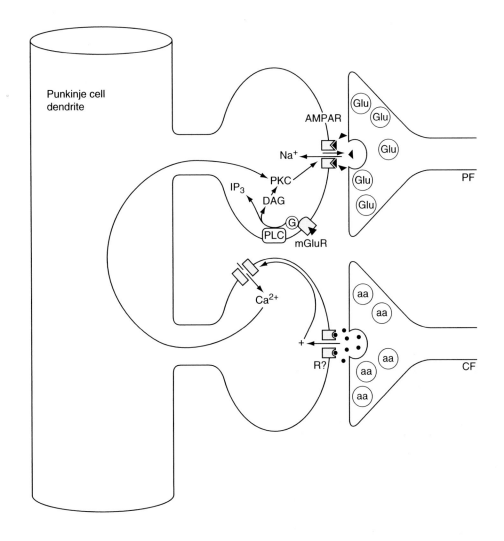

suggest that NO participates in the events leading to LTD. However, a role for NO has not yet been demonstrated for LTD induced in cultures, cerebellar Purkinje cells and in slices. The pathways leading to NO synthase activation are not yet fully understood.

19.3.5 Principal Features of LTD in Parallel Fiber–Purkinje Cell Transmission

- LTD results from a decrease of the parallel fiber-mediated EPSC or EPSP without changes in the number of afferent axons stimulated: it is a depression of the synaptic efficacy.
- LTD is a very long-lasting phenomenon since it persists for the duration of the experiment, up to several hours.
- LTD is input specific: it is restricted to those parallel fiber synapses activated at the same time as climbing fibers.
- LTD is associated with a large increase of Ca^{2+} concentration in Purkinje cell dendrites which occurs during the conjunctive stimulation of parallel and climbing fibers.

Figure 19.20   Cerebellar LTD: the different ways of induction (a–d) or blockage of induction (e–g). PC, Purkinje cell.

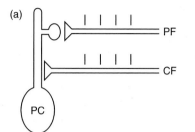

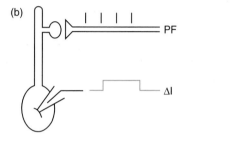

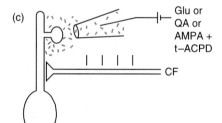

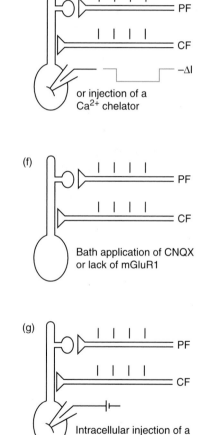

- LTD is expressed as a depression of AMPA-mediated current at the parallel fiber–Purkinje cell synapses activated at the same time as climbing fibres. It results from the long-term desensitization of AMPA receptors, which requires the activation of PKC and the production of NO (at least in intact tissues).

19.3.6 Different Ways to Induce or Block Cerebellar LTD

LTD of the response of a Purkinje cell to parallel fibre activation can be induced by (Figure 19.20a–d):

(a) conjunctive stimulation of the afferent parallel and climbing fibers;

(b) conjunctive stimulation of the parallel fibers and intracellular injection of a depolarizing current (which evokes Ca^{2+} spikes) into the Purkinje cell;

(c) conjunctive iontophoretic application of glutamate, quisqualate or AMPA + t-ACPD to the Purkinje cell dendrites and stimulation of its afferent climbing fiber;

(d) conjunctive iontophoretic application of glutamate or quisqualate or AMPA + t-ACPD to the Purkinje cell dendrites and intracellular injection of depolarizing current (which evokes Ca^{2+} spikes) into the Purkinje cell.

LTD of the response of a Purkinje cell to parallel fiber activation can be blocked by (Figure 19.20e–g):

(e) intracellular injection of a Ca^{2+} chelator into the Purkinje cell or injection of a hyperpolarizing current into the Purkinje cell during conjunctive stimulation;

(f) bath application of CNQX or the lack of mGluR1 in the cerebellum and notably in Purkinje cell membrane (mGluR1 gene-deficient mice are obtained by disrupting the mGluR1 gene);

(g) intracellular injection into the Purkinje cell or bath application of an inhibitor of PKC or NO synthase before the conditioning stimulus.

19.4 A Procedure that Induces LTD can Reverse LTP: Example of the AMPA-Mediated EPSP Recorded in CA1 Pyramidal Neurons

We have seen in Section 19.2 that in the CA1 area of the hippocampus a tetanic stimulation applied to Schaffer collaterals persistently increases the AMPA-mediated EPSP or EPSC recorded in pyramidal neurons in response to a single stimulation of Schaffer collaterals through the same stimulating electrode. In contrast, a low frequency stimulation (1 Hz for 30 min) applied to Schaffer collaterals generates a long-term depression of the AMPA-mediated (extra-cellularly recorded) field EPSP (Figure 19.21a) or (intracellularly recorded) EPSP (not shown). Application of this procedure after the induction of tetanic LTP erases LTP of the AMPA-mediated field EPSP (Figure 19.21b) or EPSP (not shown).

Tetanic stimulation-induced LTP and low frequency stimulation-induced LTD of the AMPA-mediated EPSP share common mechanisms: both require the activation of NMDA receptors, a rise of the intracellular Ca^{2+} concentration and activation of PKC. The key step that favors the induction of LTP vs. LTD is suggested to be the pattern of Ca^{2+} entry into the pyramidal cell during high or low frequency stimulation. An LTD subsequent to an LTP is proposed as a way to erase LTP when this long-term potentiation is no longer useful. If LTP is considered as a cellular basis of memory, LTD may act as an important resetting device that erases and desaturates LTP, thus allowing the potentiation of new information.

Appendix 19.1
Long-Term Depression (LTD): Pioneering Experiments of Ito *et al* (1982)

The activity of a Purkinje cell (PC) is recorded extracellularly in the rabbit cerebellum *in vivo*. The single stimulation of the contralateral vestibular nerve (CVN, a way to activate granule cells, Figure A19.1a) at a frequency of 2/s excites Purkinje cells with a latency of 3–6 ms. This early excitation represents activation through vestibular mossy fibers (MF), granule cells (GC) and their axons, parallel fibers (PF) (Figure A19.1b, control). Then, the conjunctive stimulation of this CVN at 20/s and of the inferior olive (IO, a way to activate climbing fibers, CF) at 4/s is applied for 25 s to 10 min (conditioning stimulation). After this conditioning stimulus, the early excitatory response of the Purkinje cell to the ipsilateral vestibular nerve stimulation is depressed below the control level for at least several tens of minutes (Figure A19.1b, after). The depression is specific to the early excitatory response evoked by the stimulation of the vestibular nerve involved in the conjunctive stimulation: the response to the ipsilateral vestibular nerve is not affected.

This revealed that conjunctive vestibular–olivary stimulation depresses the early excitation of Purkinje cells to vestibular mossy afferent fibers. The depression

Figure 19.21   LTD and LTP of the AMPA-mediated EPSP can be evoked in the same neurons. The activity of a population of CA1 pyramidal neurons is recorded extracellularly in hippocampal slices. (a) In response to the stimulation of Schaffer collaterals (pulse: 50 μs, 5–50 μA every 30 s), the control AMPA-mediated field EPSP is recorded (1). Its amplitude (2) and initial slope (diagram and 4) are stable over 30 min. A low frequency stimulation (LFS: a pulse every 1 s for 15 min) applied through the same electrode evokes a long-term depression of the field EPSP (3). In (4), the first 500 μs of the field EPSPs 1, 2 and 3 are superimposed in order to show the changes or absence of changes of the initial slope. (b) In another experiment, the control AMPA-mediated field EPSP (1) is recorded in response to the same stimulation of Schaffer collaterals as in (a) (pulse: 50 μs, 5–50 μA, 0.33 Hz). Its amplitude (2) and initial slope (diagram and 5) are stable over 30 min. A tetanic stimulation (TS: four trains of 10 pulses at 100 Hz every 1 s) applied through the same electrode evokes a long-term potentiation of the field EPSP (3). A low frequency stimulation (LFS: a pulse every 1 s for 15 min) given through the same electrode 30 min after the tetanus persistently reverses the LTP (4). In (5) the first 500 μs of the field EPSPs in 1, 2, 3 and 4 are superimposed in order to show the changes or absence of changes of the initial slope. (Adapted from Bernard C, Hirsch J and Ben Ari Y, 1995. Non-involvement of the redox site of NMDA receptors in bidirectional synaptic plasticity in the CA1 area of the rat hippocampus *in vitro*, *Neurosci. Lett.* **193**, 197–200, with permission.)

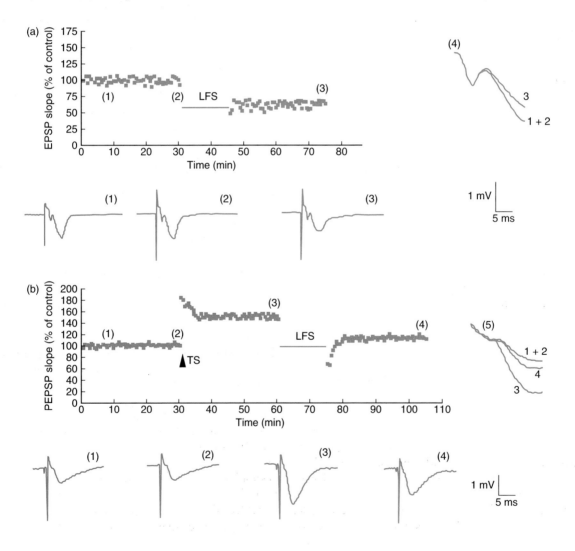

Figure A19.1 Cerebellar LTD induced *in vivo* by conjunctive stimulation of a vestibular nerve and the inferior olive. (a) Experimental arrangement for recording and stimulation. (b) Peristimulus histograms constructed before (control) and after the conditioning stimulation. Arrows mark the time of stimulation of the ipsilateral vestibular nerve (CVN). Bin width 0.5 ms, calibration 10 impulses/bin/100 sweeps. (Adapted from Ito M, Sakurai M and Tongroach P, 1982. Climbing fibre induced depression of both mossy fibre responsiveness and glutamate sensitivity of cerebellar Purkinje cells, *J. Physiol.* **324**, 113–134, with permission.)

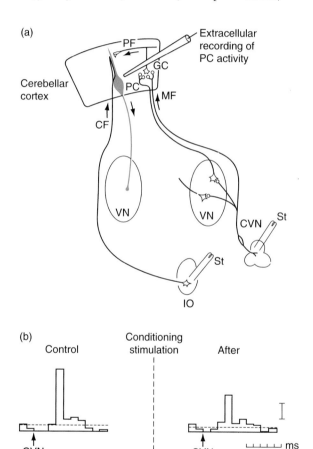

is induced by co-stimulation of the inferior olive at a relatively low frequency (4/s), which mimics climbing fiber activity in alert rabbits.

Further Reading

Aiba, A., Kano, M., Chen, C. *et al.* (1994) Deficient cerebellar long-term depression and impaired motor learning in mGluR1 mutant mice. *Cell* **79**, 377–388.

Ben Ari, Y., Aniksztejn, L. and Bregestovski, P. (1992) Protein kinase C modulation of NMDA currents: an important link for LTP induction. *Trends Neurosci.* **15**, 333–340.

Bliss, T.V.P. and Collingridge, G.L. (1993) A synaptic model of memory: long term potentiation in the hippocampus. *Nature* **361**, 31–39.

Conquet, F., Bashir, Z.I., Davies, C.H. *et al.* (1994) Motor deficit impairment of synaptic plasticity in mice lacking mGluR1. *Nature* **372**, 237–243.

De Schutter, E. (1995) Cerebellar long term depression might normalize excitation of Purkinje cells: a hypothesis. *Trends Neurosci.* **18**, 291–295.

Hammond, C., Crépel, V., Gozlan, H. and Ben Ari, Y. (1994) Anoxic LTP sheds light on the multiple facets of NMDA receptors. *Trends Neurosci.* **17**, 497–503.

Ito, M. (1989) Long-term depression. *Ann. Rev. Neurosci.* **12**, 85–102.

Ito, M. (1991) The cellular basis of cerebellar plasticity. *Curr. Opin. Neurobiol.* **1**, 616–620.

Lev-Ram, V., Makings, L.R., Keitz, P.E. *et al.* (1995) Long term depression in cerebellar Purkinje neurons results from coincidence of nitric oxide and depolarization-induced Ca²⁺ transients. *Neuron* **15**, 407–415.

Linden, D.J. and Connor, J.A. (1995) Long-term synaptic depression. *Ann. Rev. Neurosci.* **18**, 319–357.

McNaughton, B.L. (1993) The mechanism of long term enhancement of hippocampal synapses: current issues and theoretical implications. *Ann. Rev. Physiol.* **55**, 375–396.

Nakazawa, K., Mikawa, S., Hashikawa, T. and Ito, M. (1995) Transient and persistent phosphorylation of AMPA-type glutamate receptor subunits in cerebellar Purkinje cells. *Neuron* **15**, 697–709.

Wang, S.S.H. and Augustine, G. (1995) Confocal imaging and local photolysis of caged compounds: dual probes of synaptic function. *Neuron* **15**, 755–760.

Index

Note – Page numbers in *italic* refer to illustrations and tables; **bold** page numbers indicate a main discussion.